THE EVALUATION HANDBOOK

THE EVALUATION HANDBOOK

An Evaluator's Companion

■ ■ ■ ■ ■

edited by
Debra J. Rog
Leonard Bickman

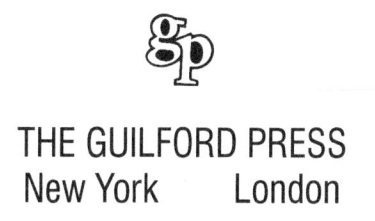

THE GUILFORD PRESS
New York   London

Copyright © 2025 The Guilford Press
A Division of Guilford Publications, Inc.
www.guilford.com

All rights reserved

No part of this book may be reproduced, translated, stored in a retrieval system, or transmitted, in any form or by any means, electronic, mechanical, photocopying, microfilming, recording, or otherwise, without written permission from the publisher.

Printed in the United States of America

This book is printed on acid-free paper.

For product and safety concerns within the EU, please contact *GPSR@taylorandfrancis.com*, Taylor & Francis Verlag GmbH, Kaufingerstraße 24, 80331 München, Germany.

Last digit is print number: 9   8   7   6   5   4   3   2   1

Library of Congress Cataloging-in-Publication Data is available from the publisher.

ISBN 978-1-4625-3734-1 (cloth)

This book has been a long time coming. Conceptualized before the COVID-19 pandemic and not long after the American Evaluation Association developed its evaluator competencies, this handbook encountered several challenges that lengthened its development, with the pandemic as one of the largest challenges. We are happy that our editor, C. Deborah Laughton, and our authors persevered with us in putting together what we hope will be a resource for evaluators for many years to come.

We have lost a number of evaluation giants over the years who have made outsized contributions to the field of evaluation through their scholarship, leadership, and noteworthy practice of evaluation. We hope this handbook is a testament to the fundamental impact they have had on our profession. We dedicate this volume to all who have passed, and specifically note a few of those colleagues who touched the editors' lives personally as well as professionally: Terry Hedrick, George Julnes, Will Shadish, and Joe Wholey

Preface

This handbook is designed as an evaluator's companion, providing expert advice to enhance the competencies evaluators need to perform exemplary evaluations. The chapters are organized according to foundational principles, designs, and methods, and address the challenges evaluators encounter in a range of situations. Rather than foster a step-by-step mentality to the work, the *Handbook* emphasizes creativity in practice and conducting evaluations with sensitivity to the specific context. Chapters are authored by evaluators with expertise in balancing rigor with practical application and who can offer direction on how to tailor evaluations to different situations. The *Handbook* is not intended to be a textbook, but rather an insiders' guide to applying evaluation theories, methods, and principles to both domestic and international evaluations.

WHY THIS BOOK IS NEEDED, ITS AUDIENCE/INTENDED READERSHIP, AND ITS APPROACH TO EVALUATION

The *Handbook* fills a void in the current literature. Although there are other handbooks and textbooks that focus on evaluation, this handbook is unique in its focus on the essential competencies evaluators need to do their work. We have envisioned this handbook as a companion to the evaluator, with each chapter serving as an advisor in how to apply and tailor the method or principle to each evaluation situation. It is as if the reader has a seasoned evaluator standing near them, distilling what a developing (or "apprentice") evaluator needs to know. The chapters aim to provide readers with a "how-to" perspective to implement each chapter's content creatively in their own evaluation situation.

The *Handbook* is a resource for evaluators who are new to the field, professors who teach evaluation, and practicing evaluators. For the novice evaluator, especially the "accidental" evaluator who has not had formal training in evaluation, the *Handbook* is designed to be an off-the-shelf guide for basic evaluation approaches, as well as offering ideas for addressing the nuances involved in designing and implementing an evaluation. For professors who teach novice evaluators, the *Handbook* spans the range of competencies and skills required by evaluators and ideally helps them infuse into their courses key content areas that may be missing or lean. Finally, for the practicing evaluator, the *Handbook* provides up-to-date information on key topics they may be familiar with but need refreshing. As evaluators often move across different evaluation settings over time and in different areas, they may need additional information on competencies necessary in these roles and contexts that are new to them.

Although we anticipate that most of our readers have had no more than one or two courses in evaluation, we do expect that most have at least a master's degree in one of the behavioral or social sciences. Therefore, the chapters are written in a manner that assumes that readers have had basic graduate-level courses in research methods and statistics. Each chapter discusses the core concepts that would be addressed in a specialized course or workshop in the area the chapter covers. Given the page limitations of each chapter, authors point readers to other supplementary material on the subject to build on the foundation of the chapter.

The *Handbook*'s design is driven by what the American Evaluation Association (AEA) has identified as core competencies that evaluators need to have to address the broad range of evaluation questions, in the variety of settings in which we work, and in the multitude of content areas that are involved. The competencies aim to improve the quality of evaluation performance, the effectiveness of evaluation education, and the shaping of evaluation outcomes to be aligned with social justice (Hall, 2020; Tucker et al., 2023). Forty-nine competences are in the AEA Evaluator Competencies, falling into five domains ordered according to how directly they are related to evaluation (King & Stevahn, 2020): Professional Practice, Methods, Context, Planning and Management, and Interpersonal Skills.

As noted by those involved in the process, not all competencies apply to every evaluator and some competencies may apply only in specific situations. As Jean King notes in Chapter 2, "the evaluator competencies provide a framework for thinking about evaluation practice, one that practicing evaluators must examine and shape to their own settings." We use the framework of the competencies as an organizing tool for the *Handbook*, highlighting some of the major sections as described below.

ORGANIZATION

The *Handbook* is organized into five sections, followed by a glossary of terms that support all chapters. We have shaped the content and organization of the *Handbook* on the competencies AEA has identified as critical for evaluators, regardless of where they work. These include those professional competencies that distinguish evaluators from other professionals; technical competencies, including designs and methods that are specific to evaluation, as well as shared by other professions; practical skills, such as planning and budgeting for evaluation; and cross-cutting competencies, such as communication, data visualization, and bringing these different roles for evaluators together in exemplary practice. Although there are not specific sections in this handbook dealing with the Context and Interpersonal Skills domains, these competencies are woven through other chapters in the examples provided.

Part I. Foundation for the Volume

Part I includes two chapters that frame the overall handbook. The first chapter by the editors provides a rationale for a handbook on competencies and how it can be used by evaluation professionals at different stages in their careers, as well as by evaluation academics in ensuring that novice evaluators are provided instruction in the range of competencies expected. The chapter also describes emerging designs, methods, and analyses becoming available to evaluators, and their implications for the competencies the next generation of evaluators may need to navigate in the ever-changing context of evaluation. The second chapter, by Jean A. King, sets a framework for the *Handbook*. She summarizes the development of AEA's core competencies, and how they can inform the education and work of evaluators.

Part II. Evaluation Theories, Foundations, Principles, and Purpose

In Part II, we commissioned chapters that highlight features of evaluation that are unique to the practice of evaluation:

- Fostering evaluative thinking (Thomas Archibald, Jane Buckley, and Guy O'Grady Sharrock)
- Using theories specific to evaluation to guide our work (Melvin M. Mark)
- Having expertise in systematically deriving the value of what we are evaluating (Emily F. Gates and Thomas A. Schwandt)
- Centering equity in our work so that our studies are fair and just (Donna Durant Atkinson)
- Anticipating and addressing ethical challenges that emerge in the work (Michael Morris)
- Taking specific actions that can foster evaluation use (Marvin C. Alkin and Anne T. Vo)
- Guiding the ways in which we design our studies with certain principles of practice in the variety of contexts in which we work (Michael Quinn Patton)

Part III. Answering Evaluation Questions: Designs, Methods, and Analyses

In Part III, evaluators are asked to address a wide range of evaluation questions that, in turn, need a variety of systematic inquiry approaches. The chapters herein offer designs, methods, and analytic strategies to answer several questions:

- How do we involve community interest holders in the design and implementation of the evaluation? (David M. Fetterman, Liliana Rodríguez-Campos, and Ann P. Zukoski)
- When is a program ready to be evaluated? (Debra J. Rog)
- How well is the program being implemented? (Byron J. Powell, Leonard Bickman, and Kimberly Eaton Hoagwood)
- How do we understand and assess the outcomes and impacts of programs? (Laura R. Peck and R. Bradley Snyder)
- How do we understand if the program was effective relative to cost? (Robert Shand, A. Brooks Bowden, and Henry M. Levin)

To address the variety of questions that are posed to evaluators, we include chapters that offer multiple approaches to qualitative, quantitative, and mixed methods studies:

- Storytelling as a systematic qualitative approach (Sharon F. Rallis and Janet Usinger)
- Planning quantitative analysis, and collecting and preparing quantitative data for analysis (Erica Harbatkin, Gary T. Henry, and Lam D. Pham)
- Conducting quantitative analysis (Lam D. Pham, Gary T. Henry, and Erica Harbatkin)
- Integrating both qualitative and quantitative designs in one evaluation (Tarek Azzam and Natalie D. Jones)

Part IV. Planning, Managing, and Implementing Evaluations

Part IV focuses on important aspects of how program evaluation is planned, managed, and implemented, some of which are not usually taught in graduate courses or presented in evaluation textbooks. Three chapters focus on planning and management, including:

- An overview of the evaluation planning process (Darlene F. Russ-Eft)
- The different types of resources that need to be considered in planning and evaluation (Leonard Bickman)
- Guidance in conducting evaluations under budget, time, and data constraints (Michael Bamberger)

A fourth chapter, by Joy Frechtling, describes how program theories and logic models can frame an evaluation and focus the evaluation questions. Finally, two chapters highlight two roles for evaluators not often described:

- The role of an internal evaluator who is a member of the program or organization staff conducting the evaluation (Arnold Love)

- The role of the independent consultant and the requirements needed to be successful in that role, including personality traits, ethics, and business planning and process to achieve financial stability (Gail Vallance Barrington)

Part V. Crosscutting Issues

We provide resources for strengthening three crosscutting competencies and issues:

- A systematic and strategic approach to communications for evaluators that can be tailored to each evaluation context (Glenn O'Neil)
- A how-to guide for developing and using different types of data visualization grounded both in understanding the purpose and audience for the communication and in good data visualization principles (Tarek Azzam, Sarah Douville, Ciara Knight, Piper Grandjean Targos, and Natalie D. Jones)
- Guidance on what it means to conduct an exemplary evaluation and putting the evaluator competencies that have been covered in all prior chapters into practice (Stewart I. Donaldson).

PEDAGOGICAL FEATURES

The *Handbook* is designed with several pedagogical features to enhance its readability and application of the concepts addressed.

- *Clarity and organization:* Each chapter begins with an opening overview to provide the reader with a concise understanding of the chapter's main concepts. Each chapter is designed to be easy for readers to navigate, with clear headings and subheadings, and a logical flow. Authors aimed to write in concise language, avoiding jargon or providing definitions for key terms within the chapter.

- *Audience focused:* As noted, the chapters are written for evaluators with little formal training but with responsibility for planning and implementing or monitoring an evaluation. Professors of evaluation also are a key audience, as are more seasoned evaluators who may benefit from having foundational chapters to refer to in their practice. Chapters highlight key glossary terms, address the core concepts in each topic, and offer ample illustrations of the topic in practice.

- *Engaging content:* The chapters are written in a "how-to" style to provide pragmatic, apprenticeship-like guidance, and often highlight the importance of cultural competence, communication, facilitation, and how to resolve differences and make decisions. All chapters have illustrations and examples, and for those chapters where it makes sense, a box example provides a more detailed example illustrating the design, method, or concept and offers a practical scenario of a real-world application to help reinforce learning. Many chapters incorporate visuals (such as diagrams, charts, or infographics) to enhance understanding. Methods chapters, in particular, include basic elements of the approaches in exhibits and boxes, outlining how key aspects of each situation and context influence how the evaluators apply the method or approach. Finally, and most important, authors are very experienced evaluators, leaders in their field, who write from their experience and expertise, drawing on it to distill what is essential for evaluators to know.

• *Resource rich:* Authors refer to other chapters in the *Handbook*, where relevant, to highlight where the writing intersects. In addition, authors realize that their chapter alone will not make an expert of the reader, but instead it will provide core issues and examples. Therefore, authors typically suggest other resources that the reader can consult for more details.

SUGGESTED READINGS

Hall, M. E. (2020). Competencies, self-awareness, and practice: Notes on my reading of Chapters 5–7. *New Directions for Evaluation, 2020*, 133–147.

King, J. A., & Stevahn, L. (2020). Presenting the 2018 AEA Evaluator Competencies. *New Directions for Evaluation, 2020*, 49–61.

Tucker, S., Peck, L. R., & Hall, J. N. (2023). Special section editors' note: A focus on the evaluation profession. *American Journal of Evaluation, 44*(3), 447–452

Acknowledgments

This handbook has had a long runway, longer than we, our authors, and The Guilford Press expected. We appreciate all who had confidence it would finally come together, and we hope you are as proud of it as we are. All authors did an incredible job of flexing with updates and revisions and providing the field with contributions that will stand the test of time. We especially want to thank Jean King for helping us understand the foundation under which the AEA competencies were established and providing an opening chapter that set the stage for the volume.

We also want to give a special shout-out to our editor for over 40 years: C. Deborah Laughton. She has been our cheerleader throughout the *Handbook* process, sticking with us through the delays and offering strategies for dealing with challenges we met. She has been our dear friend, colleague, and support from our first methods publications, and we can think of no other editor we would want to work with.

Finally, we thank our family and friends who showed patience and support as we spent another weekend or night "working on the *Handbook*."

Contents

PART I ■ FOUNDATION FOR THE VOLUME

1 ■ Setting the Stage: Supporting the Diverse Knowledge and Skills Evaluators Need in an Ever-Changing Context 3
Debra J. Rog and Leonard Bickman

2 ■ Competencies for Program Evaluators 18
Jean A. King

PART II ■ EVALUATION THEORIES, FOUNDATIONS, PRINCIPLES, AND PURPOSE

3 ■ Evaluative Thinking: Understanding and Applying the Foundations of Evaluation 35
Thomas Archibald, Jane Buckley, and Guy O'Grady Sharrock

4 ■ Evaluation Theories: Guidance to Evaluating in Various Circumstances 55
Melvin M. Mark

5 ■ Valuing in Evaluation 81
Emily F. Gates and Thomas A. Schwandt

6 ■ Equity in Evaluation 101
Donna Durant Atkinson

7 ■ Ethical Challenges 125
Michael Morris

8 ■ Fostering Evaluation Use 141
Marvin C. Alkin and Anne T. Vo

9 ■ Illuminating Evaluation's Kaleidoscope: 159
Beautiful, Diverse, Ever-Changing Manifestations
Michael Quinn Patton

PART III ■ ANSWERING EVALUATION QUESTIONS: DESIGNS, METHODS, AND ANALYSES

10 ■ Collaborative, Participatory, and Empowerment Evaluation: 181
From Community Consultation to Community Control
David M. Fetterman, Liliana Rodríguez-Campos, and Ann P. Zukoski

11 ■ Making the Most of Evaluations: Strategies for Assessing 208
Program Evaluability and Evaluation Feasibility
Debra J. Rog

12 ■ Monitoring Program Implementation 230
Byron J. Powell, Leonard Bickman, and Kimberly Eaton Hoagwood

13 ■ Examining Outcomes and Impacts: Designs and Strategies 254
in Theory and Practice
Laura R. Peck and R. Bradley Snyder

14 ■ Combining Costs and Results: Designs, Strategies, and Analysis 270
Robert Shand, A. Brooks Bowden, and Henry M. Levin

15 ■ Evaluation as Storytelling: Using a Qualitative Design 288
Sharon F. Rallis and Janet Usinger

16 ■ Planning, Data Collection, and Data Preparation 308
for Quantitative Analysis
Erica Harbatkin, Gary T. Henry, and Lam D. Pham

17 ■ Conducting a Quantitative Analysis 325
Lam D. Pham, Gary T. Henry, and Erica Harbatkin

18 ■ Mixed Methods Design 344
Tarek Azzam and Natalie D. Jones

PART IV ■ PLANNING, MANAGING, AND IMPLEMENTING EVALUATIONS

19 ■ Designing and Planning an Evaluation: Beyond Methods 365
Darlene F. Russ-Eft

20 ■ Logic Models and Program Theory 383
Joy Frechtling

21 ■ Resource Planning 398
Leonard Bickman

22 ■ The Role of an Internal Evaluator 426
Arnold Love

23 ■ The Independent Consultant: An Insider's Guide to a Consulting Career 445
Gail Vallance Barrington

24 ■ Conducting Evaluations under Budget, Time, and Data Constraints: An International Perspective 465
Michael Bamberger

PART V ■ CROSSCUTTING ISSUES

25 ■ Communicating with Interest Holders 491
Glenn O'Neil

26 ■ Information Visualization and Evaluation 509
Tarek Azzam, Sarah Douville, Ciara Knight, Piper Grandjean Targos, and Natalie D. Jones

27 ■ Exemplary Evaluations in a Multicultural World 532
Stewart I. Donaldson

Glossary 551
Author Index 574
Subject Index 581
About the Editors 604
Contributors 605

Part I

FOUNDATION FOR THE VOLUME

Chapter 1

Setting the Stage

Supporting the Diverse Knowledge and Skills Evaluators Need in an Ever-Changing Context

Debra J. Rog
Leonard Bickman

TODAY'S EVALUATION CONTEXT

Evaluation is a very diverse profession; evaluators work in a variety of capacities in many different organizations and in a wide range of topical areas. As active evaluation practitioners for more than 40 years, we have watched our field grow and change. We have seen the growth of the number of people engaged in evaluation, the types of organizations that commission and use evaluation, and the kinds of questions addressed by evaluation. In addition, we have witnessed an increasing institutionalization of evaluation in both the United States and globally, and in turn, greater needs for professional development and training.

Today, in the United States, evaluators work in all levels of government (federal, state, local, and regional), contract research organizations, universities, nonprofit and for-profit organizations, and foundations and other philanthropic organizations. For many of these organizations, evaluators are hired internally to conduct evaluations as well as serve as contract officers for evaluations that are conducted by external evaluators. Two examples in the United States that illustrate evaluation's deepening and growing influence in guiding social practice and policy come from both the federal government and philanthropy, two of the largest supporters of evaluation in the United States.

Within the federal government, the Foundations for Evidence-Based Policymaking Act of 2018 (commonly known as **the Evidence Act**) has even more firmly cemented evaluation as a critical part of federal government stewardship. The Evidence Act mandates federal agencies to implement several actions and activities to strengthen its capacity to build and use evidence, including establishing the position of an evaluation officer in the agency, engaging in a capacity assessment to evaluate the agency's ability to implement and use the data from rigorous evaluations, create learning agendas, and develop evaluation plans that include the design and implementation of evaluations (Evidence Act toolkits/Office of Evaluation Sciences; *gsa.gov*). The Evidence Act, including the standards and practices promoted with it, call for a broad range of understanding of **evaluation theory**, designs and methods, and foundational principles (such as ethics).

The federal government has had prior evaluation and data policies (e.g., **Government Performance and Results Act**, the **Program Assessment Rating Tool** review; Hart & Newcomer, 2018) and the practice of evaluation has continued to grow in federal agencies (American

Evaluation Association [AEA] Evaluation Policy Task Force, 2022). However, the Evidence Act distinguishes itself from prior evaluation movements and policies in calling for a strengthening of the government's infrastructure and its workforce to conduct evaluation and other strategies for developing and using data. As the Evidence Act continues to unfold, the federal government is expected to continue to grow and strengthen its evaluation workforce, and as noted by Epstein and colleagues (2022) from the U.S. Office of Management and Budget, "professional development and training will assume even more importance in the coming years" (p. 96).

Although not directly tied to the Evidence Act, additional guidance on developing, analyzing, and using equitable data was issued by the federal government through Executive Order 13985 on Advancing Racial Equity and Support for Underserved Communities Through the Federal Government ("Equity EO"). Three recommendations for equitable data included disaggregating survey data to understand historically underserved groups more fully, increasing public access to disaggregated data, and conducting robust **equity** assessments of federal programs.

Within philanthropy, Long (2017) notes several trends in evaluation's growth and expansion in various roles. One trend in foundations is moving toward a greater focus on accountability and learning, both within an equity framework. Long also reports a trend of foundations embedding evaluation into strategy to inform the evaluability of programs, their implementation, and impact.

Much like the federal government has explicitly described in the Evidence Act, foundations are using evaluation to provide insights for continuous improvement and learning. Of those responding to the Center for Evaluation Innovation (2023) benchmarking survey, two out of three respondents had "learning" in their job title, and over half of respondents had "evaluation" in their job title. Both measures were substantially higher than earlier surveys in 2015 and 2019. In fact, of the responsibilities that learning and evaluation staff prioritize, the top responsibility prioritized by most respondents (90%) is designing and/or facilitating learning processes or events within the foundation.

Within recent years, philanthropies have also taken a stronger equity foothold, assessing not only whether they are being successful but whether they are reaching disadvantaged and marginalized populations and addressing inequities and disparities in the system. Seventy-eight percent of the foundations surveyed in 2023 have organizationwide diversity, equity, and inclusion efforts, up from 56% of the foundations in 2019. Long (2017) notes that a growing focus is infusing into investments the perspectives of community members and other interested parties. Finally, Long notes the stronger relationship between communication and evaluation and the need for evaluators "to create a compelling narrative about *why* an investment worked, *how* it worked, and the tangible *difference* it made in people's lives"

Globally, evaluation has experienced explosive growth. As one measure of growth, over 41,500 individuals are now members of over 220 **voluntary organizations for professional evaluation** (VOPEs; national and subnational associations and societies across 129 countries) and identify as evaluators, either as practitioners, academics, or government or other officials with evaluation-related responsibilities (Rugh, 2018; International Organization for Cooperation in Evaluation [IOCE]). VOPEs help bring together evaluators across these different roles to contribute to advancing the field of evaluation.

PREPARING TODAY'S EVALUATORS

The variety of roles evaluators play and the knowledge and skills they need requires the field of evaluation to ensure that evaluation courses and training programs adequately prepare current and future evaluator generations. A cluster of recent research studies and articles (LaVelle, 2014, 2020; LaVelle et al., 2020; LaVelle & Donaldson, 2021) demonstrate that evaluation training is increasingly available, albeit not as widespread as more traditional disciplines, such as psychology. A review of university-based programs across the world (LaVelle, 2020) found, in 2017, that 87 colleges and universities in the United States were offering evaluation-specific education (two or more courses with "evaluation" in the title) across master's, doctoral, and certificate programs. Fewer programs (27) were identified in colleges and universities outside of the United States, most through master's degree and certificate programs. The number of programs has increased significantly from 2010 (with a small dip between 2014 and 2017), with the greatest growth in certificate and master's programs.

LaVelle (2020) also conducted a curriculum analysis of these university-based courses and found, consistent with previous research (LaVelle, 2014), that most programs emphasize quantitative skills, such as experimental and quasi-experimental designs, and basic and advanced statistics as well as evaluation theory. Much less common were qualitative evaluation courses, needs assessment, and data visualization. Similarly, a study of the curricula in evaluation courses in Council on Education for Public Health-accredited schools of public health and masters of public health programs (Hobson et al., 2019) analyzed the "essential competencies" for program evaluators as enumerated by Stevahn et al. (2005a, 2005b)[1] and found that the programs focus on professional practice (e.g., how to engage interest holders), systematic inquiry (e.g., design, methods), situational analysis (e.g., describing the program), and interpersonal skills (e.g., communication), but program management and reflective domains were much less covered. Also absent in most courses were **competencies** unique to evaluation, such as evaluability and meta-evaluation.

Program evaluation is also being taught at the undergraduate level (LaVelle et al., 2020). Ninety-one percent of the top 80 public and private U.S. universities offered at least one course, with an average of seven per institution and a total of 470 evaluation-specific or evaluation-related courses taught in the 2017–2018 academic year. Although still a small offering compared to other fields and disciplines, the findings indicate that evaluation principles and tools are being taught to undergraduates, though the extent to which they are being covered is less known.

Finally, evaluation courses are offered through professional development workshops, such as the Evaluators' Institute and the Minnesota Evaluation Studies Institute (LaVelle & Donaldson, 2021). These workshops, offered in person and online, span a variety of introductory and advanced topics. As with the university graduate and undergraduate courses, work is needed to assess whether these courses align with the needs of the field and with the competencies the field believes evaluators need to have.

EVALUATION COMPETENCIES

The growth in evaluation training and professional development is encouraging, but more in-depth understanding is needed of the extent to which evaluators are being adequately prepared for the range of roles in government, philanthropic, nonprofit, and contract research settings, among others. Over the last decade, in the United States and internationally, efforts have been dedicated to developing evaluation competencies (Tucker et al., 2023). Competencies are defined as the totality of knowledge, skills, attributes, behaviors, and attitudes needed to perform the role of an evaluator. In 2015, the AEA appointed a Competencies Task Force (CTF) to develop the competencies, with the aim of generating common language and criteria for distinguishing evaluation as a profession and a practice. As described by King (see Chapter 2, this volume), the CTF worked in a democratic, evolving manner to develop a set of competencies that were finalized in 2018 and published in *New Directions for Evaluation*. After the competencies project's completion, the CTF was sunsetted and, in 2021, a Professionalization and Competencies Working Group was developed to implement the task force recommendations. The work group is now gathering information on how the competencies work in practice and how they relate to the field's professionalization, defined as the process by which an occupation becomes a profession.

The competencies are intended to improve the quality of evaluation performance, the effectiveness of evaluation education, and the shaping of evaluation outcomes to be aligned with social justice (Tucker et al., 2023). The competencies developed to date are considered an initial set, building on foundational documents (the **Program Evaluation Standards, AEA Guiding Principles,** and the AEA Statement on Cultural Competence in Evaluation). Forty-nine compe-

---

[1]Prior to the summer of 2018 and before AEA endorsed professional competencies, these competencies were the most recently published peer-reviewed set of evaluation competencies.

tencies are in the AEA Evaluator Competencies, falling into five domains: professional practice, methodology, context, planning and management, and interpersonal. The domains are ordered according to how directly they are related to evaluation (King & Stevahn, 2020). As noted by those involved in the process, not all competencies apply to every evaluator. Evaluation is often a team endeavor, and others on a team may assume some of the tasks and roles. For example, teams may have specialists in qualitative evaluation and quantitative evaluation. In addition, some competencies may only apply in specific situations. As King notes (see Chapter 2, this volume), "the evaluator competencies provide a framework for thinking about evaluation practice, one that practicing evaluators must examine and shape to their own settings."

AN EVALUATOR'S COMPANION: THE WHAT AND WHY OF THE *HANDBOOK*

We have shaped the content and organization of the *Handbook* on the competencies AEA has identified as critical for evaluators regardless of where they work. These include those professional competencies that distinguish evaluators from other professionals; technical competencies, including designs and methods that are specific to evaluation as well as shared by other professions; practical skills, such as planning and budgeting for evaluation; and crosscutting competencies, such as communication and bringing these different roles for evaluators together in exemplary practice. Although specific sections in this handbook are not outlined for the context and interpersonal domains, many of these competencies are woven through the chapters in the examples provided. In addition, the chapters are written in a "how-to" style to provide pragmatic, apprenticeship-like guidance and often highlight the importance of cultural competence, communication, facilitation, and how to resolve differences and make decisions. All chapters have illustrations and examples, and for those chapters where it makes sense, a set of boxed examples provide more detail illustrating the design, method, or concept.

The *Handbook* is aimed at three audiences: the novice evaluator, professors who teach novice evaluators, and practicing evaluators. The novice evaluator, especially the accidental evaluator who has not had formal training in evaluation, can benefit from resources that prepare evaluators for the variety of roles and tasks they may need to assume. Evaluators report having anxiety in their roles, in part due to a lack of preparation and training in the areas they are being asked to work in (Renger & Donaldson, 2022). Although a handbook will not fully prepare an individual in an area they may have little background, it can provide them a foundation of knowledge to begin to navigate their way.

For professors who teach novice evaluators, the *Handbook* can also provide a guide for the span of competencies required by evaluators and ideally help infuse into their courses content that may have been missing or lean.

Finally, for the practicing evaluator, the *Handbook* provides up-to-date information on key topics they may be familiar with but want refreshing. As evaluators often move across different evaluation settings over time and in different areas, they may need additional information on competencies needed in these roles and contexts that are new to them.

OVERVIEW OF THE *HANDBOOK*

Part I. Foundation for the Volume

The first section is aimed at providing a conceptual grounding for the *Handbook*. This first chapter provides a rationale for a handbook on competencies and how it can be used by evaluation professionals at different stages in their career as well as by evaluation academics in ensuring that novice evaluators are provided instruction in the range of competencies expected of them.

In Chapter 2, Competencies for Program Evaluators, Jean King sets a framework for the *Handbook*. As she notes, "Having a set of carefully developed, comprehensive competencies that detail with some certainty what the practice of evaluation includes can help people focus on the knowledge, skills, abilities, and other characteristics that they need to become competent practitioners." King presents a background of the field of evaluation that captures why a focus on competencies is needed, what they are and what they are not, and how they can be used by novice evaluators as well as those who have been practicing evaluation for many years. She provides a brief history of the discussion of competencies and certification in evaluation and the reasons why there has been reluctance to develop them. The bulk of King's chapter describes how the current AEA competencies have been developed, as well as some context for competencies in other networks.

The remaining sections of the *Handbook* organize the chapters into four main groupings of competencies: Part II: Theories, Foundations, Principles, and Purpose; Part III: Answering Evaluation Questions: Designs, Methods, and Analyses; Part IV: Planning, Managing, and Implementing Evaluations; and Part V: Cross-cutting Issues.

Part II. Theories, Foundations, Principles, and Purpose

In this section, we commissioned chapters that highlight features of evaluation that are unique to the practice of evaluation: fostering **evaluative thinking**, using theories specific to evaluation to guide our work, having expertise in systematically deriving the value of what we are evaluating, centering equity in our work so that our studies are fair and just, anticipating and addressing ethical challenges that emerge in the work, taking specific actions that can foster evaluation use, and guiding the ways in which we design our studies with certain principles of practice. The last chapter in this section, by Michael Quinn Patton, describes the variation in evaluation practice that this chapter began with, and illustrates how evaluator's competencies are applied differently depending on the context in which the evaluator is working.

Tom Archibald, Jane Buckley, and Guy O'Grady Sharrock begin this section with Chapter 3, Evaluative Thinking: Understanding and Applying the Foundations of Evaluation. Evaluators have increasingly recognized evaluative thinking as a foundational philosophical concept in evaluation. In this chapter, the authors provide several definitions of evaluative thinking and distinguish the role that evaluative thinking plays in evaluation and in **evaluation capacity building** (ECB). As they note, evaluative thinking is critical thinking, fueled by curiosity and the quest for evidence. It involves a process of "identifying assumptions; posing thoughtful questions; marshaling evidence to make judgments; pursuing deeper understanding; and making logically aligned, contextualized decisions in preparation for action." The authors illustrate how these five components of the definition can guide the application of evaluative thinking in evaluation, incorporating reflection and multiple perspectives as they are conducted. From their own work in applying evaluative thinking in ECB, the authors outline six guiding principles for promoting evaluative thinking, including seizing opportunities that naturally occur to engage learners, incorporating it incrementally, offering opportunities to intentionally practice it, providing opportunities for identifying and questioning assumptions, offering opportunities for all to develop as evaluative thinkers and incorporating it into critical conversations involving all levels of staff, and fostering a psychologically safe and trusting environment for evaluative thinking to occur.

Mel Mark follows in Chapter 4, Evaluation Theories: Guidance to Evaluating in Various Circumstances. Theory, as Mark convincingly describes, is the evaluator's navigational tool. It guides how we do evaluation and why we do it in particular ways. It provides a basis for us to choose the methods and techniques we use in each evaluation. Mark explores the role of evaluation theory, defining what it is and the importance of theory for evaluation practice. He examines individual theorists and theories, taking a deep dive on three theories, and presents two meta-models or frameworks designed to help make sense of a multitude of evaluation theories, and how these meta-models can guide the study of evaluation theory. Mark discusses how evaluators can draw on evaluation theories as helpful guides to evaluation practice, as well as how evaluation theory might be modified or added to in the future to further influence practice.

One of the competencies of professional practice is using systematic evidence to make **evaluative judgments**. As Emily Gates and Tom Schwandt describe in Chapter 5, Valuing in Evaluation, professional evaluators bring facts and values together to make these judgments. They define **valuing** as the process of reaching warranted conclusions about value and identify it as both a responsibility and an expertise claimed by professional evaluators. The authors explain in detail this expertise and responsibility, with a particular focus on how the process of valuing should be systematic, transparent, and defensible. As they note, valuing is one of the features that distinguishes informal, day-to-day judgments of value from professionally conducted evaluation. The authors discuss a variety of values and how they influence evaluation practice, steps in valuing (i.e., selecting criteria, identifying sources of evidence, setting **standards**, and synthesis) and methods to inform them, and a checklist and questions for guiding the evaluator in navigating practical challenges in valuing.

Equity is at the center of societal discourse today and within evaluation. As Donna Atkinson describes in Chapter 6, Equity in Evaluation, evaluators have a responsibility to consider equity in the design of program evaluations to ensure that they are fair and just. To do that, we need to better understand what equity is and how to include it in our work. Atkinson aims to increase evaluators' awareness of different frameworks of equity and what it means to include it in evaluation, how to think about one's own perspectives on the topic and how those perspectives affect one's work, factors that may influence the overall approach to the evaluation when including equity, technical design topics that need to be addressed when including equity in evaluation, and strategies to incorporate equity to consider when planning an evaluation. As Atkinson states, "there is no single approach to including equity in an evaluation." As she notes, "The key to achieving equity in your evaluations is to think about it early and often, seek the support you may need, and conduct a technically solid evaluation that can determine the merits of a program *for all participants*."

In Chapter 7, Ethical Challenges, Michael Morris introduces the concept of **ethical practice** within the context of evaluation. He explores the major ethical challenges that evaluators report encountering throughout the various stages of evaluation (entry/contracting, designing the evaluation, data collection, data analysis and interpretation, reporting the results, and utilization of findings). Morris outlines professional resources evaluators can use to guide them ethically in their work (the AEA Guiding Principles, the Program Evaluation Standards), and offers strategies for planning and conducting evaluations in a way that facilitates the prevention of, and effective response to, ethical difficulties (such as establishing a foundation for dealing with ethical issues in the contracting stage, consulting with colleagues, etc.).

A foundational purpose for evaluation is to inform decision making. In Chapter 8, Fostering Evaluation Use, Marv Alkin and Anne Vo provide clear guidelines for fostering evaluation use, guided by the firm belief that evaluation use typically comes from the specific actions the evaluator takes to foster it. Extracting and examining the necessary elements for a comprehensive evaluation use theory, the authors develop guidelines for fostering use based on reviewing research on use, then identifying the evaluator actions that correspond to the research. A unique and strong "how-to" element of the chapter is the provision of examples of observable actions that both demonstrate that the evaluator action was taken and provide the novice evaluator with guidance on how to take those actions to foster change. The authors end with some practical advice to readers on how best to use the framework, either to guide their work, to teach others, or to stimulate additional research to enhance use.

Chapter 9, Illuminating Evaluation's Kaleidoscope: Beautiful, Diverse, Ever-Changing Manifestations, by Michael Quinn Patton, rounds out this section by focusing on the principles that guide evaluation practice. Through the metaphor of a kaleidoscope, Patton discusses the different roles or forms that evaluation takes: as social science method, profession, discipline, transdiscipline, science, technology, art, and evaluation practice. Using the kaleidoscope as an analogy, he illustrates how the elements of practice can combine in different ways with certain elements having more dominance than others depending on the context one is in. The kaleidoscope provides a basis for understanding the variation within evaluation discussed in the front section of this chapter and why certain aspects are more or less important in specific settings.

Part III. Answering Evaluation Questions: Designs, Methods, and Analyses

Evaluators are asked to address a wide range of evaluation questions that, in turn, need a variety of systematic inquiry approaches. In this section, the chapters offer designs, methods, and analysis strategies to answer several questions: Is the program ready to be evaluated? How is the program being implemented? How do we involve interest holders in the design and implementation of the evaluation? What are the outcomes of the program and other changes that are taking place? What is the program's impact and cost-effectiveness?

David Fetterman, Liliana Rodríguez-Campos, and Ann Zukoski begin this section with Chapter 10, Interest Holder Involvement Approaches to Evaluation: **Collaborative, Participatory,** and **Empowerment** Evaluation. The authors focus on how to engage communities in an evaluation to improve programs, build capacity, and produce credible results, especially in culturally diverse contexts and communities. They describe varying approaches that fit different program contexts and circumstances and focus on ways to empower community members to have a voice, if not control, over the design and implementation of an evaluation. The authors describe techniques to achieve involvement that are both effective and practical and offer guidance to evaluators in selecting the approach (collaborative, participatory, or empowerment) best suited to the context.

One question an evaluator should ask before embarking on an evaluation is "Is the program ready for an evaluation?" As Debra J. Rog discusses in Chapter 11, Making the Most of Evaluations: Strategies for Assessing Program Evaluability and Evaluation Feasibility, if an evaluation is conducted too soon, the program may not be sufficiently implemented to have an effect even if the conceptual basis of the program is sound. **Evaluability assessment** provides a practical approach to judging whether a program is evaluable, based on several factors that influence a program's readiness for evaluation. This chapter provides readers with a stepwise approach to judging whether an evaluation could be conducted or if an evaluation would be premature and thus not able to establish the merit and worth of a program. Rog also describes that evaluators can use evaluability assessment for more than judging evaluation readiness, including to help develop programs, select sites to use in multisite evaluations, and provide quick information on a program.

Byron J. Powell, Leonard Bickman, and Kimberly E. Hoagwood provide a comprehensive treatment of studying implementation in Chapter 12, Monitoring Program Implementation. In the last decade, the key role of the quality of **program implementation** has become the focus of not only program evaluation but any field that attempts to intervene to solve a problem. Failure to find that a program is effective can be caused by four main factors: (1) poor implementation of the program, (2) poor theory of change or program theory, (3) poor design of the evaluation, and (4) poor implementation of the evaluation. This chapter provides the reader with the perspective and techniques necessary to distinguish among these factors in the design and implementation of the evaluation, focusing on the ability to judge whether the program was sufficiently well implemented to distinguish between a program implementation failure and a program theory failure. The chapters that follow in this section provide guidance on how to design and implement the evaluation to avoid evaluation design and implementation failures.

Chapter 13, Examining Outcomes and Impacts: Designs and Strategies in Theory and Practice, by Laura Peck and Brad Snyder, focuses on the nature of cause and effect as the key consideration of **summative** or **impact** evaluations seeking to determine changes in outcomes attributable to the program. The authors embed this discussion in a classic review of **threats to internal validity** and the importance of **counterfactual comparisons**. Evaluators will benefit from the practical examples the authors provide on design options and strategies for carrying out impact evaluations as well as their discussion of how impact evaluations relate to other concepts discussed in this handbook, such as logic models, resource constraints, and quantitative design and analysis.

Robert Shand, A. Brooks Bowden, and Henry Levin focus on an important, but often neglected, aspect of program evaluation in Chapter 14, Combining Costs and Results: Designs, Strategies, and Analysis. Not only do we as evaluators want to know whether a program was successful (had an impact), as discussed in the previous chapter, but we should know whether it was effective relative to cost. The authors provide evaluators with the basic knowledge to understand how costs are allocated to a program and then the variety of methods used to analyze the cost data relative to the program. These methods include **cost-feasibility analysis, cost-effectiveness analysis, cost-utility analysis,** or **benefit–cost analysis** that all provide ways to help make decisions about the future of the program. The authors believe these methods, when combined with robust effectiveness studies, can increase the usefulness of the evidence for decision makers.

To address the variety of questions that are posed to evaluators, we have included chapters that offer multiple approaches to qualitative, quantitative, and mixed methods studies. In Chapter 15, Evaluation as Storytelling: Using a Qualitative Design, Sharon Rallis and Janet Usinger explain how to use a qualitative approach, **storytelling,** as a systematic, rigorous, criteria-guided evaluation process to develop a credible story about a program. The story can be told from different angles, including developmental, formative, and summative. As these authors illustrate, storytelling brings life to both the program and the theory underlying it, providing detail and context to generate results that enhance understanding of the program and create potential for change based on the evaluation. Rallis and Usinger base their approach on principles of systematic inquiry, which brings standards and discipline to this approach. Based on years of experience applying this approach, the authors guide evaluators in how to use storytelling to paint a compelling picture of the program using various perspectives.

Moving to a quantitative approach to evaluation in Chapter 16, Planning, Data Collection, and Data Preparation for Quantitative Analysis, Erica Harbatkin, Gary Henry, and Lam Pham provide valuable guidance on planning quantitative analysis, and collecting and preparing quantitative data for analysis. Like many of the other chapters in this handbook, this chapter focuses the evaluator on the planning that is necessary and critical before conducting an evaluation. In quantitative evaluations this preparation requires multiple steps. As the authors outline, planning a quantitative study includes the selection of a research design, sampling, power analyses, selection of measures, and other steps, such as data screening and cleaning. In addition, as the authors indicate, quantitative study planning, as with qualitative efforts (as described in Chapter 15), requires collaboration with interest holders to inform planning, including specifying the research questions, outlining the research design, organizing the data acquisition strategy, planning the data analysis approach, and determining how the findings will be communicated.

Preparing quantitative data for analysis is the last step before conducting the analysis. The same authors from Chapter 16, Lam Pham, Gary Henry, and Erica Harbatkin, offer three approaches to conducting the analysis in Chapter 17, Conducting a Quantitative Analysis. In the first approach, which they label "**exploratory,**" the evaluator develops an understanding of the patterns of the data to better understand the program and to plan more rigorous approaches to analysis in later steps. The second step, or **descriptive** analysis, attempts to describe the program, the participants, and its context more precisely. In the third step, **correlational** and **causal** analysis, the evaluator analyzes the data to see whether it had the intended effect. The authors provide several examples of each step so that the evaluator has a practical and well-informed perspective on what actions to take at each step.

In the final chapter in this section, Chapter 18, Mixed Methods Design, Tarek Azzam and Natalie Jones discuss the integration of both qualitative and quantitative designs in one evaluation, a design that is preferred by many evaluators. The design's popularity may be based on its potential to answer questions that can't be answered easily in one method. For example, focus groups, a qualitative method, is good for understanding the feelings of participants in depth, but it can't answer questions about how widespread or representative those feelings are; that can best be estimated by representative surveys. Each approach provides strengths and weaknesses to balance any single approach. However, this combined approach requires both resources and skills in both approaches, which can be more complex and demanding than any single approach. The authors walk the reader through the **mixed methods** design process, highlighting the decision points to be considered, including the priority placed on each data source, the timing of when each type of data will be collected, and where in the process the integration of the data from the different sources will occur. Using the design options as a building block, the authors then describe the ways in which different configurations of the decisions made translate into different mixed methods designs. A major strength of this chapter is the clarity in which it provides decision strategies to help the evaluator decide whether a mixed methods approach is desired and whether it is feasible.

Part IV. Planning, Managing, and Implementing Evaluations

Part IV focuses on two important aspects of program evaluation. First, we continue our focus on planning, but we consider factors that are not usually taught in graduate courses or presented in evaluation textbooks. Our focus here is on resources required to be considered in planning an evaluation. We start with an overview of the planning effort, then move to two detailed chapters on how to best use the resources available to plan an evaluation. Second, we examine roles that evaluators have in planning and conducting evaluations from two different but commonly occurring **contexts**. In the first role we consider the evaluator who is internal to the organization in which the evaluation is being conducted. Second, we carefully examine the role of the independent consultant as the evaluator. Chapters 19 and 20 show the strengths and challenges associated with conducting evaluations in these two contexts.

In Chapter 19, Designing and Planning an Evaluation: Beyond Methods, Darlene Russ-Eft provides a valuable overview of the evaluation planning process. According to Russ-Eft, the evaluator needs to consider several stages in planning an evaluation that includes but goes beyond study design. She provides important guidance for each stage, including planning and outlining the scope of the evaluation, the data collection and analysis, the work schedule, the personnel, the budget, and the risks that the evaluator may encounter. Russ-Eft provides some tools and detailed strategies for conducting these stages. Although all stages are important, attending to risks in the planning process may be the least written about but anticipating them in an explicit manner, with a risk matrix as Russ-Eft outlines, can help evaluators avoid disasters and maximize opportunities. The chapter dovetails well with two other chapters in this section, one on resource planning, by Len Bickman (Chapter 21), and the other on conducting evaluations under tight resource constraints, by Michael Bamberger (Chapter 24).

Chapter 20, Logic Models and Program Theory, by Joy Frechtling, provides a different theoretical perspective than what is found in Chapter 4 by Melvin Mark. Chapter 20 focuses on program theories, rather than evaluation theories. Frechtling describes how program theories can frame an evaluation and focus the evaluation questions. Logic models are tied to **program theory** as a way of depicting the causal relationships that are often implicit in the program developer's mind. It fell to the evaluator, almost by default, to develop the program theory to conduct a rigorous theory-based evaluation. Frechtling introduces critical tools that evaluators will need to plan and conduct evaluations based on an explicit understanding of how and why an intervention should lead to predicted outcomes. Importantly, using program theory moves an evaluation of what might be a single program being tested to a representative of the theory underlying the program being tested.

In Chapter 21, Resource Planning, Len Bickman demonstrates how careful planning for the implementation of an evaluation can be as important as the evaluation questions asked, the design and methods used, and the data collected. He discusses four types of resources to consider while planning an evaluation. These resources include the data that are needed, the time available to complete the evaluation, the people and the skills needed for the evaluation to be successful, and the funding needed to support the evaluation until completion. Because evaluations are conducted in dynamic, real-world contexts, the evaluator also must carefully consider the realistic constraints on the planning and implementation of an evaluation, many beyond the control of the evaluator. Before making decisions about the specific design to use and the type of data collection procedures to employ, the evaluator must consider the resources available and the limitations of these resources within the contextual constraints. Bickman details the steps that evaluators need to take to help ensure they have sufficient resources to complete the evaluation. Not only must these factors be considered in planning an evaluation, but they must be monitored during the evaluation for it is unlikely that no matter how carefully the evaluation was planned, things will be missed and contemporaneous changes will occur that affect the implementation of the evaluation and the resources needed.

As described at the outset of this chapter, some evaluators conduct evaluations within their own organizations, as a member of the staff of the program or the organization delivering the program. In Chapter 22, The Role of an Internal Evaluator, Arnold Love describes a position that has grown in use across the world. Love provides an understanding of what **internal evaluation** is and how it compares with other roles (such as internal audits) and describes the strengths and limitations of the conduct of an evaluation by an internal evaluator in contrast to an external evaluator. He describes the various roles internal evaluators play, including those that are valued and rewarding (such as an honest broker, navigator, management consultant, change agent, information specialist, and evaluation facilitator) as well as those that are negative (spy, number cruncher, archaeologist, publicity agent, quibbler, and terminator). Love bases many of his observations and suggestions on almost 25 years of teaching about internal evaluations as well as his role as an evaluation consultant. The chapter highlights important differences between internal evaluation and other forms of evaluation and ties those differences to specific suggestions and tips on how to manage the conflicting role an internal evaluator may have in their own organization.

In Chapter 23, The Independent Consultant: An Insider's Guide to a Consulting Career, Gail Barrington describes a different role for an evaluator, as an **independent consultant**. Her chapter describes the requirements needed to be successful in this role, which include personality traits, ethics, and business planning and processes to achieve financial stability. Independent consultants, like internal evaluators, have unique pressures in this role. Barrington describes the characteristics of the independent consultant life, often working with small organizations. She notes the need for consultants to have the intellectual capacity to be quick studies and have self-confidence, courage to face many unknowns, adaptability, and resilience. Barrington provides excellent advice and tools for starting up a new consulting practice, finding the right market niche for the evaluator's skills and interests, obtaining new business, and writing proposals. She also provides insightful advice on how to be productive and survive this challenging environment.

The final chapter in this section by Michael Bamberger, Chapter 24, Conducting Evaluations under Budget, Time, and Data Constraints: An International Perspective, provides guidance to evaluators working in less-than-ideal situations, where designing and implementing methodologically sound, meaningful evaluations are challenged by client biases, politics, unexpected budget cuts, unrealistic client expectations, shortened time frames, and denial of access to data or participants. Although Bamberger has developed his **"real-world evaluation"** approach based on his experience in conducting evaluations outside of industrialized countries, the challenges faced are frequently found in evaluations more broadly. The chapter complements Bickman's chapter on resource planning (Chapter 21) under more typical conditions as well as Russ-Eft's chapter on evaluation planning (Chapter 19) by focusing on strategies for addressing budget and resource constraints, time constraints, and data access issues. The tradeoffs Bamberger suggests in dealing with very real constraints make his chapter a practical resource for evaluators grappling with these challenges.

Part V. Crosscutting Issues

In this section, the first two chapters describe competencies that cut across evaluation practice—communications and **data visualization**. The final chapter, serving somewhat as a capstone to the handbook, describes what it means to conduct exemplary evaluation practice; that is, what counts as "competent" practice in different settings and circumstances.

As described earlier, more attention is being placed on the intersection between communication and evaluation, especially in the philanthropic sector. Glenn O'Neil, in Chapter 25, Communicating with Interest Holders, supports and describes a systematic and strategic approach to communications for evaluators that can be tailored to each evaluation context. As he accurately notes, much of the discussion and research on communications focuses on communicating evaluation findings to decision makers and other audiences. However, throughout an evaluation O'Neil notes that two-way dialogue, engagement, and interaction can heighten the effects of communication on use. He suggests a range of communication formats for presenting findings (text based, interpersonal, and audio–visual), tailoring the amounts and level of information to the needs of various interest holders and audiences. As O'Neil realistically notes, a well thought-out and implemented communication plan can foster evaluation use, but factors such as context, **organizational setting**, **decision-making characteristics**, and the **policy environment** can be countervailing forces also influencing whether results are used.

Data visualization also has emerged as a critical crosscutting skill that evaluators need to be effective, especially as clients of evaluation clamor for efficient, easy-to-follow diagrams and graphs of findings, study and program conceptual frameworks, and study designs and method. In Chapter 26, Information Visualization and Evaluation, Tarek Azzam and colleagues offer a thorough, how-to guide for developing and using different types of data visualization. Azzam and colleagues focus on first understanding the purpose and audience for the communication, and then ground the chapter in good data visualization principles that can guide effective communication. They provide the reader with an iterative process for creating visualizations, using the principles to select design choices and refine them. The authors also highlight other key topics for evaluators, such as developing **logic models**, and then outline future directions important for both novice and seasoned evaluators to consider in their work, including becoming familiar with more tools and types of data visualization, gaining skills to be sensitive to a range of audiences, understanding how to communicate qualitative and mixed methods results visually as well as quantitative findings, and using visualization as an analytic technique in addition to a vehicle for communication.

In Chapter 27, Exemplary Evaluations in a Multicultural World, Stewart Donaldson addresses what it means to conduct an exemplary evaluation and bookends this handbook with Jean King's chapter on evaluator competencies (Chapter 2). Given the diversity of what falls under the heading of evaluation, however, determining the features of what is considered exemplary practice is no small task. Donaldson uses the learnings from his year as president of AEA in 2015, the International Year of Evaluation involving over 80 evaluation conferences focused on strengthening evaluation capacity, as a springboard to outlining common themes to exemplary practice. Donaldson's query into exemplary practice found that our values determine what we see as exemplary, and that values differ by the evaluation context we are in, especially by regions of the world and across cultures. Some of the most common values for exemplary practice were consistent with the Program Evaluation Standards, AEA's Guiding Principles, and AEA's Statement on Cultural Competence. He notes that movements to develop evaluator competences, such as those developed by AEA, and the movement toward credentialing in a couple of countries signal greater emphasis in evaluation in developing the capacity for more exemplary evaluation practice. As evaluators strive for exemplary practice, Donaldson reminds us of the particular importance of evaluation theory and supports calls for more research on evaluation that can both develop more evidence-based theories to guide evaluator decisions and foster exemplary practice.

WHAT'S NEXT ON THE PLAYBILL: EMERGING DIRECTIONS IN EVALUATION

This handbook itself covers a range of topics that align with the AEA competencies. And we acknowledge that many more topics could have been included had we more space. Notable absences are **developmental evaluation**, use of **machine learning** and **natural processing language**, ethnographic methods, **complexity and systems evaluation**, **evaluation synthesis**, **performance measurement**, and **virtual data collection**, among others. Some topics are covered in one or two chapters but could have been written in several—for example, we have a chapter on interest holder approaches to evaluation and one on storytelling and qualitative evaluation, but many more chapters could be written on qualitative methods and approaches, analysis, and data collection. Similarly, Atkinson's chapter (Chapter 6) on equitable and just evaluation could have spawned more chapters digging deeper into social justice and culturally responsive evaluation. We have chapters on randomized and quasi-experimental methods but could have expanded the focus on methods that rely on secondary data sources (such as interrupted time series and synthetic control methods) that are used more prominently in other fields, as well as methods such as single-case designs that show promise in education and other areas. We therefore hope that the *Handbook* provides a starting point for evaluators, giving them some foundational principles, key designs and approaches, and planning and management tools that they can build upon with other resources.

In this section, we look ahead, identifying a few emerging trends we believe are likely to become more dominant in the field of evaluation. We have identified these trends based on our own experiences and knowledge of where the field is, rather than on a comprehensive literature review or a consensus-based process. Several of these trends support one another (e.g., **artificial intelligence** [AI] and real-time evaluation). We view these areas as likely topics, among others, to be added in a second edition of the *Handbook*. We touch on each briefly.

Artificial Intelligence

In the next few years, we expect there will continue to be tremendous growth in AI. This growth will directly impact how evaluations are conducted and conceptualized. AI will affect how both qualitative and quantitative data are collected and analyzed. The way data are collected will be expanded to include chatbots as well as using the "internet of things," which can collect data passively from sensors in the environment. Data analyses will also be influenced by AI in classifying data for qualitative analyses as well as using voice and video data to score emotional state. AI will also accelerate the use of big data, which will require evaluators to become proficient in managing and analyzing larger data sets than they are usually accustomed to (Bickman, 2020; Mason & Montrose-Moorhead, 2023).

Individuals with Lived Expertise on Evaluation Teams

Incorporating **interest holders** in evaluation and participatory approaches to evaluation are not new. However, the U.S. federal government, the largest funder of evaluations, has been slower to take up the trend. Having individuals and communities participate in evaluating the services, systems, and other interventions that affect their lives is likely to continue and become a more traditional approach to evaluation.

Evaluator Involvement in Program Development

Evaluators typically do not have a formal role in the programs they evaluate, with the exception of evaluators involved in developmental evaluation. In some situations, evaluators in a sense "back into" the issue of program development because programs often are not fully conceptualized and ready to be evaluated against their goals. In this handbook, chapters that indirectly address program development focus on evaluability assessment (see Rog, Chapter 11), and logic models and program theories (see Frechtling, Chapter 20) but are not specifically aimed at developing programs from the outset. Program development should mature into its own field, taking advantage of the skills and perspectives evaluators can bring when program and policy initiatives are first being considered and created. In lamenting what he considered the sad state of program evaluation in 1994, one of the luminaries of program evaluation, Lee Sechrest, voiced similar concerns and attributed some of the lack of advances in program development to the absence of "vigorous commitment" of the evaluation community to champion program development.

Providing Real-Time Analyses

Real-time evaluation methods are not new (Mc-Nall & Foster-Fishman, 2007) but the interest in them appears to have grown, especially with COVID-19 (e.g., Buchanan-Smith & Morrison-Métois, 2021). These methods, characterized by short time frames of generally less than 6 months, are known by a variety of terms, including *real time*, *rapid cycle*, and *rapid appraisal*. Two common terms used are described below:

- Real-time evaluation gives insight into how a program or intervention is progressing, often as the evaluation is continuing in the field

(INTRAC, 2012). The approach is associated with emergency response or humanitarian interventions, especially during their early stages when there is more flexibility to make changes.

- **Rapid cycle evaluation** generally is aimed at quickly testing program changes or specific program components or modifications. It is a formative evaluation approach that can involve different methods that range in rigor (Atukpawu-Tipton & Poes, 2020).

Rapid, real-time methods support learning, another key direction we have seen evaluation taking that goes beyond accountability purposes to those that guide direction on the intervention under study and broader. Moreover, as we move to using AI and other technological approaches in collecting and analyzing data, expectations for quick turnaround analyses and findings will grow. Evaluators need to become adept with the tools that can help them collect, analyze, and report data efficiently.

Emphasis on Personalization of Services

We expect that the influence of precision medicine and the more general move to the personalization of services will shape the way in which we evaluate health and human services (Johnson et al., 2020). There is growing recognition that the effectiveness of services is limited by the inability of program developers to personalize or design services to properly fit services to the characteristics and needs of the recipient. Among other things, this means a shift in measuring average **effect size** to individualized outcomes. There will be additional emphases to identify causal factors before conducting a randomized experiment using new methods of causal data sciences (Bickman et al., 2016; Saxe et al., 2022).

Evaluation Responsibility in Environmental Sustainability

A number of prominent leaders in evaluation across the globe (e.g., Davidson et al., 2023) have called for evaluators and sponsors of evaluation to consider environmental sustainability in their work. In their *Footprint Evaluation Guide*, Davidson and colleagues provide guidance for feasible and useful ways to infuse environmental sustainability in the planning, managing, and/or conducting of evaluations. The *Guide* shares the hope that through the emerging set of practices and principles evaluators, organizations, and governments can move to having all evaluations become "sustainability inclusive."

FINAL NOTE

As these future trends indicate, evaluation is a growing field and profession that continues to shape and change. In this handbook, we have provided a fundamental set of principles, theories, values, and methods to guide your practice. Whether you are a novice evaluator, an evaluation professor, or a seasoned practicing evaluator, we hope that this handbook becomes a resource on your shelf to strengthen the competencies you need as you move through different evaluation contexts and topics.

We especially encourage those who are novice evaluators to expand on the knowledge provided in this handbook through journals in our field: *American Journal of Evaluation* and *New Directions for Evaluation* (both supported through the AEA), *Evaluation Review, Evaluation and Program Planning, Evaluation and the Health Professionals,* and *Evaluation* (the journal of the European Evaluation Society), and *Canadian Journal of Program Evaluation* (a journal of the Canadian Evaluation Society), as well as through the variety of textbooks and other resources available. We also encourage you to build on your knowledge and fellowship in the profession by joining the evaluation association or network in your country and any local affiliate as well as seek out workshops and trainings on specific topics and methods.

Finally, we launch this handbook with 27 chapters on a range of topics and methods to align with Donald Campbell's belief in the evolution of knowledge through learning, as Mel Mark (2016) reminded us in his blog post for AEA. Quoting Campbell, Mark noted,

> In science we are like sailors who must repair a rotting ship while it is afloat at sea. We depend on the relative soundness of all other planks while we replace a particularly weak one. Each

of the planks we now depend on we will in turn have to replace. No one of them is a foundation, nor point of certainty, no one of them is incorrigible.

REFERENCES

American Evaluation Association Evaluation Policy Task Force. (2022). An evaluation roadmap for a more effective government. *New Directions for Evaluation, 2022*(173), 17–28.

Atukpawu-Tipton, G., & Poes, M. (2020). *Rapid cycle evaluation at a glance* (OPRE Report #2020-152; produced by James Bell Associates). Office of Planning, Research, and Evaluation, U.S. Department of Health and Human Services.

Bickman, L. (2020). Improving mental health services: A 50-year journey from randomized experiments to artificial intelligence and precision mental health. *Administration and Policy in Mental Health and Mental Health Services Research, 47*(5), 795–843.

Bickman, L., Lyons, A., & Wolpert, M. (2016). Achieving precision mental health through effective assessment, monitoring, and feedback processes. *Administration and Policy in Mental Health and Mental Health Services Research, 43*, 271–276.

Buchanan-Smith, M., & Morrison-Métois, S. (2021). *From real-time evaluation to real-time learning: Exploring new approaches from the COVID-19 response*. ALNAP.

Center for Evaluation Innovation. (2023). *Benchmarking foundation learning and evaluation practices 2023*. Author.

Cioffi, C. C., Hibbard, P. F., Hagaman, A., Tillson, M., & Vest, N. (2023). Perspectives of researchers with lived experience in implementation science research: Opportunities to close the research-to-practice gap in substance use systems of care. *Implementation Research and Practice, 4*.

Davidson, J., Macfarlan, A., Rogers, P., Rowe, A., & Stevens, K. (2023). *Sustainability-inclusive evaluation: Why we need it and how to do it. A Footprint Evaluation Guide*. Available at *www.betterevaluation.org/tools-resources/sustainability-inclusive-evaluation-why-we-need-it-how-do-it*

Epstein, D., Zielewski, E., & Liliedahl, E. (2022). Evaluation policy and the federal workforce. *New Directions for Evaluation, 2022*, 85–100.

Hart, N., & Newcomer, K. (2018). *Presidential evidence initiatives: Lessons from the Bush and Obama administrations' efforts to improve government performance*. Bipartisan Policy Center. Available at *https://privpapers.ssrn.com/sol3/papers.cfm?abstract_id=3786814*

Hobson, K. A., Coryn, C. L. S., Fierro, L. A., & Sherwood-Laughlin, C. M. (2019). Instruction of evaluation competencies in Council on Education for Public Health (CEPH)-accredited master of public health (MPH) degree programs. *American Journal of Evaluation, 40*(4), 590–606.

INTRAC. (2012). *Real-time evaluation*. Available at *www.intrac.org/wpcms/wp-content/uploads/2019/05/Real-time-evaluation.pdf*

Johnson, K., Wei, W.-Q., Weeraratne, D., Frisse, M. E., Misulis, K., Rhee, K., . . . Snowdon, J. L. (2020). Precision medicine, AI, and the future of personalized health care. *Clinical and Translational Science, 14*(1), 86–93.

King, J. A., & Stevahn, L. (2020). Presenting the 2018 AEA evaluator competencies. *New Directions for Evaluation, 2020*(168), 49–61.

LaVelle, J. M. (2014). *An analysis of evaluation education programs and evaluator skills across the world* (Doctoral dissertation, Claremont Graduate University).

LaVelle, J. M. (2020). Educating evaluators 1976–2017: An expanded analysis of university-based evaluation education programs. *American Journal of Evaluation, 41*(4).

LaVelle, J. M., & Donaldson, S. (2021). Opportunities and challenges ahead for university-based evaluator education programs, faculty, and students. *American Journal of Evaluation, 42*, 428–438.

LaVelle, J. M., Sabarre, N., & Umans, H. (2020). An empirical examination of evaluation's presence in the undergraduate curriculum in the United States. *American Journal of Evaluation, 41*(2), 297–310.

Long, M. (2017). *Five trends in learning and evaluation* [Blog post]. Council on Foundations.

Mark, M. (2016, May 23). *Memorial week: Mel Mark on remembering Donald T. Campbell (1996–2016), pioneer in evaluation methodology* [Blog post]. AEA365.

Mason, S., & Montrose-Moorhead, B. (Eds.). (2023). Evaluation and artificial intelligence [Special issue]. *New Directions for Evaluation, 178–179*, 1–134.

McNall, M., & Foster-Fishman, P. (2007). Methods of rapid evaluation, assessment, and appraisal. *American Journal of Evaluation, 28*, 151–168.

Ramirez, G. G., Bradley, K., Amos, L., Jean-Baptiste, D., Ruggiero, R., Marki, Y., . . . Benton A. (2022). *What is lived experience?* Office of the Assistant Secretary for Planning and Evaluation, U.S. Department of Health and Human Services.

Renger, J., & Donaldson, S. I. (2022). The prevalence of evaluator anxiety in practice: An empirical examination. *American Journal of Evaluation, 45*(2).

Rugh, J. (2018, September 23). *What are VOPEs? And how do they relate to us as evaluators?* [Blog post]. AEA365.

Saxe, G. N., Bickman, L., Ma, S., & Aliferis, C. (2022). Mental health progress requires causal diagnostic nosology and scalable causal discovery. *Frontiers in Psychiatry*, 2471.

Sechrest, L. (1994). Program evaluation: Oh what it seemed to be! *Evaluation Practice, 15*(3), 359–365.

Skelton-Wilson, S., Sandoval-Lunn, M., Zhang, X., Stern, F., & Kendall, J. (2021). *Methods and emerging strategies to engage people with lived experience: Improving federal research, policy and practice*. Office of the Assistant Secretary for Planning and Evaluation, U.S. Department of Health and Human Services.

Stevahn, L., King, J. A., Ghere, G., & Minnema, J. (2005a). Establishing essential competencies for program evaluators. *American Journal of Evaluation, 26*(1), 43–59.

Stevahn, L., King, J. A., Ghere, G., & Minnema, J. (2005b). Evaluator competencies in university-based evaluation training programs. *Canadian Journal of Program Evaluation, 20*(2), 101–123.

Tucker, S. A., Stevahn, L., & King, J. A. (2023). Professionalizing evaluation: A time-bound comparison of the American Evaluation Association's foundational documents. *American Journal of Evaluation, 44*(3), 495–512.

Chapter 2

Competencies for Program Evaluators

Jean A. King

CHAPTER OVERVIEW

This chapter begins with a rationale for the development and use of evaluator competencies and their history in the field. A brief description of formal and less formal processes for developing competencies follows, along with an explication of the program evaluator competencies in five domains that the **American Evaluation Association (AEA)** board approved in 2018. The chapter ends with thoughts on the potential use of competencies by both novice evaluators and their more experienced colleagues.

What makes an evaluator an evaluator? In one sense, everyone is an evaluator. People make judgments many times a day—for example, determining the best way to drive to a nearby community during a snowstorm, choosing to stay up late to finish a report due the following morning, or, in light of COVID-19, deciding whether to wear a face mask while running outdoors. These are evaluative decisions because they are based on "data" (traffic and weather reports, a boss's predictable response to missed deadlines, the latest health information available) that, when combined with other information, lead to a judgment and a resulting action. People also regularly make larger evaluative judgments when they, for example, decide what car to purchase, whether they should adopt a child, or accept a new job in a different city, again using the best information available to make what they believe to be the best decision. In an important way, of course, such everyday evaluative judgments—even big decisions—differ from the practice of those who conduct evaluations professionally. Professional evaluation practice systematizes **evaluative thinking** (see Archibald et al., Chapter 3, this volume), adding formal logic, rigorous social science methods, ethical commitments, and other attributes that distinguish it from the informal evaluations people make routinely. So, what, exactly, are the differences between an ordinary person's and a professional program evaluator's evaluation?[1] And why should this matter to a person considering becoming an evaluator or someone engaged in evaluation practice?

As explained below, the challenge in answering this question stems in part from the history of the field. In contrast to other professions, program evaluation is a relatively new practice. It began in the United States in response to President Lyndon Johnson's War on Poverty

---
[1]There are many types of evaluation in addition to program evaluation, including, for example, product evaluation, personnel evaluation, and policy evaluation. (For more examples, see the section on "Evaluation Practice Specializations" in Michael Patton's chapter [Chapter 9, this volume].) The competencies presented in this chapter were created specifically for program evaluators, although many of them surely apply to other types of evaluation practice.

and other Great Society programs in the 1960s when the federal government sought to assess the implementation and outcomes of millions of dollars of social programming (Fitzpatrick et al., 2011). In the 60 or so years since then, the practice of evaluation has grown and flourished around the world. There are numerous professional associations, journals, and university-based programs and professional development trainings that teach people to become evaluators. There have been standards for program evaluation since 1981; the latest edition was published in 2011 (Yarbrough et al., 2011). The AEA (2019a) also has guiding principles for program evaluators, revised most recently in 2018. Two countries (Canada and Japan) now offer a credential for professional evaluators.

But, while numerous other fields have competency frameworks and standardized procedures for developing them (Tuxworth, 1989), evaluation, until recently, did not. The perceived diversity of evaluation practice and evaluation's uncertain status among professions (Worthen, 1994), sadly coupled with a lack of resources for research on issues, such as the essential skills every evaluator needs, the actual outcomes of evaluator education, and how evaluation can contribute to the public good, have left the field in limbo for many years (King & Stevahn, 2013). This changed in May 2018, when AEA's board approved a set of **competencies** for its membership.

Three details made these competencies unique: (1) they were based on and derived from 11 sets of existing evaluator competencies from around the world carefully compared with the Program Evaluation Standards and the AEA Guiding Principles, pulling together all extant examples of English-language evaluator competencies (Tucker et al., 2020); (2) a 3-year period of extensive consultation, review, and input in a variety of forms (e.g., listening sessions at conferences, focus groups with members, a member survey) shaped two major revisions of the initial draft set; and (3) a culminating survey of the AEA membership provided strong face validity for the final set (Stevahn et al., 2018).

Why does this matter? Michael Quinn Patton (see Chapter 9, this volume) describes what he calls the "kaleidoscope" of evaluation practice—eight different ways that people describe and enact program evaluation: social science methods, a profession, a discipline, a transdiscipline, science, technology, art (craft), and practice. These eight may at first appear quite different from one another. Such diversity surely allows the field appropriate flexibility but it can also prove extremely confusing to novices and practicing evaluators alike. Having a set of carefully developed, comprehensive competencies that detail with some certainty what the practice of evaluation includes can help people focus on the knowledge, skills, abilities, and other characteristics that they need to become competent practitioners. The competencies may also help the field to make sense of its multiple forms of practice by identifying the grounding essentials that connect them all. While it is true that every set of competencies must adapt over time as professional contexts and practice evolve (Tucker et al., 2023), at the moment, they provide a good introduction to what it means to be a professional program evaluator. In this way the competencies flesh out the process of formal evaluative thinking.

This chapter begins with a rationale for the development and use of evaluator competencies and their history in the field, followed by a brief description of procedures for developing competencies, an explication of the AEA board-approved evaluator competencies, and thoughts on their potential use by both novice evaluators and their more experienced colleagues.

RATIONALE FOR THE DEVELOPMENT AND USE OF EVALUATOR COMPETENCIES

What exactly does evaluation practice look like? One way to answer this question is by considering the interpersonal participation quotient (King & Stevahn, 2013) that identifies three overlapping zones on a continuum of evaluation practice: evaluator directed, collaborative, and participant directed. Some evaluators work in seats of power, such as federal or state agencies, analyzing datasets using highly technical statistical procedures that require large N's and helping their clients make policy decisions that may affect millions. Other evaluators in such government agencies may direct well-supported studies on the implementation of programs funded across multiple sites in communities, states, regions, or countries. Evaluators working for foundations may similarly examine multiple program processes and outcomes. Typically, with less funding, others may collaborate with a small number of nonprofit staff or community members, sharing control of the process while teaching them how to continue the evaluation on their own. Yet again, some may elect to take a coaching role, perhaps with a small number of individuals, providing technical assistance and quality control to nascent evaluators in an organization.

Evaluators clearly have multiple options in shaping their practice, making the question of what all evaluators need to know perplexing. A related challenge stems from the fact that evaluation occurs in many different sectors. Think of Venn diagrams that highlight the overlap of evaluation with, for example, literacy education, HIV/AIDS programming, human rights projects, or multiple other subject-specific content (King & Stevahn, 2015). In the overlap sit the competencies required of that specific subject area (e.g., how to evaluate a literacy education program); in the evaluation part of the circle sit overarching, non-content-specific evaluator competencies. Taking all of this diversity into account, coupled with Patton's evaluation kaleidoscope, highlights the challenge of developing a common set of evaluator competencies.

As mentioned above, for many people, including Michael Patton, program evaluation is a profession. Over a quarter-century ago, Worthen (1994) analyzed the status of evaluation by applying the nine characteristics of a fully developed profession. At that time, evaluation met six of them: (1) a continuing need for evaluators; (2) unique knowledge and skills; (3) educational programs to prepare evaluators; (4) professional associations; (5) ongoing career opportunities; and (6) formal standards of practice, including, for example, the Program Evaluation Standards and the AEA Guiding Principles. However, the three characteristics that Worthen labeled unmet at that time—accreditation of preparation programs, certification or licensure of evaluators, and the exclusion of unqualified practitioners—by and large are still unmet.[2]

Jacob and Boisvert (2010) write, "After many years of debates and numerous, often passionate, discussions, the question of whether or not evaluation is indeed a profession has not yet received a definitive answer" (p. 350). The prospect of having a lawyer without legal credentials defending someone in a court case or a noncertified public accountant accountable for a complex audit seems like a terrible idea, but this is not apparently the case when it comes to evaluation. As Picciotto (2011) notes, "No one would willingly agree to have one's heart surgery performed by a plumber . . ." (p. 168). But anyone is free to call themselves an evaluator and go unchallenged because in part, until recently, there was no commonly accepted list of the competencies required in an evaluator's work.

There are two types of potential benefits of a validated and mutually accepted set of competencies. The first category of competencies benefits, given the field's history, relates to the intrinsic benefit of using competencies to establish a *distinct* field of practice and, in time, perhaps a fully established profession. As discussed, what exactly an evaluator has to do to be considered a professional remains an open question, even for many active in the field. Academics who are well trained in research methods sometimes assume that research and evaluation are indistinguishable; experienced program evaluators demur, noting distinctions owing to the source of study questions (clients rather than an academic discipline's research base) and the ultimate use of the results (by users rather than by scholars). A set of competencies makes explicit what these distinct practices have in common, enabling movement toward increased professionalization of the work and, ultimately, the possible development of accreditation for evaluator training or education programs or even individual credentialing, certification, or licensure.

Second, there are at least five potential uses of evaluator competencies that highlight the likely benefit of having them (see King, 2020):

1. Obviously, evaluators themselves, either individually or in groups, can apply competencies in self-assessments and structuring activities to promote higher-quality evaluation practice through reflection and self-education (Stevahn et al., 2020). Competencies discussions can promote reflection and community building as they may simultaneously improve the quality

---

[2] There was program evaluator licensure for a brief time in the state of Louisiana in the early 1980s (I am a Class A evaluator in Louisiana, certified for life), and currently two national evaluation societies—the Canadian Evaluation Society (CES) and the Japanese Evaluation Society (JES)—run programs that provide credentials (CES) or certification (JES) to their members (see Ayoo et al., 2020).

of practice. Members of the Minnesota Evaluation Association, for example, perceiving a need to learn about the field of project management, held a training where people both learned and discussed specific content.

2. Second, the competencies alert all evaluators to the grounding importance of social justice and racial and economic equity, which "are increasingly viewed as a foundation of (evaluation) practice, necessitating that evaluators learn how to address potential power imbalances occurring within evaluations, the larger contexts in which those evaluations occur, and the emerging profession itself" (Symonette et al., 2020, p. 117). The COVID-19 pandemic brought into stark relief the large systems issues confronting society, and the competencies may provide a way for evaluators to consider their role in addressing them.

3. Third, evaluator trainers and university-based faculty, as well as the staff of professional associations, can use competencies to structure their program curricula and professional development offerings (LaVelle & Galport, 2020). If training opportunities are designed to deliver specific preidentified knowledge or skills, evaluators can systematically build their résumés over time and address personal areas of need or growth.

4. A fourth use for competencies involves administrators responsible for commissioning evaluations and hiring or managing evaluators. They can use evidence of competencies to assess individuals' appropriateness for evaluation positions, potentially being fiscally prudent by hiring the most qualified individual for the lowest price, increasing the credibility of the process, and protecting themselves from less-than-adequate studies.

5. Ultimately, a fifth use of evaluator competencies may engage program interest holders because, on the one hand, through participation they may enhance their own understanding of and capacity to conduct an evaluation, and because, on the other hand, they may ultimately benefit from higher-quality studies of the social programs that they direct or in which they participate.

The potential for these multiple uses—and there are likely others—creates a second and powerful rationale for the development of evaluator competencies.

To be clear, while there are certainly potential advantages to the development and use of evaluator competencies, there are also several possible disadvantages:

1. A major worry relates to the prospect that increasing professionalization may limit newcomers' access to the field. Any systematizing of requirements through credentialing or certification may serve a gatekeeping function, discouraging skilled individuals from entering the field owing to a lack of awareness of options, limited opportunities for professional development, or possibly the inordinate expense of training/education. Of special concern are two groups: (a) practicing evaluators who may not have had evaluation-specific education and who fear they will be unable to continue their professional work; and (b) prospective evaluators from communities of color who may feel excluded from practice, even as explicit attention to cultural humility and issues related to power, privilege, and social justice become increasingly essential (King, 2018). The challenging evolution of diversity issues within the AEA, for example, highlights the need for explicit attention to the negative possibilities of increased gatekeeping (Shanker, 2020; Matthias, 2022).

2. A second and related disadvantage involves the possibility that mandated evaluator competencies may limit the field's access to novel strategies, techniques, and practices, privileging traditional, "approved" procedures and methods at the expense of innovations.

3. A third disadvantage stems from the possible abuses of any set of competencies. The potential of someone creating a simplistic competencies-based checklist to constrain practice, for example, cannot be overlooked. Also of concern is the naive expectation that any one individual would be required to have all competencies, especially when evaluators often work in teams with complementary skills.

4. A final disadvantage—or at least a major concern—relates to the valid measurement of competencies (i.e., the challenge of determining whether someone exhibits competence and, with that, the question of how to document it; Stevahn et al., 2020). The diversity of competency

domains (e.g., consider situational and interpersonal skills) raises multiple measurement issues, especially given the holistic nature of practice and the fact that many evaluators report gaining some competencies only on the job (Rassel, 2018). For measurement purposes, many of the competencies would require far more specificity than is currently present, a likely challenge given the context-specific nature of evaluation practice.

What, then, is the perceived value of competencies for program evaluators at this time? Patton (2010; also see Chapter 9, this volume) recommends that evaluators develop an elevator speech that explains what they do because people so rarely know what evaluation is or understand it. A helpful blog post included the following question as one of a practicing evaluator's top 10 evaluation doubts: "Will the sentence 'I'm an evaluator' . . . need no further explanation one day?" (Vaca, 2018). A set of agreed-upon competencies may help to address—finally—the enduring question of what, exactly, it means to be a program evaluator, enabling the field to break out of the "it can't be done" competencies mentality of the past 20 or so years. One thing is evident: In the past there were no competencies available, and hence there was nothing for evaluators to use. Now that competencies are commonplace, an ongoing natural experiment will occur as people apply them in improving evaluation practice and evaluator education.

THE (BRIEF) HISTORY OF AND CURRENT STATUS OF EVALUATOR COMPETENCIES

In 1999, Blaine Worthen wrote, "Evaluation competencies—skills and knowledge that enable an individual to conduct a quality evaluation study—represent the *sine qua non* in performance as an evaluator" (p. 546). But if competencies are that important and if other fields (e.g., medicine, accounting, law) have long since provided models for how to proceed, the question remains, "Why haven't competencies existed in the field of evaluation before now?" The story of their development, which is directly tied to discussions of professionalizing the field, goes back almost 30 years.

In 1995, Jim Sanders and Len Bickman wrote a memo to the AEA Board of Directors proposing a voluntary system of certification for evaluators (Altschuld, 1999a), one of the features of a profession that evaluation lacked. Building on this, Jim Altschuld led a task force that examined the prospect of developing an AEA certification system. The culminating report, summarized in Altschuld (1999b), included the word *competencies* six times, but without mention of the need to develop them for use either for certification or accreditation. The report ended with a list of eight possible actions, including as Number 1: "Maintain the status quo." As the article notes:

> In some ways this is an attractive course of action in that there are no financial costs associated with it. . . . On the other hand, it does nothing but continue the current situation, one that is not satisfactory in terms of an emerging field and profession. Continuing as we are now would allow almost anyone to say, by virtue of membership in national and/or local evaluation groups or simply by personal preference, that "I am an evaluator." In the long run this option loses its appeal. (pp. 489–490)

Two years later, returning to the theme of his 1997 AEA Presidential Address, Bickman (1999) wrote an article entitled "AEA, Bold or Timid?" in which he argued, "It is necessary to describe the unique knowledge and competencies that evaluators have if we are to exist as a profession. . . . What makes us think that evaluation is such an impossible case?" (p. 20). Twenty years later, given the current status of the field's professionalization, we know that AEA chose the timid option, and that the status quo was, indeed, the most attractive course of action, one that apparently did not lose its appeal.

Shortly after these task force activities in the late 1990s, four individuals—a group of three doctoral students and their professor at the University of Minnesota (me)—developed the first set of published evaluator competencies (King et al., 2001). Following a seminar discussion of literature that reviewed lists of proposed competencies (e.g., Covert, 1992; Ingle & Klauss, 1980; Mertens, 1994; Scriven, 1996) and explicated the difficulties of creating one set for the field (e.g., Patton, 1990), the students questioned how difficult the development process might actually be. Their complex fields (early childhood education, special education, and teacher education) all had long-standing and well-known competencies, so they wondered what made the challenge of competencies development for program evaluation so different. Undaunted by the task and building on the latest editions of the Program Evaluation Standards, AEA's Guiding Principles, and the CES's Essential Skills Series (1999), along with extant lists of proposed competencies, the group began a 2-year unfunded effort to create and initially validate a set of evaluator competencies. These were ultimately published in an article entitled "Toward a Taxonomy of Essential Evaluator Competencies" (King et al., 2001).

The initial taxonomy included four domains: systematic inquiry, competent evaluation practice, general skills for evaluation practice, and evaluator professionalism. A small exploratory study using focus groups and multiattribute utility analysis provided surprising evidence of face validity in that the 31 Minnesota evaluators who participated in the study agreed on 78% of the proposed competencies. There was near unanimous support for two competencies: "framing the evaluation questions," and "ethical conduct." The places where participants disagreed on specific competencies—for example, providing recommendations, writing literature reviews, and conflict resolution—appeared to reflect the "role- and context-specific nature of evaluation practice" (King et al., 2001, p. 245). The item that received the lowest mean, "contributes to the knowledge base of evaluation," was an activity that multiple evaluators reportedly felt was not their concern.

Once the exploratory study provided proof of concept for the creation of a set of evaluator competencies, our team of four set out to revise them, integrating comments, suggestions, and feedback from a variety of sources. Published 4 years later, this revision (Stevahn et al., 2005) presented the "Taxonomy of Essential Competencies for Program Evaluators." While many of these, given a technical definition, were not formal competencies, they nevertheless represented a well-received improvement to the original set. Expanding the categories of the initial taxonomy, the revised domains were professional practice, systematic inquiry, situational analysis, project management, reflective practice, and interpersonal competence. Even lacking formal empirical validation, this set of competencies proved practically useful. For example, the CES used them as the basis of CES competencies when formalizing their Credentialed Evaluator Program.[3] In addition, professional groups in Japan and Germany/Austria adapted them for local use.

In the roughly 15 years since the essential competencies were published, the field appears to have accepted the idea that program evaluator competencies are possible. In 2015 King and Stevahn wrote, "When considering the practical implications of the current status of competencies, one can . . . wonder if the field is nearing a tipping point that will push it to common consideration of the competencies for program evaluators" (p. 31). Indeed, two broad factors appear at this time to support more widespread use of evaluator competencies as part of the broader movement toward the field's professionalization:

1. The first such factor is extremely pragmatic and relates directly to the potential users described above. In part there is a growing need for evaluator education, training, and professional development, and competencies can provide a helpful way to structure such opportunities. Also, as the demand for evaluation increases, people commissioning and using studies want to know that the people they hire are competent to do the work and generate credible processes and products. As other fields have the means to document and verify professional competence, why shouldn't evaluation?

2. The second factor relates to the age and growing maturity of the field. As the number of practicing evaluators and voluntary organizations for professional evaluation (VOPEs) to build professional community has grown dramatically in the past decade, so, too, have discussions of how to increase the field's professionalization. In the United States, the work of the AEA Competencies Task Force and, following its conclusion, the creation of the Professionalization and Competencies Working Group were the board's responses to increased consideration of how to move AEA into a meaningful discussion of professionalization. In Canada, the Credentialed Evaluator Program of the CES (2019) requires first that evaluators assess their personal competence using a set of competencies, then respond to an expert

---

[3] The CES competencies integrated the reflective practice domain competencies into the professional practice domain, resulting in a total of five domains.

review of their portfolio. In Europe, for a time evaluators could choose to participate in a voluntary evaluation peer-review (VEPR) process grounded in self-assessment, again based on a set of "capabilities" (competencies) to improve their skills (European Evaluation Society, 2019); VEPR was ultimately phased out owing to the challenges of implementing a volunteer-based program. Importantly, the International Organization for Cooperation in Evaluation (IOCE), which "represents international, national, subnational and regional Voluntary Organizations for Professional Evaluation (VOPEs) worldwide," created a Professionalization Task Force in 2015 to "support IOCE's role and action in the professionalization of evaluation," noting that professionalization is a gradual, long term, context dependent process with many facets: (a) improved access to quality education and training; (b) dissemination of evaluation knowledge and good practices; (c) harmonization of ethical guidelines and guiding principles for evaluators; (d) *agreed evaluator capabilities or competencies frameworks*; and (e) legitimate ways of recognizing the fundamental knowledge, skills and dispositions needed to carry out work to an adequate standard of quality. (IOCE, 2019, emphasis added)

While there is visible evidence, then, that the field is moving toward increased professionalism or at least serious discussions of professionalization, at the same time it is important to note that not everyone is sanguine with these developments. Schwandt (2017), for example, raises the broader question of "what professionalism means in evaluation and what the profession itself aims to add to society, or the social good it seeks to serve," what he calls the "professional ethos of evaluation" (p. 546). The IOCE (2024) notes that its Professionalization Task Force "does not think that it is either possible or even advisable to aim for a unified approach to professionalization at this point . . ." The AEA Competencies Task Force was explicit in its presentation of the competencies that their development is only the second of three steps in professionalization, Step 1 being a review of foundational documents and global outreach to VOPEs to learn what others are doing; Step 2 being the development of competencies; and Step 3 being determining what to *do* with the competencies once created, including measuring practitioners' competence (AEA, 2018b). Next steps include determining the criteria and standards for a set of competencies that are grounded in ethics, reflective of high-quality practice, useful, achievable, and ultimately measurable.

FORMAL AND LESS FORMAL PROCESSES FOR DEVELOPING COMPETENCIES

The idea of developing competencies for a field is not new. Over the years a variety of professions and organizations have created sets of competencies, and many employers and government agencies routinely hire firms to develop competencies for specific jobs or roles. McLagan (1997) outlines three broad approaches for the development of competencies, each of which focuses on different aspects of job performance:

> The differential psychology approach emphasizes the abilities of individuals; the educational-and-behavioral approach emphasizes the developmental characteristics of competence; the management-sciences approach emphasizes job analysis rather than people. (Wilcox & King, 2014, p. 9)

There are multiple terms associated with this work. Competence is an "abstract construct describing the quality of being competent" (Wilcox & King, 2014, p. 4); it is the "habitual and judicious use of communication, knowledge, technical skills, clinical reasoning, emotions, values and reflection in daily practice for the benefit of the individual and community being served" (Epstein & Hundert, 2002, p. 226). Competence is the result of successfully demonstrating competencies. A competency is "the quality of being adequately or well qualified" for a particular task or a defined function in a specific context; it is a "more concrete concept that includes particular knowledge, a single skill or ability, or an attitude" (Wilcox & King, 2014, p. 5). Table 2.1 provides definitions for additional terms related to the competency development process, including examples from program evaluation.

The reason that evaluation professionals have not until recently engaged in formal processes for developing competencies likely stems from

TABLE 2.1. Definition and Examples of KSAOs (Knowledge/Skills/Abilities/Other Characteristics)

Term	Description	Evaluation-specific examples
Knowledge	"Knowing something with familiarity gained through experience or association"; information and facts gained through education or experience	• The Program Evaluation Standards (Yarbrough, Shula, Hopson, & Carruthers, 2011) • The philosophy that grounds qualitative methods • Facilitation techniques grounded in the principles of social psychology
Skill	"The ability to use one's knowledge effectively and readily in execution or performance; a developed aptitude or ability"	• Evaluation contract negotiation • Data analysis • Collaborative decision making
Ability	"The quality or state of being able; natural aptitude or acquired proficiency; capability"	• Interpersonal communication • Ability to work under pressure • Time management
Other characteristics	Items that do not clearly fit into the categories of knowledge, skills, or abilities; for example, personal interests, attributes, commitments, beliefs, qualities, dispositions, and attitudes	• Willingness to work long hours • A commitment to learning and self-improvement • Ten years of experience

Note. Quoted definitions are from www.merriam-webster.com.

what has been discussed previously (i.e., evaluation means different things to people who engage in the practice and the status of the field remains indefinite). If the role and tasks of evaluators are diverse or unclear, then how exactly would a competency study define performance effectiveness criteria? Another possible reason concerns the fact that someone would need to pay for such a study. Indeed, a request from the Treasury Board in Canada was partly responsible for the origin of Canada's Credentialed Evaluator Program; if the CES had not stepped up to the task, the Treasury Board might have hired a firm to develop competencies for evaluators working in the federal government (King, 2015). The government of South Africa has similarly stimulated the development of agency-specific competencies not only for evaluators but for evaluation managers (Podems et al., 2013).

Instead of a funded competencies development process, what has happened in evaluation is the development of almost a dozen sets of evaluator competencies through a less formal—but still systematic—process whereby practicing evaluators who are members of professional associations or organizations inductively create sets of competencies by assembling existing lists and subjecting them to expert review and commentary. That is how the AEA Competencies Task Force, empaneled in January 2015, developed the AEA competencies over the course of 3 years (2015–2018; see Tucker et al., 2020).

It is important to note that AEA's Task Force was explicitly charged with developing competencies for the AEA membership. Headquartered in the United States, roughly 85% of AEA's members predominantly reside and practice evaluation in the United States, and Task Force members felt that it "would be presumptuous and arrogant (even hegemonic) to assume that we could develop competencies for all evaluation practice around the world" (King, 2016, p. 2). Highlighting the importance of contextual practice, then, these competencies are *not* meant to be general evaluator competencies but rather they are competencies that evaluators can and should adapt to their personal contexts—which is why they are included in this handbook.

The AEA competencies use the simplest structure for a set of competencies (i.e., they are a general set of categorized competencies in which items are grouped into domains without additional within-domain organization; Rassel, 2018). They do not detail minimal requirements for novices or describe what eventual mastery looks like, and there is no expectation that every evaluator must be minimally skilled in every competency or expert in any given competency, again, because so much depends on where and with whom evaluators are working. At this time, these competencies provide both novice and experienced evaluators and others engaged in evaluation endeavors content for reflection and potential action.

One concern may stem from the fact that the competencies are presented in linear and numerical order for clarity and easy identification. This fails to acknowledge the overlap between and among them and risks the potential of someone creating a checklist for evaluating evaluators, which is surely not the intent. In addition, the linear order may suggest a hierarchy or an order of importance that is not intended, nor are competencies rank ordered within domains. Figure 2.1 presents the AEA Task Force's Venn diagram that is nonhierarchical and nonlinear in an attempt to capture the interrelated nature of the domains in evaluation practice.

THE AEA COMPETENCIES FOR PROGRAM EVALUATORS

As explained above, the competencies are grouped into five domains that are sufficiently broad to make them inclusive of multiple types of evaluation practice. Not only is it appropriate to adapt them to specific contexts, given the diversity of people's practice, it is essential that evaluators do so, both individually and in groups. The competencies required by an external evaluator contracted individually to build evaluation capacity in a small nonprofit organization will dramatically differ from those applicable to a team of evaluators working on a major policy study for a large government department. The phrase "as appropriate" appears several times in these competencies, noting the importance of creating a viable process for a highly specific context. But the overarching domains remain the same:

- Professional practice "focuses on what makes evaluators distinct as practicing professionals."
- Methodology "focuses on technical aspects of data-based, systematic inquiry for valued purposes."
- Context "focuses on understanding the unique circumstances, multiple perspectives, and changing settings of evaluations and their users/interest holders."
- Planning and management "focuses on determining and monitoring work plans, timelines, resources, and other components needed to complete and deliver an evaluation study."
- Interpersonal "focuses on human relations and social interactions that ground evaluator effectiveness for professional practice." (AEA, 2018b)

This section details the competencies in each domain, and the section following provides illustrations of how people might apply them in practice.

Domain 1: Professional Practice

Table 2.2 presents the competencies in the professional practice domain. This domain distinguishes evaluation from other forms of practice (like research) that require data collection, analysis, and reporting of results. Central to its content—and highlighted by its placement as Competency 1.1—is a commitment to ethical behavior, including integrity and respect for all. While ethics appear explicitly in only one competency, it literally undergirds all of the other competencies.[4] Also critical is an awareness of the professional documents in the field, including, among others, the Program Evaluation

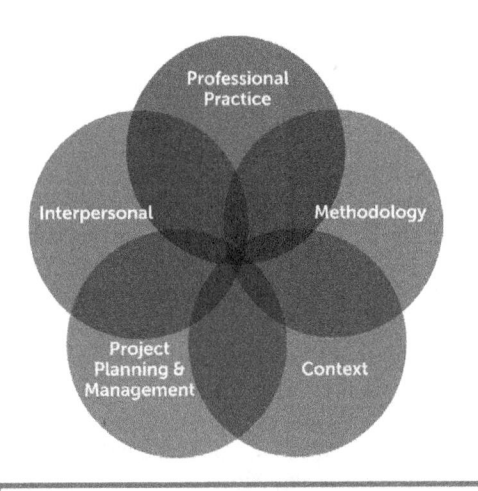

FIGURE 2.1. AEA Competency Task Force diagram showing the overlap of the competency domains.

---
[4]The initial draft of the AEA competencies included an ethical competency in each domain. Member feedback was highly critical of this redundancy, so the decision was made to have only one competency address ethics, but to make it the first one to highlight its centrality.

TABLE 2.2. Competencies in the Professional Practice Domain (Domain 1)

The competent evaluator . . .

1.1	Acts ethically through evaluation practice that demonstrates integrity and respects people from all cultural backgrounds and indigenous groups.
1.2	Knows and applies the foundational documents adopted by the American Evaluation Association that ground evaluation practice.
1.3	Knows and applies appropriate evaluation approaches and theories.
1.4	Uses evidence and logic in determining merit, worth, or value.
1.5	Engages in reflective practice and articulates personal evaluator competence, areas for growth, and implications for professional practice.
1.6	Pursues ongoing professional development to extend personal learning, stay current, and build connections in the field.
1.7	Considers how evaluation practice can promote social justice and the public good.
1.8	Recognizes the value of evaluation and advocates for the field.

Standards, the Guiding Principles for Evaluators, the AEA Statement on Cultural Competence (AEA, 2019b), and these competencies. Evaluation-specific knowledge (i.e., approaches, models, and theories specific to the field) again distinguishes practice in this field from others that may involve data collection and analysis. This is also true of the use of evidence and logic to determine "merit, worth, or value," a commitment that is distinctive of evaluation practice. Two competencies focus on the personal nature of competence; evaluators need to continually think about their own practice, know their strengths and areas for growth, and commit to ongoing learning to stay up-to-date as the field continues to evolve. Competency 1.6 also highlights the connected nature of the work as networking is an important skill.

The final two competencies may surprise people new to the field who view evaluation as an "objective," value-free activity. In fact, since the first edition of the Program Evaluation Standards in 1981, language related to benefiting the public good has been included in AEA's professional commitments. After extensive review and consultation, the Task Force developing these competencies elected to include both the terms *social justice* and *the public good* as content for professional practice (see Symonette et al., 2020). Competency 1.8 emphasizes the role of every evaluation practitioner to speak up for the field, advocating for it and encouraging its practice.

Domain 2: Methodology

The content of the second domain, methodology, includes what many would expect to see in an evaluator's toolkit. It "includes quantitative, qualitative, and mixed methods designs for understanding, decision making, and judging" (AEA, 2018b, p. 2). Table 2.3 details the 15

TABLE 2.3. Competencies in the Methodology Domain (Domain 2)

The competent evaluator . . .

2.1	Identifies evaluation purposes and needs.
2.2	Determines evaluation questions.
2.3	Determines and justifies appropriate methods to answer evaluation questions, e.g., quantitative, qualitative, and mixed methods.
2.4	Articulates values and assumptions that underlie methodologies.
2.5	Conducts reviews of the literature when appropriate.
2.6	Designs credible and feasible evaluations that address identified purposes and questions.
2.7	Identifies relevant data sources and sampling procedures.
2.8	Involves interest holders in designing, implementing, interpreting, and reporting evaluations as appropriate.
2.9	Collects data using credible, feasible, and culturally appropriate procedures.
2.10	Analyzes data using credible, feasible, and culturally appropriate procedures.
2.11	Articulates strengths and limitations of the evaluation design and methods.
2.12	Interprets findings/results in context.
2.13	Uses interpretations to draw conclusions, making judgments and recommendations when appropriate.
2.14	Communicates evaluation findings/results and conclusions.
2.15	Assesses evaluations formally or informally to improve future practice.

competencies related to methodology from beginning to end, moving from the initial steps in framing an evaluation process (purpose, needs, questions), to design and methods, to conducting the evaluation, and then to communicating results. Competency 2.8 notes that, as appropriate, interest holders can be involved throughout the process, and three adjectives—"credible, feasible, and culturally appropriate"—point to the importance of taking context into careful account during data collection and analysis. The final competency encourages meta-evaluation, either formal or informal, so that evaluators will reflect on and improve their practice over time.

Domain 3: Context

Every evaluation context is unique because it always involves a given time and place, specific individuals in that specific setting who can change over the course of a study, and numerous possible users and uses (see Table 2.4). The descriptor included with the AEA competencies (2018b) lists multiple features that are part of context: "site/location/environment, participants/interest holders, organization/structure, culture/diversity, history/traditions, values/beliefs, politics/economics, power/privilege, and other characteristics" (p. 3). The competencies in this domain require evaluators to attend to contextual issues by thoroughly understanding the program being evaluated, sometimes by developing program logic or program theory, and by interacting with a range of interest holders and facilitating mutual understanding of the program, including its grounding assumptions and its surrounding politics. The competencies also highlight context in a broader sense, including systems issues that may affect the program and its evaluation. Finally, Competency 3.9 requires evaluators to attend to what happens once the study is completed by considering its potential use or broader influence in context.

Domain 4: Planning and Management

The nine competencies in this domain focus on the nuts and bolts of planning and managing evaluations (see Table 2.5). This includes a variety of activities related to "determining and monitoring work plans, timelines, resources, and other components needed to complete and deliver an evaluation study" (AEA, 2018b, p. 3). Many specific activities are listed, including negotiating, managing, documenting, coordinating, supervising, and monitoring—all related to

TABLE 2.4. Competencies in the Context Domain (Domain 3)

	The competent evaluator . . .
3.1	Respects and responds to the uniqueness of the evaluation context.
3.2	Identifies and engages diverse users/interest holders throughout the evaluation process.
3.3	Describes the program, including its basic purpose, components, and its functioning in its broader context.
3.4	Facilitates shared understanding of the program and its evaluation in context.
3.5	Elicits program logic and program theory as appropriate.
3.6	Clarifies cultural assumptions, diverse perspectives, and political forces within the context.
3.7	Considers contexts beyond the program context that may affect the evaluation.
3.8	Addresses systems and complexity within the context.
3.9	Promotes evaluation use and influence in context.

TABLE 2.5. Competencies in the Planning and Management Domain (Domain 4)

	The competent evaluator . . .
4.1	Negotiates and manages a feasible evaluation plan, budget, resources, and timeline.
4.2	Attends to aspects of culture in planning and managing evaluations.
4.3	Manages and safeguards evaluation data.
4.4	Plans for and fosters evaluation use and influence.
4.5	Documents evaluation processes and products.
4.6	Coordinates and supervises evaluation processes and products.
4.7	Monitors evaluation progress and quality and makes adjustments when appropriate.
4.8	Uses technology appropriately to support and manage the evaluation.
4.9	Communicates evaluation processes and results in timely and effective ways.

conducting a successful evaluation. These competencies also direct attention to cultural issues, the protection of data, the potential need for adjustments in the study, and the appropriate use of technology. Finally, this domain details that a competent evaluator knows how to communicate effectively in ways that can lead to evaluation use.

Domain 5: Interpersonal

The final domain may seem the least directly related to program evaluation, but absent highly developed interpersonal skills, evaluators may be unable to even initiate studies, let alone conduct them successfully (see Table 2.6; King & Stevahn, 2013; King, 2023). These interpersonal skills include "cultural competence, communication, facilitation, negotiation, [and] conflict resolution" (AEA, 2018b, p. 3). What the competencies in this domain emphasize is an evaluator's ability to interact and work with all kinds of people in ways that are positive and trust building. The competent evaluator knows how to listen carefully and connect with others so that the diversity of perspectives in any context is brought forward. One competency requires evaluators to think explicitly about the effects of power and privilege, and another encourages purposefully structuring effective interactions. Two distinct roles are highlighted: that of evaluation team leader or member, and that of evaluation mentor or capacity builder. The final competency requires evaluators to be skillful in managing conflicts, even if they cannot be resolved.

In sum, these five competency domains and their 51 associated competencies highlight the characteristics of what it means to be a good evaluator. A good evaluator is one who engages in high-quality, ethical evaluation practice, uses appropriate and rigorous methodology, is highly sensitive to specific contexts, knows how to plan and manage an evaluation study, and responds thoughtfully to the people involved. By attending to these competencies, both novice and experienced evaluators can examine their practice and reflect on ways to identify strengths and weaknesses in hopes of emphasizing or building on the first and improving the second.

POTENTIAL USES OF THE EVALUATOR COMPETENCIES

As should be clear by now, the evaluator competencies provide a framework for thinking about evaluation practice, one that practicing evaluators must examine and shape to their own settings. In contrast to automobile ads that caution drivers from attempting risky maneuvers at home, these competencies are not presented on a closed track. Nor—to mix metaphors—are they set in stone. They are meant to be adapted to fit specific contexts, and that is where evaluators' creativity comes into play. In other words, *do* try contextualizing and adapting the competencies on the job. As people spend time with the competencies and make them their own, they are likely to identify areas of omission or find places where rewording is needed, which can be helpful. The point is to use these competencies in any way that advances your evaluation practice. Table 2.7 highlights three examples of evaluators' applying the competencies either personally or in their organization. In addition, consider these five further illustrations:

TABLE 2.6. Competencies in the Interpersonal Domain (Domain 5)

The competent evaluator . . .	
5.1	Fosters positive relationships for professional practice and evaluation use.
5.2	Facilitates shared decision making for evaluation practice.
5.3	Builds trust throughout the evaluation.
5.4	Listens to understand and engage different perspectives.
5.5	Recognizes how power and privilege affect interpersonal relationships in evaluation practice.
5.6	Communicates in ways that enhance understanding throughout the evaluation.
5.7	Facilitates constructive and culturally responsive interaction throughout the evaluation.
5.8	Collaborates and facilitates teamwork when appropriate.
5.9	Mentors and coaches others for evaluation capacity building when appropriate.
5.10	Manages conflicts constructively.

1. An experienced evaluator who graduated with a master's in evaluation 18 years ago reads Competency 1.3 ("Knows and applies appropriate evaluation approaches and theories") and elects to attend an update session on newer approaches that were not included in his earlier training, including the latest take on Chen's theory-driven evaluation and Patton's developmental, principles-focused, and blue marble evaluation.

2. Charged with developing an introductory evaluation course, an instructor requests review copies of several textbooks and uses the competencies to identify the content and skills that each cover (even minimally) and areas of emphasis. The text selected is the one that best addresses competencies the instructor believes are important for a single semester course.[5]

3. In preparation for an external review, evaluation departmental faculty review the existing graduate curriculum and course syllabi to see which domains, in their opinion, are adequately covered, which are minimally addressed, and what topics are missing. They work together to revise the courses to highlight what is well covered and to shore up areas of concern.

4. A newly hired internal director of evaluation is charged with building evaluation capacity in the agency. Working with the team of evaluators on staff, she conducts an assessment within the organization to identify areas of existing competence and areas where training is needed. Based on the results, the director develops a series of workshops and informal quizzes targeting specific competencies.

5. The new head of an evaluation association is concerned that recent attendance at the association's professional development sessions has declined. He asks his staff to poll the membership to determine which competencies would be of most interest for future training sessions and is pleased when two specific topics emerge: one related to promoting social justice and the public good and the other about the appropriate uses of innovative technology to support

---

[5]This same process can be applied to this handbook, which includes extensive content from competency Domains 1 (professional practice), 2 (methodology), and 4 (planning and management), and less from Domains 3 (context) and 5 (interpersonal).

TABLE 2.7. Examples of Evaluators Using the Program Evaluator Competencies

Who	Potential use
A novice evaluator, relatively new to the field	She uses the competencies to conduct an informal, personal self-assessment. Although thoroughly trained in methodology and well-grounded in program contexts, she is unaware of the Program Evaluation Standards, the AEA Guiding Principles, and other foundational documents, so she decides to study the documents and then determine how to apply them in her projects. She also revises her resume to highlight what she now knows are areas of strength.
The head of an internal evaluation for a multi-million-dollar program	He is tasked with putting together an effective, well-balanced evaluation team for a 5-year effort. He asks his colleagues to identify the competencies that they consider their major strengths and those where they feel less comfortable, then uses that information to identify people who will join the team and assign initial tasks. At the first team meeting, they discuss each person's areas of strength.
A program officer at a family foundation	The foundation is about to launch a major initiative that will seek to "move the needle" nationally on a major social issue. She needs to craft a meaningful RFP and job descriptions to hire a consulting firm to conduct an ongoing developmental evaluation of the effort. Since a sizeable amount of funding is available, she can envision a full complement of evaluators working for 3–5 years on the effort.

and manage evaluations. He works with the association leadership to plan trainings on these topics.

At this time, the value of the competencies for program evaluators stems from evaluators' ability to apply them in highly personalized ways unique to their individual practice or to the collective practice of an evaluation team. As the field becomes accustomed to the use of competencies, there may well be movement toward more formal professionalization, but that is a topic for future editions of this handbook.

SUMMARY AND CONCLUSION

This chapter has provided an overview of competencies in the field of program evaluation, including a rationale for their development and use, a description of their history and current status, and a discussion of processes for developing them. It also detailed one specific set of competencies—the board-approved competencies of the AEA—and gave examples of their potential uses. Remember these three key takeaways:

1. There are five domains of competencies with which evaluators should be familiar: professional practice, methodology, context, planning and management, and interpersonal.

2. A viable set of evaluator competencies now exists, and evaluators should take advantage of this by adapting them for personal and organizational use.

3. There is an opportunity to foster the use of competencies in program evaluation in a helpful and productive manner, with hopes of avoiding potential negative possibilities.

REFERENCES

Altschuld, J. W. (1999a). The case for a voluntary system for credentialing evaluators. *American Journal of Evaluation, 20*, 507–517.

Altschuld, J. W. (1999b). The certification of evaluators: Highlights from a report submitted to the Board of Directors of the American Evaluation Association. *American Journal of Evaluation, 20*(3), 481–493.

American Evaluation Association. (2018). *The 2018 AEA Evaluator Competencies.* Handout distributed at the 2018 Annual Conference, Cleveland, OH. Available at *www.eval.org/p/us/in*

American Evaluation Association. (2019a). *Guiding principles for evaluators.* Available at *www.eval.org/p/cm/ld/fid=51*

American Evaluation Association. (2019b). *Statement on cultural competence in evaluation.* Available at *www.eval.org/p/cm/ld/fid=92*

Ayoo, S., Wilcox, Y., LaVelle, J. M., Podems, D., & Barrington, G. V. (2020). Grounding the AEA competencies in the broader context of professionalization. *New Directions for Program Evaluation, 168*, 13–30.

Bickman, L. (1999). AEA, bold or timid? *American Journal of Evaluation, 20*(3), 19–20.

Canadian Evaluation Society. (1999). *Essential skills series.* Available at *www.evaluationcanada.ca/essential-skills-series-evaluation*

Canadian Evaluation Society. (2019). *About the CE designation.* Available at *https://evaluationcanada.ca/ce*

Covert, R. W. (1992). *Successful competencies in preparing professional evaluators.* Paper presented at the annual meeting of the American Evaluation Association, Seattle, WA.

Epstein, R. M., & Hundert, E. M. (2002). Defining and assessing professional competence. *Journal of the American Medical Association, 287*(2), 226–235.

European Evaluation Society. (2019). *The VEPR initiative.* Available at *www.europeanevaluation.org*

Fitzpatrick, J. L., Sanders, J. R., & Worthen, B. R. (2011). *Program evaluation: Alternative approaches and practical guidelines* (4th ed.). Pearson.

Ingle, M. D., & Klauss, R. (1980). Competency-based program evaluation: A contingency approach. *Evaluation and Program Planning, 3*, 277–287.

International Organization for Cooperation in Evaluation. (2024). Professionalization. Available at *www.ioce.net/professionalization.*

Jacob, S., & Boisvert, Y. (2010). To be or not to be a profession: Pros, cons and challenges for evaluation. *Evaluation, 16*(4), 349–369.

King, J. A. (2015). From the outside, looking in: Implications of CES's Credentialed Evaluator Program. *Canadian Journal of Program Evaluation, 29*(3), 134–153.

King, J. A. (2016). *Introductory content to accompany draft competencies* [Unpublished manuscript]. Department of Organizational Leadership and Policy Development, University of Minnesota.

King, J. A. (2018). *Presenting the AEA Program Evaluator Competencies.* Presentation at the Annual Meeting of the American Evaluation Association, Cleveland, OH.

King, J. A. (Ed.). (2020). The American Evaluation Association's Program Evaluator Competencies [Special issue]. *New Directions for Evaluation, 2020*, 1–172.

King, J. A. (2023). Evaluator education for the twenty-first century: The centrality of developing evaluators' interpersonal competencies. *Journal of Multidisciplinary Evaluation, 19*(46), 10–22.

King, J. A., & Stevahn, L. (2013). *Interactive evaluation practice: Mastering the interpersonal dynamics of program evaluation.* Sage.

King, J. A., & Stevahn, L. (2015). Competencies for program evaluators in light of adaptive action: What? So what? Now what? *New Directions for Evaluation, 145*, 21–37.

King, J. A., Stevahn, L., Ghere, G., & Minnema, J. (2001). Toward a taxonomy of essential evaluator competencies. *American Journal of Evaluation, 22*(2), 229–247.

LaVelle, J. M., & Galport, N. (2020). Using the 2018 AEA competencies for evaluator education and professional development. *New Directions for Evaluation, 168*, 99–116.

Matthias, C. (2022). *Practicing evaluators' visions of social justice: Definitions, theories, approaches, and problem framing* [Unpublished doctoral dissertation]. University of Minnesota.

McLagan, P. A. (1997). Competencies: The next generation. *Training and Development, 51*(5), 40–47.

Mertens, D. M. (1994). Training evaluators: Unique skills and knowledge. *New Directions for Program Evaluation, 62,* 17–27.

Patton, M. Q. (1990). The challenge of being a profession. *Evaluation Practice, 11,* 45–51.

Patton, M. Q. (2010). *Utilization-focused evaluation* (4th ed.). Sage.

Picciotto, R. (2011). The logic of evaluation professionalism. *Evaluation, 17*(2), 165–180.

Podems, D., Goldman, I., & Jacobs, C. (2013). Evaluator competencies: The South African government experience. *Canadian Journal of Program Evaluation, 28*(3), 71–85.

Rassel, S. M. (2018). *The development and use of interpersonal competencies by evaluators* [Unpublished doctoral dissertation]. University of Minnesota.

Schwandt, T. A. (2017). Professionalization, ethics, and fidelity to an evaluation ethos. *American Journal of Evaluation, 38*(4), 546–553.

Scriven, M. (1996). Types of evaluation and types of evaluator. *Evaluation Practice, 17*(2), 151–161.

Shanker, S. (2020). *Definitional tension: The construction of race in and through evaluation* [Unpublished doctoral dissertation]. University of Minnesota.

Stevahn, L., Berger, D. E., Tucker, S., & Rodell, A. (2020). Using the AEA evaluator competencies for effective program evaluation practice. *New Directions for Evaluation, 168,* 75–97.

Stevahn, L., King, J. A., Ghere, G., & Minnema, J. (2005). Establishing essential competencies for program evaluators. *American Journal of Evaluation, 26*(1), 43–59.

Stevahn, L., Tucker, S., & King, J. A. (2018). *The final results of the 2017 AEA membership survey on competencies.* Presentation at the 2018 conference of the American Evaluation Association, Cleveland, OH.

Symonette, H., Miller, R. L., & Barela, E. (2020). Power, privilege, and competence: Using the AEA competencies to shape socially just evaluation practice. *New Directions for Evaluation, 168,* 117–132.

Tucker, S., Barela, E., Miller, R. L., & Podems, D. (2020). The story of the AEA Competencies Task Force (2015–2018). *New Directions for Evaluation, 168,* 31–48.

Tucker, S. A., Stevahn, L., & King, J. A. (2023). Professionalizing evaluation: A time-bound comparison of the American Evaluation Association's foundational documents. *American Journal of Evaluation, 44*(3), 495–512.

Tuxworth, E. (1989). Competency based education and training: Background and origins. In J. W. Burke (Ed.), *Competency based education and training* (pp. 10–25). Falmer Press.

Vaca, S. (2018, November 10). *Sharing my top 10 evaluation doubts.* Available at *https://aea365.org/blog/?s=sara+vaca*

Wilcox, Y., & King, J. A. (2014). A professional grounding and history of the development and formal use of evaluator competencies. *Canadian Journal of Program Evaluation, 28*(3), 1–28.

Worthen, B. R. (1994). Is evaluation a mature profession that warrants the preparation of evaluation professionals? *New Directions for Program Evaluation, 62,* 3–15.

Worthen, B. R. (1999). Critical challenges confronting certification of evaluators. *American Journal of Evaluation, 20,* 533–555.

Yarbrough, D. B., Shulha, L. M., Hopson, R. K., & Caruthers, F. A. (2011). *The program evaluation standards: A guide for evaluators and evaluation users* (3rd ed.). Sage.

Part II

EVALUATION THEORIES, FOUNDATIONS, PRINCIPLES, AND PURPOSE

Chapter 3

Evaluative Thinking

Understanding and Applying the Foundations of Evaluation

Thomas Archibald
Jane Buckley
Guy O'Grady Sharrock

CHAPTER OVERVIEW

Evaluative thinking is central not just to the field of evaluation but to all human thought. Yet despite its centrality, the concept has not been widely studied or discussed in the evaluation literature until recently. In this chapter, we describe and define evaluative thinking, demonstrating that it can be framed both as a fundamental philosophical concept at the heart of evaluation and as an approach to evaluation capacity building designed to unleash the power of inquiry within programs and organizations, in service of learning and adaptive management. Then, focusing on this second framing, we share practical case examples whereby the core elements of evaluative thinking—identifying assumptions, posing thoughtful questions, reflecting and taking multiple perspectives, and making informed decisions in preparation for action—are used to guide evaluation capacity building processes. We conclude by reviewing some principles and practices to promote a culture of evaluative thinking. We posit that understanding and applying evaluative thinking as a foundational evaluation concept is a core competency needed to perform exemplary evaluations that are creative, adaptive, and sensitive to diverse contexts, and thus is an important consideration for readers of this handbook and for all evaluators alike.

In this chapter, we present the notion of **evaluative thinking**, a concept at the heart of evaluation practice. Evaluative thinking has been around for a long time. It is as old as evaluation itself, much older than the field of professional evaluation—as Scriven (2013) points out, it likely emerged around 2.25 million years ago along with the evolution of early hominids. In terms of Kahneman's (2011) *Thinking, Fast and Slow*, predicated on the evolution of human cognition, both System 1 (fast) and System 2 (slow) thinking are evaluative, according to House (2015): "evaluative thinking constitutes the core of cognitive processes. Human thought is fundamentally evaluative" (p. 18). Yet until recently, despite its essential importance at the heart of evaluation, the concept of evaluative thinking has strangely not been the subject of sustained and explicit attention, possibly because it appears so deceptively self-evident as to be invisible. As Vo and Archibald (2018) suggest, it is worthwhile—or perhaps imperative—to think carefully and intentionally about evaluative thinking, in spite of (or because of) its centrality to the practice of evaluation:

> Evaluative thinking is perhaps so ubiquitous as to be mundane. "It's what we do," an evaluator might say. Yet too often it is used without explanation, ironically relying on an assumption that we all know what we mean when we speak and write about evaluative thinking. Further, as an ever-present concept, it is troublingly easy to fall into the trap of circular logic when describing or defining evaluative thinking: "Evaluative thinking is how we think when we are evaluating." (p. 7)

Elsewhere, Patton (2010) warned, "As attention to the importance of evaluation culture and evaluative thinking has increased, we face the danger that these phrases will become vacuous through sheer repetition and lip service" (p. 162). That is why, in the first section of this handbook, it is important to pause and reflect on the nature of evaluative thinking.

Throughout this increased attention in recent years, conversations about evaluative thinking tend to fall into two overlapping categories, depending on how the concept is framed. On one hand, evaluative thinking is a foundational philosophical concept at the heart of what sets evaluation apart as a discreet professional domain or, alternatively, as a **transdiscipline**—that is, a discipline (like statistics or logic) "that has standalone status as a discipline *and* is also used as a methodological or analytical tool in several other disciplines" (Scriven, 2008b, p. 65, emphasis in original). From this perspective, evaluative thinking is a unique cognitive and values-informed reasoning process that evaluators do (or that anyone does when evaluating something).

On the other hand, evaluative thinking is framed as a new horizon in the panoply of ways to decentralize and democratize evaluative inquiry, such as developmental, collaborative, participatory, and empowerment evaluation (see Fetterman et al., Chapter 10, this volume), and **evaluation capacity building** (ECB). ECB is "the intentional work to continuously create and sustain overall organizational processes that make quality evaluation and its uses routine" (Stockdill et al., 2002, p. 14). A more recent definition describes ECB as "an intentional process to increase individual motivation, knowledge, and skills, and to enhance a group or organization's ability to conduct or use evaluation" (Labin et al., 2012, p. 308). From this perspective, evaluative thinking is what King (2007) described as the ultimate goal of ECB practice: "free-range evaluation," or evaluative thinking that lives unfettered in an organization (p. 46).

In the first conceptualization, the role of values and valuing is paramount, a topic covered in much more detail by Gates and Schwandt (see Chapter 5, this volume), in House (2015), and in a special issue of the *Evaluation Journal of Australasia* (Gullickson et al., 2019). In the second conceptualization, the emphasis is on unleashing the power of inquiry throughout all of an organization's practices and processes, even if the result of that inquiry is not necessarily a formal, explicit judgment claim about the value (i.e., merit, worth, or significance) of something. The first centers mostly on evaluative thinking among professional evaluators, whereas the second is focused on how ECB facilitators help program implementers, administrators, and others (i.e., non-evaluators) become better evaluative thinkers.

Amid these varied perspectives on evaluative thinking's contours and boundaries, some questions remain even about whether the term itself is the right one—Schwandt (2018) suggested we ought to be talking about "evaluative reasoning" rather than evaluative thinking, while Delahais and colleagues translated evaluative thinking into French as *la posture evaluative* (Quadrant Conseil, 2018), more akin to an "evaluative stance." Years prior, Weiss (1998) described something similar as "an evaluative cast of mind" (p. 25). Even our own definition of evaluative thinking presented below raises questions about the overlap between critical thinking and evaluative thinking, and emphasizes that evaluative thinking is not a mere cognitive activity—thinking for thinking's sake—but rather one that involves both an affective element (i.e., an evaluative attitude) and a call to action (i.e., better-informed decision making). Below, we first provide a broad view of the current thinking on evaluating thinking, then go more in depth into some practical case examples of efforts to intentionally foster evaluative thinking as a way to do ECB.

DESCRIBING AND DEFINING EVALUATIVE THINKING

Although evaluative thinking is an ancient human practice, the term only began to appear in the evaluation literature with much frequency around 2005. In her 2007 presidential address to the American Evaluation Association, Preskill (2008) highlighted the construct's importance, asking, "How do we build the capacity of individuals, teams, and organizations to think evaluatively and engage in evaluation practice?" (p. 129). In an interview with the International Development Research Centre (IDRC) in Canada, Patton (2005) described evaluative thinking as "a willingness to do reality testing, to ask the question: how do we know what we think we know? . . . Evaluative thinking is not just limited to evaluation projects. . . . It's an analytical way of thinking that infuses everything that goes on" (para. 10). Elsewhere, Patton (2014) makes a strong connection between evaluative thinking and evaluation use: "Evaluation is an activity. Evaluative thinking is a way of doing business. This distinction is critical. It derives from studies of evaluation use. Evaluation is more useful—and actually used—when the program and organizational culture manifests evaluative thinking" (p. 1).

Also based on work at the IDRC, Carden and Earl (2007) described how evaluative thinking was infused into that organization's culture, primarily through changes made to their reporting structure. They echo Patton's (2005) description of evaluative thinking:

> Evaluative thinking shifts the view of evaluation from only the study of completed projects and programs toward an analytical way of thinking that infuses and informs everything the center does. Evaluative thinking is being clear and specific about what results are sought and what means are used to achieve them. It ensures systematic use of evidence to report on progress and achievements. Thus, information informs action and decision making. (p. 72, no. 2)

For Wind and Carden (2010), "Evaluative thinking involves being results oriented, reflective, questioning, and using evidence to test assumptions" (p. 31). Bennett and Jessani (2011) agree; they define evaluative thinking as a "questioning, reflecting, learning, and modifying . . . conducted all the time. It is a constant state-of-mind within an organization's culture and all its systems" (p. 24).

In addition to the IDRC, the Bruner Foundation is another leading organization in working with evaluative thinking. They also emphasize the necessity that evaluative thinking (ideally) be ubiquitous within an organization, not limited solely to evaluation tasks. They discuss how helping grantees think more evaluatively can ultimately increase positive impacts in communities. In their report on "Integrating Evaluative Capacity into Organizational Practice," Baker and Bruner (2012) describe evaluative thinking as a type of **reflective practice** that integrates the same skills that characterize good evaluation—"asking questions of substance, determining what data are required to answer specific questions, collecting data using appropriate strategies, analyzing collected data and summarizing findings, and using the findings"—throughout all of an organization's work practices (p. 1). Their description, however, raises a question about the boundary of evaluative *thinking* and evaluative *doing*.

Along these lines, Volkov (2011) discusses evaluative thinking as an important component of the work of internal evaluators (see also Love, Chapter 22, this volume). Volkov proposes the notion of "the evaluation meme" to help conceptualize how ideas, behaviors, and styles of evaluation can spread through an organization:

> Modern internal evaluators will understand how to integrate evaluation into programs and staff development in a way that reinforces the importance of evaluation, contributes to its habituation, but at the same time prevents its harmful routinization (senseless, repetitive use of the same techniques or instruments). Evaluative thinking is not only a process, but also a mind-set and capacity, in other words, a person's or organization's ability, willingness, and readiness to look at things evaluatively and to strive to utilize the results of such observations. A challenging role for the internal evaluators

will be to promulgate such a mind-set throughout the entire organization. (p. 38)

Volkov's point is echoed by Griñó et al. (2013): "the antithesis of evaluative thinking is treating evaluation as a check-it-off compliance activity" (p. 2).

Davidson et al. (2004) also articulate the multidimensionality of this construct. They define evaluative thinking as "a combination of commitment and expertise, involving an understanding of the performance gap [between the current level of performance and a desired level of performance] and knowing how to gauge it" (pp. 260–261). Essentially, they focus on two distinct components of evaluative thinking: evaluative know-how and passion for improvement (or an evaluative attitude, emphasizing the affective and motivational dimensions of evaluative thinking).

All of these descriptions of evaluative thinking are helpful, but it was not until recently that more explicit efforts were undertaken to clearly define what it is. For instance, based on the results of a Delphi study with evaluation thought leaders, Vo (2013) proposed that:

> Evaluative thinking is a particular kind of critical thinking and problem-solving approach that is germane to the evaluation field. It is the process by which one marshals evaluative data and evidence to construct arguments that allow one to arrive at contextualized value judgments in a transparent fashion. (p. 107)

From our experience as ECB practitioners, informed by Brookfield's (2012) work on teaching critical thinking, we have elsewhere proposed that:

> Evaluative thinking is critical thinking applied in the context of evaluation, motivated by an attitude of inquisitiveness and a belief in the value of evidence, that involves identifying assumptions, posing thoughtful questions, pursuing deeper understanding through reflection and perspective taking, and informing decisions in preparation for action. (Buckley et al., 2015, p. 378)

Building on these earlier definitions of evaluative thinking, and informed by the theoretical framings and practice-based experiences described in this chapter, we propose this updated definition: Evaluative thinking is a cognitive and relational process, motivated by an attitude of inquisitiveness and a belief in the value of evidence, that involves identifying assumptions, posing thoughtful questions, marshaling evidence to make judgments, pursuing deeper understanding, and making logically aligned, contextualized decisions in preparation for action.

Evaluative thinking can happen outside of formal evaluation, just as evaluation can happen without any evaluative thinking (see Figure 3.1). In the first case, using a Scrivenesque definition of "evaluation," whereby it is a cognitive process that far exceeds the bounds of professional program evaluation (see Scriven, 1998; cf. Trochim, 1998), we practice evaluative thinking when buying toothpaste or a new car, for example. The second case—all too common—is when evaluation activities occur only as technical, compliance-oriented, check-the-box protocols within an organization's administrative functioning, what Dahler-Larsen (2017) has called "an institutionalized autopilot" (p. 243), or what Volkov (2011) described as "harmful routinization (senseless, repetitive use of the same techniques or instruments)" (p. 38). In these cases, evaluation activities (e.g., creating surveys, collecting data) can occur but without any evaluative thinking. As suggested by early empirical studies on this subject, when evaluation activities are informed and inspired by evaluative thinking, better evaluation occurs (Archibald et al., 2016; Griñó et al., 2013).

Below, reflecting on our own ECB practice, plus new lessons and insights shared in a 2018 *New Directions for Evaluation* volume on evaluative thinking (Vo & Archibald, 2018), we

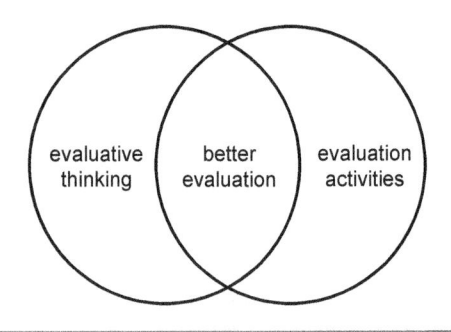

FIGURE 3.1. Overlap of evaluative thinking and evaluation activities.

focus on how to promote, learn, and apply evaluative thinking across diverse contexts. But first we consider in slightly more detail the framing of evaluative thinking as a foundational philosophical concept for the field of evaluation.

EVALUATIVE THINKING AS A FOUNDATIONAL PHILOSOPHICAL CONCEPT

Some of the first writing on what we now call evaluative thinking was provided by Scriven, especially in *Reasoning* (1976) and *The Logic of Evaluation* (1980). Other contributions are found in House's (1977, 1980) writing on the logic of the evaluative argument and Fournier's (1995) paper on working logic for establishing evaluative conclusions. These foundational theoretical writings are summarized by Nunns (2011; see also Nunns et al., 2015): "No matter the sophistication of our evaluation design, our attention to methodological rigor, our strategies and tools to encourage evaluation use, *an evaluation will lack impact without sound evaluative reasoning and argument*" (Nunns, 2011, slide 3; emphasis in original).

Another important part of understanding evaluative thinking as a foundational philosophical concept has to do with differentiating it from the more familiar notion of critical thinking. In 1987, the National Council for Excellence in Critical Thinking (which included Scriven) defined critical thinking as "the intellectually disciplined process of actively and skillfully conceptualizing, applying, analyzing, synthesizing and/or evaluating information gathered from, or generated by, observation, experience, reflection, reasoning or communication, as a guide to belief and action" (Scriven & Paul, 1987, para. 1). Note that this definition contains the phrase "evaluating information,"

so it seems that critical thinking may require evaluative thinking, making it difficult to distinguish clearly between the two. On this point, Vo and colleagues (2018) propose, "Making a reasoned choice about value and being able to defend it is what distinguishes evaluative thinking from critical thinking" (p. 40).

One of the most fruitful ways to translate these fundamental philosophical notions into the practical application of evaluative thinking in an ECB intervention is through the idea of "alignment." Reflecting on the four component parts laid out in our original definition of evaluative thinking (i.e., identifying assumptions, posing thoughtful questions, pursuing deeper understanding through reflection and perspective taking, and making informed decisions in preparation for action), we focus on the need for a common logical thread that aligns and links the different elements. For every assumption there is one or more aligned question. In turn, based on how the question is posed, there is an implied method of pursuing understanding, which leads to a claim that eventually can inform an implied decision. Figure 3.2 presents an example of alignment (albeit an overly simplistic one), in this case in the context of a needs assessment inquiry. By using a needs assessment example, we demonstrate how the logic of evaluative thinking applies much more broadly than just to the context of making formal formative or summative evaluation conclusions.

Misalignment between one or more of these components is in practice all too common. Yet, maintaining alignment is critical to high-quality evaluation. Figure 3.3 depicts a situation in which misalignment is present, which would render the evaluative inquiry invalid and unhelpful. For example, the main idea, or "construct," at the heart of the evaluation question is *knowledge*, yet the claim is about *behavior*.

Assumption	Question	Method	Evidence	Claim	Decision
Intended program participants have a need for a program like ours.	Do our intended participants have a need for a program like ours?	Focus groups with people drawn from the population of intended participants for the program.	Reported perspectives of intended participants about their need for a program like this.	Intended program participants have a need for a program like ours.	Pursue the development of the program based on intended participants' reported need.

FIGURE 3.2. An example of alignment between the elements of an evaluative claim.

Assumption	Question	Method	Evidence	Claim	Decision
If youth participate in 6 hours of nutrition education, they will eat a healthier diet.	Does the program cause an increase in the knowledge of nutrition among participants?	Online post-survey of participants with items about nutrition knowledge.	Descriptive statistics of the nutrition knowledge scores of some program participants.	The program caused youth to eat a healthier diet.	Scale up the program to other schools and contexts.

FIGURE 3.3. An example of misalignment between the elements of an evaluative claim.

Also, the claim is causal in nature, whereas the methods and analysis do not provide any evidence of causation.

Alignment, with methodological and logical appropriateness at its heart, should be considered one of the "gold standards" in evaluation. To reiterate, it is not the methodology alone that makes an evaluation high quality or "rigorous"—it is the alignment among the program model (i.e., logic model), evaluation question, the methods, the evidence, the claims, and the eventual use.

Attending to alignment is an application of evaluative thinking to **meta-evaluation**, because it involves thinking evaluatively about the processes and products of one's initial evaluative thinking and evaluation activities. For example, imagine a program team, well-versed in the intentional practice of evaluative thinking, conducting an assumption audit—that is, "a quick recap or clarification of the assumptions [their] arguments are based on, the assumptions that lie behind the way [they] respond to specific questions" (James & Brookfield, 2014, p. 31). Each person is thinking evaluatively and taking turns identifying assumptions about how and why their program works. Among them, the meta-evaluative thinkers are already reflecting on each of the assumptions, thinking about the questions they might ask related to each assumption, how those questions might be answered, and how useful those answers might be. This "alignment thinking" is the first step in determining on which assumptions to focus; it allows an activity such as an assumption audit (which can at times feel overwhelming) to feel purposeful, systematic, and generative in the process of program development and adaptive management.

In focusing on alignment, we also broach the subject of what counts as credible evidence (Archibald, 2015; Donaldson et al., 2014), which is yet another way of applying evaluative thinking as a meta-evaluative lens. One early dominant (and still persistent) fallacy about credible evidence is that the randomized controlled trial (RCT) is the "gold standard" for producing credible evidence about "what works" (see Baron, 2018; Mosteller & Boruch, 2002), despite Scriven's (2008a) claim that the RCT design "has essentially zero practical application to the field of human affairs" (p. 12). And while Baron, Mosteller, Boruch, and others advocating for the preeminence of RCTs do admit the importance of nonrandomized designs (including observational, qualitative studies) for purposes other than establishing causal claims of "impact" with high internal validity, the political economy of the RCT movement in evaluation and applied social science (e.g., economics) has often obscured that nuance (Bédécarrats et al., 2019; Chambers, 2017; Deaton & Cartwright, 2018). Yet, to regain some of that missing nuance, when applying an evaluative thinking lens—informed by the need for alignment and by the primacy of the logic of evaluative reasoning—it becomes obvious that the true gold standard is methodological appropriateness and rigorous thinking, not strict adherence to one prescribed design or method among many others (Bickman & Reich, 2014; Greene, 2014; Scriven, 2008b).

EVALUATIVE THINKING IN PRACTICE: UNLEASHING THE POWER OF INQUIRY

Now that we have defined and described evaluative thinking and touched on its place as a fundamental philosophical concept in evaluation, the remainder of this chapter is focused on how to promote evaluative thinking, and as such is likely of greatest interest to those evaluation practitioners who see ECB as part of their job (an ever-growing community). However, even for evaluators who are not explicitly interested in ECB—if we are to heed Schwandt's (2008) call to "educate for an intelligent belief in evaluation" among the field of professional evaluators, among program implementers and administrators, and in society at large—the following section may be salient to all. Promoting evaluative thinking across all of an organization's processes can unleash the power of inquiry for continuous learning, adaptation, and improvement. In this section, we share some principles and practices from our experience as ECB facilitators in diverse settings; for those who want to go deeper into this aspect, much more information on these ECB approaches informed by evaluative thinking can be found elsewhere (Archibald et al., 2016; Archibald, Sharrock, et al., 2018; Buckley et al., 2015; Sharrock et al., 2017).

In workshops with program staff, administrators, evaluators, and others, it is helpful to teach evaluative thinking by proceeding in a relatively sequential fashion through the components of the definition presented above. As a reminder, those components are:

1. Identifying assumptions.
2. Posing thoughtful questions.
3a. Reflection.
3b. Taking multiple perspectives.
4. Making informed decisions in preparation for action.

In addition to providing a framework for teaching or building capacity on evaluative thinking, these steps can also serve as a heuristic device or reminder to structure an organization's application of evaluative thinking in their day-to-day program work.

Identifying Assumptions

One of the most powerful ways to use evaluative thinking to enhance people's capacity to do quality evaluation is to help them identify and rethink assumptions in their program planning and evaluation work (Nkwake, 2012; Nkwake & Morrow, 2016). Program planning and evaluation are replete with assumptions, for example, about:

- The way activities are purported to contribute to producing outcomes ("causal" assumptions).
- The need for a given program or activity, or what "ought" to happen in a given situation ("prescriptive" assumptions).
- How the problem undergirding the need for the program is framed ("diagnostic" assumptions; see also Archibald, 2020).
- The underlying worldview informing the program's approach, often linked to assumptions on any existing data or theory undergirding the program as well ("paradigmatic" assumptions).
- What should serve as a good indicator for a given outcome.
- What counts as credible evidence of that indicator.
- What methods are best suited to garner such credible evidence.
- How different interest holders, including program participants, should have a role in the evaluation.
- The ways in which power dynamics affect program planning and evaluation decisions, and much more.

While this list is by no means exhaustive, it represents the ubiquity and centrality of assumptions in program planning and evaluation. Going deeper, paradigmatic assumptions can be **ontological** (about the nature of reality), **epistemological** (about the nature of knowledge), **axiological** (about the nature of ethics), **methodological** (about systematic means to ascertaining or generating knowledge), or **praxeological** (about the nature of human action) (Brookfield, 2012; Biesta, 2015; Mertens & Wilson, 2012; Nkwake & Morrow, 2016).

Above, we described an "assumption audit" (James & Brookfield, 2014), which is one practical and tangible way of intentionally and explicitly working with assumptions in an evaluation context. Another device that works well in ECB practice is a scenario analysis (Brookfield, 2012), in which people read a hypothetical scenario (ideally one that is close to their real context, but not about their actual organization or program). Then, working as a collaborative group, they (i.e., the program implementors, guided by the evaluator or ECB facilitator) respond to the following prompts:

1. What assumptions—explicit and implicit—do you think the characters in the story are operating under? List as many as you can.
2. Of the assumptions you've listed, which ones could the characters check by simple inquiry? How could they do this?
3. Give an alternative interpretation of this scenario—a version of what's happening that is consistent with the events described but that you think the character would disagree with or has not noticed (from Brookfield, 2012; see also Archibald et al., 2016).

Helping people diagram their thinking, especially by working collaboratively to create a schematic or graphical depiction of their program's theory of change, is also a fruitful way to unearth buried assumptions and thus to practice evaluative thinking (Archibald et al., 2016; see also Frechtling, Chapter 20, this volume, on logic modeling).

Posing Questions: The Spectrum of Inquiry

The most obvious and central role of questioning in evaluation pertains to posing what are broadly referred to as evaluation questions (Davidson, 2005; Wingate & Schroeter, 2007). According to Wingate and Schroeter, such questions should be evaluative, pertinent, reasonable, specific, and answerable. Yet, with an evaluative thinking lens, other important types of questions also arise—the less formal, quicker-to-answer, reflective questions that good practitioners ask all the time.

Reflective practice is a hallmark of an evaluative thinker (Tovey & Archibald, 2023); but, like evaluative thinking, it is not often "counted" as evaluation or even as inquiry. To more explicitly admit reflective questions into the realm of valid evaluative questioning, it is helpful to conceptualize a "spectrum of inquiry" (see Figure 3.4). On the left end of the spectrum are the most frequently asked questions. Such questions are informal, although they can also be systematic and intentional. These questions can focus on implementation or outcomes, and include, for example: "What is your sense of how that went?"; "Did we have the materials we needed to complete that task?"; and "Do you think more people would have come if we offered the program on a weekend instead of a weekday?" Good evaluative thinking practitioners should be posing these thoughtful questions continuously. At the other end of the spectrum are the most formal, hardest-to-answer questions, which require more planning, time, complex methodologies, and resources to address—as such, they are naturally posed with far less frequency. These questions include, for example: "Did our intervention cause a long-term change?" and "Is our program effective across contexts and participant groups?" Where one falls on the spectrum of inquiry is also a function of the developmental stage of the program (Urban et al., 2014).

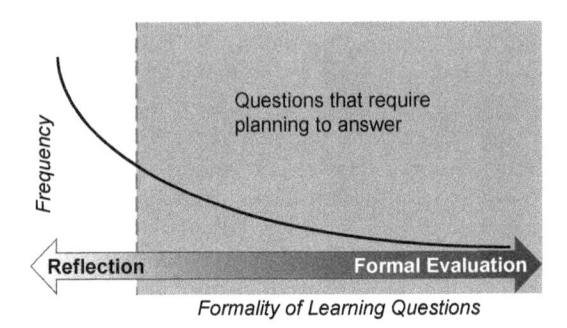

In between, there are questions that represent every shade of formality. Such questions could be clarifying questions (to help us better understand something), adjoining questions (to explore related aspects of the problem that may be otherwise ignored, such as "How would this concept apply in a different context?"), elevating questions (to raise broader issues and highlight the bigger picture), or funneling questions (to dive deeper; Pohlmann & Thomas, 2015). The shaded box on the right side of Figure 3.4 illustrates that most of the questions on the spectrum of inquiry require some amount of systematic planning to answer. For many, this is how they define evaluation. However, evaluative thinking includes and values all of the questions on the spectrum, and the phrase "posing thoughtful questions" in the definition of evaluative thinking is intended to include the full spectrum of inquiry—again, even if the questions do not necessarily lead to a formal, *explicit* judgment claim about the value of something.

FIGURE 3.4. The spectrum of inquiry.

Reflection

In his book *Evaluation Foundations Revisited: Cultivating a Life of the Mind for Practice*, Schwandt (2015) positions reflective practice as an antidote to overly mechanistic understandings of the role of knowledge in professional practice:

> The idea that dominates most thinking about knowledge for the professions is that practice is the site where this theoretical knowledge is *applied* to solutions to problems of instrumental choice . . . a matter of applying a toolkit or following a pre-approved set of procedures or practices. (p. 32, emphasis in original)

This idea is a manifestation of "**technical rationality**," a positivist epistemology of professional knowledge and practice in which "professional activity consists of instrumental problem solving made rigorous by the application of scientific theory and technique" (Schön, 1983, p. 21). Technical rationality is the dominant epistemology of practice, "the view of professional knowledge which has most powerfully shaped both our thinking about the professions and the institutional relations of research, education, and practice" (p. 21). However, due to the messiness of "'wicked problems,'" practitioners more often engage in "reflection-in-action, a kind of ongoing experimentation, as a means to finding a viable solution to such problems" leading to "a particular kind of craft knowledge (or the wisdom of practice)" (Schwandt, 2015, p. 32). Such **practical wisdom** plays an important role in ensuring an ethical evaluation practice (House, 2023; Hurteau & Archibald, 2023). Framing the importance of reflection in this way, evaluative thinking can be seen as a praxis to demystify theory and remystify practice (Lederach et al., 2007).

Taking Multiple Perspectives

The most obvious way of taking multiple perspectives in evaluation is through the myriad approaches for working with interest holders (Bryson et al., 2011). Tools such as a power/interest matrix, where interest holders can be classified as subjects (high interest and low power), crowd (low interest and low power), context setters (low interest and high power), or players (high interest and high power), can allow an evaluative thinker to try to see the program or the evaluation from any or all of those varied perspectives. Such a tool can be helpful at all stages of the program cycle—for example, during design to ensure that potential disrupters have their concerns addressed, and later on, as part of ongoing monitoring processes to determine whether course corrections are necessitated. Also in the vein of role-play activities, the Six Thinking Hats approach (De Bono, 1985) can help facilitate taking multiple perspectives; in this activity—for example, in a project evaluation meeting—program staff and other participants may be assigned to breakout groups to discuss the initial findings of the evaluation team. In so doing they are invited to adopt the perspective of one of six different character types or viewpoints (optimistic, discerning, emotional, creative, information based, or managerial). The discussion allows time for each perspective to be given "air time" and discussed, so that all sides of the topic are considered.

One final consideration that we have found to be salient when taking multiple perspectives is the role of power dynamics. To help people think about how power relations may influence one's perceptions of a problem, program, evaluation, or other object of inquiry, one useful tool is the Power Cube, developed by Gaventa (2006) and colleagues. This tool helps analyze various dimensions of power, such as its levels (global, national, and local), forms (visible, hidden, and invisible), and spaces (closed, invited, and claimed or created). Thus, it is a helpful tool for evaluative thinking, especially since critical reflection requires being attuned to power dynamics—always asking, Who benefits, Who loses, Who decides, Why, and How?

Making Informed Decisions in Preparation for Action

The final part of the definition of evaluative thinking helps move from thought to action. Sometimes, new information aligns easily with a plan of action. For example, if a simple inquiry activity (i.e., semistructured focus groups using a convenience sample drawn from community members) suggested that community members are unaware of available resources, there is a decision to be made about whether there is a need to learn more about why they are not aware, or if enough is already understood, to modify current efforts to increase awareness about available resources. Other times, the "correct" action is less clear. The lack of clarity can result from ambiguity, uncertainty, or lack of consensus on either technical or social terms (Stacy, 1996; Zimmerman, 2001). For example, there may be relatively high apparent technical certainty about the benefits of a conservation agriculture practice, but social norms and other less-apparent sociocultural considerations may impede uptake of that practice.

Making decisions is closely linked to the preceding step of posing thoughtful questions. There are some questions for which the bar for credible evidence is set higher, and the question is to the right on the spectrum of inquiry (e.g., whether a state should fund an early childhood literacy intervention for another 10 years). Yet other questions require only informal evidence and little planning (e.g., whether a program should be offered on Wednesdays or Saturdays), and thus can lead to rapid cycles of inquiry and action. This is where a probe–sense–act approach and many small "safe-to-fail" experiments (Snowden, 2002, 2005) may be warranted justification for decision making. In short, cost, effort, time, judgment, and experience all serve as determinants of decisions regarding future action.

Also, from their various perspectives and positions, different interest holders may experience asymmetries in information and evidence. Facilitated evaluative thinking processes can help surface those asymmetries and weigh the strengths and weaknesses of each person's evidence that might inform the decision. Then together, the team can collaboratively follow these five steps: (1) describe what you are seeing, (2) brainstorm plausible alternative explanations behind what you are seeing, (3) brainstorm plausible courses of action, (4) weigh alternative explanations and actions, and (5) make an action plan.

PRINCIPLES AND PRACTICES TO PROMOTE A CULTURE OF EVALUATIVE THINKING

Buckley et al. (2015, pp. 380–381) proposed five guiding principles aimed at ECB practitioners, teachers of evaluation, professional development facilitators, and anyone else involved in intentional educational efforts to promote evaluative thinking. Below, we revisit and extend these principles. In doing so, we also provide examples of evaluative thinking practice from our own practical applications of this work in real-world settings, both in the United States and internationally. In particular, we draw examples and lessons from our many years of offering a program of ECB rooted in evaluative thinking to various community development programs within Catholic Relief Services (CRS), a large international nongovernmental organization that implements social transformation projects worldwide. Our approach with CRS and other similar organizations consists of a workshop series designed for three participant groups (field-based staff, supervisors, and national leadership) sequentially implemented over a 3-year period.

The Opportunist Principle

Promoters of evaluative thinking should be opportunistic about engaging learners in a way that builds on and maximizes intrinsic motivation and sets out clear implementation intentions. Promoting evaluative thinking works best when it builds on what is already naturally occurring. Where conversations are already taking place regarding the merits or otherwise of an intervention, there is an opportunity to introduce evaluative thinking. Doing so will bring intentionality and structure to the process. This is applicable at all levels in an organization in which decisions can benefit from being informed by a review and critique of all reasonably accessible evidence.

One practical example from CRS is its incorporation of the "Learning to Action Discussions" (LADs) tool in guidance for the design of project monitoring systems. The focus of LADs, facilitated via the use of prompt questions (see Box 3.1), is the explicit intention to deliberate about what a given dataset may be implying for project management decision making. As such, the LAD is also an example of the element of evaluative thinking focused on posing thoughtful questions.

In so doing, "staff are encouraged to use the data they have been collecting to reflect on their own work. This active use of data serves to reinforce the collection of data and the appreciation staff have for M&E [monitoring and evaluation]" (Hahn & Sharrock, 2010, p. 43). One example from Sierra Leone involved project field staff discussing school registration data with their supervisors at their fortnightly meet-

> **BOX 3.1. Example Prompt Questions from the CRS LADs Tool**
>
> 1. What did we plan for the month? Quarter? Six months?
> 2. What did we achieve?
>   a. Review the data on the monthly data reports.
>   - What do these data tell us?
>   - What don't the data tell us?
>   - Who do the data represent?
>   - Who don't the data represent?
>   - What else do we need to know?
>   b. Are these data consistent with our observations on field visits?
>   c. Review of successes and challenges. Focus on the facts!
>   *Successes*
>   - What is going well?
>   - Why did it happen?
>   - So, what does this mean?
>   - How does it affect us?
>   *Issues/Challenges*
>   - What problems/issues are we having?
>   - Why is this happening?
>   - So, what does this mean?
>   - How does this affect us?
> 3. What happened (both good and bad) that we did not expect?
> 4. How are these results contributing to our objectives?
>
> *Note.* From Hahn and Sharrock (2010).

ings. Topics for discussion included seeking to understand why registration numbers might be different from previous occasions, and whether girls or boys were particularly implicated in any trend. Determining *who* to involve in evaluative thinking discussions is driven by context, and by the objective, scope, and significance of the topic. It is a managerial decision that balances time, cost, effort, and motivational considerations.

Another approach adopted by CRS has been the use of checklists. Staff are emboldened to use checklists to redesign and strengthen existing processes and systems in a manner that intentionally incorporates evaluative thinking. For example, a district supervisor in a project in Zambia developed a checklist to help her incorporate evaluative thinking into her monthly meetings with field staff. Inspired by the work of Gawande (2011), the checklist was restricted to one page, and indicated how to prepare, manage, and then report on the monthly meeting with prompts to ensure evaluative thinking was integrated at each stage. The value of the checklist is that the desire (or "goal intention") to apply evaluative thinking is supported by the act of setting out in advance—via the checklist—details of how the goal will be achieved, defined as "implementation intentions" (Wieber & Gollwitzer, 2010).

The Scaffolding Principle

Promoting evaluative thinking should incorporate—in both ECB activities and subsequent applications in the field—incremental experiences, following the developmental process of scaffolding. In pedagogy, "scaffolding" refers to a progressive strategy of instruction to help participants advance stepwise toward stronger understandings and, ultimately, greater independence in learning (Wood et al., 1976). The facilitator establishes successive exercises progressing from the most basic, or easiest to perform, to the most complex and challenging. In the case of evaluative thinking, it is easiest to think evaluatively about something that is different from one's own work or was developed by an unknown or anonymous person. In this case, the participant has little at stake and less bias, which allows them to think more freely and directly identify an area of need without a sense of vulnerability or risk. The next step is to practice thinking evaluatively about something that is more similar to, but not the same as their own work, and so on. The most difficult exercises involve the consideration of one's own, real work. This is both because our own assumptions (especially our paradigmatic assumptions) are the most difficult to identify, and because our deep knowledge of the context and the demands placed on the program complicate our ability to pose questions, seek evidence, and make decisions. As participants work through this progression of exercises, they gain evaluative thinking knowledge, skills, and confidence and, in turn, the amount of instructional support decreases. As with physical scaffolding, the supportive strategies are incrementally removed, and the facilitator gradually shifts more responsibility over the learning process to the participant.

One of the goals of scaffolding is to reduce the negative self-perceptions and feelings that participants may experience if an evaluative way of thinking is novel and is producing too much cognitive dissonance. It is intended to address those emotions of discouragement and vulnerability, since attempting a new, challenging thought process can sometimes feel critical and complex.

For CRS, scaffolding is embedded in the evaluative thinking workshop structure. The training is split over three rounds and progresses from simple to complex as well as from neutral to more personal. This admittedly longer process enables the content to be parsed out between the rounds and, during the intervening periods, for participants to reflect on the knowledge and skills they have acquired during each ECB cycle. Different forms of the workshops can be tailored to fit with time and other constraints. Research—using evidence gathered in 10 experimental studies with a sample of over 4,000 individuals, conducted across different environments, geographies, and populations—suggests that purposeful reflection on one's accumulated experience leads to greater learning than the accumulation of additional experience (Di Stefano et al., 2016).

Another approach to scaffolding involves using a "sandwich" ECB model in which face-to-face training is followed by a period of coaching leading to a final in-person reflection event. This approach enables the evaluative thinking promoter to track postworkshop uptake of the ideas, tools, and techniques introduced in the initial event, and to address participants' issues and concerns as they surface. While this approach is more resource intensive, there are opportunities via knowledge management and lessons sharing processes to widen the learning audience, thereby improving opportunities for scaling the impact of evaluative thinking ECB activities.

The Practicing Principle

Evaluative thinking is not a born-in skill nor does it depend on any particular educational background or job title or position; therefore, promoters should offer opportunities for it to be intentionally practiced by all who wish to develop as evaluative thinkers. Evaluative thinking does not rely on academic prowess. Drawing from Brookfield's (2012) experiences with teaching critical thinking, we posit that evaluative thinking can be instilled in five ways: (1) as a social learning process in which assumptions are surfaced and tested among peers; (2) by observing competent evaluative thinkers applying it in practice; (3) through informal experimentation using examples drawn from the world in which learners operate; (4) responding to an unanticipated event that obliges a novel way of thinking because the findings are so unexpected; and (5) as discussed with the Scaffolding Principle earlier, through a process of scaffolded learning. CRS's experiences of promoting evaluative thinking suggest that the five themes presented above do not depend on innate skill or educational attainment. Often, junior staff are quick to understand and apply evaluative thinking, while more senior staff, often locked into long-established conceptual frameworks, find it much harder to "remystify" their conventional thinking processes (Lederach et al., 2007).

Improved evaluative thinking capacity among *all* individuals throughout all of an organization's processes—programmatic, human resource, financial, logistical, and so on—can enable operations to be more open to inquiry, learning, and adaptation. Such adaptations may include recalibrating statements of expected results and redefining the intervention strategies employed to both achieve and evaluate results. The very process of doing evaluative thinking necessitates greater involvement of those of individuals working at the ground level in a more participatory and collaborative way. When monitoring data suggest that the interventions of a project are not being adopted to the extent that was originally expected, it is at the field level where plausible explanations are most likely to be identified. This paradigmatic shift toward listening more carefully to those most often ignored in the organizational hierarchy is corroborated by the wealth of literature on participatory development approaches (Anderson et al., 2012; Chambers, 1997, 2017).

The Assumptions and Belief Preservation Principle

Evaluative thinkers must be aware of—and work to overcome—assumptions and belief preservation (see Kahneman, 2011). Our work promoting evaluative thinking has demonstrated that a better understanding of assumptions helps program staff and administrators improve program quality, do more transparent reporting, and make more grounded decisions in response to actual project performance (see Hahn & Sharrock, 2010, for evidence of these effects). As discussed above, Brookfield (2012) is unequivocal about the central importance of assumptions:

> Trying to discover what are our assumptions are, and then trying to judge when, and how far, these are accurate is something that happens every time critical thinking occurs. You cannot think critically without hunting assumptions; that is, without trying to uncover assumptions and then trying to assess their accuracy and validity, their fit with life. (p. 7)

Buckley et al. (2015) noted the need for a "variety of structured and informal learning opportunities to help people identify and question assumptions" (p. 381). Underlying this suggestion is the understanding that evaluative thinking and, specifically, identifying assumptions, is a habit that must be adopted and then intentionally maintained and practiced.

We have found workshop participants to be both surprised and delighted by their newfound heightened awareness of implicit assumptions; once let loose, participants have no problem in collectively surfacing multiple possible "real-world" reasons that might have caused, for example, a lower than expected adoption rate of a technology or practice that the program was promoting with farmers. When this aspect of evaluative thinking is applied by professional evaluators, it is often done so by using methodological design or logic, such as Scriven's (2008b) general elimination method (GEM) or Campbell's attention to plausible alternative explanations (Bickman, 2000). The GEM is a theory-driven qualitative evaluation method that improves understanding of cause-and-effect relationships by systematically identifying and then ruling out causal explanations for an outcome of interest, which is similar in some ways to Campbell's plausible alternative explanations notion that

> the presumed cause must be the only reasonable explanation for changes in the outcome measures. If there are other factors which could be responsible for changes in the outcome measures we cannot be confident that the presumed cause–effect relationship is correct. (Trochim & Land, 1982, p. 1)

Once levels of awareness have been raised, the issue then becomes one of ensuring that the prevailing organizational culture intentionally accommodates opportunities for discussing assumptions in an ongoing way. Like any habit, evaluative thinking has to be attended to and maintained over time. Morell (2018) summarized this well:

> The goal is to include a consideration of assumptions with all the other considerations that go into planning discussions. It is not necessary to always pay attention to assumptions. Just as it may be unnecessary to consider budgets or staffing, it sometimes may be unnecessary to discuss assumptions. But the possible relevance of budgets and staffing will always be latent in whatever discussions people have, and they have the mindset to know when budgets and staffing should be part of a discussion. Moreover, an appreciation of budgets and staffing exists at a group level. Any single person who brings up these topics can be confident that the legitimacy of talking about these subjects will be accepted by all. Also, people have the technical and experiential knowledge needed to discuss budgets and staffing in a meaningful way. So too should it be with the topic of "assumptions." (p. 7)

Group conversations that are intentionally designed and managed to optimize learning around assumptions can provide an effective bridge between individuals' field-based learning, through group discussion, and organizational learning (Preskill et al., 2017). Intentionality in such meetings is critical for enabling participants to feel comfortable to share opinions and ideas, hear multiple perspectives, and create a climate in which the collective desire is aimed at taking action to improve the status quo. There are numerous techniques for facilitating such intentional group learning meetings (e.g., Preskill et al., 2017; Lipmanowicz & McCandless, 2014; Ramalingam, 2006). These can be brief, to be conducted within the span of 20 minutes, such as the "One Question" activity, described here:

> To address questions that participants may have about the state of something, a concern, or an opportunity, invite participants (this could be a rotating opportunity) to bring one question to

a meeting. For example, a participant might be wondering about a trend they are seeing in the field and might be curious whether others are also noticing it. They may bring the following question (or multiple questions related to the larger question) to be discussed: *In conversations I've been having with our colleagues and partners, I've started sensing that XX is happening. Are any of you seeing this as well? If yes, what do we think it might mean?* Start by describing the goal of the conversation, stating the question(s), and describing how answers will be used. Spend the first 15 to 20 minutes of the meeting reflecting on and discussing this question. Don't save it until the end; you likely won't get to it if you save it for last on the agenda! (Preskill et al., 2017, p. 12)

Or they might be more in-depth facilitated approaches, such as creating and using data placemats (Pankaj & Emery, 2016), after-action reviews (Cronin & Andrews, 2009), or a world café (Brown & Isaacs, 2005). The ultimate goal is that program staff and leadership will adopt these techniques and use them on their own in a regular, ongoing way.

The Social Learning Principle

Learning to think evaluatively is a social learning process; it requires all levels of staff to apply and practice the skill together, through intentionally facilitated "critical conversations," continuously and in multiple contexts. As Brookfield (2012) notes,

> social learning is not chatting comfortably and letting the conversation follow whichever way chance takes it. No, social learning for critical learning focuses on listening carefully to each other, asking questions of each other that uncover assumptions, and offering new perspectives or ideas. (p. 59)

Though one person can think evaluatively on their own, when done in conversation with a peer or colleague, the power and value of that thinking is multiplied. This is supported by a long history of research from the field of adult education that has framed learning as a fundamentally relational, social process (Bandura, 1977; Lave, 1988; Leeuwis & Pyburn, 2002; Niewolny & Wilson, 2011). At the same time, the best evaluative thinkers are those that do not limit their thinking practice to one area of work. Using evaluative thinking in multiple contexts allows the motivation to think evaluatively emerge more easily and naturally across those contexts, making evaluative thinking a "habit of mind" (Katz et al., 2002).

There are three recognizable misconceptions associated with the Social Learning Principle: (1) applying evaluative thinking is best achieved as a separate activity, (2) the application of evaluative thinking should be targeted to specific areas of activity, and (3) evaluative thinking is an "expert" activity applicable only to intermittent formal evaluations. We discuss each of these misconceptions briefly in turn below.

Concerning the first point, an ever-present risk in using the term *evaluative thinking* is that what should be a modus operandi firmly embedded in all ongoing activities ends up becoming isolated, viewed as a separate add-on activity. CRS has worked to encourage the view that the most cost-effective approach is to be intentional about embedding evaluative thinking into existing learning and reflection events. While accommodating evaluative thinking requires resources, time, and effort, an approach that integrates it into day-to-day work practices is likely to generate the most benefit, leading to more informed decisions. CRS has successfully integrated evaluative thinking in settings ranging from field staff monthly monitoring meetings, to large project design workshops, to annual project review events, and more.

Turning to the second misconception above (i.e., the application of evaluative thinking should be targeted to specific areas of activity), it is important to note that evaluative thinking activities are not the exclusive purview of programmatic discussions. Thinking evaluatively can enrich evidential conversations equally well when applied to other areas of operations in which assumptions can play a critical role, such as logistics, operations management, supply chain management, human resources, and financial management.

The third misconception concerns the sense of "otherness" that can sometimes be associated with evaluative thinking. This perception often implies that evaluative thinking is viewed as an activity that only experts can undertake, typically when they are applying it in the context of a formal evaluation, and that it adds no value to ongoing project monitoring; both views are misplaced. Evaluative thinking can be thought of as "the deliberate exploration of experience for a purpose" (De Bono, 1976, p. 33), within the sphere of monitoring, evaluation, and program management activities. In this vein, the voices of so-called non-experts in evaluation can serve as very powerful contributions to the project management decision-making process, all along the spectrum of inquiry described earlier in this chapter.

The Social Learning Principle has the expressed aim of normalizing the use of evaluative thinking in all situations. In undertaking its internal ECB work regarding evaluative thinking, part of CRS's process has been to involve nonprogram staff. For example, with the CRS Mawa project in eastern Zambia, a mixed team comprising field staff and experts complemented each other to use evaluative thinking to address a specific challenge that arose following the introduction of a new approach to farming (Baldridge & Sharrock, 2017).

The Psychological Safety Principle

For evaluative thinking to thrive, the right enabling conditions must exist, particularly a psychologically safe and trusting environment. Such an environment is characterized by mutual respect, authenticity, humility, clearly established roles, acknowledgment of feelings, trust, shared purpose, reciprocity, co-ownership, open communication, mutual questioning and feedback, and acceptance of failure and mistakes (Buckley et al., 2021). Other performance pressures—meeting deadlines, hitting targets, getting caught up in the general push and pull of everyday work—can distract from allocating time for reflection and learning. Leadership at all levels has a key role in influencing the right enabling conditions. As mentioned above, CRS's evaluative thinking ECB activities were undertaken at three different levels of the hierarchical system: (1) field-based staff, (2) senior program staff, and (3) country leadership (including nonprogrammatic leaders from human resources, finance, etc.). This reflected a view that for evaluative thinking to take hold, a simultaneous bottom-up and top-down approach was needed.

Beyond simple statements of support from leadership, there is a need for an intentional commitment to modeling, motivating, and managing in a manner that encourages and rewards quality evaluative thinking. Leaders should encourage all staff to value alternative explanations about surprising project results, even when they run contrary to received wisdom. This can be challenging, since individuals are wary of having opinions that differ from those to whom they report, or across topic-area boundaries. Also, many of us do not necessarily have the skills to offer or take and accept constructive criticism.

Leaders must appreciate the importance of establishing and sustaining an environment of psychological safety for interpersonal risk taking (Edmondson & Lei, 2014). Staff should know and appreciate that their opinions will be heard and valued and not used to humiliate or punish them. Becoming aware of the assumptions that underpin our projects can often be puzzling. Thus, creating a working environment that encourages different perspectives, viewpoints, sources of information, and even critique is essential. Such a working environment provides a sense of liberation to speak up in good faith and offer opinions that may run contrary to all other previously articulated opinions, or to ask seemingly naive questions that no one else has dared ask. CRS has trained some of their staff on approaches that have been shown to promote psychological safety, suggesting that leaders should (1) frame all work as a learning opportunity, not merely an execution issue, to open up the space for collaborative inquiry; (2) acknowledge their own fallibility so that colleagues feel safe in articulating their thoughts; and (3) model curiosity so that others can follow suit (Edmondson & Lei, 2014).

To question is not to criticize. Evaluative thinking is about figuring out the "why," not a simplistic binary choice of "right" or "wrong," or "good" or "bad." Relatedly, it takes some time for staff to feel comfortable acknowledging that they do not always have the answers. As Wheatley (2002) stated, "we live in a complex world, we often don't know what is going on, and we won't be able to understand its complexity unless we spend more time not knowing. . . . Curiosity is what we need" (pp. 34–35). For example, program monitoring, too often viewed as a bean-counting exercise, is increasingly viewed as an evaluative process; this shift in perception has invaluable implications. Programs operate in contexts that shape and challenge them and, despite the preparatory analyses, often find that initial assumptions are either no longer valid, or at the very least do not apply to all evaluands. Evaluative thinking that embodies mindfulness and values multiple perspectives applied in complex contexts—that is, those where outcomes cannot be known with certainty in advance, only after the fact, is key. As Langer (2014) says, "Mindfulness is the process of actively noticing new things. When you do that, it puts you in the present. It makes you more sensitive to context and perspective. It's the essence of engagement" (p. 68). Done well, evaluative thinking encourages staff to accept that there is little certainty along the originally mapped development pathway. That is not to say that the ultimate ambition of a given project will be necessarily open to renegotiation—for example, reducing food insecurity or improving the health of women and children would remain unchanged. It is the route to achieving those aims that is likely to end up being much more convoluted.

Encouragingly, the value of establishing a culture that enables collaborating, learning, and adapting has been recognized by the U.S. Agency for International Development and other large development agencies and organizations (Archibald, Sharrock, et al., 2018). There is movement toward

> being comfortable sharing opinions and ideas, hearing different perspectives, taking action on different ideas . . . [creating] safe spaces to have candid conversations no matter who is in the room . . . [and having] strong relationships and networks throughout the system we operate in that are based on trust, knowledge sharing, and good communication. (Ziegler, 2016)

There is a mutually constitutive and supporting relationship between the conditions described by Ziegler and a culture of evaluative thinking—that is, the more those conditions are in place, the more evaluative thinking can flourish, and vice versa, in a virtuous cycle. In such settings, one might begin to see and hear indicators of evaluative thinking, such as those listed in Box 3.2.

When these indicators of evaluative thinking increasingly appear, the ultimate goal of ECB has been attained: free-range evaluation, or evaluative thinking that lives unfettered in an organization (see Box 3.3; King, 2007). Even beyond the organizational level, reflecting on Schwandt (2008), as we face the erosion and degradation of the role of thoughtful evaluative thinking and reasoning in the achievement, maintenance, and enhancement of "the good life," we hope that evaluative thinking can also play an important part in educating for an intelligent belief in evaluation, and thus contribute to making the world a better place.

BOX 3.2. Indicators of Evaluative Thinking in an Organization

Things you may hear:

- Why are we assuming X?
- How do we know X?
- What evidence do we have for X?
- What is the thinking behind the way we do X?
- How could we do X better?
- Interest holder X's perspective on this might be Y.
- How might we be wrong?

Things you may see:

- More evidence gathering and sharing.
- More feedback (in all directions).
- Reflective conversations among staff, beneficiaries, leadership, etc.
- More illustrating of thinking.
- Evolution in the way people do things.
- More effective and efficient work.

REFERENCES

Anderson, M. B., Brown, D., & Jean, I. (2012). *Time to listen: Hearing people on the receiving end of international aid.* CDA Collaborative Learning Projects.

Archibald, T. (2015). "They just know": The epistemological politics of "evidence-based" non-formal education. *Evaluation and Program Planning, 48,* 137–148.

Archibald, T. (2020). What's the problem represented to be? Problem definition critique as a tool for evaluative thinking. *American Journal of Evaluation, 41*(1), 6–19.

Archibald, T., Sharrock, G., Buckley, J., & Cook, N. (2016). Assumptions, conjectures, and other miracles: The application of evaluative thinking

BOX 3.3. Tying It All Together: Key Takeaways

- Evaluative thinking (ET) is both a fundamental philosophical concept at the heart of evaluation and an approach to evaluation capacity building designed to unleash the power of inquiry within programs and organizations, in service of learning and adaptive management.
- Understanding and applying ET as a foundational evaluation concept is a core competency needed to perform exemplary evaluations that are creative, adaptive, and sensitive to diverse contexts.
- ET consists of both evaluative know-how and an evaluative attitude, an important affective dimension of ET.
- ET helps ensure logical alignment among questions, evidence, and claims; it can be applied as meta-evaluation to judge the alignment and trustworthiness of evaluations and claims.
- ET can and should be fostered and promoted among non-evaluators (e.g., program implementers and evaluators) by operationalizing the key components of Buckley et al.'s (2015) definition:
  - Identifying assumptions—through assumption audits, scenario analysis, etc.
  - Posing thoughtful questions—in a way sensitive to the variety of questions along the spectrum of inquiry.
  - Reflection—against technical rationality, the critically reflective aspect of ET can help bring the practical wisdom of evaluators and evaluative thinkers to the fore.
  - Taking multiple perspectives—in ways sensitive to power dynamics, using tools like interest holder analysis, Six Thinking Hats, and the Power Cube, among others.
  - Making informed decisions in preparation for action—not thinking for thinking's sake.
- Evidence-informed principles for promoting ET include:
  - The opportunist principle—promoters of ET should be opportunistic about engaging learners in a way that builds on and maximizes intrinsic motivation and sets out clear implementation intentions.
  - The scaffolding principle—promoting ET should incorporate, in both ECB activities and subsequent applications in the field, incremental experiences following the developmental process of scaffolding.
  - The practicing principle—ET is not a born-in skill nor does it depend on any particular educational background or job title or position; therefore, promoters should offer opportunities for it to be intentionally practiced by all who wish to develop as evaluative thinkers.
  - The assumptions and belief preservation principle—evaluative thinkers must be aware of—and work to overcome—assumptions and belief preservation.
  - The social learning principle—learning to think evaluatively is a social learning process; it requires all levels of staff to apply and practice the skill together, through intentionally facilitated "critical conversations," continuously and in multiple contexts.
  - The psychological safety principle—for ET to thrive, the right enabling conditions must exist, particularly a psychologically safe and trusting environment.

to theory of change models in community development. *Evaluation and Program Planning, 59,* 119–127.

Archibald, T., Sharrock, G., Buckley, J., & Young, S. (2018). Every practitioner a "knowledge worker": Promoting evaluative thinking to enhance learning and adaptive management in international development. *Evaluative Thinking, 158,* 73–91.

Baker, A., & Bruner, B. (2012). *Integrating evaluative capacity into organizational practice.* Bruner Foundation. Available at *www.evaluativethinking.org/docs/Integ_Eval_Capacity_Final.pdf*

Baldridge, E., & Sharrock, G. (2017). *Making connections, measuring results: CLA in a food security program in Zambia.* USAID CLA Case Competition. Available at *https://usaidlearninglab.org/library/making-connections-measuring-results-cla-food-security-program-zambia*

Bandura, A. (1977). *Social learning theory.* Prentice Hall.

Baron, J. (2018). A brief history of evidence-based policy. *Annals of the American Academy of Political and Social Science, 678*(1), 40–50.

Bédécarrats, F., Guérin, I., & Roubaud, F. (2019). All that glitters is not gold: The political economy of randomized evaluations in development. *Development and Change, 50*(3), 735–762.

Bennett, G., & Jessani, N. (Eds.). (2011). *The knowledge translation toolkit: Bridging the know-do gap: A resource for researchers.* SAGE.

Bickman, L. (Ed.). (2000). *Research design: Donald Campbell's legacy.* SAGE.

Bickman, L., & Reich, S. M. (2014). Randomized controlled trials: A gold standard or gold plated? In S. I. Donaldson, C. A. Christie, & M. M. Mark (Eds.), *Credible and actionable evidence: The foundation for rigorous and influential evaluations* (pp. 83–113). SAGE.

Biesta, G. (2015). On the two cultures of educational research, and how we might move ahead: Reconsidering the ontology, axiology and praxeology of education. *European Educational Research Journal, 14*(1), 11–22.

Brookfield, S. D. (2012). *Teaching for critical thinking: Tools and techniques to help students question their assumptions.* Jossey-Bass.

Brown, J., & Isaacs, D. (2005). *The world café: Shaping our futures through conversations that matter.* Berrett-Koehler.

Bryson, J. M., Patton, M. Q., & Bowman, R. A. (2011). Working with evaluation stakeholders: A rationale, step-wise approach and toolkit. *Evaluation and Program Planning, 34*(1), 1–12.

Buckley, J., Archibald, T., Hargraves, M., & Trochim, W. M. (2015). Defining and teaching evaluative thinking: Insights from research on critical thinking. *American Journal of Evaluation, 36*(3), 375–388.

Buckley, J., Hargraves, M., & Moorman, L. (2021). The relational nature of evaluation capacity building: Lessons from facilitated evaluation partnerships. *New Directions for Evaluation, 169*, 47–64.

Carden, F., & Earl, S. (2007). Infusing evaluative thinking as process use: The case of the International Development Research Centre (IDRC). *New Directions for Evaluation, 116*, 61–73.

Chambers, R. (1997). *Whose reality counts? Putting the last first.* Intermediate Technology.

Chambers, R. (2017). *Can we know better? Reflections for development.* Practical Action.

Cronin, G., & Andrews, S. (2009). After action reviews: A new model for learning. *Emergency Nurse, 17*(3), 32–35.

Dahler-Larsen, P. (2017). Critical perspectives on using evidence in social policy. In B. Greve (Ed.), *Handbook of social policy evaluation* (pp. 242–262). Elgar.

Davidson, E. J. (2005). *Evaluation methodology basics: The nuts and bolts of sound evaluation.* SAGE.

Davidson, E. J., Howe, M., & Scriven, M. (2004). Evaluative thinking for grantees. In M. Braverman, N. Constantine, & J. K. Slater (Eds.), *Foundations and evaluation: Contexts and practices for effective philanthropy* (pp. 259–280). Jossey-Bass.

De Bono, E. (1976). *Teaching thinking.* Smith.

De Bono, E. (1985). *Six Thinking Hats: An essential approach to business management.* Little, Brown.

Deaton, A., & Cartwright, N. (2018). Understanding and misunderstanding randomized controlled trials. *Social Science and Medicine, 210*, 2–21.

Di Stefano, G., Gino, F., Pisano, G. P., & Staats, B. (2016). *Making experience count: The role of reflection in individual learning.* Harvard Business School NOM Unit Working Paper No. 14-093. Available at *https://ssrn.com/abstract=2414478*

Donaldson, S. I., Christie, C. A., & Mark, M. M. (Eds.). (2014). *Credible and actionable evidence: The foundation for rigorous and influential evaluations.* SAGE.

Edmondson, A. C., & Lei, Z. (2014). Psychological safety: The history, renaissance, and future of an interpersonal construct. *Annual Review of Organizational Psychology and Organizational Behavior, 1*(1), 23–43.

Fournier, D. (1995). Establishing evaluative conclusions: A distinction between general and working logic. *New Directions for Evaluation, 68*, 15–32.

Gaventa, J. (2006). Finding the spaces for change: A power analysis. *IDS Bulletin, 37*(6), 23–33.

Gawande, A. (2011). *The checklist manifesto: How to get things right.* Penguin Books.

Greene, J. (2014). How evidence earns credibility in evaluation. In S. I. Donaldson, C. A. Christie, & M. M. Mark (Eds.), *Credible and actionable evidence: The foundation for rigorous and influential evaluations* (pp. 205–220). SAGE.

Griño, L., Levine, C., Porter, S., & Roberts, G. (2013). *Embracing evaluative thinking for better outcomes: Four NGO case studies.* InterAction and the Centre for Learning on Evaluation and Results for Anglophone Africa. Available at *www.interaction.org/document/embracing-evaluative-thinking-better-outcomes-four-ngo-case-studies*

Gullickson, A. M., Hassall, K., Hannum, K. M., & Roorda, M. (2019). Editorial. *Evaluation Journal of Australasia, 19*(4), 159–161.

Hahn, S., & Sharrock, G. (2010). *ProPack III: The CRS project package: A guide to creating a SMILER M&E System.* Catholic Relief Services. Available at *www.crs.org/our-work-overseas/research-publications/smiler-guide*

House, E. R. (1977). *The logic of evaluative argument* (Monograph No. 7). Center for the Study of Evaluation, UCLA Graduate School of Education, University of California.

House, E. R. (Ed.). (1980). Logic of evaluative argument. In *Evaluating with validity* (pp. 67–96). SAGE.

House, E. R. (2015). *Evaluating: Values, biases, and practical wisdom.* Information Age.

House, E. (2023). The practical wisdom of evaluators. In M. Hurteau & T. Archibald (Eds.), *Practical wisdom for an ethical evaluation practice.* Information Age.

Hurteau, M., & Archibald, T. (Eds.). (2023). *Practical wisdom for an ethical evaluation practice.* Information Age.

James, A., & Brookfield, S. D. (2014). *Engaging imagination: Helping students become creative and reflective thinkers.* Jossey-Bass.

Kahneman, D. (2011). *Thinking, fast and slow.* Macmillan.

Katz, S., Sutherland, S., & Earl, L. (2002). Developing an evaluation habit of mind. *Canadian Journal of Program Evaluation, 17*(2), 103–119.

King, J. A. (2007). Developing evaluation capacity through process use. *New Directions for Evaluation, 116*, 45–59.

Labin, S. N., Duffy, J. L., Meyers, D. C., Wandersman, A., & Lesesne, C. A. (2012). A research synthesis of the evaluation capacity building literature. *American Journal of Evaluation, 33*(3), 307–338.

Langer, E. (2014). Mindfulness in the age of complexity. *Harvard Business Review, 92*(3), 68–73.

Lave, J. (1988). *Cognition in practice: Mind, mathematics, and culture in everyday life*. Cambridge University Press.

Lederach, J. P., Neufeldt, R., & Culbertson, H. (2007). *Reflective peacebuilding: A planning, monitoring and learning tool kit*. Joan B. Kroc Institute, University of Notre Dame and CRS.

Leeuwis, C., & Pyburn, R. (Eds.). (2002). *Wheelbarrows full of frogs: Social learning in rural resource management*. Van Gorcum.

Lipmanowicz, H., & McCandless, K. (2014). *The surprising power of liberating structures: Simple rules to unleash a culture of innovation*. CreateSpace.

Mertens, D. M., & Wilson, A. T. (2012). *Program evaluation theory and practice: A comprehensive guide*. Guilford Press.

Morell, J. (2018). *Revealing implicit assumptions: Why, where, and how?* Catholic Relief Services Report. Available at *www.crs.org/sites/default/files/report_revealing_assumptions.pdf*

Mosteller, F., & Boruch, R. (Eds.). (2002). *Evidence matters: Randomized trials in education research*. Brookings Institution.

Niewolny, K. L., & Wilson, A. L. (2011). "Social learning" for/in adult education? In S. B. Merriam & A. P. Grace (Eds.), *The Jossey-Bass reader on contemporary issues in adult education* (pp. 340–349). Jossey-Bass.

Nkwake, A. M. (2012). *Working with assumptions in international development program evaluation*. Springer.

Nkwake, A. M., & Morrow, N. (2016). Clarifying concepts and categories of assumptions for use in evaluation. *Evaluation and Program Planning, 59*, 97–101.

Nunns, H. (2011). The "heart" of evaluation influence: A compelling evaluative argument. Presentation to the Australian Evaluation Society conference [PowerPoint presentation]. Available at *https://slideplayer.com/slide/7678560*

Nunns, H., Peace, R., & Witten, K. (2015). Evaluative reasoning in public-sector evaluation in Aotearoa New Zealand: How are we doing? *Evaluation Matters—He Take Tō Te Aromatawai, 1*, 137–163.

Pankaj, V., & Emery, A. K. (2016). Data placemats: A facilitative technique designed to enhance stakeholder understanding of data. *New Directions for Evaluation, 2016*(149), 81–93.

Patton, M. Q. (2005). In conversation: Michael Quinn Patton. Interview with Lisa Waldick, from the International Development Research Center. Available at *www.idrc.ca/en/ev-30442-201-1-DO_TOPIC.html*

Patton, M. Q. (2010). Incomplete successes. *Canadian Journal of Program Evaluation, 25*(3), 151–163.

Patton, M. Q. (2014). Preface. In L. Griñó, C. Levine, S. Porter, & G. Roberts (Eds.), *Embracing evaluative thinking for better outcomes: Four NGO case studies*. InterAction and the Centre for Learning on Evaluation and Results for Anglophone Africa. Available at *www.interaction.org/document/embracing-evaluative-thinking-better-outcomes-four-ngo-case-studies*

Pohlmann, T., & Thomas, N. M. (2015, March 27). Relearning the art of asking questions. *Harvard Business Review*. Available at *https://hbr.org/2015/03/relearning-the-art-of-asking-questions*

Preskill, H. (2008). Evaluation's second act: A spotlight on learning. *American Journal of Evaluation, 29*(2), 127–138.

Preskill, H., Gutiérrez, E., & Mack, K. (2017). *Facilitating intentional group learning: A practical guide to 21 learning activities*. FSG. Available at *www.fsg.org/tools-and-resources/facilitating-intentional-group-learning*

Quadrant Conseil. (2018). *Consultation sur le bilan de Mieux Légiférer*. Available at *www.quadrant-conseil.fr/ressources/documents/Quadrant_Mieux_Legiferer.pdf*

Ramalingam, B. (2006). *Tools for knowledge and learning: A guide for development and humanitarian organisations*. Overseas Development Institute.

Schön, D. (1983). *The reflective practitioner: How professionals think in action*. Basic Books.

Schwandt, T. (2008). Educating for intelligent belief in evaluation. *American Journal of Evaluation, 29*(2), 139–150.

Schwandt, T. (2015). *Evaluation foundations revisited: Cultivating a life of the mind for practice*. Stanford University Press.

Schwandt, T. (2018, November). *Evaluative thinking, Part 1*. Panel discussion at the American Evaluation Association Conference, Cleveland, OH.

Scriven, M. (1976). *Reasoning*. McGraw-Hill.

Scriven, M. (1980). *The logic of evaluation*. Edgepress.

Scriven, M. (1998). Minimalist theory: The least theory that practice requires. *American Journal of Evaluation, 19*(1), 57–70.

Scriven, M. (2008a). The concept of a transdiscipline: And of evaluation as a transdiscipline. *Journal of MultiDisciplinary Evaluation, 5*(10), 65–66.

Scriven, M. (2008b). A summative evaluation of RCT methodology: An alternative approach to causal research. *Journal of Multidisciplinary Evaluation, 5*(9), 11–24.

Scriven, M. (2013). *The past, present and future of evaluation*. Keynote presented at the Australasian Evaluation Society Conference, Melbourne, Australia. Available at *www.youtube.com/watch?v=MN6v1\An\2g*

Scriven, M., & Paul, R. (1987). *Defining critical thinking*. Statement presented at the 8th Annual International Conference on Critical Thinking and Education Reform. Available at *www.criticalthinking.org/pages/defining-critical-thinking/766v*

Sharrock, G., Buckley, J., & Archibald, T. (2017). *Evaluative thinking facilitator's guide*. Catholic Relief Services. Available at *www.crs.org/our-work-overseas/program-areas/monitoring-evaluation-accountability-and-learning/key-tools-and-inititatives*

Snowden, D. (2002). Complex acts of knowing: Paradox and descriptive self-awareness. *Journal of Knowledge Management, 6*(2), 100–111.

Snowden, D. (2005). Multi-ontology sense-making: A new simplicity in decision-making. *Management Today Yearbook 2005*.

Stacy, R. (1996). *Strategic management and organizational dynamics* (2nd ed.). Pitman.

Stockdill, S. H., Baizerman, M., & Compton, D. W. (2002). Toward a definition of the ECB process: A conversation with the ECB literature. *New Directions for Evaluation, 93,* 7–26.

Tovey, T. L., & Archibald, T. (2023). The relationship between reflective practice, evaluative thinking, and practical wisdom. In M. Hurteau & T. Archibald (Eds.), *Practical wisdom for an ethical evaluation practice* (pp. 87–101). Information Age.

Trochim, W. M. (1998). An evaluation of Michael Scriven's "minimalist theory: The least theory that practice requires." *American Journal of Evaluation, 19*(2), 243–249.

Trochim, W., & Land, D. (1982). Designing designs for research. *The Researcher, 1*(1), 1–6.

Urban, J. B., Hargraves, M., & Trochim, W. M. (2014). Evolutionary evaluation: Implications for evaluators, researchers, practitioners, funders and the evidence-based program mandate. *Evaluation and Program Planning, 45,* 127–139.

Vo, A. T. (2013). *Toward a definition of evaluative thinking* [Unpublished doctoral dissertation]. Graduate School of Education, Division of Social Research Methods, University of California, Los Angeles.

Vo, A., & Archibald, T. (Eds.). (2018). Editors' notes. *New Directions for Evaluation, 158,* 7–9.

Vo, A. T., Schreiber, J. S., & Martin, A. (2018). Toward a conceptual understanding of evaluative thinking. *New Directions for Evaluation, 158,* 29–47.

Volkov, B. B. (2011). Beyond being an evaluator: The multiplicity of roles of the internal evaluator. *New Directions for Evaluation, 132,* 25–42.

Weiss, C. H. (1998). Have we learned anything new about the use of evaluation? *American Journal of Evaluation, 19,* 21–33.

Wheatley, M. J. (2002). *Turning to one another: Simple conversations to restore hope to the future*. Berrett-Koehler.

Wieber, F., & Gollwitzer, P. M. (2010). Overcoming procrastination through planning. In C. Andreou & M. D. White (Eds.), *The thief of time: Philosophical essays on procrastination* (pp. 185–205). Oxford University Press.

Wind, T., & Carden, F. (2010). Strategy evaluation: Experience at the International Development Research Centre. *New Directions for Evaluation, 128,* 29–46.

Wingate, L., & Schroeter, D. (2007). Evaluation questions checklist for program evaluation. Available at *http://wmich.edu/evaluation/checklists*

Wood, D., Bruner, J. S., & Ross, G. (1976). The role of tutoring in problem solving. *Journal of Child Psychology and Psychiatry, 17*(2), 89–100.

Ziegler, J. (2016, October 4). Lucky #7: Meet the updated CLA framework, Version 7. USAID Learning Lab. Available at *https://usaidlearninglab.org/lab-notes/lucky-7-meet-updated-cla-framework%2C-version-7*

Zimmerman, B. (2001). *Edgeware-aides: Ralph Stacy's agreement and certainty matrix*. York University. Available at *www.betterevaluation.org/en/resources/guide/ralph_staceys_agreement_and_certainty_matrix*

Chapter 4

Evaluation Theories
Guidance to Evaluating in Various Circumstances

Melvin M. Mark

CHAPTER OVERVIEW

The idea of "theory" can be off-putting to some people, perhaps especially in a field such as evaluation. Evaluation is premised on the belief that its practice can make a positive difference in the world. Evaluators who want practical guidance may think that theory is abstract, overly general, and not sufficiently practical. This chapter asserts that, despite some people's skepticism about theory, fluency in evaluation theory can enhance evaluation practice. One major way that fluency in theory can be helpful is by improving judgments about which evaluation approach to employ in different contexts. This chapter discusses what evaluation theory is; considers multiple reasons why evaluation theory matters; examines two meta-models, or theories about evaluation theories; and reviews a small, select set of classic evaluation theories, with an example from practice for each theory and an update on the theory's influence. The chapter also briefly describes aspects of several more recent evaluation theories, explicates different ways that evaluation theory can guide evaluation practice, and offers suggestions for the future of evaluation theory.

For newcomers to the field of evaluation, it does not take long to discover that a vast array of methods are used under the umbrella of evaluation. Scanning through evaluation journals, or reviewing **evaluation reports** from different sources, or even reading the chapters in a volume such as this handbook, the fledgling evaluator encounters a wide, perhaps even bewildering variety. One article might use a randomized experiment, where prospective program participants are assigned by a flip of the coin either to the program or to a wait list, and the two groups are compared on outcomes of interest. In another case, the evaluator may conduct analyses of existing datasets to try to answer questions put forward by program managers. Yet another evaluation report may summarize the evaluator's efforts to engage program staff as collaborators, coaching them to collect and interpret data about the program. And another may summarize the use of in-depth interviews and observations to try to understand the lived experience of program participants.

The list of possible methods used by evaluators extends well beyond these few examples. Given such a rich set of alternatives, one of the most challenging tasks facing an evaluator is not *how* to do the evaluation but *why* to do the evaluation *in a particular way*. In other words, on what basis should the evaluator (or whoever is deciding) choose from among the myriad options that evaluators use?

Evaluation theory is an important possible answer to this question, or at least a part of the answer. This is not a new suggestion. In a classic book on evaluation theory, Shadish et al. (1991) stated,

> Evaluation theories are like military strategy and tactics; methods are like military weapons and logistics. The good commander needs to know strategy and tactics to deploy weapons properly or to organize logistics in different situations. The good evaluator needs theories for the same reasons in choosing and deploying methods. (p. 34)

Will Shadish, one of the authors of that book, made a similar point while commenting on evaluation training in the mid-1990s. Shadish (1996) said,

> It is probably fair to say that most courses in program evaluation emphasize methods. Indeed, courses on theory are often seen as being of secondary relevance to the practical needs of evaluators. In my view nothing could be further from the truth. What the field lacks most is people who know something about when, where, why and how different methods could and should be used in evaluation practice. Theory tells us that. (p. 553)

In this chapter, we (i.e., you, the reader, and me, the author) explore the role of evaluation theory. We consider what an evaluation theory is, and why practicing evaluators should be concerned about evaluation theory. We look at a pair of meta-models—that is, frameworks that are designed to help make sense of a multitude of evaluation theories, and we briefly consider how these meta-models can guide the study of evaluation theory. Using the two meta-models as a guide, we compare and contrast a small, select set of (mostly) classic evaluation theories and more selectively review others, including some more recent ones. Then we turn explicitly to a key, and underexamined, question: How exactly can evaluators draw on evaluation theories as helpful guides to evaluation practice? In that context, we explore portions of a larger number of evaluation theories. Finally, we look at possible developments in evaluation theory for the future.

WHAT IS EVALUATION THEORY?

Years ago, I was teaching a workshop on evaluation theory to a group of practicing evaluators—some novice, and others not. I spent a bit of time early in the workshop talking about why it was important for evaluators to be familiar with evaluation theory before I turned to what an evaluation theory is. I noticed two people in the back of the room who seemed to grimace and whisper to each other every time I used the phrase "evaluation theory." I tend to spread introductions of workshop participants over time, so had not yet learned that these two were college professors from the physical sciences. As I recall, one of them taught physics and the other may have taught chemistry. They had gotten involved at their college with interventions that were intended to improve student success in the sciences, and especially to increase the participation of students from traditionally underrepresented groups. This involvement in turn led to their engagement in evaluation, a field relatively foreign to them. Especially foreign to them was my use of the word *theory* in the phrase "evaluation theory." To them, theories were highly formalized, usually mathematically, with aspirations of wide applicability and generalizability. In contrast, others in the room from fields such as sociology and education were not so obviously bothered by my use of the term.

As I pointed out to those two workshop participants years ago, no one owns the word **theory**, and different people use it in different ways. Shadish et al. (1991) said, "*What do we mean by theory?* No single understanding of the term is widely accepted. *Theory* connotes a body of knowledge that organizes, categorizes, describes, predicts, explains, and otherwise aids in understanding and controlling a topic" (p. 30). Shadish et al. went on to indicate that a good **evaluation theory** would describe the activities to be engaged in while doing an evaluation, the goal(s) that the evaluation is intended to achieve, and the processes that are supposed to link the evaluative activities to the intended goals. Examples to come in this chapter will put some proverbial flesh on the bones of this description.

For the moment, perhaps it helps to note that a good evaluation theory contains more than a simple description of methods to use in doing an evaluation. A good evaluation theory also addresses such questions as what the goal of evaluation should be and why, as well as whether and how this should vary across situations. An evaluation theory should also clarify what counts as legitimate evidence, and also where the questions to address in an evaluation should come from and why. Additionally, a complete evaluation theory lays out a stance on what the key characteristics are of social programs (or whatever it is that's being evaluated). And a good evaluation theory highlights the implications of these various attributes for how evaluation should be done. An experienced evaluator who is unfamiliar with evaluation theory will nevertheless have views regarding at least some of the issues that a good evaluation theory should address. But a good evaluation theory will be more systematic and more explicit, including in the sense of suggesting linkages across its different elements (e.g., indicating how the goal of evaluation emphasized by that theory helps determine which/whose questions should have priority for an evaluation). Familiarity with evaluation theory, especially with multiple evaluation theories, should enrich evaluators' perspectives on the field, broaden their understanding of options that might be considered, and enhance their ability to match an evaluation to the circumstances.

The two physical science faculty members at my workshop are not the only people who have qualms with the term *evaluation theory*. Some evaluators also prefer different terminology, or at least are ambivalent about what the best label is. For example, Marv Alkin (2004) said that "In some ways, rather than theories it would be more appropriate to use the term *approaches* or *models*" (p. 4). Still, Alkin settled on using the term *evaluation theory* in his classic volume that traced the roots of a set of major theorists. Another notable evaluator, Dan Stufflebeam, wrote that his "monograph [which was published as an issue of the quarterly publication *New Directions for Evaluation*] uses the term *evaluation approach* rather than *evaluation model*" (2001, p. 9). Stufflebeam was concerned that the term *model* might be taken as implying that a particular approach was a good one. (For a touch of irony, check the reference section to see what the title of that issue of *New Directions for Evaluation* is.) Given that even people in evaluation differ in terms of their preferred terminology, it might be better to refer to "evaluation theories, models, or approaches." But that phrase is cumbersome and would likely grow old over the course of the chapter. Thus, for the most part in the rest of the chapter I refer to evaluation theories, which seems consistent with fairly common usage. And I invite you to substitute your preferred term, if you have one (perhaps keeping in mind that Smith, 2010, has encouraged different meanings for theory, model, and approach).

At the risk of adding confusion, I should note that some evaluators differentiate between different kinds of evaluation theories. We return to one important distinction of this sort later in the chapter, when we consider the future of evaluation theory.

WHY EVALUATION THEORY MATTERS

Evaluation is a practice-oriented enterprise. One might ask therefore, Why should evaluators care about theory? Theories are often esoteric—and perhaps are viewed as esoteric even when they are not. A popular stereotype is that theorists travel at 30,000 feet, while the real action is taking place on the ground. We have already seen the primary rationale for attending to evaluation theory, which is that theory can serve as a guide to evaluation practice. We return to this rationale in a subsequent section, which describes different ways of translating from evaluation theory to evaluation practice.

In this section we first attend to some other reasons evaluators should be attentive to evaluation theory. Two additional reasons are related to the idea of evaluation theory as a guide to practice. One is that evaluation theories are a way of consolidating lessons learned, of synthesizing prior experience, and of facilitating future progress. Years ago, Madaus et al. (1983) indicated that evaluators who lack the kind of knowledge that is embedded in evaluation theory "are doomed to repeat past mistakes and, equally debilitating, will fail to sustain and build on past successes" (p. 4). An old expression refers to the inefficiencies of reinventing the wheel. Even more problematic is the possibility of reinventing the square wheel—that is, of adopting an approach that others had already learned does not work. There is also a relevant elaboration of the familiar expression that we should learn from our mistakes. Told in various ways and attributed to sources including Oliver Wendell Holmes, Eleanor Roosevelt, Admiral Hyman Rickover, and Groucho Marx, it goes something like this: "You need to learn from the mistakes of others, because you don't live long enough to make them all yourself." Familiarity with evaluation theory helps us learn the lessons of the past—after all, theorists tend not to advocate practices that in their experience have failed—and in this way evaluation theory can guide us away from repeating others' mistakes—that is, reinventing the square wheel.

A related reason for learning about evaluation theories is that comparing across theories is a way of identifying key debates in the field and, correspondingly, identifying unsettled or disputed practice issues. Newcomers to evaluation sometimes encounter rationales within their organizations of the "but that's the way it's done" variety. Very often, the way it's always been done in one's organization has support in some quarters but not all. Being able to point to alternative theoretical perspectives that support a different way of doing things can be helpful, at least in facilitating consideration of future change or of fitting alternative evaluation practices to different circumstances. Understanding the points of disagreement between evaluation theories can also be valuable for those who want to contribute to the evaluation literature. These fault lines are often fertile territory for research on evaluation, or for trialing new approaches in an evaluation.

Yet another reason for attending to evaluation theory is that it should be a central part of our identity as evaluators and of our shared community and culture. In the words of Will Shadish (1998), from his presidential address at the American Evaluation Association in the mid-1990s, "Evaluation theory is who we are" (p. 1).

Beyond being an important aspect of our professional identity, evaluation theory can have a more tangible benefit, related to the observation that applied social researchers from various disciplines have methods expertise that overlaps with the methods an evaluator would use. What is it that makes an evaluator different from any applied social researcher who happens to conduct an evaluation? One answer is that it is the knowledge and skill sets embodied in evaluation theory. Skillful use of evaluation theory, as already stated, can help guide judgments about what methods to use, when and why. In addition, familiarity with multiple evaluation theories, and with the different rationales they provide for alternative approaches to evaluation practice, can provide an awareness and appreciation for options that might not be apparent to an evaluator unfamiliar with evaluation theory. For example, familiarity with multiple evaluation theories can sensitize an evaluator to the varied possible sources of value judgments, as illustrated in a later section. Indeed, a case can be made that familiarity with evaluation theory, and the enhanced judgments that result, is the value proposition that makes it advisable for funders to hire an evaluator rather than a skilled research methodologist who is not an evaluator (or who claims the title of evaluator but is unaware of the range of options embedded in alternative evaluation theories).

META-MODELS

This section describes two versions of what can be called a **meta-model** or a theory of evaluation theories. By way of preview, I view one of the meta-models as describing in general terms the issues that a comprehensive evaluation theory should address. The other is an attempt to characterize the lay of the land, in the sense of grouping evaluation theories into something akin to families.

In the first of these meta-models, Shadish et al. (1991) contend that good evaluation theories need to address five general issues. Alternatively phrased, Shadish and colleagues claim that a comprehensive program evaluation theory would include **five components**. These are:

1. *Social programming*, which involves a view of how programs operate, what the external forces are that constrain programs, and the role programs play in social change.

2. *Knowledge construction*, such that the theory takes a stance on how to construct knowledge and justify knowledge claims.

3. *Valuing*, in the sense that an evaluation theory indicates how to explicate value issues and select the values to which an evalu-

ation should attend (such as which possible program outcomes to measure, and whether and how to weight each in the face of mixed findings). Foreshadowing some subsequent discussion in this chapter, Shadish and colleagues include matters of social justice in the valuing component of their meta-model.

4. *Use*, whereby the theory specifies what kind of evaluation use matters and, if the theory addresses multiple forms of use, under what conditions each is more important, as well as what the evaluator ought to do to facilitate use (under various conditions).

5. *Practice*, that is, more specific methods and techniques regarding how to do evaluation, including on-the-ground issues involving evaluation purpose; evaluator role; and selection of questions, design, and activities related to use.

Examples to come should help illustrate and clarify these five components. Additional clarification and discussion on various components can also be found in other chapters of this volume, such as in Alkin and Vo's (see Chapter 8) discussion of use and Gates and Schwandt's (see Chapter 5) presentation of valuing. Archibald et al.'s (see Chapter 3) discussion of evaluative thinking is also relevant.

Shadish (1996) used the circles of a Venn diagram to show the idea that these components overlap, with the practice component in the middle and overlapping with and drawing on each of the other four. If we were to apply this kind of graphical representation to individual evaluation theories, using a convention that the size of each circle corresponds to the amount of attention that component receives, we would see that theories differ in terms of their attention to a given component. For example, the utilization-focused evaluation approach of Patton (2008) gives a great deal of attention to use, while the approach associated with Campbell (1969) pays far less attention to use while dealing extensively with knowledge construction.

Shadish et al. (1991) used the five-component model to organize discussion of the work of seven evaluation theorists: Michael Scriven, Donald Campbell, Carol Weiss, Joseph Wholey, Robert Stake, Lee Cronbach, and Peter Rossi. This equating of an evaluation theory with an evaluation theor*ist* has been common to date. We return to this matter later in the chapter.

A second meta-model, Alkin and Christie's (2004) evaluation theory tree (Christie & Alkin, 2023), is based on a similar idea—that is, that evaluation theories vary in terms of the *relative degree of emphasis* on three key issues: methods, valuing, and use/users. This is not to say that any evaluation theory addresses only one of these issues. Rather, the idea is that theories tend to emphasize one of these issues *more* than the others.

The evaluation theory tree has been revised several times, including different versions in the three editions of the book *Evaluation Roots* (Alkin, 2004, 2013; Alkin & Christie, 2023). The origin of the theory tree lies in the efforts of Alkin and his students to trace the analog of academic genealogies within program evaluation. In other fields, such as psychology, people have traced mentor–mentee relationships in ways that resemble family trees (see, e.g., *https://academictree.org/psych*). The short history of evaluation as a distinguishable scholarly and practice field does not lend itself to a family tree. Evaluation does not have decades of one faculty member mentoring multiple students, some of whom go on to mentor others. Instead, in a relatively short period of time, many people who were trained in other fields entered evaluation, and some of them came to be labeled as evaluation theorists. In addition, because evaluation has been multidisciplinary, some major evaluation figures have trained students who focus on their home discipline, while others who trained in evaluation enter applied settings that may have limited opportunities for training the next generation. Thus, the family tree model does not work as well as it does in older disciplines such as psychology—for example, Len Bickman's mentors came from two major lines in social psychology: (1) Stanley Milgram, who was trained by Gordon Allport, who had been trained by Solomon Asch; and (2) Hal Proshansky, who was trained by Morton Deutsch, who had been trained by Kurt Lewin, the latter widely considered the "father" of social psychology. Instead, in classes on evaluation theory, Alkin and his students discussed different representations and ended with the metaphor of a tree. Unlike an academic family tree, the evaluation theory tree is not based on advisor–advisee relationships. And unlike a traditional family tree, the evaluation theory tree does not widen as you move back in time, with one set of parents, two sets of grandparents, and so on. Instead, the theory tree has three main branches, which are defined by *relative focus* and organized in terms of patterns of influence. Like the Shadish et al. (1991) book, the evaluation theory tree and the Alkin (2004, 2013) book has been organized in terms of evaluation theorists. This is explicit in the book's original subtitle: *Tracing Theorists' Views and Influences* (Alkin, 2004). This linkage of theory and theorist is evolving, however, as noted in a subsequent section of the chapter on the future of evaluation theory.

Figure 4.1 is one version of the **evaluation theory tree**. There have been several versions of the tree, including one or two in each edition of the *Evaluation Roots* book. Figure 4.1 came from an article that revisited the version of the tree that had been presented in the first edition of *Evaluation Roots*. Later in the chapter, we see a more recent version, which includes revisions aimed at addressing some of the criticisms of the original tree.

As shown in Figure 4.1, there are **three branches** on the Alkin and Christie evaluation theory tree, each associated with one of three issues: "(a) issues related to the methodology being used, (b) the manner in which the data are to be judged or valued, and (c) the user focus of the evaluation effort" (Alkin, 2004, p. 7). Each theorist is located on one branch, based on which of these three issues they emphasize(d) the most.

In addition, a theorist who tended to influence other theorists is located closer to the trunk of the tree. In the first edition of *Evaluation Roots*, Alkin (2004) asked the theorists who contributed chapters to comment on their placement on the evaluation tree and to list the main influences on their work. The structure of the tree was in some sense validated, in that most of the volume contributors were satisfied with

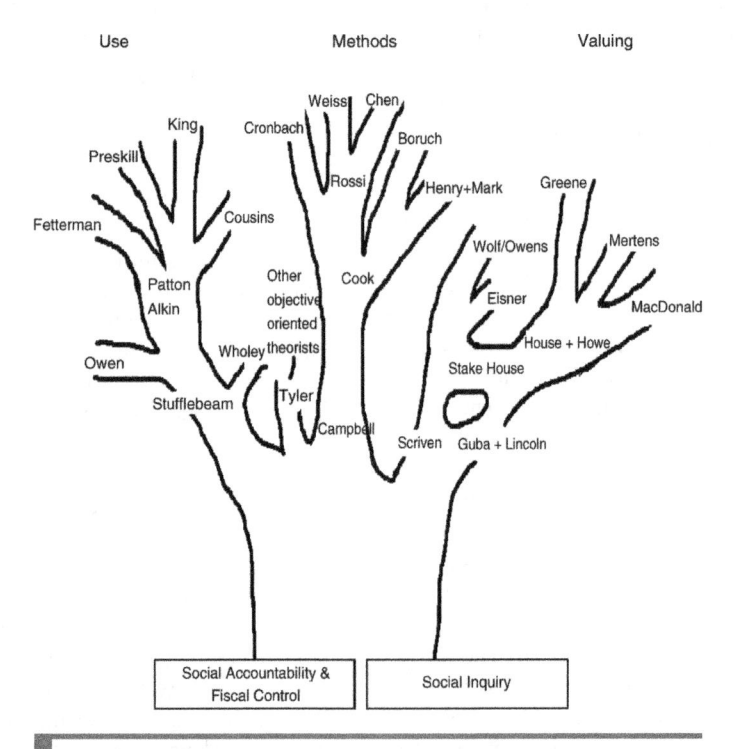

FIGURE 4.1. Earlier version of evaluation theory tree, with branches named after theorists. From Christie and Alkin (2008). Copyright © 2008 Elsevier, Ltd. Reprinted by permission.

their placement, and in that there appeared to be more influence within, rather than across the branches of the tree. For instance, in revisiting the tree in the last chapter of the first edition of *Evaluation Roots*, Alkin and Christie (2004b, p. 391) note that "On the methods branch, Cook, Weiss, Rossi, and Chen all indicate the strong influence of Donald Campbell." They also note that Cronbach, who was represented in the *Roots* book by Jennifer Greene, a former student, clearly "was influenced in the way in which he reacted to Campbell's writing. (p. 391)

As illustrated in subsequent sections, the two meta-models can be used to help frame a review of evaluation theories. They also can be used to guide one's own thinking and reading or, if you prefer, to inform one's professional development activities regarding evaluation. In numerous workshops, I have asked people to identify a handful of big-picture issues or questions that they would like an evaluation theory to address. Many of the answers translate reasonably well into one or more of the five components of evaluation theory identified by Shadish and his colleagues (usually when an issue involves two components, one of them is practice). However, people often do not generate questions that correspond to social programming. Despite this common omission, attention to the thing that we are evaluating (or as Michael Scriven has labeled it, the "evaluand") can be quite important. Archimedes is supposed to have said something to the effect of "give me a lever and a place to stand, and I can move the world." To know where there are leverage points, one must know something about the thing being evaluated. Is a yes-or-no, go-or-no-go, thumbs-up-or-thumbs-down kind of decision foreseeable? Or are only smaller, more incremental changes feasible? Are there times when program change is more (or less) likely to take place? An evaluation may be poorly positioned to make a difference if the evaluator (or someone, such as the commissioner of the evaluation) has not thought about what kind of information is likely to be actionable, and when, given the program that is being evaluated and its environment.

More generally, self-assessment in relation to the five components of the Shadish and colleagues' meta-model can guide one's personal learning agenda for the future. So, for example, if you have no idea what a given component of the model refers to, then it would probably be valuable to do readings, attend talks, or participate in workshops that include a heavy dose of that component. The theory tree can be used in a similar fashion, to guide continuing professional development regarding a branch with which you are unfamiliar or, alternatively, to dig deeper into the writings associated with a branch with which you have an affinity. In short, although they are used in the remainder of this chapter to guide our selection and review of a limited set of evaluation theories, the two meta-models have value in and of themselves.

Evaluation Theory Is Not the Same as Program Theory

To avoid a potential source of confusion, evaluation theory needs to be differentiated from program theory, a concept used widely in evaluation literature and practice. **Program theory** (Bickman, 1987; Chen, 1990) refers to a conceptual model, often presented schematically, that describes the anticipated operations of a program. Many variants exist. Some have boxes that show the components of the program on the left, the long-term anticipated outcomes (or goals of the program) on the right, intermediate steps or underlying processes in the middle, and arrows representing anticipated cause-and-effect relationships among the components, processes, and outcomes. Developing or uncovering a program theory or one of its cousins, such as a logic model (see Frechtling, Chapter 20, this volume), is widespread in evaluation practice. It is also a central part of what was originally labeled theory-driven evaluation (Chen, 1990), which for the sake of clarification has also been labeled as program theory-driven evaluation (Donaldson, 2007).

Program theory-driven evaluation can be considered as one example of what we are calling evaluation theory. But "program theory" is a more specific term than evaluation theory. Evaluation theories *can* attend to program theory, but they need not do so. At the risk of repeating words too often in a single sentence: Program theories are central to the evaluation theory called program theory-driven evaluation; on the other hand, there is no requirement for all evaluation theories to attend to what is widely called program theory.

Criticisms and Comparisons of the Meta-Models

The original version of the evaluation theory tree was dominated by theorists who were North American, male, and White. Not surprisingly, this has been a cause for criticism. In response, the second edition of the Alkin (2013) book includes an expanded list of theorists, as does the final version of the tree in that book. And the third edition has an even larger and more diverse set of theories and theorists represented (as we shall see in a subsequent figure). Nevertheless, in anticipation of the third edition an online petition called for additional changes, including increased representation of indigenous and global south figures (*https:// docs.google.com/forms/d/e/1FAIpQLSeNojhY I2RWIlqaKXfGGe97m5mcCwrywXuedcaOJ lw4_YNAgg/viewform*).

In a related criticism, Donna Mertens has argued that the evaluation tree should be expanded to include a fourth branch: social justice (e.g., Mertens & Wilson, 2019). There has indeed been a proliferation of evaluation theorists who emphasize social justice, especially since the heyday of the early theorists who were reviewed in Shadish et al. (1991). Mertens and Wilson support the idea of four branches by tying each one to a different philosophical stance, with the social justice branch tied to a transformative paradigm. This is a defensible position, though one can question whether the relationship between espoused paradigms and evaluation theories is so strong that all the theorists on a branch follow a common paradigm, distinct from paradigms associated with the other branches. An alternative to the Mertens and Wilson approach, as Alkin and Christie (2004b) suggest, is that the evaluation theories emphasizing social justice can be included on the valuing branch. One can argue that this makes sense, given that an emphasis on social justice has implications primarily for the values/bases that are to be imbued within an evaluation. In any case, the most recent version of the Alkin and Christie (2023) theory tree includes social justice-oriented theories as a major subbranch of the values branch, as we shall see later. Regardless of whether one supports a three- or four-branch theory tree, it is an important, positive development to see a larger number of social justice-focused theories and a more diverse set of theorists represented on the tree.

The theory tree was also criticized by Shadish and Luellen (2004), who wrote a chapter representing Campbell for the original *Evaluation Roots* volume. Shadish argued against the three-branch structure of the tree, and in favor of the five-component structure he developed with Cook and Leviton. One perspective, adopted here, is that both meta-models are useful. The theory tree gives a comparative map, across multiple evaluation theories, based on relative emphasis and on sources of influence over time. In contrast, the five-component model of Shadish et al. provides an aspirational outline for any individual theory of evaluation that attempts to be comprehensive. (For further discussion related to Shadish's criticism of the evaluation theory tree, and some further thoughts on what the differences between the two meta-models might reveal, see Appendix 4A, located at the end of the chapter).

A FEW EVALUATION THEORIES, REVIEWED

In a semester-long class on evaluation theories, it would be common to review several evaluation theories. In a 15-week semester, a dozen or more theorists might be reviewed. In selecting theorists for review, the evaluation tree can serve as a kind of sampling frame, with one or more theories drawn from each major branch. A more in-depth review than in the current chapter could include both older, influential theories near the trunk of the tree, newer theories toward the tips of each branch, and some theories that fall in between. For each theory, the five components from Shadish et al. (1991) might be used to organize discussion. In this chapter, however, only a few seminal evaluation theories are summarized in relation to all five components, with a theorist near the trunk from each of the three branches. A few more will subsequently be reviewed more selectively. Readers interested in further exploration of evaluation theories should see the references listed at the end of the chapter.

As previously noted, the literature on evaluation theories has often been presented in terms of the work of individual evaluation theorists. For example, the Shadish et al. (1991) and Alkin (2004, 2013) books are organized around evaluation theorists. Mertens and Wilson (2019) also summarize the views of numerous evaluation theorists. I follow that tradition of organizing this section and the next around evaluation theorists. Descriptions of the approaches associated with Donald Campbell, Joseph Wholey, and Michael Scriven follow, as does a newer approach: culturally responsive evaluation (which is associated with multiple theorists). In the final section of the chapter, I comment on the tradition of equating evaluation theories with evaluation theorists, expressing the hope that things will be different in the future and pointing out a notable step in that direction. Now, on to the individual theorists.

Donald Campbell was a social psychologist, though he is probably most widely known and remembered for his contributions to research methodology. Much of his writing fits within Shadish and colleagues' knowledge construction component of evaluation theory and within the methods branch of the evaluation theory tree. With various collaborators, Campbell developed and popularized the distinction between internal and external validity, created lists of validity threats, and detailed alternative quasi-experimental designs and examined their susceptibility to various validity threats.

Internal validity, in the context of program evaluation, refers to the accuracy of one's inferences about whether (or to what extent) the program caused a difference in some outcome(s) of interest. **External validity**, in contrast, refers to the accuracy of one's inferences about whether (or to what extent) the findings of an evaluation can be generalized to other settings, to other people, and to other times.

With his list of internal validity threats, Campbell helped sensitize others to the idea of considering and trying to rule out plausible alternative explanations. In the context of a program evaluation, the evaluator of a preschool program would need to rule out the possibility that children score better on outcome measures simply because they are older than when they enrolled; this would be an example of the internal validity threat of **maturation**. Ruling out the threat of maturation might best be done by using a comparative research design, with some children in the preschool program and others in the no-treatment comparison group. But everyday processes, whereby some children end up in preschool and others do not, could lead to qualitatively different groups—a threat called **selection bias**—which would make it harder to tell whether preschool is making a positive difference. Campbell's writings sensitize evaluators to the possibility of such biases, while also indicating which are better ways to try to deal with them. Pham et al. (see Chapter 17, this volume) discuss some of the design options associated with the Campbellian tradition as well as more contemporary analysis techniques.

At a more abstract level, Campbell espoused the philosophical stance of **critical realism** (Bhaskar, 1978; Shadish et al., 1991, Ch. 4). By critical realism, he meant to suggest that there is indeed a world that exists apart from the social construction of it, and that accordingly it was meaningful to talk about such things as the causal effect of an educational program on student achievement. At the same time, Campbell recognized that our understanding of this external reality is imperfect, mediated by human knowledge processes that may be biased. His philosophical view of knowledge construction fit well with his emphasis on preferred research methods as a means of trying to reduce biases in evaluation findings. As Bhaskar noted, "to be a fallibilist about knowledge, it is necessary to be a realist about things" (p. 43). In other words, to believe our knowledge may not be perfect, but that better versus worse answers exist, you also must believe that there is an answer that exists apart from human construction.

Although Campbell's major emphasis was on knowledge construction and methods, his approach also had a particular focus when it came to the social programming component of Shadish et al.'s (1991) meta-model. His emphasis was on identifying relatively effective program options. The idea was that good information about whether a program was effective, or about which of two or more programs was more effective, could help inform judgments by policymakers and others when they make decisions about whether to implement a new program, or about whether to expand a small-scale program, or about whether an existing program should be replaced or continued. Colloquially speaking, Campbell's model of evaluation fits with the decision-making context when there is a fork in the road—for example, when Congress faces reauthorization of major educational or social welfare legislation. In such a circumstance, better choices can be made if sound answers are available to the following question: Which, if any, alternatives to the current arrangements lead to better outcomes?

Regarding use in Campbell's approach, the focus was on evaluative information informing decision makers who made judgments about program adoption, continuation, expansion, or cessation. This form of use illustrates what is sometimes called **direct or instrumental use**—that is, identifiable action or decisions. Campbell did not go very far, however, when it came to the use component. His focus was far more on how to get the best, least biased answer to the question about the relative effects of program or policy alternatives—not on how to try to ensure that these results were used in actual decision making. He sometimes referred to evaluators as methodological servants of the experimenting society (Campbell, 1991).

Similarly, Campbell did not go extensively into the issue of valuing. Instead, he seemed to assume that matters such as deciding what indicators to use when assessing the effectiveness of an intervention, or how to weight different criteria when a program does well on some indicators but poorly on others, is best left in the hands of others. Often in practice this appears to translate into adopting official program goals as the criteria to be used in evaluating a program. My view is that it is a principled, defensible stance to say that valuing should be the responsibility of those who are in legitimate decision-making positions. As we shall see, however, this is far from the only view of valuing within evaluation theories, and other perspectives exist that are also principled and defensible (see Gates & Schwandt, Chapter 5, this volume) and more likely to seem appropriate to many, perhaps most, contemporary evaluators and others involved in evaluation.

Having provided a summary of one notable evaluation theorist's views, I hasten to add a set of caveats. It is impossible to do justice to decades worth of writings in such a brief summary. A theorist's views may change over time, and such changes or other nuances are hard to capture in a page or two. Nevertheless, even a brief description, such as those here, can clarify the similarities and differences associated with various evaluation theories. In addition, even a brief overview such as this covers more territory than the typical truncated view of Campbell and other early theorists today. The view that many current evaluators have of Campbell (assuming they have one) is simply of a methodologist who advocated for the use of randomized experiments and strong quasi-experiments in evaluation. One benefit of studying program theorists is to gain a richer view of their perspectives, thereby enriching our own.

By way of an update, Campbell's approach to program evaluation has continuing influence in the field today. Evaluations using experimental and quasi-experimental designs to estimate the effects of a program are fairly commonplace in various programming areas (e.g., Gopalan et al., 2020). In addition, descendants of Campbell's theory appear on the theory tree and in practice. One of these, generally known as theory-driven evaluation (Chen, 1990, 2014; Coryn et al., 2011), is perhaps better labeled program theory-driven evaluation (Donaldson, 2007) to clarify that it is an evaluation approach that emphasizes program theory. Much of program theory-driven evaluation draws on Campbell, especially with respect to knowledge construction, concern for validity threats, and experimental and quasi-experimental methods. However, in terms of the social program, program theory-driven evaluators emphasize the rationale underlying the program—that is, the program theory—and they use the program theory to guide the evaluation, for instance, in the identification of interim and long-term measures. More generally, Campbell remains influential to many approaches that attempt to identify how and when a program works (Lemire et al., 2020).

Compared to Campbell, program theory-driven evaluation is more sensitive to program stage. For example, early in a program's life, the evaluator may focus more on surfacing the program theory and on examining whether the program is operating as the program theory suggests, including changes in the more proximal indicators. For a more mature program, these evaluators often use a Campbell-like comparative design to test whether the program causes improvements in the long-term outcomes. But going beyond Campbell, this is likely to be ac-

BOX 4.1. An Evaluation Using a Quasi-Experimental Design

Among the quasi-experiments that Campbell advocated is the **interrupted time-series (ITS) design**. Michielutte and colleagues (2000) used an ITS to complement a pretest–posttest comparison group design in their evaluation of an education and support program designed to increase screening for breast and cervical cancer among women ages 40 and older in low-income housing in Winston-Salem, North Carolina. Figure 4.2 shows the ITS portion of the evaluation, with the number of mammograms per 100 patient visits shown over time across 19 two-month intervals (data were aggregated into 2-month intervals to avoid instability from smaller numbers and from short-term closures of the mammography unit). Data are reported separately for women 40–49, for whom the official screening recommendations had varied over time, and for women 50 and above, for whom screening recommendations had been consistent. As shown in the solid line, for women ages 40–49, mammogram rates are fairly steady prior to the intervention, with values ranging from 6 to 7 per 100 patient visits.

Just after the program started, the rate increased linearly for the next several observations, plateauing at a rate of 8.5–8.75 mammograms per 100 patient visits. Statistical analysis showed that the increase following the introduction of the program was significant. Note that the time-series data give more information about the intervention's effect across time than would a typical pretest–posttest comparison (i.e., that after an initial increase, the rate plateaued). As shown in the dotted line in Figure 4.2, for women 50 and older there was not a similar increase immediately following the intervention. However, mammogram rates among women 50 and older increased later, roughly 2 months after the start of the intervention. The evaluators speculate that this is a delayed effect of the program, with the 40- to 49-year-olds being more immediately susceptible to information in the intervention because of the previously conflicting recommendations about screening in that age group. Uncertainty about the findings for those 50 and older is a good reminder about the benefits of having design adjuncts beyond the simple ITS (Reichardt, 2019), such as (1) implementation assessment, which could indicate whether women of different ages received somewhat different treatment over time; (2) qualitative data from the women, which could have been informative about the processes of change; and (3) time-series data from outside the treatment area, which should show no increase in mammogram rates in either age group—*if* Figure 4.2 is showing an immediate and a delayed treatment effect, respectively, among women 40–49 and 50 and above.

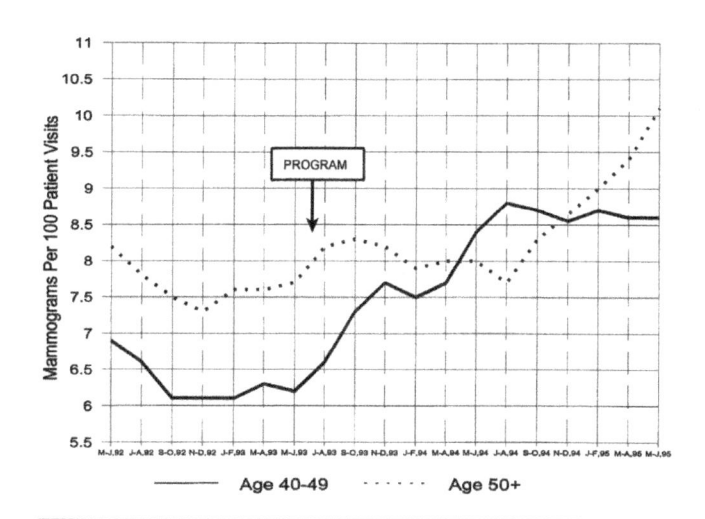

FIGURE 4.2. Mammograms per 100 patient visits; 12-month moving averages. From Michielutte et al. (2000). Copyright © Oxford University Press. Reprinted with permission.

BOX 4.2. A Performance Measurement System

Sawhill and Williamson (2001) describe the development and use of a performance measurement system that is consistent with Wholey's approach. The Nature Conservancy is a nonprofit organization committed to conserving biodiversity. For much of its existence, it did so primarily by acquiring land thought vital for the survival of at-risk species. It focused on two indicators—"bucks and acres"—that is, the total of the donations received and the amount of land acquired. Although the Conservancy was growing annually at double digits, the old bucks and acres approach contributed to some dysfunctions, such as buying land, especially in states rich in donors, rather than dealing with broader ecosystem issues. This is not surprising to those familiar with the mantra "What gets measured gets managed," an expression that in part serves as a warning about the possible dysfunctional effects of excessive attention to imperfect performance measures. So, the Nature Conservancy went to work on a revised system. A first attempt at an improved performance system failed, however, revealing a valuable lesson. In a yearlong process, the Conservancy developed a system with 98 measures. It "promptly collapsed under its own weight" (p. 374) due to the record-keeping burden and the fact that managers could not tell which portions of the extensive information were most important. Subsequently, drawing on a form of strategic planning, a usable set of performance indicators was developed, with the nine measures falling within three general categories: capacity, activity, and impact. Sawhill and Williamson report that the revised system had effects. For example, it motivated line managers to initiate activities other than land purchases, and guided staff to do more in terms of identifying threats to species in their area and seeking ways to abate them. Notably, evaluative judgments are embedded in such changes. And over time, a performance measurement system like this should enhance managers' ability to adjust program activities based on the impact measures.

BOX 4.3. A Culturally Responsive Evaluation Example

Manswell-Butty et al. (2004) describe a culturally responsive evaluation of a school-to-career intervention program implemented in an urban junior high school. The program provided a "career breakfast club," with eight 1-hour sessions. Among other things, these sessions included information and discussion on such topics as pathways to college, completing job applications, and the array of available education, training, and career options. Manswell-Butty and colleagues illustrated the way CRE informed their evaluation, organized in terms of the eight phases as presented by Frierson et al. (2002). With respect to preparing for the evaluation and engaging those with an interest in the evaluation, the evaluators held multiple initial meetings with various groups, striving to develop genuine collaboration and to freely debate ideas and plans (which was enhanced by the support of key school leaders). In terms of identifying the goals and purpose of the evaluation, the evaluators sought to obtain and respond to interest holder input, and as a result engaged in both formative and summative evaluation activities with a mixed methods design. The formative component drew heavily on student feedback after each session to guide improvements with the goal of enhancing participants' engagement. The summative component included qualitative and quantitative measures and a pretest–posttest design with a nonprogram comparison group. Question framing and the design of the evaluation were also guided by input from the relevant groups and, throughout the process, a desire to be culturally responsive. For example, Manswell-Butty et al. report that the students preferred discussions and other interactive activities, rather than completing surveys, which the evaluators took into account in the data collection plan. Considerable attention also went into the selection and development of measures, to ensure they were culturally sensitive.

In the case of one instrument that had been developed and normed on a population unlike that of the participating school, supplementary data were collected. Regarding data collection, members of the evaluation team, by virtue of their intensive engagement with and sensitivity to the context, strove to be aware of the program's cultural context. The evaluators' cultural awareness (aided by team members' own backgrounds) probably also aided them in drawing conclusions from the findings, but also important was obtaining input from students and staff on how to disaggregate the data and what the findings meant. Findings were reported to the full range of interested parties, including a reporting out to students in what we are told was a student-friendly manner.

companied by efforts to see whether changes occur as expected along the various steps in the program theory, often using **mediational analyses**. Advocates of program theory-driven evaluation say their approach not only shows whether a program is bringing about the desired change but also why it is (or is not), thereby opening the door to possible improvements. More generally, those following in Campbell's footsteps tend to address a wider array of questions, including about implementation, **mediators**, and **moderators**, assuming resources and practicalities allow.

The continuing influence of Campbell's approach to program evaluation is also the subject of considerable criticism. The criticisms focus largely on overstated claims by advocates of randomized experiments, often referred to as **randomized controlled trials (RCTs)**. RCT advocates, sometimes referred to as "randomistas" are criticized for treating experiments as an unqualified gold standard, indicating they "clinch" a conclusion, and ignoring or at least downplaying the challenges of generalizing such findings elsewhere (Bickman & Reich, 2014; Deaton & Cartwright, 2018). The overstated claims of some advocates of RCTs seem ironic, given Campbell developed the concept of external validity and cataloged various quasi-experimental designs, some of which approach RCTs in terms of internal validity.

For the next evaluation theorist, we consider **Joseph Wholey**. The initial focus is on one portion of Wholey's approach, specifically on the development of **performance measurement systems**. We turn subsequently to another aspect of Wholey's work, **evaluability assessment (EA)**.

Wholey worked for many years at the Urban Institute, where he and his colleagues spent considerable time observing ongoing programs. They noticed that, although program managers played a vital role in the operations of the program, they often lacked quality information about how well things were going. In contrast, in the private sector, business managers typically at the very least had relatively good and timely feedback about the proverbial bottom line—that is, about how the business or their unit was doing from a profit–loss perspective. Unlike the private sector, public sector managers typically lacked comparable information about the extent to which program activities were successful in leading to program objectives. Given the shortage of information available to the public sector managers at that time, Wholey (2004) and his colleagues became leading advocates for the development of information systems, sometimes called performance monitoring or performance measurement systems.

These data systems typically include information about program activities, such as the extent to which various program services were delivered. They track client outcomes, ideally starting with measures from when the client entered the program and continuing as far downstream as feasible. Such systems should be constructed with managers' information needs in mind. Thus, if managers anticipate needing aggregate data by regions or sites, this should be accommodated. Ideally, information systems provide reports on a regular schedule suited to managers' needs but can also be queried if desired. They may also have some form of red flag system so that unusual or problematic scores on an indicator result in a report even if one is not scheduled.

In contrast to Campbell and his focus on go/no-go decisions and on the kind of information policymakers would find useful in choosing the better option, Wholey focused on social programs that are ongoing and on the kind of information program managers would find useful for improving ongoing program operations. Metaphorically, Campbell was concerned about occasions when there are forks in the road, while Wholey's concern focused on situations in which a program will be moving on down the road for quite some time. Neither is right or wrong. Instead, they focus on different periods in the life cycle of a social program, and correspondingly on the information needs of different parties (policymakers vs. program managers). And importantly, these contrasting views of social programming and evaluation users are associated with very different-looking approaches to evaluation.

Wholey had a clear focus with respect to use. He identified a primary intended user group—that is to say, program managers. Information systems were to be developed with their information needs in mind. If the desired use took place, it would mean that managers drew upon the results from the information systems to evaluate how things were going, to implement modifications when and where things were not going well, and to track whether outcomes improved following those modifications. As with Campbell, this is a kind of direct, instrumental use. However, Campbell focused on full-scale programs being adopted or not, while Wholey's use would likely involve more minor program modifications, and perhaps many such modifications tried over time. Using language from Michael Scriven, Campbell's evaluations are **summative** and Wholey's performance measurement-based evaluative judgments are **formative**.

The preceding description of Wholey's approach to evaluation actually pulls out one part from the richer landscape of his work. That portion, using performance measurement for what has come to be known as results-oriented management, is what Wholey is best known for today in some circles, such as in public policy and management. At least in part, this is because of the codification of performance measurement into U.S. law, especially in the Government Performance and Results Act (GPRA) of 1993 and the GPRA Modernization Act of 2010. The widespread development of and attention to performance measurement systems in the wake of these laws followed in the footsteps of Wholey and his colleagues. Originally, however, Wholey's attention to performance measurement systems was a portion of a multistep set of options.

Another of Wholey's options was EA (see, e.g., Wholey, 2004; Rog, Chapter 11, this volume; Trevisan & Walser, 2015). This contribution is what Wholey is best known for among some evaluators. An EA involves the evaluator, program managers and staff, and key policymakers if possible. It creates a kind of map of a program—that is, a form of program theory, often in the form of a **logic model** (see Frechtling, Chapter 20, this volume). If agreement exists about program goals, if a plausible set of linkages connects program activities to the desired goals, and if further evaluation could address potential users' information needs, then the EA would conclude that further evaluation activity is warranted. On the other hand, if one or more of these conditions were not met, then the EA would suggest that this problem should be addressed before other evaluation activities take place. For example, if general agreement did not exist about a program's goals—as might be the case in a multicomponent program that evolved willy-nilly over time—this problem would need to be addressed first, perhaps by streamlining the program or by facilitating a shared vision of what the program aims to do. EA and the possibility of next steps illustrates what Wholey called the sequential purchase of evaluative information. Colloquially, he encouraged that the right bite-size of evaluation be found.

Another option Wholey endorsed was rapid feedback evaluation. The premise is that often organizations already have plenty of data with evaluative implications but they lack individuals with the time and perhaps the ability to make sense of it. In essence, rapid feedback evaluation involves parachuting in a couple of expert evaluators to review and offer recommendations based on observations, interviews, and existing data. The kind of results-oriented management via performance measurement systems, which we have already discussed, is another of Wholey's options. So too is what Wholey called intensive evaluation, which he defined less explicitly but might involve an approach such as Campbell's.

Wholey's approach has held considerable sway in government, especially the U.S. federal government, where the development and use of performance measurement systems is a key element of what has come to be called results-based management (Holzer & Ballard, 2021). Though the approach has limits, including the inability to attribute a change in outcomes to the program (De Lancer Julnes, 2006), it has grown, in no small part due to the mandates of GPRA and the GPRA Modernization Act of 2010. Those involved in the development and use of the performance measurement systems stimulated by these laws follow in the footsteps of Wholey and his colleagues. With respect to EA, reviews have shown a resurgence of its use early in this century (Trevisan & Walser, 2015), including for program development and revision (Lam & Skinner, 2021) and in program areas including public health (Leviton et al., 2010) and international development (Davies & Payne, 2015).

Although the writings of a third evaluation theorist, **Michael Scriven**, are plentiful and rich, we review his work only briefly here. As to knowledge construction, Scriven believes there are real, knowable answers to the question of whether a program (or other evaluand) has merit and worth. But Scriven also believes that a person's perspective can bias their evaluations. As a result, he generally prefers an external (vs. an internal) evaluator, especially for summative evaluations. Scriven also endorses **meta-evaluation**—that is, the evaluation of an evaluation. As related to bias control, the idea is that if evaluators know their judgments will be reviewed by a knowledgeable third party, they will be better at laying out the bases for their judgments and at fairly calling balls and strikes, so to speak.

Scriven has been especially lauded for his approach to valuing, which has been described as involving four general steps (Shadish et al., 1991). The first is to identify criteria of merit—that is, the characteristics by which the evaluand is to be judged. For example, the criteria of merit for a preschool program might include children's language skills, self-regulation, and interpersonal skills. Second, performance standards should be set. Will success be judged relatively (e.g., compared to a control group), or is there an absolute level of performance required for a judgment of success—and if so, what is it? Third, performance must be measured. This should be done using whatever measurement techniques are appropriate (e.g., evaluating running shoes calls for different methods than evaluating preschool programs). Fourth, results should be synthesized into an evaluative judgment. How, for example, should a preschool program with moderate positive effects on interpersonal skills and self-regulation but no effect on language skills be rated, relative to another program with strong positive effects on language skills only?

It is hard to point to an archetypical Scriven-style evaluation, given that he is open to whatever way of measuring performance makes sense for a given evaluand. The commonalities involve the steps of the evaluation, including where the criteria of merit originate. Scriven (1974) does *not* see criteria of merit as coming from public officials, managers, or other decisions makers. Indeed, he has advocated for "goal-free evaluation," in which evaluators avoid even familiarizing themselves with official statements about what a program is intended to do, such as would be found in enabling legislation or program documentation. Instead, Scriven suggests that the evaluator should attend to a kind of **needs assessment**, identifying the real needs that a program was intended to address. Scriven assumes a stronger role for the evaluator in identifying needs than most evaluators would. Scriven would approve of the identification of needs being informed by sources such as program clients or developers but would not hand the identification of needs to them. Many other evaluators would instead rely primarily on judgments from such parties, though various techniques exist that can be used to identify needs (Russ-Eft & Sleezer, 2019).

In any case, the identified needs would then inform valuing, such as selection of the indicators to be measured and the way to integrate across multiple indicators to generate a single, bottom-line judgment (regarding the synthesis step, according to Scriven the weighting should reflect the extent to which the indicators are related to basic needs). Many other evaluation theorists do not include in their approaches the synthesis of findings from multiple criteria of merit into a single evaluative judgment. Campbell, for example, would leave this to others, such as the decision makers in a democracy. But for Scriven, evaluating requires getting to a judgment, a grade, a rating—to some form of an evaluative conclusion. For Scriven, the evaluation results are then made available to the consumer, policymaker, or whomever, with the idea that the evaluation results can help them make better choices if they choose.

In the first edition of the *Evaluation Roots* book, other theorists on the valuing branch, including Stake, Guba and Lincoln, and House, mentioned the influence of Scriven on their work (Alkin, 2004, p. 391). In a sense, the influence of Scriven today is partially mediated by his influence on these and other influential figures. In other ways, it is difficult to update Scriven's influence, largely because he did not espouse particular research designs, specific engagement processes, or the like. His logic is flexible in the sense of being applicable across a wide array of areas and techniques. The work of Davidson (2004, 2013), a past student of Scriven's, is perhaps the most notable example of his direct ongoing influence.

The evaluation theories reviewed so far, from Campbell, Wholey, and Scriven, can be characterized as classics. When talking about endeavors such as literature, movies, or rock music, a classic is typically one that is of high merit, comes from an earlier era, and has stood the test of time. There is also the idea of an "instant classic," a work that, while more recent, is of such quality that it deserves the accolade "classic" even without the usual passage of time. We can think of the next evaluation theory, **culturally responsive evaluation (CRE)**, as an instant classic.

CRE, unlike the approaches identified so far, is not affiliated with one single theorist. Instead, this theory is more generally credited to a number of developers, several of whom have collaborated at times. The term *culturally responsive evaluation* is credited to Stafford Hood (Hood, 1998) in a presentation honoring the work of Robert Stake (1976), who had developed "responsive evaluation" (Hood et al., 2015). In short, Stake had argued against preordinate evaluation designs, calling instead for the evaluator to immerse in, and subsequently plan evaluation activities that were responsive to the actual program as implemented and its context. In introducing CRE, Hood (1998) emphasized the importance of responsiveness to cultural features, including race. Since that initial reference to CRE, several key contributions have taken place, including Frierson et al. (2002, 2010), Hopson (2009), and Hood et al. And it is important to note that, even though I have labeled CRE an instant classic, it has drawn on and acknowledged important precursors and contributions, including scholars of color, such as Reid E. Jackson and Asa Grant Hilliard, III as highlighted in the "nobody knows my name" project (Hood & Hopson, 2008).

CRE addresses all five components of the Shadish et al. (1991) model of evaluation theory. With respect to social programming, CRE is premised on the idea that programs take place within a cultural context and that efforts to evaluate a program without adequate consideration of that context will fall short. Part of accounting for the cultural context, according to CRE, involves recognition of relevant power dynamics. More generally, CRE calls on evaluators to describe the history of the program, including its cultural context.

With respect to the valuing component, a culturally responsive evaluator seeks to include within an evaluation's focus the questions and concerns held by the intended program beneficiaries, along with those of other key parties with an interest in the evaluation. Notice the contrast with the previously discussed theories. Also related to valuing, a culturally responsive evaluation explicitly addresses dynamics of power, privilege, and inequity as they arise in the program and its context. This requires having and/or developing an understanding and appreciation of intended beneficiaries' lived experience.

Drawing on social constructivism, CRE emphasizes that knowledge construction takes place in a social and cultural context. Accordingly, who is at the table, or put differently, what voices are included in the processes of knowledge construction matters greatly. Program participants and those from traditionally underserved communities should participate in the shaping of evaluative conclusions, and they should be asked to weigh in on the accuracy of those conclusions. From the moment of the evaluator's initial engagement, the process of building trust is critical, including in terms of the quality of the conclusions that are drawn from an evaluation. Culturally responsive evaluators also tend to eschew deficit-based explanations of the problems a program is designed to address, and instead acknowledge both strengths in the relevant community and the systems factors that contribute to the problem.

Regarding use, a key contention of CRE is that being culturally responsive throughout the evaluation process will result in evaluation findings (and processes) that are both more credible and more useful. Reasons for this include the emphasis on developing trust and the involvement of key parties in question formulation and in the review of preliminary findings. CRE encourages dissemination to a range of interested groups, certainly including intended program beneficiaries, in culturally appropriate ways, and perhaps with different communication procedures for different groups. Where feasible, feedback to the various groups should be done in an ongoing basis.

In terms of practice, CRE calls for bringing a culturally responsive lens to all stages of an evaluation, from preparing to enter the context in which the evaluation will be conducted, to the framing of questions, and to the dissemination of findings and facilitation of use (to mention but a few of the stages of evaluation highlighted by Hood et al., 2015). Given its emphasis on the lived experience of program participants, early versions of CRE tended to emphasize qualitative methods. Recent writings about CRE have taken more of a mixed methods approach.

Given its more recent development and status here as an instant classic, talking about CRE's current influence is less relevant than it is for older evaluation theories. However, one notable point of influence is in the development of "equitable evaluation," which provides a framework and support for foundations that fund various initiatives and their evaluation (Center for Evaluation Innovation, 2017). Second, CRE's influence is consistent with the first Executive Order from President Joe Biden: Advancing Racial Equity and Support for Underserved Communities through the Federal Government (Executive Order 13985) and with evaluation-related responses to the racial reckoning stiavmulated by the murder of George Floyd. It is also worth noting that CRE has overlap with other contemporary evaluation approaches that Mertens and Wilson (2019) place upon the social justice branch of the expanded evaluation theory tree. These approaches include but are not limited to indigenous evaluation theory, such as that based on evaluation by and for the Maori people (e.g., Cram, 2009), disability rights and deaf rights theory (e.g., Munger & Mertens, 2011), and feminist evaluation theory (e.g., Sielbeck-Bowen et al., 2002).

WAYS FOR EVALUATION THEORY TO GUIDE EVALUATION PRACTICE

In the previous section we examined a small number of evaluation theories, with a classic one from each of the three branches of the original theory tree. We also examined a newer, instant classic evaluation theory from, if you prefer, the social justice branch of the revised tree or the social justice subbranch of the valuing branch. We looked at each theory from the lens of Shadish and colleagues' (1991) five-component model. We now turn to a critical question that is less frequently addressed in the literature on evaluation theory—that is, how exactly are these theories supposed to guide practice? How might a practicing evaluator translate from the generalities of an evaluation theory to the specific activities to be implemented for a particular evaluation?

Adhering to a Theory

One approach, arguably employed too frequently, is to identify an evaluation theory to use as a guide, and then implement it in most, if not all, of one's evaluations. This is the approach people often take when they identify themselves as a **realist evaluator**, or an **empowerment evaluator**, or as an adherent to some other theory. This would be fine if the chosen evaluation theory fits well with all the varied circumstances in which evaluations takes place but this seems unlikely for most evaluation theories. It would also be acceptable if an adherent of theory X did evaluations only when that theory fit well to the circumstances. This sorting could occur either if the evaluator was able to take assignments only in circumstances in which theory X fits well, or if the market effectively selected evaluators only for situations in which their preferred theories fit well. While this is possible, especially for evaluators who work in a narrow niche, it does not seem likely for the most part. Moreover, one of the risks of strong identification with a particular evaluation theory is the possibility that you will assume it fits well with a broader range of circumstances than it does.

Matching Theory to Situation, Based on Comparison of Theories

An alternative way to translate from evaluation theory to evaluation practice involves using multiple theories to enable a kind of matching function. By thinking about the assumptions and (perhaps implicit) context and purposes embedded in each theory, the evaluator may be able to do a better job selecting an appropriate evaluation approach to the specific case. For example, as noted in the previous section, Campbell and Wholey focused on very different aspects of programs. Campbell emphasized evaluative evidence that could inform the selection (or retention or expansion) of a program, while Wholey focused on information to help managers better manage existing programs. These different emphases led to very different perspectives on what evaluation would look like. A familiarity with evaluation theories that allows this kind of comparisons can aid in the selection of an evaluation approach method that fits the particular circumstances. Context is an important consideration for evaluation practice (Rog et al., 2012) but evaluators often do not have a good sense of which of the countless contextual attributes should be attended to. Being multilingual with respect to evaluation theories helps point an evaluator to key aspects of context, as illustrated by the juxtaposition of Campbell and Wholey.

Still, a problem can arise from overadherence to a single evaluation theory, especially when following that theory across situations, but even when applying it after matching theory to the situation. Existing evaluation theories were developed in light of the experiences (as well as readings and other influences) of the evaluation theorist, and these may not match all of the specific details of the case at hand—that is, a single theory may provide a general guideline but probably is not nuanced enough to guide all the decisions for the multifaceted context of a given evaluation. An evaluation theory should not be treated as a paint-by-number template or an Ikea-like set of instructions. Admittedly, painting by numbers is easier and takes less judgment but it is less likely to lead to evaluations that bring benefits, especially if the evaluator only has one paint-by-number template.

Combining Theories I: Fully Integrating Two Theories

An alternative to situational matching is to combine evaluation theories. One version of this involves an attempt to fully integrate two approaches, so that neither predominates. Thomas and Parsons (2017) discussed the integration of two theoretical perspectives, one addressed earlier in the chapter and the other not: CRE and systems-oriented evaluation, respectively. Thomas and Parsons also illustrated an evaluation based on this integration, specifically, an evaluation of a science, technology, engineering, and mathematics (STEM) education program.

In addition to the characteristics of CRE sketched earlier in this chapter, the systems-oriented approach brought attention to topics such as the systems, both formal and informal, that are part of the context within which the project operates; the broader history of STEM instruction and learning relevant to the project; the connections among people, perspectives, and the like that influence the power dynamics in and around the project; and the formal and informal systems and their elements that foster or inhibit program operations. Thomas and Parsons (2017) did not try to bring one element of Theory A into an evaluation primarily shaped by Theory B. Instead, they sought a thorough combination and integration.

Complete, equal integration of two approaches may be challenging. It probably requires a team with expertise in each approach (which Thomas & Parsons, 2017, provided), as well as patience, teamwork, and likely more time and resources than if one theory were in the lead. In addition, aspects of some theories appear not to be compatible. To take but one example, Campbell's view of the evaluator as servant to the experimenting society might be hard to mesh seamlessly with Scriven's view that the evaluator needs to synthesize findings into a comprehensive evaluative judgment.

Combining Theories II: Mixing and Matching

Yet another approach is not to consider evaluation theories in whole but to think of theories as having parts or modules that might be combined in various ways. For example, various evaluation theories provide widely differing guidance for selecting the values that are embedded in an evaluation. Campbell, as suggested by his description of evaluators as servants of the experimenting society, implied that valuing was the business of others—that is, matters such as what program outcomes to measure, or how to draw a conclusion about a program in the face of mixed results, should be the responsibility of the duly elected or appointed officials who are charged with making decisions about the program. Wholey took a similar stance, relying largely on program managers and perhaps policymakers. In contrast, as indicated in goal-free evaluation, Scriven does not give the same standing to public officials or other decision makers. Instead, Scriven contends that the evaluator should identify the real needs that a program was intended to address. One could, however, imagine an evaluation generally consistent with any of these three theories, but with a different approach to valuing substituted. For example, several of the practices of CRE could be combined with what otherwise would look like an evaluation inspired by Campbell or Wholey.

A broader review of evaluation theories suggests even more options for mixing and matching. Another evaluation theorist, Ernie House, has advocated over time for two different positions regarding valuing. Indeed, the version of the evaluation theory tree shown in Figure 4.1 (Christie & Alkin, 2008) lists House in two places on the values branch! Earlier in his career, House (1976) was influenced by the philosopher John Rawls's (1971) book *A Theory of Justice*. A philosophical tome that was as deep as it was long (560 pages), the book addressed the topic of the fair distribution of resources. One of the principles Rawls argued for was that inequalities were fair only if they were to the benefit of the least well-off. Drawing on Rawls's argument, House contended that evaluations should reflect the vantage point of the least well-off. From this perspective, knowing that a program brings benefits on average is not sufficient. Instead, one must know whether the program benefits the most disadvantaged, such as by closing performance gaps. One of the notable things about House's Rawlsian perspective is that it brings a values stance to evaluation that comes from outside the programming or decision-making world. House does not suggest that evaluators should apply Rawls because it serves the stated information needs of managers, policymakers, or other interest holders. He advocates that this principle, drawn from philosophy, should apply generally to evaluation. This differs from Campbell's position that valuing is the job of someone, as the phrase goes, at a higher pay grade than evaluators, or from Scriven's view that real client needs are the basis for valuing. Familiarity with multiple evaluation theories can broaden an evaluator's perspectives on the range of options that exist for various tasks.

House, along with his collaborator Ken Howe (1999), is also associated with another evaluation theory. In brief, House and Howe's "deliberative democratic evaluation" specifies a set of procedures for adjudicating value issues in evaluation. In essence, House and Howe provide a set of methods for selecting and engaging representatives from multiple groups with an interest in the evaluation and facilitating discussion to hash out values issues, such as which possible outcomes to measure and how to draw conclusions in the face of mixed results. House and Howe fall on the social justice branch as articulated by Mertens and Wilson (2019), along with CRE, indigenous evaluation, and other approaches. These share a general emphasis on inclusion of often-overlooked voices in determining the values and questions that drive an evaluation.

This kind of cross-comparative review of the positions of several evaluation theories could be expanded, adding ideas from evaluation theories not reviewed in this chapter to our comparative examination of perspectives on where and why the questions that guide an evaluation are supposed to come from, beyond those of House and Howe, House's earlier Rawlsian approach, CRE, Campbell, Wholey, and Scriven. More importantly, such comparisons can be useful in several ways. At the least, considering the array of options can be a kind of mental "stretching exercise," expanding one's views about the available options. It might provide you with support if you want to argue within your organization, or in a proposal, or with a program officer, about doing something different from past practice. Or, again, such a comparison across evaluation theories might guide an effort to merge one portion of one evaluation theory onto another. For instance, an evaluator following Campbell's or Wholey's approach in general might add on House and Howe's extensive engagement of representatives of interested groups for valuing or add the lens CRE brings throughout the evaluation. Related to this, an aspect of one theory might serve as an ancillary to another. For instance, an evaluation contract may be written with the (perhaps implicit) assumption that valuing is the responsibility of certain decision makers but the evaluators might nevertheless be able to engage in a Scriven-based needs assessment to see if other criteria of merit emerge, which the evaluator could suggest also should be considered.

In short, one approach to translating from evaluation theory to evaluation practice involves eclecticism, or a kind of integrative effort.

Applying a Contingency Theory

Several evaluation theories emphasize criteria for choosing from among alternative ways of doing evaluation. For some evaluation theories, which can be called **contingency models**, this issue is central. It is at the very core of the theory. At least three different kinds of contingency models exist.

One kind of contingency model is based on the idea that **program stage**—that is, where a program is in its life cycle, should be a key driver of the kind of evaluation to be done. A relatively simple and early form involves the suggestion that one starts with more program-improvement or formative evaluation, and then shifts toward more thumbs-up/thumbs-down, or summative evaluation later in the life of a program (Cronbach, 1980). Wholey also suggested a kind of stage model, as implied by his advocacy of the sequential purchase of evaluation. More detailed forms of program stage models have been proposed by Chen (2014) and by Scheirer (2012). In addition to program stage, Chen considers whether the anticipated use of the evaluation is internal to the program or its broader organization, or for external accountability purposes.

Michael Quinn Patton's popular utilization-focused evaluation illustrates another kind of contingency model based on intended use. Central to this kind of contingency model is the idea that the choice of what an evaluation should look like should be driven by the kind of use that is sought. The key phrase for Patton is **intended use by intended users**. Utilization-focused evaluation can include virtually any kind of evaluation, whether it looks like Campbell, Wholey, Scriven, CRE, any other evaluation theorist's approach, or is an eclectic mix, as long as doing the evaluation like that will facilitate intended use by whomever the intended users may be. Key to the practice of utilization-focused evaluation are techniques for identifying intended users and then presenting and considering options with them to identify the intended use.

A third kind of contingency model involves a more **policy-analytic** assessment of the potential contribution of different kinds of evaluation. An example of this kind of contingency theory is given by Mark et al. (2000). Rather than identifying and interacting with intended users, it involves an analysis as to which kinds of decisions about the program are more (or less) feasible in the circumstances at hand. Sometimes, for example, it is clear that a program will not be discontinued for the foreseeable future. The political winds may be too strong, or the timing wrong. But at the same time there may be room to look for opportunities for program improvement, or to test the relative effectiveness of program variants. In contrast, under other circumstances, it may be predictable that consideration will be given to replacing the current program, such as when a program is scheduled for reauthorization, or the organization includes sunset clauses. These two different circumstances, according to this third kind of contingency model, call out for different forms of evaluation. More generally, this contingency theory calls for a form of situational analysis of the relative feasibility (and potential payoff) of different forms of actions that might be taken regarding a program and then drawing preferences about types of evaluation activities accordingly.

I suggest that there are benefits, not only of being familiar with a contingency theory but also of being "multilingual" with respect to such models. The relative fit of the different kinds of contingency models is likely to vary across situations. A slogan might be "even the contingencies are contingent." For example, it may be easy to engage in discussions with an intended user in some cases, but quite infeasible in others (e.g., when evaluation is intended to inform the U.S. Congress). To take another example, a desire to engage in extended formative evaluation prior to summative evaluation, as would be encouraged by a program stage-based theory, might be overridden by a need to be responsive to the decision-making timeline specified in legislation. The templates provided by contingency theories of evaluation might fit more situations than simpler evaluation theories but probably not all. Judgment is still required.

THE FUTURE OF EVALUATION THEORY

In this final section of the chapter, a few suggestions are offered for the future development and application of evaluation theory.

Theory Testing, Theory Building, and Research on Evaluation

As noted earlier, some evaluators differentiate evaluation theories into different kinds. For example, according to Alkin (2004),

> there are two general types of models: (1) *a prescriptive model*, the most common type, is a set of rules, prescriptions and prohibitions, and the guiding frameworks which specify what a good or proper evaluation is and how evaluation should be done. Such models serve

as *exemplars*; (2) *a descriptive model* is a set of statements and generalizations which describes, predicts, or explains evaluation activities. Such a model is designed to offer an *empirical theory*. (p. 4)

The evaluation theories that have been described in this chapter are predominantly prescriptive models. Shadish et al. (1991) referred to something akin to Alkin's (2004) notion of empirical theory. In describing "The ideal (never achievable) evaluation theory," Shadish and colleagues indicated that, among other characteristics, it would "empirically test propositions to identify and address those that conflict with research or other critically appraised knowledge about evaluation" (pp. 30–31). In other words, the developers of both of our meta-models advocate for the increased use of empirical research to test tenets of evaluation theories.

Notable examples of such empirical testing of evaluation theories already exist in the evaluation literature. One focused on empowerment evaluation, a form of collaborative evaluation that was developed by David Fetterman (e.g., 1994; see also Fetterman et al., Chapter 10, this volume). Miller and Campbell (2006) examined 47 cases described by their authors as empowerment evaluations. Miller and Campbell examined two issues. First was whether the evaluations followed the principles of empowerment evaluation, and thus could be differentiated from other related approaches. Second, Miller and Campbell asked what evidence existed that the empowerment evaluations actually resulted in increased empowerment for those who participated in the evaluation process or for the intended beneficiaries of the program being evaluated. They reported that collectively the 47 case examples did not do well with respect to either issue. The review by Miller and Campbell addressed a key issue for those who conduct research on evaluation: Do evaluation theories, models, or approaches actually result in the benefits they claim will result (Mark, 2008)?

A second notable example comes from a 2012 book by Brad Cousins, an advocate and developer of another collaborative approach to evaluation, practical participatory evaluation, and his ex-student and colleague, Jill Anne Chouinard. Like Fetterman, Cousins falls on the use branch of the evaluation theory tree. In their 2012 book, Cousins and Chouinard synthesize the research by Cousins and others on practical participatory evaluation, with a key lesson being that engaging interest holders can in fact increase evaluation use. Related to the topic of engagement, another empirical contribution to a future descriptive theory of evaluation comes from Shulha et al. (2016), who, in a multiphase inquiry, drew on the responses of those experienced in conducting collaborative evaluation to derive and validate a set of principles for collaborative evaluation practice. Cousins (2020) draws on both of the contributions just mentioned in an edited volume. As yet another example, Mark et al. (2021) showed that those with an interest in an evaluation prefer that multiple groups be involved in providing input to guide the program.

Not only should there be increased research that tests the propositions embedded in one or more evaluation theories but in addition, those developing a new evaluation theory should emphasize the research (as well as practice) base from which they draw. We should remember that empirical findings from an earlier period of research on evaluation, sometimes called the "golden age" of research on evaluation, had a strong impact on evaluation theory and concepts. To take one example, Michael Patton found that when direct, instrumental use occurred, there often was an individual in the organization who had served as an advocate for evaluation use. This finding led to the concept of the "personal factor" and served as an underpinning of Patton's (1978, 2008) influential utilization-focused evaluation. In a second example, the idea of "enlightenment" or conceptual use of research was a research finding (Oral History Project Team, 2006). It arose when Carol Weiss (1977) found that although only a minority of her study participants reported engaging in direct, instrumental use, most also indicated that an evaluation affected the way they thought about the underlying social problem or its potential solutions. This finding helped broaden evaluators' conception of use, was part of Weiss's legacy as an evaluation theorist, and has influenced subsequent approaches, such as program theory-driven evaluation.

Evidence suggests that research on evaluation is increasing in frequency (Coryn et al., 2017). However, much remains to be done to tie empirical findings back to evaluation theory and practice. This would be a worthwhile area of contribution that readers of this chapter might make prior to the next edition of this handbook.

More People Shaping Evaluation Theory, Often with Less Comprehensive Scope

Elsewhere I have suggested the value of encouraging more members of the evaluation community to be actively involved in evaluation theory, perhaps with the slogan "Evaluation theory is too important to be left in the hands of a few people labeled as evaluation theorists" (Mark, 2018). It would be a sign of the field maturing, I believe, if we shift away from seeing evaluation theory as the realm of a few people who end up on a theory tree. As in other fields, some individuals might elect to specialize in theory building, but many others might participate in testing and refining a given theory or cluster of theories. And even more are likely to try to apply the lessons in practice.

The latest version of the evaluation theory tree (Alkin & Christie, 2023) is a notable step in that direction. As shown in Figure 4.3, the tree now lists theory names. Further progress remains, however, given that almost every chapter is authored by a single theory developer or, in the case of theorists no longer living, the best available proxy. (Another notable change in the tree is the inclusion of additional social justice-oriented theories on the valuing branch.) Perhaps future editions of the tree will include more contributions from people other than the original theory developer, these being individuals who have continued to modify, update, and test an evaluation theory or set of related theories. This would be another sign of growing maturation of evaluation theory, similar to developments over time in other fields. In various areas of psychology, for example, many theories initially were named after the original developers but over time have come to be referred to by a theory name.

Another potentially beneficial step would be to shift, at least partially, away from such extensive focus on relatively comprehensive, five-component evaluation *theories* as detailed by

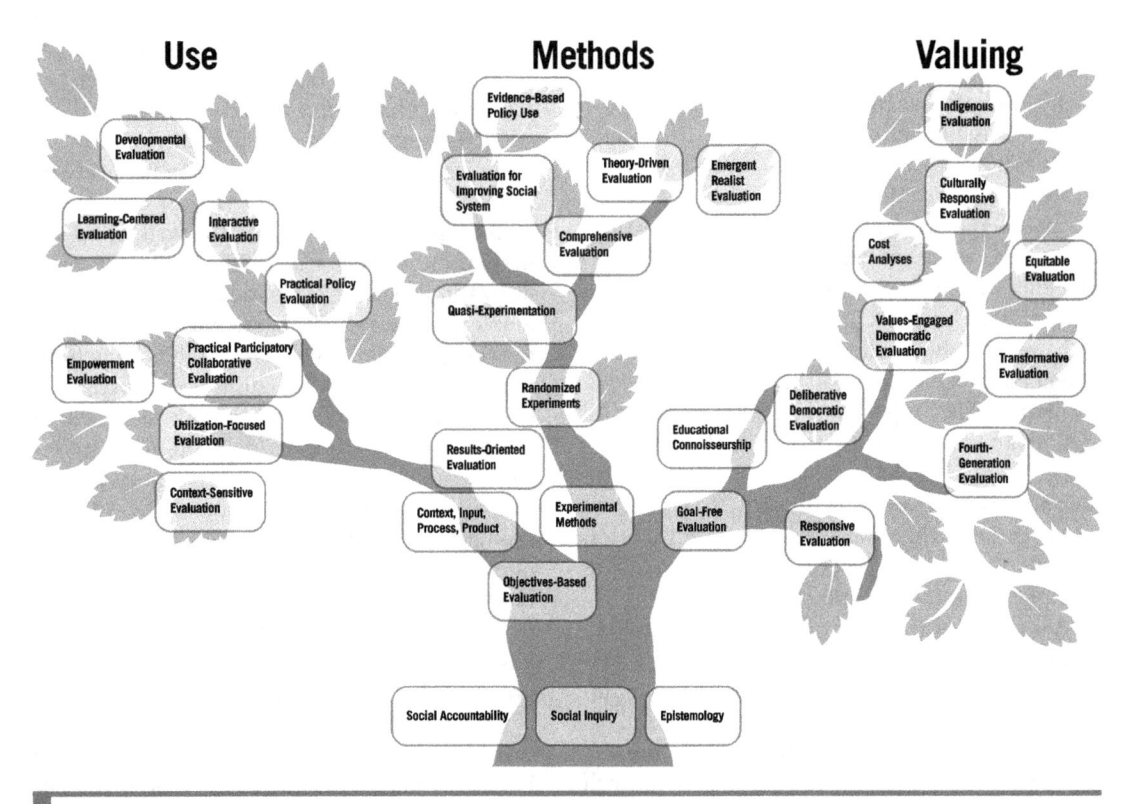

FIGURE 4.3. Latest version of evaluation theory tree, with branches named after theories.

Shadish et al. (1991). Instead, both theory developers and theory testers could increasingly concentrate on one or more theoretical *issues*. Some people might specialize broadly, with an interest such as valuing or one of the other five components of the Shadish et al. model. Others might specialize more narrowly, such as on facilitating participation by program clients, staff, or other interested parties, or even more specifically on such participation within, say, empowerment evaluation. If people specialize in specific issues within an evaluation theory, not only is depth of expertise encouraged but also the cost of entry into theory testing and theory formulation becomes smaller. Additionally, it would be valuable to have more people involved in developing and trialing evaluation theories, and in conducting and synthesizing research on evaluation theory. Over time, then, sharable evidence, more than assertion, would undergird the guidance that comes from evaluation theories.

Evaluation Theory and Lessons for Non-Evaluators

This chapter has for the most part sidestepped a very important constraint on the potential application of evaluation theory to evaluation practice—that is, the shape of an evaluation is often specified, not by an evaluator but by the staff of the agency that houses a program, or the oversight body, or a funder. A potentially important future project might be to try to consolidate lessons from evaluation theory for evaluation practice, and to disseminate them in formats and venues that could inform those, other than the evaluator, who influence the practice of evaluation.

Multilingualism, Contingency Models, and Theory as an Aid to Judgment

Adherence to a single evaluation theory is probably not the best way forward. True believers in a theoretical approach may bring some benefits, such as pushing a single evaluation approach as far as it can go. But the alternative kinds of contributions that evaluation can bring, and the disparate nature of programs and their broader contexts, are so varied that a single approach to evaluation is not likely to optimize the contributions that the practice of evaluation can bring. Instead, in the ideal, evaluators should be multilingual with respect to evaluation theory. And they should treat evaluation theories as a potential aid to judgment about practice, not as a recipe book that replaces judgment.

BOX 4.4. A Happy Marriage

Claire started the morning in a familiar way, checking her work emails with a cup of coffee. She had really been triaging these for more than a week, having been distracted by her stepson's wedding. As she scanned the long queue in her inbox, Claire was pleased to see the increase in requests for proposals (RFPs) and other notices about upcoming evaluations. As she started digging into the emails and links, she flashed back to the chapter she'd read some time ago about evaluation theory and the online class it had led her to take. One of the first emails Claire opened was from a regional foundation she had done some work for in the past. The email announced a fairly open-ended call for proposals. Claire's first thought was about proposing an EA about the foundation's grant making as a whole. The foundation's grants had evolved in various directions as program officers came and went. Hmm, another thought was to try to help lay out a variety of evaluation activities the foundation may use, and why, working with the foundation's new director of monitoring, evaluation, and learning. Claire next turned her attention to an email from a colleague at a large contract research firm. The firm had considerable expertise in randomized experiments and quasi-experiments, and planned to go after a contract for a large RCT. From what her friend said, it seemed to Claire like the circumstances suited such an evaluation. The friend mentioned he knew Claire had never done an RCT, but he and his colleagues liked what she had brought conceptually to the evaluation she had partnered on with them before. The RFP specified the design as well as some outcome measures. But Claire wondered whether there would be value added in proposing additional effort to consider other measures, drawing on the values components of several evaluation theories she'd studied. As she reviewed the rest of her emails, and as she started making some notes about a couple of possible proposals, Claire mused occasionally about how much she enjoyed her stepson's marriage. And she thought, as another smile appeared, the marriage of evaluation theory and evaluation practice isn't too bad either.

REFERENCES

Alkin, M. C. (Ed.). (2004). Comparing evaluation points of view. In *Evaluation roots: Tracing theorists' views and influences* (pp. 3–11). SAGE.

Alkin, M. C. (Ed.). (2013). *Evaluation roots: A wider perspective of theorists' views and influences* (2nd ed.). SAGE.

Alkin, M. C., & Christie, C. A. (2004a). An evaluation theory tree. In M. C. Alkin (Ed.), *Evaluation roots: Tracing theorists' views and influences* (pp. 12–65). SAGE.

Alkin, M. C., & Christie, C. A. (2004b). Evaluation theory tree revisited. In M. C. Alkin (Ed.), *Evaluation roots: Tracing theorists' views and influences* (pp. 381–392). SAGE.

Alkin, M. C., & Christie, C. A. (Eds.). (2023). *Evaluation roots: Theory influencing practice* (3rd ed.). Guilford Press.

Bhaskar, R. A. (1978). *A realist theory of science*. Humanities Press.

Bickman, L. (Ed.). (1987). The importance of program theory. In *Using program theory in evaluation* (pp. 5–18). Jossey-Bass.

Bickman, L., & Reich, S. (2014). Randomized controlled trials: A gold standard or gold plated? In S. I. Donaldson, C. A. Christie, & M. M. Mark (Eds.), *What counts as credible evidence in applied research and evaluation practice?* (2nd ed., pp. 83–118). SAGE.

Campbell, D. T. (1969). Reforms as experiments. *American Psychologist, 24*, 409–429.

Campbell, D. T. (1991). Methods for the experimenting society. *Evaluation Practice, 12*(3), 223–260.

Center for Evaluation Innovation. (2017, July). *Equitable evaluation framework (EEF) framing paper*. Equitable Evaluation Initiative. Available at www.equitableeval.org

Chen, H. T. (1990). *Theory-driven evaluations*. SAGE.

Chen, H. T. (2014). *Practical program evaluation: Theory-driven evaluation and the integrated evaluation perspective* (2nd ed.). SAGE.

Christie, C. A., & Alkin, M. C. (2004). An evaluation theory tree. In M. C. Alkin (Ed.), *Evaluation roots: A wider perspective of theorists' views and influences* (pp. 11–57). SAGE.

Christie, C. A., & Alkin, M. C. (2008). Evaluation theory tree re-examined. *Studies in Educational Evaluation, 34*(3), 131–135.

Christie, C. A., & Alkin, M. C. (2023). An evaluation theory tree. In M. C. Alkin & C. A. Christie (Eds.), *Evaluation roots: Theory influencing practice* (3rd ed., pp. 13–65). SAGE.

Coryn, C. L., Noakes, L. A., Westine, C. D., & Schröter, D. C. (2011). A systematic review of theory-driven evaluation practice from 1990 to 2009. *American Journal of Evaluation, 32*(2), 199–226.

Coryn, C. L. S., Wilson, L. N., Westine, C. D., Hobson, K. A., Ozeki, S., Fiekowsky, E. L., Greenman, G. D., & Schröter, D. C. (2017). A decade of research on evaluation: A systematic review of research on evaluation published between 2005 and 2014. *American Journal of Evaluation, 38*(3), 329–347.

Cousins, J. B. (2020). *Collaborative approaches to evaluation: Principles in use*. Sage.

Cousins, J. B., & Chouinard, J. A. (2012). *Participatory evaluation up close: A review and integration of the research base*. Information Age Press.

Cram, F. (2009). Maintaining indigenous voices. In D. Mertens & P. Ginsberg (Eds.), *The handbook of social research ethics* (pp. 308–322). SAGE.

Cronbach, L. J. (1980). *Toward reform of program evaluation*. Jossey-Bass.

Davidson, E. J. (2004). *Evaluation methodology basics: The nuts and bolts of sound evaluation*. SAGE.

Davidson, E. J. (2013). *Actionable evaluation basics: Getting succinct answers to the most important questions*. Real Evaluation.

Davies, R., & Payne, L. (2015). Evaluability assessments: Reflections on a review of the literature. *Evaluation, 21*(2), 216–231.

De Lancer Julnes, P. (2006). Performance measurement: An effective tool for government accountability? The debate goes on. *Evaluation, 12*(2), 219–235.

Deaton, A., & Cartwright, N. (2018). Understanding and misunderstanding randomized controlled trials. *Social Science and Medicine, 210*, 2–21.

Donaldson, S. I. (2007). *Program theory-driven evaluation science: Strategies and applications*. Erlbaum.

Fetterman, D. M. (1994). Empowerment evaluation. *Evaluation Practice, 15*(1), 1–15.

Frierson, H., Hood, S., & Hughes, G. (2002). A guide to conducting culturally responsive evaluation. In J. Frechtling (Ed.), *The 2002 user-friendly handbook for project evaluation* (pp. 63–73). National Science Foundation.

Frierson, H., Hood, S., Hughes, G., & Thomas, V. (2010). A guide to conducting culturally responsive evaluation. In J. Frechtling (Ed.), *The 2010 user-friendly handbook for project evaluation* (pp. 75–96). National Science Foundation.

Gopalan, M., Rosinger, K., & Ahn, J. B. (2020). Use of quasi-experimental research designs in education research: Growth, promise, and challenges. *Review of Research in Education, 44*(1), 218–243.

Holzer, M., & Ballard, A. (Eds.). (2021). *The public productivity and performance handbook* (3rd ed.). Routledge.

Hood, S. (1998). Responsive evaluation Amistad style: Perspectives of one African American evaluator. In *Proceedings of the Stake symposium on educational evaluation* (pp. 101–112). University of Illinois at Urbana–Champaign.

Hood, S., & Hopson, R. K. (2008). Evaluation roots

reconsidered: Asa Hilliard, a fallen hero in the "Nobody Knows My Name" project, and African educational excellence. *Review of Educational Research, 78*(3), 410–426.

Hood, S., Hopson, R. K., & Kirkhart, K. E. (2015). Culturally responsive evaluation. In K. E. Newcomer, H. P. Hatry, & J. S. Wholey (Eds.), *Handbook of practical program evaluation* (4th ed., pp. 281–317). Wiley.

Hopson, R. K. (2009). Reclaiming knowledge at the margins: Culturally responsive evaluation in the current evaluation moment. In K. E. Ryan & J. Bradley Cousins (Eds.), *The Sage international handbook of educational evaluation* (pp. 429–446). SAGE.

House, E. R. (1976). Justice in evaluation. In G. V. Glass (Ed.), *Evaluation studies review annual* (Vol. 1, pp. 75–100). SAGE.

House, E. R., & Howe, K. R. (1999). *Values in evaluation and social research.* SAGE.

Lam, S., & Skinner, K. (2021). The use of evaluability assessments in improving future evaluations: A scoping review of 10 years of literature (2008–2018). *American Journal of Evaluation, 42*(4), 523–540.

Lemire, S., Peck, L. R., & Porowski, A. (2020). The growth of the evaluation tree in the policy analysis forest: Recent developments in evaluation. *Policy Studies Journal, 48,* S47–S70.

Leviton, L. C., Khan, L. K., Rog, D., Dawkins, N., & Cotton, C. (2010). Evaluability assessment to improve public health policies, programs, and practices. *Annual Review of Public Health, 31*(1), 213–233.

Madaus, G. F., Scriven, M., & Stufflebeam, D. L. (1983). *Evaluation models.* Kluwer-Nijhoff.

Manswell-Butty, J.-A. L., Reid, M. D., & LaPoint, V. (2004). A culturally responsive evaluation approach applied to the talent development school-to-career intervention program. *New Directions for Evaluation,* 37–47.

Mark, M. M. (2008). Building a better evidence-base for evaluation theory. In P. R. Brandon & N. L. Smith (Eds.), *Fundamental issues in evaluation* (pp. 111–134). Guilford Press.

Mark, M. M. (2018). Strengthening links between evaluation theory and practice, and . . . Comments inspired by George Grob's 2017 Eleanor Chelimsky forum presentation. *American Journal of Evaluation, 39*(1), 133–139.

Mark, M. M. (2022). Engaging with program adaptations in evaluation: A range of existing options and a new opportunity. *American Journal of Evaluation, 43*(3), 314–334.

Mark, M. M., Allen, J. B., & Goodwin, J. L. (2021). Stakeholder involvement in evaluation: Does it affect observers' perceptions of an evaluation? And which stakeholder group(s) do people think should to participate? *Evaluation Review, 45*(3–4), 166–190.

Mark, M. M., Henry, G. T., & Julnes, G. (2000). *Evaluation: An integrated framework for understanding, guiding, and improving policies and programs.* Jossey-Bass.

Mertens, D. M., & Wilson, A. T. (2019). *Program evaluation theory and practice: A comprehensive guide* (2nd ed.). Guilford Press.

Michielutte, R., Shelton, B., Paskett, E. D., Tatum, C. M., & Valez, R. (2000). Use of an interrupted time-series design to evaluate a cancer screening program. *Health Education Research, 18,* 615–623.

Miller, R. L., & Campbell, R. (2006). Taking stock of empowerment evaluation: An empirical review. *American Journal of Evaluation, 27*(3), 296–319.

Munger, K. M., & Mertens, D. M. (2011). Conducting research with the disability community: A rights-based approach. *New Directions for Adult and Continuing Education, 132,* 23–33.

Oral History Project Team. (2006). The oral history of evaluation, part 4: The professional evolution of Carol H. Weiss. *American Journal of Evaluation, 27*(4), 475–484.

Patton, M. Q. (1978). *Utilization-focused evaluation.* SAGE.

Patton, M. Q. (2008). *Utilization-focused evaluation* (4th ed.). SAGE.

Rawls, J. (1971). *A Theory of Justice.* Harvard University Press.

Reichardt, C. S. (2019). *Quasi-experimentation: A guide to design and analysis.* Guilford Press.

Rog, D. J., Fitzpatrick, J. L., & Conner, R. F. (Eds.). (2012). *Context: A framework for its influence on evaluation practice* (New Directions for Evaluation, No. 135). Jossey-Bass.

Russ-Eft, D., & Sleezer, C. (2019). *Case studies in needs assessment.* SAGE.

Sawhill, J. C., & Williamson, D. (2001). Mission impossible? Measuring success in nonprofit organizations. *Nonprofit Management and Leadership, 11*(3), 371–386.

Scheirer, M. A. (2012). Planning evaluation through the program life cycle. *American Journal of Evaluation, 33*(2), 263–294.

Scriven, M. (1974). Pros and cons about goal-free evaluations. In W. J. Popham (Ed.), *Evaluation in education: Current applications* (pp. 34–67). McCutchen.

Shadish, W. R. (1996, June). Teaching evaluation theory. *Evaluation News and Comment, 5*(1), 553.

Shadish, W. R. (1998). Evaluation theory is who we are. *American Journal of Evaluation, 19*(1), 1–19.

Shadish, W. R., & Luellen, J. K. (2004). Donald Campbell: The accidental evaluator. In M. C. Alkin (Ed.), *Evaluation roots: A wider perspective of theorists' views and influences* (pp. 80–87). SAGE.

Shadish, W. R., Jr., Cook, T. D., & Leviton, L. C. (1991). *Foundations of program evaluation: Theories of practice.* SAGE.

Shulha, L. M., Whitmore, E., Cousins, J. B., Gilbert, N., & al Hudib, H. (2016). Introducing evidence-based principles to guide collaborative approaches to evaluation: Results of an empirical process. *American Journal of Evaluation, 37*(2), 193–215.

Sielbeck-Bowen, K. A., Brisolara, S., Seigart, D., Tischler, C., & Whitmore, E. (2002). Exploring feminist evaluation: The ground from which we rise. *New Directions for Evaluation, 2002*(96), 3–8.

Smith, N. L. (2010). Characterizing the evaluand in evaluating theory. *American Journal of Evaluation, 31*(3), 383–389.

Stake, R. E. (1976). A theoretical statement of responsive evaluation. *Studies in Educational Evaluation, 2*(1), 19–22.

Stufflebeam, D. L. (Ed.). (2001). *Evaluation models* (New Directions for Evaluation, No. 89). Jossey-Bass.

Thomas, V. G., & Parsons, B. A. (2017). Culturally responsive evaluation meets systems-oriented evaluation. *American Journal of Evaluation, 38*(1), 7–28.

Trevisan, M., & Walser, T. (2015). *Evaluability assessment*. SAGE.

Weiss, C. H. (1977). Research for policy's sake: The enlightenment function of social research. *Policy Analysis, 3*, 531–543.

White House. (2021, January 21). *Executive order on advancing racial equity and support for underserved communities through the federal government*.

Wholey, J. S. (2004). Evaluability assessment. In J. S. Wholey, H. P. Hatry, & K. E. Newcomer (Eds.), *Handbook of practical program evaluation* (2nd ed., pp. 33–62). Wiley.

Appendix 4A

As noted elsewhere in this chapter, in a chapter in the *Evaluation Roots* book on behalf of Campbell (who had died years earlier), Will Shadish argued against the theory tree with its three branches, arguing instead for the five-component Shadish et al. (2001) model. The two meta-models overlap a great deal, of course. Both include use and valuing. In addition, the evaluation theory tree includes a methods branch, which corresponds generally to the knowledge construction component of Shadish et al.—that is, the methods proclivities of an evaluation theorist are for the most part the more specific, practice-oriented techniques of knowledge construction. (An evaluation theory can include methods that align with other components, such as methods for valuing or for facilitating use, but it is methods related to knowledge construction that are emphasized in the methods branch of the theory tree.)

Regarding the practice component, perhaps it is not surprising that Alkin and Christie did not include this as a branch on the tree. After all, evaluation theories almost inevitably include a strong emphasis on evaluation practice. At the risk of taking the tree metaphor too far, perhaps one can think of practice as the acorns that fall to the ground from the tree.

On reflection, it also may not be surprising that social programming is not a separate branch on the evaluation theory tree. After all, the theorists represented in the *Evaluation Roots* book are all involved in *program* evaluation (although Scriven aspires to be a more general theorist of the evaluation of anything). On the other hand, *if* Alkin had included chapters by theorists of personnel evaluation, theorists of policy evaluation, and theorists of product evaluation, then the subject of the evaluation, or as Scriven has called it, the evaluand, might have appeared as part of the graphical representation. It seems likely that, rather than adding another branch to the current program evaluation tree, this would have involved drawing multiple trees, one for each kind of evaluand (program, policy, personnel), with each tree having branches (containing theorists who might appear on only that tree).

Alternatively, one could imagine the development of other approaches to program evaluation, with each premised on a different view of social programs, their role and operation. For example, one evaluation theory view might assume a competitive market of privately owned programs and center that feature of the evaluand, while another evaluation theory might focus on government-run programs that rarely are discontinued and give priority to the characteristics of such programs in laying out its approach to evaluation. Or an evaluation theory could give major focus to the way programs vary in their complexity/adaptability, such as in the number of distinct components and the expected or allowed adaptability (Mark, 2022), laying out alternative evaluation approaches based on the degree of complexity of the program. In such an alternative world, there may have been the need for a social program branch on the evaluation theory tree. But given the absence of different schools of thought about social programs as underpinnings of evaluation theories, Alkin and Christie's theory tree has three main branches.

Chapter 5

Valuing in Evaluation

Emily F. Gates
Thomas A. Schwandt

CHAPTER OVERVIEW

Valuing—the process of reaching warranted conclusions about value—is both a responsibility and an expertise claimed by professional evaluators. One of the features that distinguishes informal, day-to-day judgments of value from professionally conducted evaluation is that the latter is a form of systematic, objective, disciplined inquiry in which facts and values are brought together to construct an argument about the value of objects, plans, strategies, projects, programs, policies, and so forth. In this chapter, we explain in great detail this expertise and responsibility with a particular focus on how the process of valuing should be systematic, transparent, and defensible.

People routinely make judgments about value—for example, in reviewing a local restaurant, critiquing a colleague's work, deciding which school or college to attend, determining where to invest one's money, and choosing which candidate to vote for. Evaluation as a professional practice requires an intentional, systematic, and transparent process for making judgments about the value of an intervention. In the *Encyclopedia of Evaluation*, Fournier (2005) explains that:

> Evaluation is an applied inquiry process for collecting and synthesizing evidence that culminates in conclusions about the state of affairs, value, merit, worth, significance, or quality of a program, product, person, policy, proposal, or plan. Conclusions made in evaluations encompass both an empirical aspect (that something is the case) and a normative aspect (judgment about the value of something). It is the value feature that distinguishes evaluation from other types of inquiry, such as basic science research, clinical epidemiology, investigative journalism, or public polling. (pp. 139–140)

Reaching warranted conclusions about value is both a responsibility and an expertise claimed by professional evaluators (Grob, 2012; Davidson, 2012; Scriven, 2016b).

In this chapter, we explain in greater detail this expertise and responsibility with a particular focus on how the process of valuing should be systematic, transparent, and defensible. We begin by explaining how values are at work in multiple ways in evaluation drawing on some basic distinctions between the concepts of values and valuing. We then discuss the activity of valuing and explain the logic of valuing (Scriven, 1994, 2007, 2012; Davidson, 2005, 2014; Fournier, 1995). In that discussion we highlight several methods used in the activity of valuing. We conclude with considerations for creative and responsible valuing in evaluation practice.

VALUES IN THE EVALUATION FIELD

Values are deeply held convictions about what matters to both individuals and groups. They are expressions of the regard that something is held to deserve. Highly respected values in the field of evaluation are readily evident in statements of standards and ethics adopted by professional evaluation associations and societies, including, for example, the Program Evaluation Standards (Yarbrough et al., 2011), the American Evaluation Association (AEA) Guiding Principles for Evaluators (2018), the Aotearoa/New Zealand Evaluation Association Evaluator Competencies (Wehipeihana et al., 2014), and the United Nations Evaluation Group Ethical Guidelines (2008). Professional values include moral values that serve as norms for what is good or right in terms of human conduct, including honesty, truthfulness, respect for persons, cultural sensitivity, and kindness, among others. Cherished professional values also include epistemic or cognitive values, such as a commitment to evidence and criticism, systematic inquiry and justified belief, empirical grounding of claims, and objectivity as guides to the characteristics of good evaluation research.

Political values reflect views of what the government ("We, the people") ought to be doing or promoting, such as equality, social justice, democratic deliberation, and gender equity. Broadly speaking, commitments on the part of individual evaluators to various political values "underlie the justification and conduct of evaluation as an important social practice" (Schwandt, 2015, p. 45). Moral, epistemic, and political values (often intertwined) influence evaluators' understandings of their professional roles. Greene (1997) labels these as "regulative ideals" (p. 3) that inform (often conflicting) purposes of evaluation, such as serving rational decision making, developing interpretive meaning, empowering program beneficiaries, engaging in community activism, and facilitating democratic debate. Political values are manifest in all versions of evaluation practice whether informed by a philosophy of experimentalism, results-based management, critical theory, feminist standpoint methodologies, culturally responsive professional practice, or any other set of commitments.

What political values an individual evaluator may cherish can influence the way they conceive of serving the public interest and their sense of responsibility for the general and public welfare as an evaluation professional (Schwandt, 1997; Gates, 2018). For example, some evaluators maintain an impartial, value-neutral role arguing that evaluators should provide unbiased, fair information as input to public debate about social direction. **Value neutrality** means that the evaluation should be conducted without any influence of the evaluator's (or an evaluation team's or evaluation organization's) social, moral, or political values. Others argue that the public interest is better served if evaluators specifically attend to and prioritize the voices and experiences of historically underrepresented and disenfranchised groups (Datta, 2011; Schwandt, 2003). For example, culturally responsive approaches, particularly indigenous-led evaluations, underscore the embeddedness of values in culture and the necessity and benefits of centering indigenous values within evaluative processes (Wehipeihana & McKegg, 2018; Hepi et al., 2021).

Other kinds of values are at play in evaluation practice in ways that may be less readily apparent. For example, Chelimsky (2014) has argued that social and environmental interventions are designed by planners, policymakers, and public administrators to address a wide variety of public interest values. Some of which she identifies as arguably being supported by relative consensus, such as liberty from foreign control, public safety, and equality of citizens before the law. Others she says are clearly controversial, such as the scope and limits and recourse to secrecy in governmental affairs and the specific governmental role in pursuing equality of results among its citizens. Chelimsky argues that evaluators working in the public sector ought to be involved in assessing whether the stated goals of any given intervention are well aligned with public interest goals and "how, based on this analysis, might [an] intervention be structured or restructured to achieve the best test of its potential in the immediate, and to make program sustainability more achievable, over the longer term" (p. 531). Of course, not all evaluators are working in the public sector. Many examine initiatives, policies, programs, and practices in the private sector where return on investment, contribution to the bottom line, cost savings, market reach, customer satisfaction, and other economic considerations are considered most critical to organizational success. Evaluators in these environments often are involved in examining the alignment of initiatives with these kinds of valued outcomes.

In a somewhat similar vein, institutional values evident in what we call "valuing schemes" (Schwandt & Gates, 2021) often direct the way an evaluation is commissioned and conducted. These schemes include the value of social impact investing and social return on investment that drives the choice of programming of many philanthropic foundations; promotion of the value of accountability as a cornerstone of government policies; the routine use of the Organisation for Economic Co-operation and Development's Development Assistance Committee (OECD/DAC) criteria of relevance, effectiveness, efficiency, sustainability, and impact to evaluate development initiatives (Peersman, 2014); and the results-based management frameworks characteristic of many nongovernmental and multilateral organizations. The values held and promoted by an organization that an evaluator works for, coupled with the values that an organization's clients embrace, often serve to structure or frame an evaluation. Value perspectives also underlie the design and purposes of various initiatives that are to be evaluated—for example, Housing First (2016), as an effective response to homelessness preferred by multiple audiences, transformational versus transactional development, restorative versus criminal justice, charter schools and school voucher policies versus public education, anti-immigration policy, and so forth.

The foregoing might be considered as special cases of interest holder values and how they can influence an evaluation. Program and policy planners, designers, funders, managers, administrators, and beneficiaries all promote and defend their stakes in a given evaluation. **Stakes** can be understood as role-specific concerns and interests that, in turn, reflect what interest holders value (Reynolds, 2010, 2014). For example, frontline aid workers might place highest value on practicality and success of implementation of an initiative in highly complex, real-life circumstances, while policymakers might assign greatest value to assessing the relationship between the financial investment in an initiative and achievement of predefined outcomes.

The ways in which values—other than the customary focus on professional ethical values—influence practice are important areas for empirical research on evaluation and discussion among evaluation practitioners. As Michael Scriven (2016a) noted, the field of evaluation has largely treated ethics as a matter of professional ethical behavior, ignoring the more knotty issues surrounding the ethical aspects of practices and interventions worthy of study and discussion. In a systematic review of research on evaluation published between 2005 and 2014, Coryn and colleagues (2017) found that "very few Research on Evaluation investigations in the published literature explicitly address values or valuing in evaluation (3.50%)" (p. 339). They suggest possibilities for empirical investigations of values in evaluation, such as "how evaluators identify and validate relevant values for use in an evaluation" and "how evaluators reconcile competing values (e.g., those of different interest holder groups)," among others. In addition to formally studying values in evaluation, evaluators can consider the ways in which values influence and should influence their practices. Greene (2012) focuses on evaluation commonplaces, such as evaluation questions and variables or constructs of interest, as practice areas that are influenced by values (see also Teasdale, 2021, for discussion of evaluation commonplaces). Greene argues for an educative role in which evaluators facilitate discussions and deliberations about whose and which values influence an evaluation, which Boyce (2017) and Reid (2020) practically illustrate in science, technology, engineering, and mathematics (STEM) contexts. Box 5.1 provides an illustrative vignette of the ways evaluators can thoughtfully and ex-

> **BOX 5.1. Vignette: How Do Values Influence Evaluation? A Conversation among Three Evaluators**
>
> The multiple ways in which values are at work in evaluations is illustrated in this brief exchange among three evaluators. Key considerations in this exchange include which values are legitimate, when, and how.
>
> - Nicholas, an independent consultant who contracts with international nongovernmental organizations to conduct multisite evaluations for development
> - Irina, a federal employee of the U.S. government who oversees commissioning of evaluations of policies mandated by Congress
> - Malika, an academic evaluator and evaluation professor who conducts evaluations of community-based initiatives and social service organizations
>
> *Malika:* "Nicholas and Irina, as fellow evaluators, I'm hoping you can help me. A colleague recently asked me how I justify advocating for social justice in my evaluation work. I responded that *all* evaluations advance some (and not other) values, but they were unconvinced claiming that evaluation ought to be impartial. What values influence your evaluation work and how so?"
>
> *Nicholas:* "Well, I work internationally, and we try to make sure that whatever we are evaluating is in line with the United Nations' Universal Declaration of Human Rights. Beyond that, we don't take stances on values in our evaluation work as our evaluations need to be considered rigorous and credible by a wide variety of interest holders, from government officials to wealthy donors to the actual people and communities who are supposed to benefit from the projects."
>
> *Irina:* "I can relate to what you're saying Nicholas. In my work at the government, we commission independent firms to carry out evaluations. When reviewing proposals and selecting evaluators, we try to pick those that have sufficient social science research expertise and experience to conduct rigorous, objective studies. That said, we know evaluation is different than research and so we also look for firms that uphold the Joint Committee Standards for Educational Evaluation and the American Evaluation Association's guiding principles."
>
> *Malika:* "That's different than my work. A lot of the organizations I work for specifically focus on social justice and reducing inequities between majority and minority groups. So, I always bring a social justice lens and also tend to use evaluation approaches like culturally responsive evaluation and deliberative democratic evaluation that focus on social justice."

plicitly reflect on values in evaluation. For ideas of further readings on values in evaluation, see Hassall (2020).

VALUING IN THE EVALUATION FIELD

In the previous section we emphasized that *values* influence the way in which evaluators conceive of their responsibility as professionals and the role that evaluation plays or ought to play in society. We also suggested that the values embedded in the context and design of programs and policies, as well as in institutions that commission and conduct evaluation, can shape the purpose and design of an evaluation, and that how that happens (and the consequences of that influence) is a proper subject for evaluative investigation. In this section, we turn specifically to the professional evaluation responsibility of **valuing** defined as the activity of reckoning or determining the value of something that takes the form of an **evaluative judgment** (Schwandt & Gates, 2021).[1]

Several kinds of evaluative judgments are made in planning and conducting evaluations. Some of which occur during the evaluation process and may not, at first, appear to involve valuing, such as the following:

- Judging the appropriateness of particular means of data collection and analysis to answer specific evaluation questions.
- Judging the relevance, sufficiency, and probative force of different types of evidence in support of claims.

---

[1] There is some evidence that evaluators do not systematically engage in making evaluative judgments. A meta-analysis conducted by Hurteau et al. (2009) examining the legitimacy and justification of judgments made by program evaluation practitioners found that just 20 out of 40 reports included judgments. Even though "elements required to support legitimate and justified judgments were present in the reports in similar proportions, whether the reports generated a judgment or not" (p. 307).

- Judging the ethics of interventions (this includes the ethical conduct of program managers and frontline personnel delivering the intervention, as well as whether the intervention itself is ethical).

Each of these involves an assessment or appraisal of value that can be done in a more or less explicit way. Other evaluative judgments are related to the purpose (or type) of evaluation and the questions being examined within an evaluative process, such as the following:

- Judging how an intervention can be improved—as in formative evaluations.
- Judging whether an intervention (e.g., project, policy, program, strategy) is being implemented as planned—as in implementation evaluations.
- Judging the extent to which an intervention achieves desired outcomes or results and minimizes negative consequences—as in outcome evaluations.
- Judging whether an intervention causes or contributes to desired impacts and, therefore, whether such intervention is of value as compared to no or alternative interventions—as in impact evaluations.
- Judging an intervention on its performance relative to specific objectives, criteria, standards, indicators, benchmarks, and so on—as in performance evaluation, measurement, or monitoring.
- Judging whether (or the extent to which) a group of social innovators work together to develop, implement, adapt, improve, or otherwise support an innovation—as in developmental evaluations.
- Rendering an overall (synthesis) judgment of the value of a given intervention by examining performance across multiple criteria and standards—for example, is intervention X designed and implemented in such a way that it is cost-effective, culturally responsive, impactful, and sustainable over time—as in summative evaluations.

All warranted or defensible evaluative judgments have four distinguishing characteristics:

1. They are the outcome of **evaluative reasoning**. Evaluative reasoning relies on skills of critical thinking that involve identification and careful appraisal of assumptions, pursuing evidence for claims, and developing justifications for inferences. Evaluative judgments are inferences based on a combination of facts and values that come in the form of statements like "Thus . . . ," "Because . . . ," Consequently . . . ," or "It follows that . . . "

2. Evaluative judgments require criteria or principles as bases for inferences. For example, in the statements of types of judgments noted above, the terms *appropriateness*, *relevance*, *sufficiency*, *benefits in terms of costs*, *cultural responsiveness*, and *sustainability* are all examples of criteria that can be used in rendering an evaluative judgment. Some criteria are capable of being expressed in quantitative and measurable ways (e.g., efficiency, effectiveness), whereas others are expressed qualitatively (e.g., relevance, responsiveness). Criteria are, of course, themselves subject to interpretation and based on some normative ideals or values.

3. Evaluative judgments can be *objectively determined and debated*, where "objectively" means working toward an unbiased statement by means of employing the procedures of the professional practice and observing the norms of proper argument (House & Howe, 1999; Schwandt, 2005; Scriven, 2012).

4. Evaluative judgments are not merely declarations or assertions that such and such is the case (e.g., X caused Y; X had the following outcomes and impacts) but are framed as *arguments* intended to convince a particular audience (e.g., commissioners, funders, managers, beneficiaries, the public) of a particular conclusion or claim about what is being evaluated. The claim that evaluative judgments are arguments signifies that there is something more involved than making a diagnosis or determination of value. Arguments are sets of reasons for why a particular audience ought to be persuaded of a value claim; they "may be more or less technical, more or less sophisticated, but they must persuade if they are to be taken seriously in the forums for public deliberation" (Majone, 1989, p. 8).

VALUING LOGIC AND RELATED METHODS

While there is general agreement that the purpose of evaluation is to establish the value of something, there is disagreement on how that should be done. One point of debate, or at least differing views, has to do with whether making evaluative judgments is more or less a matter of expert clinical judgment involving automatic, intuitive reasoning relying on knowledge acquired through past experiences or whether it is an analytic and reflective reasoning process that is rule or procedure governed. In actuality, these types of reasoning are not mutually exclusive; judgment strategies likely depend on the circumstances an evaluator confronts. Because the cognitive processes involved in evaluative judgment are complex, they are prone to various cognitive errors, such as faulty heuristics/cognitive biases and affective influences. We acknowledge that many evaluative judgments are made on the basis of experience, practice wisdom, and situated knowledge, yet contend that the core process of making evaluative judgments ought to be as explicit and transparent as possible. Furthermore, in practice, evaluative judgments may be made by and through group discussion and deliberation rather than by an individual evaluator or evaluation team. The question then becomes whether the grounds for evaluative judgments are a summing up of individual expert judgments or a rendering through some explicit process guided by rules or principles (Schwandt & Gates, 2021).

A related point of difference has to do with whether value (merit, worth, significance, quality, etc.) is something that is best understood and represented through narrative accounts of firsthand experience or quantitative renderings in terms of measurement (Stake et al., 1997); expressed in Stake and Schwandt (2006, pp. 407–408) as "quality-as-experienced" compared to "quality-as-measured." We presume that a dichotomous choice here is not necessary—both ways of accounting for value (as experienced *and* measured) and of rendering value (as expert, clinical judgment *and* as a rule-governed, explicit process) can contribute to valuing in specific evaluation circumstances.

In the view of some evaluation practitioners and scholars (Scriven, 1994, 2007, 2012; Davidson, 2005, 2014; Fournier, 1995), a particular **logic of evaluation** serves to distinguish the field from related practices in applied social research. The logic generally involves four steps: (1) identifying and selecting criteria, (2) identifying sources of evidence to use in assessing performance on each criterion, (3) determining merit by comparing evidence of performance and with established standards, and (4) rendering a judgment across performance on multiple criteria. Not all evaluators are attentive to this logic, yet Davidson (2005, 2014) argues that evaluation requires evaluation-specific logic and methodology. She outlines nine steps for this process, which incorporate these four steps with others within an evaluation process. For our purposes, we use the four steps—selecting criteria, identifying evidence, setting standards, and synthesis—as the general valuing logic. Evaluation-specific methodologies are those that facilitate combining descriptive data and empirical evidence with relevant values to draw explicitly evaluative judgments (Davidson, 2005). In what follows, we discuss each step of the logic in greater detail along with several methods and procedures that may be used to carry out that step.

Selecting Criteria

Criteria refer to "aspects, qualities, or dimensions that distinguish a meritorious or valuable evaluand from one that is less meritorious or valuable" (Davidson, 2005, p. 91). Evaluative judgments of all kinds—for example, about the design and implementation of a policy or program, the achievement of intended outcomes and impacts, the benefits compared to costs, and comparative effectiveness—require criteria as a basis for that judgment. In some evaluations, all of these types of judgments are required. In others, an evaluation may be focused on a single type of judgment, as for example, one finds in impact evaluation where the primary judgment is one of causal inference—that is, whether observed outcomes are attributable to the intervention in question. See Box 5.2 for potential criteria to use in an evaluation.

There are several important considerations in the identification of criteria. First, there is no one correct way to identify, select, and justify criteria (Hall et al., 2011; Henry, 2002; Julnes, 2012a; Schwandt, 2015). The choice and justification of criteria is subject to multiple influences including evaluator preferences based on past experience with similar objects of evaluation, institutional norms prescribing valued outcomes, interest holders' perceptions of what criteria should receive the greatest attention, and so forth. Hence, the choice and prioritization of criteria is often something negotiated in each evaluation situation. This is the case even when there are highly recommended criteria. For example, almost all development initiatives reference the OECD/DAC criteria of relevance, effectiveness, efficiency, sustainability, and impact. Yet, in practice, agencies that employ them in evaluations—for example, the United Nations Development Programme, the U.K. Foreign Commonwealth and Development Office, formerly known as the Department of International Development, the U.S. Agency for International Development, and so on—emphasize some over others, sometimes neglect one or more, sometimes add additional criteria, and so forth. The use of these criteria has been the subject of recent critical examination (see, e.g., Zenda Ofir's 2017 blog, as well as the views of the former director of the Independent Evaluation Group at the World Bank, Caroline Heider, in *Rethinking Evaluation*, 2017) and have been moderately revised (OECD, 2021).

Second, criteria are themselves subject to interpretation. In reference to measuring social value, Mulgan (2010) emphasizes not assuming that social value is something that is "objective, fixed, and stable" but instead viewing social value as something that is "subjective, malleable, and variable" (p. 1). Operationalizing social value and particular criteria requires a process of identifying, deliberating, negotiating, and reaching some agreement on how the criteria will be defined (and perhaps measured) in a specific evaluation situation. For example, in an evaluation of a professional development initiative for mathematics teachers, the evaluation team developed a set of evaluative criteria based on goals of the funding agency and project leaders, the project description and logic model, and interviews with participating teachers. This generated many potential criteria, which they refined and defined as a cohesive set in conversation with project leadership (see Teasdale et al., 2023, for this case description).

Third, although as much as possible one wishes to specify relevant criteria in advance of conducting an inquiry, it is not uncommon that relevant criteria might emerge during the course of an evaluation. This could be due to unforeseen circumstances, such as when an educational program's capacity to adapt to online formats became an important criterion due to school closures during the COVID-19 pandemic. This could also be due to the ways in which what is valuable or meaningful about a program gets discovered through its implementation, such as when home caregiving for physical health gener-

---

BOX 5.2. Evaluation Criteria

- *Stated program objectives:* to what extent and in ways an intervention accomplished what it set out to accomplish
- *Efficacy:* extent to which an intervention does more good than harm when delivered under optimal conditions
- *Effectiveness:* extent to which an intervention does more good than harm when delivered under actual real-world conditions
- *Relevance:* extent to which intervention objectives are consistent with specific priorities, needs, policies, and so on
- *Equity:* whether and how much the intervention reduced inequities, benefited those considered those least well-off in a given context
- *Efficiency:* extent to which monetary costs, time, and effort are well used
- *Social impact:* measurement of social, public, and/or civic value created by some intervention(s)
- *Sustainability:* whether intervention can continue to exist and/or outcomes/impacts can continue to exist beyond period of funding and other initial supports
- *Cultural relevance and responsiveness:* whether design and implementation of an intervention and its defined value adequately address the culture of target groups, communities, and so on
- *Established requirements:* extent to which intervention adheres to guidance or requirements in laws, policies, and/or other formal requirements
- *Expert opinion:* how well an intervention meets norms, procedures, standards, and so on set by experts in a given field or intervention area
- *Needs assessment:* whether and how much an intervention reduces or addresses a gap identified with regard to specific needs of target population or organization

Note. Adapted from Schwandt (2015).

ates a sense of mattering and connectedness for caregivers and receivers. Using the analogy with dating, Davies (2018) emphasizes that some criteria regarding what one finds valuable in a relationship come about through the experience of the relationship. In the context of evaluation, this translates to "coming up with good criteria that are shared across interest holders . . . involves balancing what can be easily measured with the more important criteria that can only be discovered over time and deep engagement with all participants" (p. 125).

With these caveats in mind we can point to some widely used approaches for identifying criteria. Because values are the basis for criteria, some evaluators advocate using *values inquiry*—social science research methods, such as surveys, focus groups, and document analysis—to identify value positions of interest holders and the public (Mark et al., 2000). The purpose of such inquiry is to identify and prioritize those values (and hence the criteria and outcomes) most prized by interest holders and the public and then designing the evaluation to address those concerns. Based on an empirical review of evaluations in informal science, Teasdale (2021) provides an *integrated model* that identifies widely used domains and sources of criteria. Domains are the focuses or substantive areas (e.g., effectiveness, cultural responsiveness) of criteria; sources are the people, places, and/or materials from which criteria may be identified (e.g., grant proposals, intended beneficiaries). This model provides a useful guide for practitioners and students of evaluation to explicitly and systematically consider, discuss, and select criteria (Teasdale et al., 2023). Harman and Azzam (2018) conducted a study to examine the feasibility and reliability of setting criteria and standards using *crowdsourcing*, enlisting members of the public to complete research tasks for small fees:

> Research shows that when the responses of a diverse and independent group of people using only their personal knowledge of a topic are averaged by an independent mechanism, the solution will be more accurate than the response of the smartest individual. Using this logic, crowdsourcing has been shown to produce better results than using subject matter experts for a growing pool of tasks. (p. 70)

While identifying criteria using traditional research methods, an integrated model and crowdsourcing are relatively feasible approaches; measuring multidimensional social values using multiple criteria comes with challenges. With regard to the construction of a well-being index, the Overseas Development Institute found that identification of relevant dimensions across interest holder groups was achievable—however, assigning weights to these dimensions required further support. Takeuchi (2014) contrasts advantages and disadvantages of normative, data-driven, and elicited weighting systems. One of the challenges with assigning weights to criteria discussed is the way people's current life circumstances, limited information, and internalization of sociocultural and religious expectations can influence their ratings such that they do not express ideal value preferences. Identification, measurement, and weighting of values should consider this and other challenges in incorporating people's values in the selection of criteria. Takeuchi illustrates this with reference to efforts to use well-being as a criterion. In the Human Development Index, for example, all aspects of well-being (health, education, income, etc.) are weighted equally. Takeuchi suggests more empirical investigation of values attached to these different aspects by eliciting people's values via a variety of empirical methods and then assigning weights based on their responses. In some circumstances, it may not be necessary to combine and weigh criteria, particularly when evaluation audiences and users may weight criteria differently and, subsequently, render different evaluative judgments.

Other options for determining criteria include *needs and values assessments* (Altschuld & Kumar, 2010) as well as *checklists* proposed by evaluation theorists for the range of criteria that should be considered, including Stufflebeam's (2001) "Evaluation Values and Criteria Checklist" and Scriven's (2007) "Key Evaluation Checklist." Stufflebeam's (2001) checklist includes societal values (e.g., equity, conservation, citizenship), criteria inherent in the definition of evaluation (e.g., merit, worth), institutional values (e.g., mission, goals, priorities), technical requirements (e.g., codes, standards), duties of personnel (e.g., professional competence, job performance), and criteria that are identified as the evaluation unfolds. Scriven's (2007) checklist outlines the evaluation process and within that the types of values that an evaluation might consider, as summarized below. These checklists provide a handy reference to identifying criteria but do not provide guidance on selecting criteria. See Box 5.3 for a list of potential criteria.

Another option is to identify values in conjunction with development of a *logic model* or program theory. For example, Renger and Bourdeau (2004) discuss how the antecedent conditions, target antecedent conditions, and measurement approach to logic model development can incorporate values inquiry to identify the relevant values and outcomes to the program being evaluated. (See Frechtling, Chapter 20, this volume, on logic models.) Or similarly, one could use *theories or models that guide the design of the intervention* and suggest quality. For example, Martz (2013) examines how various models of organizational performance—goal model, systems model, process model, strategic constituencies model, and competing values framework—offer different bases for selecting criteria.

Criteria may also be identified and prioritized using *evaluation frameworks* recommended by agencies overseeing, commissioning, or sponsoring evaluations—examples include the OECD/DAC criteria for international development initiatives (i.e., relevance, effectiveness, efficiency, impact, sustainability) and the comparative evaluation framework of 10 general criteria for evaluating children's programs developed by the U.S. Government Accountability Office (GAO) at the request of Congress (GAO, 1988; Shipman, 1989). Similarly, there are evaluation frameworks espousing specific criteria within intervention areas, such as a human rights-based approach to programming that focuses on five principles (i.e., normativity, nondiscrimination, participation, transparency, accountability) and criteria used in humanitarian assistance (i.e., coverage, coordination, protection, coherence; Peersman, 2014). Selecting criteria might also be informed by the evaluation framework or approach used by the evaluator as, for example, found in the values-engaged, educational approach to evaluating STEM education initiatives that examine program quality at the intersection of content, pedagogy, and attention to diversity and equity (Greene et al., 2006). What is most critical in the selection of criteria is developing a justification for any specific selection for the audiences with immediate stakes in what is being evaluated as well as taking responsibility, as the evaluator, for explaining why some criteria may have been omitted from consideration. Box 5.4 provides a practical example of several ways to select and justify criteria.

Identifying Sources of Evidence

Both qualitative (narrative) and quantitative (statistical) data as well as multiple sources of information (e.g., documentation, observation, input from multiple groups of interest holders, previous evaluations of similar objects, literature reviews) can all serve as potential sources of evidence. It is necessary to identify the evidence required by the specific evaluative questions and criteria and to systematically collect this evidence in a rigorous and defensible way. Two examples of tying methods to specific evaluation questions follow.

BOX 5.3. Sources of Possible Values Used in Evaluative Judgments

- Values that follow from the definition of the evaluand
- Needs of the target population, intended beneficiaries, and so on
- Logical requirements that follow from the goals or purposes of the evaluand
- Legal requirements or sublegal guidance
- Cultural values held by those involved or affected by the evaluand
- Personal, group, and organizational goals/desires
- Fidelity to implementation plans or procedures
- Professional standards or expert input on standards
- Historical or traditional standards (e.g., from similar prior interventions)
- Scientific merit/worth/significance
- Marketability or resource economy
- Political merit, potentially established through cross-party agreement
- Likelihood (or probability) of failure or success and the potential losses/gains or intended/unintended consequences associated with failure or success

Note. Adapted from Scriven's (2007) Key Evaluation Checklist.

> **BOX 5.4. Examples of How Evaluators Could Select Criteria**
>
> Evaluators' approaches to selecting criteria vary in part by their own value stances, the institutions they work for and with, and their professional judgments about appropriate criteria that suit the intervention and evaluation context. Three evaluations that explicitly describe and justify the selection of criteria are summarized below.
>
> **Example 1: Criteria and Value for Money**
>
> In international development contexts, King and Allan (2018) discuss how they used these five criteria—economy, efficiency, effectiveness, cost-effectiveness, and equity—to define "value" in a value-for-money evaluation of a subnational governance program in Pakistan to support reforms in public financial management, planning, and service improvement. These criteria were required by the evaluation commissioner. Evaluators paired these criteria with use of evaluation rubrics to make the evaluative reasoning explicit.
>
> **Example 2: Public Input with Crowdsourcing**
>
> Crowdsourcing uses online platforms, such as Amazon MTurk, to recruit and pay a group of workers to complete specified tasks within a short timeframe. Harman and Azzam (2018) conducted a study comprising four phases to examine how a crowd can set stable and high-quality evaluation criteria and standards. Researchers concluded that the crowd was able to set stable, high-quality criteria and did so at a minimum cost and time investment. Harman and Azzam suggest that crowdsourcing may be a practically feasible way for evaluators to select criteria as well as weight, and set standards for performance on these criteria. This approach may be most appropriate for areas where there is a clear consensus on what a "good" program means. For programs that lack consensus, other approaches that involve deliberation may be more appropriate.
>
> **Example 3: Evaluation Approach/ Evaluator Stance**
>
> A values-engaged, educative evaluation approach (Greene et al., 2006, 2011) specifically considers program quality along three dimensions: content, pedagogy, and equity. In the words of Greene et al. (2011), "In values-engaged, educative evaluation, the evaluator attends to the contextual quality of the program's content and pedagogy, and further defines educational quality at the intersection of high-level and current content, appropriate pedagogy, and equity" (p. 48). This approach has been most widely used in evaluations of STEM education programs (e.g., see Boyce, 2017).
>
> *Note.* Foreign Commonwealth and Development Office (FCDO), U.K.

There is a family of economic methods used to gather evidence when the key evaluative question is about return on investment or value for money—"How well are we using resources, and are we using them well enough to justify their use?" (King, 2016, p. 7; King & Oxford Policy Management [OPM], 2018). These include cost-effectiveness, cost–benefit, and cost–utility analysis as well as social return on investment (King, 2016; King & OPM, 2018; Gargani, 2017). These methods utilize financial and resource data combined with quantitative outcome data, which may be supported by qualitative data capturing interest holder conceptions of outcomes and their value.

When the evaluative question of interest focuses on the causal relationship between an intervention and its effects, evidence can be particularly contested. Some evaluators subscribe to the view that when impact evaluations are required of interventions with high stakes and investments, the best evidence for that kind of evaluative judgment comes from experiments or quasi-experiments. These designs focus on the evaluative questions of whether observed outcomes/impacts can be attributed to a particular intervention. Typically, quantitative, standardized measurement of outcomes at multiple time points is necessary evidence. Other evaluators argue that other forms of investigation (e.g., contribution analysis, process tracing) can yield other types of evidence from which to infer causation. Gates and Dyson (2017) discuss how the conversation about causality in the evaluation field has broadened such that a wider array of causal questions and sources of evidence are often relevant. These may include narrative accounts of an intervention's influence in beneficiaries' lives, theory-based explanations of causal processes, evidence of multiple interventions working together to produce outcomes/impacts, or causal loop diagramming of data-based and hypothetical variables to model causal processes. See Gates and Dyson and Stern et al. (2012) for a range of approaches to generate evidence of causal relationships.

Setting Standards

Determining the merit, value, worth, or significance of what is being evaluated requires setting standards of performance on criteria—the standards are guides to deciding whether performance on a given criterion is poor, satisfactory, good, outstanding, and so forth. In the *Encyclopedia of Evaluation*, Mathison (2005) says, "there is much mystery associated with standard setting" (p. 398). Some of this mystery has to do with the inevitable sociopolitical influences and professional judgment involved in setting standards. "The quality of the judgment about what constitutes an appropriate standard or level of performance is determined as much by who is making the determination as by any particular method used" (p. 398). That said, Mathison identifies methods from achievement testing that are used to set cut scores that could be adapted by evaluators to set standards. These include the *Angoff procedure* that uses expert judgment about the probability of a minimally competent person answering a question correctly and then summing probabilities to arrive at a cut score; the *contrasting groups procedure* that "compares expected and actual performance among different ability groups" and uses the score that best distinguishes a group; and the *bookmark procedure*, developed by CTB/McGraw-Hill, that involves ordering questions in difficulty level and then having experts individually and collectively set the cutoffs for levels of performance (p. 398).

One way of managing standard setting is to develop *rubrics* that provide an evaluative description of what performance looks like at two or more defined levels. Rubrics readily align with the logic of valuing and have been used by some evaluators to guide and make transparent the valuing process in evaluation (Dickinson & Adams, 2017; Oakden, 2013; King et al., 2013). According to Dickinson and Adams,

> there are two basic elements to a rubric—the evaluation criteria to be rated and the performance standards. The evaluation criteria serve as identifying the dimensions of interest that will be used as the basis for judging how well the programme has performed on particular interventions or outcomes. (p. 114)

As Davidson et al. (2011), Davidson (2014), and Martens (2018) advise, rubrics can be used to build detailed descriptions of what performance means at different levels and to "paint the broad picture of what performance looks like regardless of what evidence is available" (Davidson, 2014, p. 6). See Oakden (2013) for an example of using rubrics to evaluate a program for first-time principals in New Zealand schools.

The technique known as *most significant change* (Davies & Dart, 2005) has also been used when there is a great diversity and conflicting views on what criteria and standards are most important. In its most basic form the technique involves collecting stories of what are regarded as the most important change in practice or outcomes (including a process to generate and collect stories from the extremes of little or negative change) and then sharing and discussing those stories as a means to come to a better understanding of what is valued by whom and why. *Outcome harvesting* offers another example of a method that does not use predefined criteria or standards but, instead, uses the processes of gathering and analyzing evidence of outcomes to discern desirability of outcomes (Wilson-Grau, 2018).

Another technique of growing importance in the field is *critical systems heuristics*, first introduced by Ulrich (1983) and elaborated by Ulrich and Reynolds (2010) and Williams and van 't Hof (2016). The heuristic consists of a set of 12 questions that help make explicit the judgments of what facts and values are considered to be relevant (and irrelevant) in understanding a situation and designing an intervention for improving it. The questions address four areas (i.e., purpose, decision making, knowledge, and legitimacy) and are typically posed in descriptive (i.e., what is) and normative (i.e., what should be) modes. The framework can be used throughout the valuing process to set criteria within different ways of framing the object of evaluation, determine a relevant mix of evidence, identify normative standards, and inform overall synthesis (Gates, 2018).

Synthesis

The last step in the process of valuing is **evaluation synthesis**—drawing an overall evaluative judgment about performance on multiple criteria, or quite simply, "piecing together information to create a whole" (Mathison, 2005, p. 405). The rendering of synthesis judgments is controversial and disputed in the field of evaluation. Schwandt (2015) argues that "the processes by which synthesis judgments are made is not well understood, and there is little consensus in the field of evaluation about how to aggregate findings across multiple criteria or across interest holders' differing perspectives on important criteria" (p. 59). Shipman (2012) claims that synthesis judgments require prioritizing criteria and in the case of evaluations conducted by the U.S. GAO that is, in essence, a political decision, which the GAO ought to avoid. Davidson (2015, p. v) has repeatedly argued that many evaluators fail to employ "evaluation-specific methodologies" required to reach synthesis judgments. Scriven (1994, p. 367) has claimed that the lack of explicit justification for evaluation syntheses is the "Achilles' heel" of the practice.

The four most common approaches to making a synthesis judgment are (1) rule-governed, algorithmic, and rubric-based approaches; (2) non-algorithmic, intuitive-based holistic judgment approaches; (3) all-things-considered approaches; and (4) deliberative approaches (Schwandt, 2015). *Rule-governed* approaches, often called weight and sum, involve assigning importance weights to each criterion and performance scores for each standard and then adding or combining the scores to render an overall conclusion. Rubrics follow this approach specifying, for example, what "excellent," "good," "adequate," and "inadequate" performance levels look like for multiple criteria. The process of rating the performance levels of various aspects of an intervention as well as synthesizing across ratings may be carried out deliberately as a group with evaluator(s) facilitating the process. Numerical weight and sum follow this process but typically involve a set of mathematical calculations. *Non-algorithmic*, *intuitive-based* approaches assume that the overall value of an intervention cannot be sufficiently understood or captured using the analytic process of rating, weighting, and summing. Stake (2004) discusses his pushback to the latter approach:

> Some evaluators try hard to be explicit. But I am wary of using a single or even just a few criteria, wanting to become experientially acquainted with the collection of aspects of the program . . . one cannot squeeze the summary of program quality into a single rating or descriptor, such as A- or Barely Acceptable or Smashing, but to ignore the complexity of the evaluand's activity and merit is to misrepresent the truth to shortchange audiences. (p. 6)

The approach Stake prefers involves firsthand experience of the program being evaluated, full consideration of a diversity of perspectives and evidence, and bringing these together into a holistic portrayal that leads to a narrative conclusion (Schwandt, 2015). *All-things-considered* approaches involve bringing together the relevant facts, values, criteria, and interests within specific evaluation circumstances and rendering an evaluative conclusion that generally considers all of those factors. *Deliberative approaches* are those that bring together public reasoning of multiple people or groups with contrasting perspectives or arguments and empirical evidence to render evaluative judgments. These may be combined with rubrics, as is described by Oakden (2013) and King et al. (2013), or with an all-things-considered approach. For the same reason that one cannot literally rate or rank the importance of different techniques for gathering data, these different approaches to making a synthesis judgment cannot be weighted in terms of importance. Much like research methods, each synthesis method has advantages and disadvantages. The choice of an approach depends on an evaluator simultaneously considering their own abilities and skills, client preferences, and what an evaluator believes interest holders in the situation at hand will find most acceptable and convincing. Box 5.5 illustrates four different approaches to valuing within an evaluation scenario to show the differences.

BOX 5.5. Illustration: One Case, Four Approaches to Valuing

Several foundations, school districts, and a local university fund a program for school principals to build leadership capacity within schools and across the leadership network to improve equitability of student learning and experiences. The program theory, in short, is this: "If the program develops leadership capabilities within and across schools, then leaders foster more equitable school and classroom environments, and if leaders make changes toward equity in their schools, then students will have more equitable opportunities and, ultimately, more equitable outcomes." Program staff want an evaluation to examine whether the program has successfully reduced inequities in student outcomes. Ideally, the program would like to use the evaluation findings in a proposal for significant funding to sustain and expand the program to two neighboring states. The program has a variety of existing data, including longitudinal surveys of participating leaders, school-level student demographics, and student state assessment data. Program staff send out a request for proposals that identifies the evaluation purpose of determining the successfulness of the program. Four submissions stand out, but staff cannot agree on which one to select because each determines successfulness differently:

- **Proposal 1** focuses on the questions of what success means from the perspectives of leaders and emphasizes collecting the stories of a sample of successful and nonsuccessful leaders and learning about the contextual challenges that help or hinder success. The team proposes a design centered around a success case method that uses a survey to all leaders followed by in-depth interviews with a purposive sample of leaders who reported highest and lowest on success metrics.
- **Proposal 2** focuses on the question of value for money acknowledging that since scarce resources were pooled together to support this program and further funding from a new source is desired, the key question is whether the investment was worthwhile. The researchers seek to use social return on investment that considers the financial and human capital inputs and examines the cost per leader participating over time in relation to leader self-reported changes in schools and student assessments on state tests. To identify the various relevant outcomes and define performance levels, the team pairs social return on investment with a participatory rubric-based process.
- **Proposal 3** reframes the question posed from whether the program was successful to how well the program worked to influence equitability of student experiences and outcomes via school leaders and a leadership network. Using a theory-based framework, they proposed to conduct a literature review and interviews with a variety of involved interest holders to construct the theory of the program's design and then empirically examine the extent to which this theory was implemented or adapted. They paired this theory-based component with an examination of changes in student outcomes over time arguing that without a comparison group, the theory verification would be necessary to support internal validity.
- **Proposal 4** reframes the question "successfulness compared with what?" Prior to the leadership program, there was no other leadership program in place but since the program's implementation, other leadership professional development and support opportunities have been initiated. The authors proposed setting up a study focused on the incoming cohort of leaders that would randomly assign leaders who met selection criteria to one of three conditions: this leadership program, an alternative program, and a wait-list condition. Each group would complete standardized leadership surveys before, during, and after their participation and these would be linked with student data.

CONSIDERATIONS FOR VALUING: A GUIDING CHECKLIST AND QUESTIONS

Thus far in this chapter, we discussed a variety of values and their influences on evaluation practice and discussed the logic of valuing (i.e., criteria, standards, evidence, synthesis) and some valuing methods that can inform each step. In this concluding section we discuss practical challenges and offer a checklist and a set of questions to provide guidance on creative and responsible valuing.

If there is a distinctive professional ethos for evaluators that distinguishes the practice and the public good it serves from other related professional endeavors in social research and program auditing, then it most likely centers on the responsibility for making systematic, transparent, and defensible evaluative judgments. Scriven (2016b) discusses the centrality of valuing to evaluation as well as its unavoidable challenges:

> In the applied branches of social research disciplines, it is evaluation that carries the burden

of dealing proactively, rather than reactively, with the human problems and values typically involved or presupposed, that is, dealing in a way that leads to evaluative answers to evaluative questions rather than just to reports on the answers of other people and to purely nonevaluative reports on the phenomena they are evaluating. These evaluative questions usually are requests for improvements or ranking or critique of options . . . but dealing seriously with these problems and the relevant values in order to answer the questions society needs answered requires not only identifying the relevant values, and not only just rejecting the illegitimate values, for example, valuing publicity at the expense of validity, but also justifying the choice of the legitimate ones, for example, the importance of long-term follow-ups in drug evaluation, and combining the values with each other, and with the nonevaluative data that social science is so well equipped to determine, in order to draw the correct evaluative conclusions. (pp. 30–31)

One of the key challenges to valuing is that there is no one "right" way (Alkin et al., 2012)—rather, evaluators must work out how to conceive of and carry out valuing given specific evaluation circumstances and audiences.

To provide some general guidance on valuing, we synthesize our discussion in this chapter into a brief checklist of decision points in Box 5.6. These include but are not limited to the following: primary audiences; mode of valuing; key valuing questions and judgments; key value and criteria; standards for performance; whether a synthesis judgment is necessary; whether and which methods to guide synthesis judgments, roles, and responsibilities; how to represent, communicate, and/or facilitate valuing; and alignment of the valuing process. We encourage evaluators to consider options at each of these decision points; invite deliberation on options among the evaluation team and interest holders; make selections transparent to others; and, within reason, make the valuing process explicit in evaluation communications (e.g., contracts, plans, reports).

While having a brief checklist might provide some structure and guidance to the valuing process, we encourage readers to pair this checklist with reflection and consideration on several questions to help them tailor the valuing process to the particular evaluation context.

> **BOX 5.6. Checklist for Valuing to Be Used during Evaluation Planning**
>
> - Identify the *primary audiences* for valuing process and judgments.
> - Consider *which values and sources of evidence* are to be considered or not considered within the scope of the evaluation.
> - Frame the *key valuing questions and judgments*.
> - Identify and *define the values and criteria* that will inform the valuing processes and judgments.
> - Set *standards for performance* in relation to these criteria.
> - Determine *whether a synthesis judgment* will be reached and by whom or whether results will be presented in relation to different criteria without a synthesis judgment.
> - Consider which *synthesis methods or practices* will be used to reach a synthesis judgment.
> - Identify *roles and responsibilities* for evaluators, interest holders, and the public in valuing.
> - Craft ways to *represent and communicate evaluative judgments* to various interest holders (e.g., narrative account, numerical index) or *facilitate valuing* among interest holder groups (e.g., data parties, structured deliberation).
> - *Align the valuing process* with the evaluation purposes, audiences, and intended uses.
> - Make the *valuing process explicit* by explaining the rationale and each aspect of the process (as listed here) in evaluation plans, reports, and other communications.

Which Valuing Processes Suit the Evaluation Context?

Choices about valuing are inevitably contextual. Moreover, evaluative claims about the value of an intervention are often contextually bound such that an intervention deemed valuable in one context may not be valuable at all or to the same extent in another context. When considering context, important considerations include the nature of the decisions confronting interest holders, the degree of contestability around the goals of a proposed initiative, audiences to whom evaluative arguments are directed, and the "needed complexity and precision of valuation" (Julnes, 2012a, p. 109; Julnes, 2012b; Patton, 2012) required. Evaluative judgments are matters of inference and there is always some uncertainty in deciding what to make of the evidence (Douglas, 2014). In circumstances where criteria are uncontested and precisely defined, where performance on criteria can be accurately measured, and where all variables affecting the reasoned judgment are subject to control, evaluative judgment might be amenable to algorithmic support tools, such as a decision tree that models decisions, and their possible outcomes, costs, and utility. However, in the world of realpolitik where evaluations are subject to multiple and often-contested interpretations of criteria, evidence, and performance, the making of evaluative judgments is a practical matter and the decisions that a judgment represents are not decisions best modeled in terms of decision theory but reasoned judgments that are more accurately framed in the language of prudential arguments.

How Do (Might) Sociopolitical Factors Influence the Valuing Process?

Just as evaluations are influenced by sociopolitical factors in the institutional societal contexts in which they are conducted, so are evaluative judgments. One way in which these matter for evaluators has to do with the aspiration for nonpartisan evaluations. Partisanship, conceived here as advocacy for specific perspectives, interests, or values, inevitably influences the valuing process. Datta (2000) distinguishes nonpartisan evaluation as that which is "regarded by partisans of all persuasions as balanced, fair, and faithful, so that if methodological quality is high, debates focus on the implications of the findings for practice or policy, not on the credibility of the findings themselves" (p. 1). In constructing a valuing process, consider whether the evaluation strives to be nonpartisan and/or partisan to particular perspectives and interests and how this might shape valuing choices.

Another way sociopolitical consideration can matter has to do with the ways in which valuing is (or ought to be) set up to address the public interest or common good. There is broad consensus on the notion that evaluation ought to serve the public good. The recently revised AEA Guiding Principles for Evaluators (2018) includes the principle "Evaluators strive to contribute to the common good and advancement of an equitable and just society." But how exactly that contribution is to be made is debated. Some evaluators are content with rendering evaluative judgments about the value of means to given ends—for example, the effectiveness of international aid in delivering food, shelter, water, medicine, and so on to those living in poverty, or the relative effectiveness of an antismoking campaign using Strategy A (warnings and pictures of disease on the package of cigarettes) versus Strategy B (public service announcements). Other evaluators (Schwandt, 2017, 2018a; Scriven, 2016a, 2016b) argue that evaluative judgments are also appropriate about the intended aims or ends of the intervention itself. This falls under the broad topic of the ethics of intervention, which focuses on examining the values and ethics that underlie policies and programs (e.g., early childhood programs, parent education programs, smoking cessation programs) that are deliberately designed to change behaviors, feelings, and attitudes of targeted individuals or groups (Sigel, 1983). This is a critical and underexplored issue in evaluation that has direct bearing on how evaluators understand their professional responsibility.

What Roles Do (Should) Evaluator(s), Interest Holders, and the Public Play in Valuing?

Evaluators should consider what role they play with regard to valuing and, relatedly, what roles various interest holders and members of the public have in the process. Alkin et al. (2012) distinguish between valuing rendered by interest holders alone, interest holders and evaluators, and evaluators only. Based on their review of the role of valuing within various evaluation theories and theorists' work, they discuss three primary roles evaluators might take. Evaluators might provide the empirical evidence for interest holders while leaving the valuing process and rendering of evaluative judgments to them; they might serve as facilitators, setting up processes to guide interest holders in reasoning their way to evaluative judgments; or the evaluator(s) could take the sole role of valuing and rendering evaluative judgments.

Additionally, evaluators ought to consider what, if any, role members of the public play in valuing as well as how the valuing process may attend to those potentially negatively affected by it. Incorporating public input could be carried when identifying criteria—for example, by using crowdsourcing (Harman & Azzam, 2018) or incorporating public interest values (Chelimsky, 2014). Gates (2018) draws on critical systems heuristics as a way to

> incorporate a witness role for groups, interests, and worldviews potentially affected by the situation of interest an evaluand (and evaluation) addresses to participate directly or be represented in the valuing process. Witnessing means identifying and calling attention to who or what may be negatively affected and fostering responsibility in an evaluation for mitigating further exclusion and marginalization. (p. 215)

Beyond who is involved and how, evaluators will want to consider potential imbalances in power and legitimacy (Mark & Shotland, 1985).

Davidson (2014) identifies five considerations when determining who should be involved: (1) validity (i.e., whose expertise is needed to get it right), (2) credibility (i.e., whose involvement will ensure that evaluative conclusions are believable to various groups), (3) utility (i.e., who will use the evaluative conclusions and, therefore, who should be involved in producing them), (4) voice (i.e., whose perspectives and experiences need to be considered, especially considering who or what have historically been excluded or marginalized), and (5) cost (i.e., are the time and resources of involving various people worthwhile; p. 8).

What Are the Potential Benefits and Risks of Valuing? How Might Evaluation Mitigate These?

When carrying out valuing, it is imperative that evaluators consider the potential benefits and risks as well as possible ways to support or mitigate these. As mentioned, there is no "right" way to carry out valuing and, ultimately, the process is a matter of evaluators' professional judgment. Furthermore, valuing can result in consequential decisions, such as continuing or not continuing to fund an intervention, privileging accountability for and demonstration of some outcomes over others, or highlighting the perspectives of some interest holder groups and interests (e.g., intended beneficiaries) while overlooking others (e.g., surrounding natural environment). These are real-life practical, political, and ethical consequences. As Schwandt (2018b) points out, drawing on Ulrich (2017), "evaluators and social researchers more generally cannot justify their claims about what should be done, about social improvements, about the ethical correctness of their proposals of value, and so forth on the basis of their theoretical and methodological expertise" (p. 133). Rather, careful consideration of choices and potential consequences and professional rationalization and justification of these choices are a basis for enacting the ethical responsibility of valuing. For example, an evaluation team working in partnership with a nongovernmental group in the Amazon explicitly considered ethical issues when establishing a monitoring, evaluation, and learning system for efforts to ecologically and culturally protect the Amazon. They argue that this ethical analysis provides the grounds for the legitimacy of their work (and not claims of technical expertise; Gates et al., 2023).

When valuing occurs in circumstances where there is considerable diversity in and potentially conflicting values among those involved and/or affected, evaluators might want to consider setting up valuing as a matter of *stakeholding development*. From the point of view of developmental evaluation and some forms of systems practice, situations marked by complexity, uncertainty, interdependencies, and multiple interest holders and their perspectives can be transformed through concerted action by interest holders who build their stakeholding (interests as well as specific issues, problems, concerns associated with roles) in the process of boundary setting (Ison, 2010, p. 10). Martin Reynolds (2010) refers to this as evaluation focused on "stakeholding development" versus simply accounting for various kinds of stakes (i.e., role-specific concerns of various interest holders; Schwandt, 2018b, p. 132). Such an approach is well aligned with evaluations that incorporate considerable interest holder participation and deliberation, as well as those that seek to facilitate collective learning and action. One inspiring example of stakeholding development comes from the work of Pinzon-Salcedo and Torres-Cuello (2018), who used a participatory multimethodology design incorporating problem-structuring methods (i.e., interactive planning, critical systems heuristics, soft systems methodology) to facilitate dialogue between those who had perpetrated and been victim to violence to inform a systemic peace education program in Colombia.

CONCLUDING THOUGHTS

We began by noting that people routinely make judgments about value but it is evaluators who uniquely claim professional expertise and responsibility for valuing. While this may be the case, the line between evaluators and ordinary people asking and answering questions about value is often blurry (Grob, 2012). Moreover, there are plenty of social researchers, economists, policy analysts, and others who conduct objective, disciplined inquiries about the value of various interventions using well-established research designs. The question of how evaluators and the evaluation field can contribute to these valuing processes—whether in terms of objectivity, transparency, critical partiality, and so on—and the actual material consequences of various approaches to valuing remains open.

On one hand, as we have discussed here, the evaluation field has made considerable progress in its recognition of values and their influences on the evaluation process; development of approaches to identify, select, and incorporate various interest holder and public values in evaluations; and, perhaps currently, growing agreement on the need for explicit evaluative reasoning and use of value bases (criteria, standards) to guide valuing (Davidson, 2014). On the other hand, there has been minimal empirical research on values and valuing (Coryn et al., 2017) and few examinations of evaluation-specific methodologies beyond practical guidance and case applications. Some scholars are concerned that those commissioning evaluations have more influence over the values considered relevant—the evaluative questions that should be asked and the preferred designs and methodologies for answering them (Julnes, 2012a, 2012b; Chelimsky, 2012).

In conclusion, this chapter provides an abbreviated synthesis of the state of the field at the moment with the aim of providing some guidance to those looking to creatively and responsibly address values and valuing in their practices. However, if the practice of evaluation is continually defined by the centrality of values and valuing, then further work is needed to offer practical guidance and to develop empirical and moral bases for how we as evaluators handle (and should handle) questions of value.

REFERENCES

Alkin, M. C., Vo, A. T., & Christie, C. A. (2012). The evaluator's role in valuing: Who and with whom? *New Directions for Evaluation, 2012*(133), 29–41.

Altschuld, J., & Kumar, D. (2010). *Needs assessment: An overview.* SAGE.

American Evaluation Association. (2018). *Guiding principles for evaluators.* Available at *www.eval.org/p/cm/ld/fid=51*

Boyce, A. (2017). Lessons learned using a values-engaged approach to attend to culture, diversity, and equity in a STEM program evaluation. *Evaluation and Program Planning, 64,* 33–43.

Chelimsky, E. (2012). Valuing, evaluation methods, and the politicization of the evaluation process. *New Directions for Evaluation, 2012*(133), 77–83.

Chelimsky, E. (2014). Public-interest values and program sustainability: Some implications for evaluation practice. *American Journal of Evaluation, 35*(4), 527–542.

Coryn, C. L. S., Wilson, L. N., Westine, C. D., Hobson, K. A., Ozeki, S., Fiekowsky, E. L., . . . Shroeter, D. C. (2017). A decade of research on evaluation: A systematic review of research on evaluation published between 2005 and 2014. *American Journal of Evaluation, 38*(3), 329–347.

Datta, L. (2000). Seriously seeking fairness: Strategies for crafting non-partisan evaluations in a partisan world. *American Journal of Evaluation, 21*(1), 1–14.

Datta, L. (2011). Politics and evaluation: More than methodology. *American Journal of Evaluation, 32,* 273–294.

Davidson, E. J. (2005). *Evaluation methodology basics: The nuts and bolts of sound evaluation.* SAGE.

Davidson, E. J. (2012). *Actionable evaluation basics: Getting the most succinct answers to the most important questions.* Real Evaluation.

Davidson, E. J. (2014). *Evaluative reasoning* [Methodological briefs: Impact evaluation No. 4]. UNICEF. Available at *www.unicef-irc.org/publications/749-evaluative-reasoning-methodological-briefs-impact-evaluation-no-4.html*

Davidson, E. J. (2015). Question-driven methods or method-driven questions? How we limit what we learn by limiting what we ask. *Journal of Multi-Disciplinary Evaluation, 11*(24), i–x.

Davidson, J., Wehipeihana, N., & McKegg, K. (2011, September). *The rubric revolution.* Paper presented at the meeting of the Australasian Evaluation Society, Sydney, Australia.

Davies, R. (2018). Dating and the need for establishing evaluation criteria. *New Directions for Evaluation, 2018*(157), 125–127.

Davies, R., & Dart, J. (2005). The most significant change technique (MSC): A guide to its use. Available at *https://europa.eu/capacity4dev/iesf/document/%E2%80%98most-significant-change%E2%80%99-technique-davies-dart-2005*

Dickinson, P., & Adams, J. (2017). Values in evaluation—the use of rubrics. *Evaluation and Program Planning, 65*, 113–116.

Douglas, H. (2014). Values in social science. In N. Cartwright & E. Montuschi (Eds.), *Philosophy of social science* (pp. 162–182). Oxford University Press.

Fournier, D. M. (1995). Establishing evaluative conclusions: A distinction between general and working logic. *New Directions for Evaluation, 1995*(68), 15–32.

Fournier, D. M. (2005). Evaluation. In S. Mathison (Ed.), *Encyclopedia of evaluation* (pp. 139–140). SAGE.

Gargani, J. (2017). The leap from ROI to SROI: Farther than expected? *Evaluation and Program Planning, 64*, 116–126.

Gates, E. F. (2018). Towards valuing with critical systems heuristics. *American Journal of Evaluation, 39*(2), 201–220.

Gates, E. F., & Dyson, L. (2017). Implications of the changing conversation about causality for evaluators. *American Journal of Evaluation, 38*(1), 29–46.

Gates, E. F., Page, G., Crespo, J. M., Oporto, M. N., & Bohórquez, J. (2023). Ethics of evaluation for socio-ecological transformation: Case-based critical systems analysis of motivation, power, expertise, and legitimacy. *Evaluation, 29*(1), 23–49.

Government Accountability Office. (1988, August). Children's programs: A comparative evaluation framework and five illustrations (Reprint). Available at *www.gao.gov/assets/80/77183.pdf*

Greene, J. C. (1997). Evaluation as advocacy. *Evaluation Practice, 18*(1), 25–35.

Greene, J. C. (2012). Values-engaged evaluations. In M. Segone (Ed.), *Evaluation for equitable development results* (pp. 192–206). United Nations Children's Fund.

Greene, J. C., Boyce, A., & Ahn, J. (2011). *A values-engaged, educative approach for evaluating education programs: A guidebook for practice.* Available at *https://rmcresearchcorporation.com/denverco/wp-content/uploads/sites/4/2016/05/31-Values-Engaged-Educative-Guidebook-.pdf*

Greene, J. C., DeStefano, L., Burgon, H., & Hall, J. (2006). An educative, values-engaged approach to evaluating STEM educational programs. *New Directions for Evaluation, 2006*(109), 53–71.

Grob, G. F. (2012). Evaluators in a world of valuators. *New Directions for Evaluation, 2012*(133), 91–96.

Hall, J. N., Ahn, J., & Greene, J. C. (2011). Values engagement in evaluation: Ideas, illustrations, and implications. *American Journal of Evaluation, 33*, 195–207.

Harman, E., & Azzam, T. (2018). Incorporating public values into evaluative criteria: Using crowdsourcing to identify criteria and standards. *Evaluation and Program Planning, 71*, 68–82.

Hassall, K. (2020). Exploring values in evaluation: A guide to reading. *Evaluation Journal of Australasia, 20*(2), 109–115.

Heider, C. (2017). *Rethinking evaluation.* Available at *http://ieg.worldbankgroup.org/sites/default/files/Data/RethinkingEvaluation.pdf*

Henry, G. T. (2002). Choosing criteria to judge program success: A values inquiry. *Evaluation, 8*, 182–204.

Hepi, M., Foote, J., Ahuriri-Driscoll, A., Rogers-Koroheke, M., Taimona, H., & Clark, A. (2021). Enhancing cross-cultural evaluation practice through Kaupapa Māori evaluation and boundary critique: Insights from Aotearoa New Zealand. *New Directions for Evaluation, 2021*, 51–65.

House, E. R., & Howe, K. R. (1999). *Values in evaluation and social research.* SAGE.

Housing First. (2016). *What is Housing First?* Available at *https://endhomelessness.org/resource/housing-first*

Hurteau, M., Houle, S., & Mongiat, S. (2009). How legitimate and justified are judgments in program evaluation? *Evaluation, 15*(3), 307–319.

Ison, R. (2010). *Systems practice: How to act in a climate change world.* Springer-Verlag.

Julnes, G. (2012a). Developing policies to support valuing in the public interest. *New Directions for Evaluation, 2012*(133), 109–129.

Julnes, G. (2012b). Managing valuation. *New Directions for Evaluation, 2012*(133), 3–15.

King, J. (2016). Value for investment: A practical evaluation theory. Available at *www.julianking.co.nz/wp-content/uploads/2014/09/160527-VFI-jk8-web.pdf*

King, J., & Allan, S. (2018). Applying evaluative thinking to value for money: The Pakistan subnational governance programme. *Evaluation Matters—He Take Tō Te Aromatawai, 4*, 207–233.

King, J., McKegg, K., Oakden, J., & Wehipeihana, N. (2013). Evaluative rubrics: A method for surfacing values and improving the credibility of evaluation. *Journal of Multidisciplinary Evaluation, 9*(21), 11–21.

King, J., & Oxford Policy Management. (2018). The OPM approach to assessing value for money:

A guide. Available at *www.opml.co.uk/files/Publications/opm-approach-assessing-value-for-money.pdf?noredirect=1*

Majone, G. (1989). *Evidence, argument, & persuasion in the policy process*. Yale University Press.

Mark, M. M., Henry, G. T., & Julnes, G. (2000). *Evaluation: An integrated framework for understanding, guiding, and improving public and nonprofit policies and programs*. Jossey-Bass.

Mark, M. M., & Shotland, R. L. (1985). Stakeholder-based evaluation and value judgments. *Evaluation Review, 9*(5), 605–626.

Martens, K. S. R. (2018). How program evaluators use and learn to use rubrics to make evaluative reasoning explicit. *Evaluation and Program Planning, 69*, 25–32.

Martz, W. (2013). Evaluating organizational performance: Rational, natural, and open system models. *American Journal of Evaluation, 34*(3), 385–401.

Mathison, S. (Ed.). (2005). Evaluation. In *Encyclopedia of evaluation* (p. 140). SAGE.

Mulgan, G. (2010). *Measuring social value*. Available at *http://data.theeuropeanlibrary.org/BibliographicResource/3000087785485*

Oakden, J. (2013). Evaluation rubrics: How to ensure transparent clear assessment that respects diverse lines of evidence. Available at *www.betterevaluation.org/sites/default/files/Evaluation%20rubrics.pdf*

Ofir, Z. (2017, November 18). Updating the DAC evaluation criteria: Part 1. Their enduring and endearing influence. Available at *http://zendaofir.com/updating-the-dac-evaluation-criteria-part-1*

Organisation for Economic Co-operation and Development. (2021). *Applying evaluation criteria thoughtfully*. Author.

Patton, M. Q. (2012). Contextual pragmatics of valuing. *New Directions for Evaluation, 2012*(133), 97–108.

Peersman, G. (2014). *Evaluative criteria* [Methodological briefs: Impact evaluation 3]. UNICEF Office of Research.

Pinzon-Salcedo, L. A., & Torres-Cuello, M. A. (2018). Community operational research: Developing a systemic peace education programme involving urban and rural communities in Colombia. *European Journal of Operational Research, 268*(3), 946–959.

Reid, A. M. (2020). Applying an educative approach to engage stakeholder values in evaluations of STEM research and education programmes. *Evaluation Journal of Australasia, 20*(2), 103–108.

Renger, R., & Bourdeau, B. (2004). Strategies for values inquiry: An exploratory case study. *American Journal of Evaluation, 25*(1), 39–49.

Reynolds, M. (2010, October). *Evaluation and stakeholding development*. Paper presented at the meeting of the European Evaluation Society, Prague, Czech Republic.

Reynolds, M. (2014). Equity-focused developmental evaluation using critical systems thinking. *Evaluation, 20*(1), 75–95.

Schwandt, T. A. (1997). The landscape of values in evaluation: Charted terrain and unexplored territory. *New Directions for Evaluation, 1997*(76), 25–39.

Schwandt, T. A. (2003). In search of the political morality of evaluation practice. *Studies in Educational Policy and Educational Philosophy, 2*, 1–6.

Schwandt, T. A. (2005). The centrality of practice to evaluation. *American Journal of Evaluation, 26*(1), 95–105.

Schwandt, T. A. (2015). *Evaluation foundations revisited: Cultivating a life of the mind for practice*. Stanford University Press.

Schwandt, T. A. (2017). Professionalization, ethics, and fidelity to an evaluation ethos. *American Journal of Evaluation, 38*(4), 546–553.

Schwandt, T. A. (2018a). Acting together in determining value: A professional ethical responsibility of evaluators. *Evaluation, 24*(3), 306–317.

Schwandt, T. A. (2018b). Evaluative thinking as a collaborative social practice: The case of boundary judgment making. *New Directions for Evaluation, 158*, 125–137.

Schwandt, T. A., & Gates, E. F. (2021). *Evaluating and valuing in social research*. Guilford Press.

Scriven, M. (1994). The final synthesis. *Evaluation Practice, 15*(3), 367–382.

Scriven, M. (2007). Key evaluation checklist. Available at *https://wmich.edu/sites/default/files/attachments/u350/2014/key%20evaluation%20checklist.pdf*

Scriven, M. (2012). The logic of valuing. *New Directions for Evaluation, 2012*(133), 17–28.

Scriven, M. (2016a). The last frontier of evaluation: Ethics. In S. I. Donaldson & R. Picciotto (Eds.), *Evaluation for an equitable society* (pp. 11–48). Information Age.

Scriven, M. (2016b). Roadblocks to recognition and revolution. *American Journal of Evaluation 37*(1), 27–44.

Shipman, S. (1989). General criteria for evaluating social programs. *Evaluation Practice, 10*(1), 20–26.

Shipman, S. (2012). The role of context in valuing federal programs. *New Directions for Evaluation, 2012*(133), 53–63.

Sigel, I. E. (1983). The ethics of intervention. In I. E. Sigel & L. M. Laosa (Eds.), *Changing families* (pp. 1–21). Springer.

Stake, R. E. (2004). *Standards-based and responsive evaluation*. SAGE.

Stake, R. E., Migotsky, C., Davis, R., Cisneros, E. J., Depaul, G., Dunbar, C. J., . . . Chaves, I. (1997). The evolving syntheses of program value. *Evaluation Practice, 18*(2), 89–103.

Stake, R. E., & Schwandt, T. A. (2006). On discerning quality in evaluation. In I. F. Shaw, J. C.

Greene, & M. M. Mark (Eds.), *Handbook of evaluation* (pp. 404–418). SAGE.

Stern, E., Stame, N., Mayne, J., Forss, K., Davies, R., & Befani, B. (2012). *Broadening the range of designs and methods for impact evaluations* (Report of a study commissioned by the Department for International Development, Working paper 38). Available at *www.dfid.gov.uk/Documents/publications1/design-method-impact-eval.pdf*

Stufflebeam, D. (2001). Evaluation models. *New Directions for Evaluation, 89*, 7–98.

Stufflebeam, D. L. (2001). Evaluation values and criteria checklist. Available at *https://wmich.edu/sites/default/files/attachments/u350/2014/values_criteria.pdf*

Takeuchi, L. (2014). *Incorporating people's values in development: Weighting alternatives* [Overseas Development Institute Project Note]. Available at *www.odi.org/publications/8501-development-participation-well-being*

Teasdale, R. M. (2021). Evaluative criteria: An integrated model of domains and sources. *American Journal of Evaluation, 42*(3), 354–376.

Teasdale, R. M., Pitts, R. T., Gates, E. F., & Shim, C. (2023). Teaching specification of evaluative criteria: A guide for evaluation education. *New Directions for Evaluation, 2023*(177), 31–37.

Ulrich, W. (1983). *Critical heuristics of social planning: A new approach to practical philosophy.* Swiss National Science Foundation.

Ulrich, W. (2017). *If systems thinking is the answer, what is the question? Discussions on research competence* (Expanded and updated version of Working Paper No. 22, Lincoln School of Management, University of Lincoln, Lincoln, UK, 1998). *Ulrich's Bimonthly*, May–June (Part 1) and July–August (Part 2).

Ulrich, W., & Reynolds, M. (2010). Critical systems heuristics. In M. Reynolds & S. Holwell (Eds.), *Systems approaches to managing change: A practical guide* (pp. 243–292). Springer.

United Nation's Evaluation Group. (2008). *Ethical guidelines*. Available at *www.unevaluation.org/document/detail/102*

Wehipeihana, N., Bailey, R., Davidson, E. J., & McKegg, K. (2014). Evaluator competencies: The Aotearoa New Zealand experience. *Canadian Journal of Program Evaluation, 28*(3), 49–69.

Wehipeihana, N., & McKegg, K. (2018). Values and culture in evaluative thinking: Insights from Aotearoa New Zealand. *New Directions for Evaluation, 158*, 93–107.

Williams, B., & van 't Hof, S. (2016). Wicked solutions: A systems approach to complex problems. Available at *www.researchgate.net/publication/263110523_Wicked_Solutions_A_Systems_Approach_to_Complex_Problems*

Wilson-Grau, R. (2018). *Outcome harvesting: Principles, steps, and evaluation applications.* Information Age.

Yarbrough, D. B., Shulha, L. M., Hopson, R. K., & Caruthers, F. A. (2011). *The program evaluation standards* (3rd ed.). SAGE.

Chapter 6

Equity in Evaluation

Donna Durant Atkinson

CHAPTER OVERVIEW

Equity is at the center of societal discourse today. As evaluators we have a responsibility to consider it as we design our program evaluations. To be clear, including equity in our evaluations should not solely be based on societal influences but on conducting evaluations that are fair and just. How this is accomplished may vary depending on the evaluation. This chapter begins by defining equity and what it means to include equity in evaluation, and encourages evaluators to engage in deep reflection before engaging in equitable work. The chapter then delves into laying the foundation for conducting an evaluation with an equity perspective, including sharing frameworks that can provide useful guidance, and walking through steps to consider when infusing equity in each stage of the evaluation.

The goal of this chapter is to discuss **equity** in program evaluation from the perspective of the evaluator and includes potential implications for the evaluand. The objectives of the chapter are to (1) describe what equity is in order to enhance evaluators' awareness of it, (2) discuss what it means to include equity in evaluation, (3) prompt evaluators to think about their personal perspectives on the topic, (4) identify factors that may influence the overall approach to the evaluation when including equity, (5) identify technical design topics that need to be addressed when including equity in evaluation, and (6) offer strategies to consider when planning an evaluation.

The concept of equity plays a significant role in the work conducted by evaluators, other social science researchers, and scientists. This is especially true today when equity is also front and center in our societal discourse and is at the root of many challenges we face as a society. These challenges exist often due to the lack of equity or not having an equitable perspective. Since it is often a central theme of these discussions, it remains a challenge that we are pressed to address. As evaluators, we should look to ensure that program evaluation, which attempts to determine the merit or worth of something (Scriven, 1991), is fair and just and considers merit and worth for all involved.

Equity is a broad concept and is not limited to program evaluation. It can be seen as a component of **comparative effectiveness research (CER)**. The heightened use of CER studies over the past few decades has led the medical field to look for and apply ways to better understand how to provide effective treatments for patients with specific characteristics. The desire to make informed decisions about treatments that are tailored for specific individual groupings are supported by the development of CER protocols to improve health outcomes (Armstrong, 2012; Sox & Goodman, 2012). This work could not have been done properly without attention to specific population characteristics and more specifically, attention to individual groupings of patients. This means that the central tenet of CER is a focus on the diversity of individuals who participate in CER studies, and that to achieve equitable outcomes for all individuals, this diversity is a significant goal. The concepts at the basis of CER, to focus on and meet the needs of specific groups of individuals to improve outcomes, can translate to program evaluation. Similarly, there would be a focus on the characteristics of individuals participating in the program in order to achieve an equitable approach to the evaluation and improve the probability of identifying improvements in program outcomes for all participants.

WHAT IS EQUITY?

Multiple Definitions of Equity

Let's start at the beginning, as you would in any conversation, and go over definitions; and answer the question: What is equity and how is it defined? As Table 6.1 shows, multiple definitions of equity exist, from a standard dictionary definition to definitions used by the federal government, the nation's large health foundations, and others. Though many of these definitions use different words, they all describe a similar concept: justice. Note that though most definitions of equity do not mention a specific discipline, when a discipline is mentioned, it is most often described in reference to health or education.

Equity and Equality

It is important to distinguish between equity and **equality** and note that they are not synonyms.

TABLE 6.1. Definitions of Equity

Source	Definition	Reference
Merriam-Webster Dictionary	"**Equity** is justice according to natural law or right, *specifically*: freedom from bias or favoritism."	Equity Definition & Meaning—Merriam-Webster, 2022
White House *Executive Order on Advancing Racial Equity and Support for Underserved Communities through the Federal Government*	**Sec. 2. Definitions.** For purposes of this order: (a) The term "equity" means the consistent and systematic fair, just, and impartial treatment of all individuals, including individuals who belong to underserved communities that have been denied such treatment, such as Black, Latino, and Indigenous and Native American persons, Asian Americans and Pacific Islanders and other persons of color; members of religious minorities; lesbian, gay, bisexual, transgender, and queer (LGBTQ+) persons; persons with disabilities; persons who live in rural areas; and persons otherwise adversely affected by persistent poverty or inequality.	Executive Order on Advancing Racial Equity and Support for Underserved Communities through the Federal Government—The White House, 2021
George Washington University Milken Institute School of Public Health	"Equity recognizes that each person has different circumstances and allocates the exact resources and opportunities needed to reach an equal outcome."	Equity vs. Equality: What's the Difference? | Online Public Health (*gwu.edu*), 2020
Annie E. Casey Foundation	"The state, quality or ideal of being just, impartial and fair." The concept of equity is synonymous with fairness and justice. It is helpful to think of equity as not simply a desired state of affairs or a lofty value; it needs to be thought of as a structural and systemic concept.	Equity vs. Equality and Other Racial Justice Definitions—The Annie E. Casey Foundation (*aecf.org*), 2021
Robert Wood Johnson Foundation (RWJF)	"Health equity means that everyone has a fair and just opportunity to be as healthy as possible."	RWJF, 2022, Health Equity: Everyone Counts, 2022
National Equity Project	"Educational equity means that each child receives what they need to develop to their full academic and social potential."	Educational Equity Definition—National Equity Project, 2022

The George Washington University Milken Institute School of Public Health (2020) makes a critical distinction between these two words and describes equity as "just" treatment, not equal treatment. More specifically, equity means that individuals in a group receive the resources they specifically need to achieve a set of outcomes; each person may receive *different resources* to achieve the same set of outcomes. And equality means that individuals in a group receive the *same resources* to achieve a set of outcomes.

In regard to equality, assuming that everyone will have commensurate benefit from the same resources may be incorrect thinking. Giving everyone the same resources may mean that someone is not getting what they need to achieve their outcomes. For example, giving everyone the same pair of eyeglasses (reference to equality) is insufficient if the prescription is not tailored to each individual's visual needs (equity would mean everyone gets the eyeglasses based on their own prescription). A reference in an article in *Teacher Magazine* states that we may indeed want *inequality* in order to achieve equity (Masters, 2018). In this way, resources are tailored to each individual to achieve the same outcomes as the group.

The distinction between understanding how a program was designed and conducting an equitable evaluation is essential to recognize when assessing a program, defining appropriate measures, and collecting and analyzing data to determine outcomes. If, for example, there is an evaluation of an educational program for students with disabilities and there is no accommodation made for any student, then the outcomes may be called into question. The educational outcomes may not reflect the true assessment of the students' abilities since they were not provided with the resources needed to perform at their best. As evaluators, we must think about designing evaluations that are equitable and where all participants have an "equitable opportunity" to be seen fairly and justly. Providing a level playing field for all participants to be seen, heard, and understood would be an equitable approach. As visualized in Figure 6.1, though everyone has a bicycle, which would be considered equality, not everyone can appropriately ride the bicycle they have (Robert Wood Johnson Foundation, 2017). It is in the second row where the bicycle is tailored to the riders' needs where everyone is in an equitable situation (they were seen, heard, and understood).

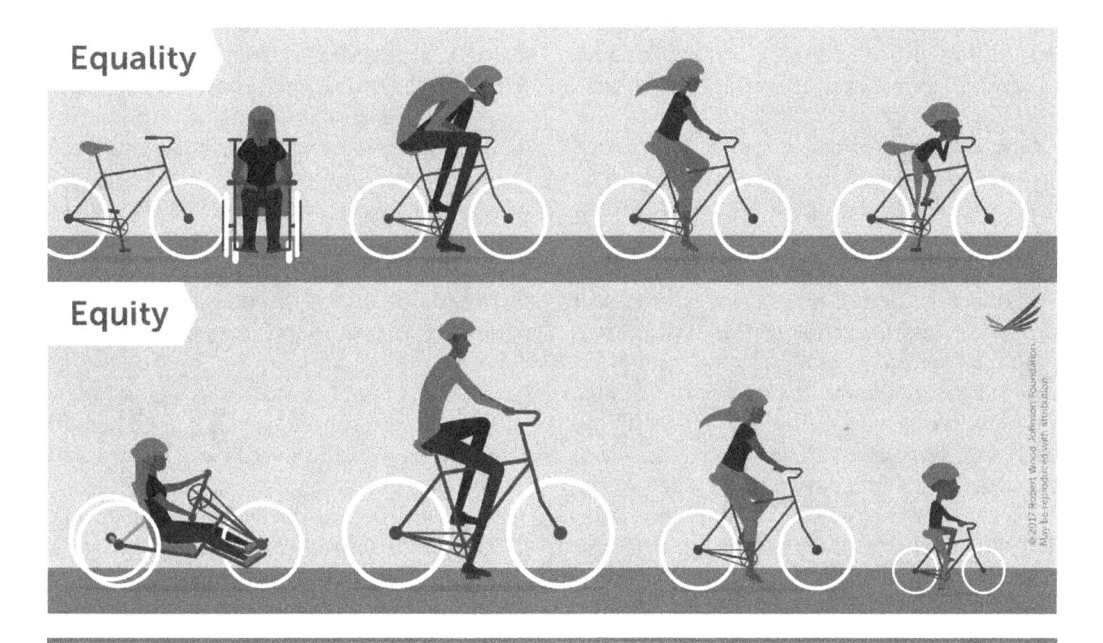

FIGURE 6.1. Equality versus equity. From Robert Wood Johnson Foundation (2017). Visualizing Health Equity: Diverse People, Challenges, and Solutions Infographic (*rwjf.org*)

IT'S TIME FOR DEEPER REFLECTION IN EVALUATION

Program evaluation was born and bred to address social policies and programs; some introductory evaluation texts even describe evaluation as the "scientific study of social problems" (Rossi et al., 2004, p. 2). It is indeed time for deeper reflection in the evaluation world we work in due in part to a keen focus on equity all around us. This focus is extremely relevant as current policies and programs are being called into question regarding their merit or worth for *all* targeted populations. Evaluation work has continued over the decades to address social problems and issues.

The breadth and depth of information readily available now to support us in incorporating equity into our work and to make evaluation responsive to social problems, is tremendous and almost overwhelming. The number of these reports, publications, statements, and other documents continue to grow. The content of this information is often reflective of the current social issues we face and can serve as resources in the work evaluators are doing to address social issues. Having this information available creates a responsibility for us to act on it and contemplate including it in our work. Reading about the evaluations our colleagues conduct can inform us of innovative strategies and techniques that are being applied in this work and in turn makes us more knowledgeable to improve our own evaluations. We can discover how to enhance the traditional designs that we learned about in Cook and Campbell (1979) with a focus on equity as well as look to create new designs with equity at their core. In addition, we can discover strategies on how best to collect and analyze data that will yield useful information to improve programming for the groups included in the evaluation. It is not only available from work produced by other evaluators (Hood et al., 2015; Frierson et al., 2002) but also from select federal government agencies, such as the U.S. Centers for Disease Control and Prevention (CDC; 2023), that are focused on equity (Rudiger, 2022).

Evaluators need to assess the information these resources present to determine their relevance and value for their evaluations. This information includes publications and reports on program evaluations, conceptual documents and statements on equity and equity frameworks, and methodological publications on equity in program evaluation and other types of social science research. The availability of this information is more possible and timelier now due to technological advances that make information dissemination easier and more widespread (Shonhe, 2017).

A few sources on equity are particularly influential for program and policy as well as evaluation. For example, the White House issued an executive order communicating the administration's position on equity (White House [2021] Executive Order on Advancing Racial Equity and Support for Underserved Communities through the Federal Government). White House policy statements on equity can be very influential as they shape how federal agencies address equity and can impact whether it is on an agency's agenda as a priority. In addition, when organizations such as the Robert Wood Johnson Foundation (RWJF) take a stand on equity and reshape their programming and funding to address equity, it is notable (RWJF, 2023b). The RWJF is well recognized as a leader in funding programs that address social issues. Their vision is "building a Culture of Health that provides everyone in America a fair and just opportunity for health and wellbeing" (RWJF, 2023a). Other foundations, such as the Kresge Foundation (2023), also place a major focus on equity in their core programming. The Kresge Foundation's "North Star is the expansion of opportunity in America's cities, to be achieved through our correlated values of creativity, equity, respect, partnership and stewardship."

In addition to the types of resources mentioned here that are available to better understand what equity is and who is supporting it, there are other types of resources available to evaluators. These resources include documents that describe how to share and present information analyzed from an equity perspective, and how to support an equity lens (Feng & Schwabish, 2021; Schwabish & Feng, 2021). It is possible to let the data speak for themselves through illustrative graphics (Ogden, 2010). More platforms and graphics are available to promote the utilization of findings than there were in 1983 when Graphics Press published Edward Tufte's

(1983) first book on data visualization: *The Visual Display of Quantitative Information*. Visualizations help to make the data clearer and visually represent the differences that are found between groups when equity is included in the data collection and analysis plan.

Evaluation Is Influenced by Society

While the plethora of information we study about conducting program evaluations relates to methodologies, we understand that it should not just be about conducting a technically solid evaluation but it should also be about the impact the evaluation and its results can have in our society. As program evaluators we have professional and self-defined responsibilities to make improvements and offer recommendations to better programs—their objectives, their outcomes, and possibly their missions.

The intersection between how we conduct program evaluation and society is where we continue to find ourselves. We are more aware now about the need to acknowledge this intersection and how important it is to consider in our work as evaluators. As a result, the intersection compels us to simultaneously consider *what we do* with *what is happening around us*. And, even more importantly, we should consider (1) what the findings, from an evaluation that considers how variables intersect, can yield, (2) what the implications can be for applying recommendations, and (3) the impact this can have on future directions. As Shadish and Luellen (2005) have stated, "evaluation has clearly been influenced over the years by the social and political climates of the day" (p. 186).

While program evaluation has been grounded in social policies and programs, there is a different intensity to it now. The increased awareness of equity is making a stronger impact on the evaluations we conduct. We can take what we are learning through current events, digest it, and use it in our work as appropriate. We can educate ourselves both technically and culturally and secure the requisite resources needed to perform culturally appropriate work to help improve individual and community outcomes. Being aware of what is needed to conduct a culturally appropriate evaluation should result in the better identification, measurement, and analysis of outcome variables that may not have previously been considered. Reflecting on equity in evaluation work and how it can be thought about when conducting an evaluation *is a philosophy and starts very early in the process.*

Let's Go Back in Time Just a Little to Understand Why and How We Should Move Forward

Over the course of the past few decades, our work as program evaluators has been influenced by our culture and principles used in evaluation practice that were pertinent at the time (*Encyclopedia of Evaluation*, 2011). These perspectives were often not influenced by a multicultural perspective. Ideas and practices were based on recognizing the majority population as the standard. While the research often included participants from other nonmajority groups, they were not always seen as dominant or playing an impactful role in the evaluation nor singled out to examine. Many aspects of evaluation from design through analysis and reporting were viewed from the perspective of someone from the dominant culture as the norm given that many evaluators were from that culture. Some would say that even with the recognition of the need to reference different cultures it was not done (Frierson et al., 2002). That is why there is a growing awareness and also a wealth of information now acknowledging the need for culturally appropriate evaluation; the ideological position has shifted toward diversity in evaluation. The American Evaluation Association (2018) has addressed this in its Guiding Principles for evaluators. The guidance is to include cultural perspectives and address equity in our evaluations.

To be clear on the messaging for this chapter, our position is not solely based on societal influence but what we think is fair and just. From that perspective, equity should be included in all evaluations. While race/ethnicity is the more common variable that people think about when reflecting on diversity, equity, and inclusion due to a history of racial discrimination in this country, this goes beyond race. Evaluations conducted decades ago may have been based on societal influences but those evaluations may not have been fair and just. The message now is to conduct evaluations that are fair and just. The way you do that is to infuse equity in the evaluation.

There Is an Updated Approach to Conducting Program Evaluations with Revised Terminology

A revised approach to program evaluation is evident and is having an impact on our work right now (Kellogg, 2021; Dean-Coffey, 2018; CDC, 2014). This approach includes inclusivity, justice, and equity for all populations. It takes into consideration both the majority population and population subgroups as both being relevant to evaluation work. Current expectations are to conduct technically solid evaluations while being inclusive of the populations involved and ensuring that their perspectives are included in a just way. Some previous approaches resulted in evaluations that did not always fully consider the perspectives of all participants/evaluands and evaluators. In this new day, that approach would be questioned. For example, conducting an equitable evaluation involving the merits or benefits of nutrition programs and diet in predominantly Jewish communities means also considering the role and importance of traditional Jewish diets. Not considering the role and importance of a Jewish diet would be culturally questionable but it would be possible if you did not have an equity perspective.

A second example focuses on conducting an evaluation in a predominantly Black school district to explore the impact of innovative teaching techniques. These techniques were normed on non-Black students and did not include the perspectives of Black educators on how students in their district learn in comparison to other districts with predominantly non-Black students. In this case the evaluation may miss key factors important to the learning process for Black students. The evaluation may not include the variables that influence outcomes for these students. Because of these reasons, as well as the general cultural affront to not including those involved and affected by the interventions in the evaluation, evaluators are becoming increasingly aware of the importance of grounding evaluation with the perspectives of those who are impacted as well as others with a stake in the outcomes. This grounding increases sensitivities that can affect the implementation of the evaluation. For example, understanding that target populations may come from different cultures and have different worldviews of interpersonal dynamics increases the likelihood that the evaluation of behavioral health interventions based on family dynamics will need to take the participants' cultures into consideration. Evaluating the interventions without recognizing culture would not only be inappropriate but misleading. Infusing evaluation with cultural sensitivity is not only appropriate but may lead to more valid findings (Inouye et al., 2005). Applying these perspectives in the evaluation design ultimately helps make the findings more appropriate and useful for program improvements (Dean-Coffey, 2018).

LAYING THE FOUNDATION TO ESTABLISH AN OVERARCHING EQUITY FRAMEWORK IN EVALUATION WORK

What Does It Mean to Conduct an Evaluation with an Equity Perspective?

By now you realize what it means to consider conducting an evaluation with an equity perspective: It means to think about the nuances and experiences that each individual or group of individuals bring to an evaluation and as appropriate, integrate those factors into the design and give them the same level of consideration as other factors in the evaluation. Individuals who can bring beneficial perspectives to an evaluation include program participants, program management staff, **persons with lived experiences** relevant to the program being evaluated, interested parties concerned for their communities and participant outcomes, and evaluators. If you include and incorporate these multiple perspectives, you increase the probability of conducting a more thorough, sensitive, and relevant evaluation. Having the input of these individuals upfront as you prepare for the evaluation by engaging in such tasks as creating a suitable design and determining the right questions to ask, contributes to making the work more meaningful for the participants and the program. The evaluation results will likely produce a more accurate reflection of the program's impact on all participants due to a better understanding of how the program does or does not work for them, generating a more sensitive measurement process, and conducting a thoughtful analysis of program outcomes.

Consider what it would mean to a group of participants if their culture, customs, and/or standards were not reflected in any aspect of the evaluation because they were not seen as unique, not considered significant enough to be studied, or were just overlooked—with "neutral" intentions on the part of the evaluator. Reflect on the following scenarios.

Think about conducting an evaluation of educational programs in a culturally diverse school district where students speak dozens of languages. This requires the evaluator to do a little preliminary work to assess the number of students whose first language is not English and may result in the need for the evaluator to modify data collection strategies. As a first step, the evaluator may want to collect data on what the students' first languages are and what other languages they speak. Once these results are obtained, the evaluator may find that there is a need to translate data collection tools into multiple languages. Not considering language as a potential impact of student learning when English is not a student's first language may limit not only the understanding of the program's impact on all students but what needs to be done to improve educational outcomes for students who are bilingual. While being bilingual may not impact the educational attainment of some students, it may be impactful for others, and therefore should be considered as a part of the evaluation. How bilingual students are influenced by teaching and learning styles needs to be understood when exploring how programs are designed and when assessing program outcomes. When evaluators explore the educational outcomes from these programs, they can use what they find to make recommendations on improving the programs' designs. These recommendations may lead to equitable outcomes for all students. It is about offering a level playing field for all students to achieve in order to provide equity in educational outcomes. It is about first acknowledging that an equitable approach is needed, and then applying research strategies that ensure this equitable approach is implemented.

In another example, think about conducting an evaluation of programs offered at a community-based health clinic in a diverse neighborhood where diversity includes gender and sexual orientation. In this case, the evaluator needs to consider how the health clinic meets the needs of everyone they serve, an obvious statement. But if the evaluation is conducted without considering sexual orientation as a part of the design, then that oversight is significant for a comprehensive evaluation of clinic programs and recommendations for program improvement. It could be as simple as including the appropriate items and terminology on the data collection instruments, such as including current and appropriate gender and sexual orientation response options for participants to select so that they know that the clinic acknowledges who they are. It can also include an analysis plan where the results can speak to whether the clinic is meeting the needs of everyone they serve, including the lesbian, gay, bisexual, transgender, queer or questioning, plus (LGBTQ+) communities.

How Does Using an Equity Lens Impact My Work?

At a minimum, including an equity lens in your evaluation increases the probability that it will be more thoughtful and comprehensive. This approach also may yield more useful recommendations to improve the program and increase the chances for better outcomes for program participants. Acknowledging differences in program participants based on their cultural identities can produce more meaningful results for the target populations than conducting the evaluation without recognizing these critical variables (Stern et al., 2019).

There are a few questions that you might be asking right now:

- *What does including equity mean exactly for the evaluations that I conduct?* It means that your evaluations will dig deeper into the characteristics of the target populations, research the environments in which the program operates and where the evaluation is conducted, and bring those factors out in the evaluation.
- *Can I do it?* Yes. You may be able to do it without additional support but if support is needed, you should identify consultants or persons who can support your team and fill in any gaps in content knowledge and expertise that you need.
- *If I need experts in equity to advise me, how*

do I identify and engage them? If you do decide to engage experts, be sure to bring the right ones on board so they can provide the type of input you need. The right ones will have the content expertise you need, will work well with other members of your team, and may have experience with the target populations and/or program that will be evaluated. You may want to identify consultants or persons with lived experiences to bring on board so that they can lend that perspective to the discussion.

- *Will it take longer to complete the evaluation?* Possibly, but the "generalizability" of your results may take on new meaning and may be more far-reaching.
- *Will it cost more when I include an equity approach?* There are components that might require additional costs. For example, if you bring on consultants (e.g., persons with lived experiences who are relevant to the evaluation or advisory panel members with the types of experiences your team is lacking), you need to compensate them for their time. Another potentially expensive component of an evaluation is the number of participants included, especially when you plan to disaggregate the data for each of the identified subgroups. More participants often means higher costs. This is where innovation is required to keep costs down. Specific ideas are offered in upcoming sections.

What's Needed to Include Equity in Program Evaluation?

What's needed is very straightforward but can be challenging. While it is not rocket science, there is a science to it. Decisions need to be systematic and thoughtful to maximize your results. It is more the psychology of understanding what's needed than the behavioral component of making it happen. First, you need to maintain an open mind to include a variety of perspectives beyond those you may traditionally have. And for those evaluators who have previously included equity in your evaluations, you still need to keep an open mind. Be open to learn something from each evaluation; make sure to acknowledge and capture that. You may need to think about conducting your evaluation in a slightly different way than you have done before, or you may just need to make enhancements to approaches previously used. For example, for those seasoned evaluators who have conducted numerous evaluations on a specific topic, they too need to assess the status of equity for each new evaluation. While an evaluator may have conducted many evaluations on homelessness, for example, they will still need to assess how to include equity in each new evaluation, assess how the interested parties will receive it, and determine the feasibility of including persons with lived experiences to help shape the evaluation design. Each new evaluation will have its own unique characteristics and be conducted in its own context and therefore, should be considered from a fresh perspective.

An open mind allows you to design an evaluation that has a more comprehensive set of evaluation questions and be more inclusive of all target groups than it would be without it. Without an equity lens, evaluation results will be constrained by the limitations of the evaluation, and the outcomes and findings may be less applicable to the groups the results are intended to help. And when designing your evaluation, being receptive to new ideas allows you to ask more questions about what you are evaluating. It may also allow you to better understand how what you are evaluating was designed and what impact those design features have on the program and the ensuing evaluation.

What Frameworks Provide Useful Guidance When Conducting Equity-Focused Program Evaluation?

While more programs today are designed with equity in mind and built on equity frameworks, many others are not. As described below, this distinction plays a role in the evaluation design you select. There are a number of equity frameworks that have been developed and that can explicitly guide a program evaluation. Evaluators should be aware of two types of frameworks: a program equity framework and an evaluation equity framework. The ones I offer here are just a few examples to get started with.

Evaluating programs designed to produce equitable outcomes takes on a different lens than evaluating those that were not. When a program is designed with equity in mind, the evaluation is to determine whether the programs were indeed successful in their design and in achieving equitable outcomes for participants. When a program is not designed with equity in mind, the task is to first ensure that the evaluation is equitable and allows for exploring equity in the evaluation itself and then given that lens, determine whether the program achieved equitable outcomes.

A **program equity framework** is used for program development and not necessarily for evaluation, though it can inform an evaluation. When designing an evaluation for a program that was built using an equity framework you can look at it as having a head start. The U.S. Department of Health and Human Services Centers for Medicare and Medicaid Services (CMS), for example, uses an equity framework that supports *building* programs focused on equity (CMS, 2023). Program components designed with this framework have already considered equity. Take for example, just one component: data collection. The first priority for the CMS framework for **health equity** is on data. There is a high probability that the program has already collected the data elements needed for an equity-focused analysis and that they will be available for the evaluation. For example, if a program is designed to serve diverse religious groups of people including those who are Christian, there is a good chance that the questions about religion break down the religious groups to include multiple subgroups, such as Baptist and Methodist. There may be no need to develop plans to ensure that religion is captured for all participants. The program's identification of subpopulations in this example guarantees that the data can be disaggregated to the appropriate levels for analysis. In another example, exploring how cultural groups may interact with an intervention may be possible if the needed data are already included in the program's data collection plan identifying various cultural groups. The evaluation will be able to note if there are any differences between Asian population subgroups since the data needed to conduct such an analysis will be available. The evaluator can explore and discuss findings about the effectiveness of the program for individual participant subgroups, such as Chinese, Japanese, and Korean, when participants are able to identify their specific identity as opposed to checking a box that only designates "Asian" as the category.

Program equity frameworks are based on understanding the need for equity in programming, where programmatic changes are needed, and the potential for addressing and linking equity with policy needs. These frameworks are useful for thinking about how programs are designed, and how equity is infused into organizational processes and strategies. General program equity frameworks are versatile and may have components that are relevant for an evaluation; they may also be applied in different settings. For example, when evaluating programs that were designed on equity principles, the evaluation questions may more easily focus on aspects of equity that were built into the program. For example, an evaluator might ask if an intervention is more effective when it is tailored to the target populations' cultural groups than when it is not. In another example, it is appropriate to take culture into account when evaluating programs that serve multicultural youth in metropolitan areas. For those youth who are from immigrant families, an important factor is whether youth are from first- or second-generation immigrant families. Programs built around equity have probably taken immigration status into account, understanding that first- and second-generation families likely differ in how they integrate into the predominant culture. Immigration status would be easily acknowledged in the evaluation design since it was most likely a component of the program. Differences between first- and second-generation status can be included in the evaluation questions and used to better understand the effectiveness of the interventions for these groups.

While program equity-focused frameworks may differ in what they emphasize, some are more general than others, some are based specifically on the goals and work an organization does, and some are more discipline specific, but they all have the same goal. This goal is to keep equity at the forefront of the work being done and integrate it into the program development process to ultimately produce outcomes and results that will be useful to the targeted communities.

Box 6.1 highlights three program equity frameworks that focus on program development but are useful for thinking about designing an equity-focused evaluation. The frameworks share the same raison d'être but each has unique

BOX 6.1. Examples of Program Equity Frameworks and Their Usefulness for Evaluation

The CMS Framework for Health Equity

CMS's framework for infusing equity into its programming is organized into five priority areas. This is an example of a framework that is discipline specific—in this case, health. A description is provided along with how the priority relates to conducting an equitable evaluation.

1. **Expand the collection, reporting, and analysis of standardized data**—The CMS states that it is committed to reporting and improving health conditions through the use of high-quality data. Data addressing demographic characteristics including race, ethnicity, sexual orientation, and social determinants of health variables are important to better serve the health care needs of individuals. (*Synergy to an equitable evaluation: Evaluation collects and analyzes high-quality data that can be disaggregated appropriately to identify and explain potentially meaningful results. There is a higher probability that the data will be detailed enough to allow for disaggregated analyses of the target populations when a program is set up to examine participants' demographic characteristics.*)

2. **Assess causes of disparities within CMS programs, and address inequities in policies and operations to close gaps**—The CMS is committed to engaging in actions to address health disparities. (*Synergy to an equitable evaluation: Evaluation is action oriented and designed to be able to identify appropriate recommendations to address disparities. With objectives to identify and close gaps of inequity, data need to be available to address those issues.*)

3. **Build capacity of health care organizations and the workforce to reduce health and health care disparities**—The CMS is committed to building the capacity of organizations to support the delivery of needed services to improve health status. (*Synergy to an equitable evaluation: Evaluation is action oriented with appropriate recommendations to support capacity building to address disparities. With objectives to improve health status and reduce disparities data need to be available to address disparities.*)

4. **Advance language access, health literacy, and the provision of culturally tailored services**—The CMS supports making services available to all individuals in need and that they are language appropriate, and individuals are able to understand communications and they are culturally appropriate. (*Synergy to an equitable evaluation: Evaluation assesses availability of services for all individuals and makes recommendations for improvements as required to improve access. With a focus on language and the delivery of culturally relevant services, the program will be set up to accommodate participants' languages and other culturally specific characteristics that can then be included in the analyses.*)

5. **Increase all forms of accessibility to health care services and coverage**—The CMS strongly encourages equal access to health care services for all individuals. (*Synergy to an equitable evaluation: Evaluation addresses access as a major variable and is already focused on tailoring services to all individuals.*)

The United Way Framework

The United Way's framework guides its programming. The framework includes six components viewed by the United Way as actionable items to support its work and function as "levers" in what it does. These components are:

1. **Data**—Equity can be supported by the active use of collecting, analyzing, and sharing data in order to better understand needs. (*Synergy to an equitable evaluation: Evaluation collects and analyzes high-quality data that can be disaggregated appropriately to explain meaningful results.*)

2. **Community mobilization and engagement**—Prioritize equity through mobilization and engagement. (*Synergy to an equitable evaluation: Evaluation explores supporting community engagement and includes interested parties in most all aspects of the evaluation.*)

3. **Communications and awareness building**—Delivering effective communications to inform others of equity issues. (*Synergy to an equitable evaluation: Evaluation explores factors in knowledge transfer and effective communication strategies tailored to target populations.*)

4. **Policy and advocacy**—Promoting equity through policy and advocacy. (*Synergy to an equitable evaluation: Evaluation provides information to support the exploration of the need for targeted policies and advocacy work; this information will support the elimination of disparities.*)

5. **Fundraising, resource allocation, and grant making**—Promoting equity through fundraising and increasing budgets. (*Synergy to an equitable evaluation: Evaluation explores diversity in funding sources that may expand and or shape expectations and in turn expand the need for an equitable approach.*)

6. **Local capacity building**—Promoting a shared vision for equity at the United Way and sharing that with partners to continue the vision. (*Synergy to an equitable evaluation: Evaluation promotes the inclu-*

> sion or enhancement of a shared vision for equity and includes interested parties in the evaluation design.)
>
> **The National Equity Project Framework (Leading for Equity Framework)**
>
> This framework has three components: See, Engage, and Act. The framework is based on the idea that "Equity leadership moves from the "inside out," as different from traditional leadership, which tends to move top-down. The premise is that how we *See* informs how we *Engage*, which informs how we *Act*. While this appears straightforward, it has some complexities. What is it that we actually "see," who do we "engage," and then what do we do ("act")? Those are the basics of much of the thinking about an equitable perspective; the catch is the application. (*Synergy to an equitable evaluation: This framework encourages evaluators to gather information from colleagues and other sources to conduct a useful evaluation and to make sure that they, as evaluators, understand their own biases.*)

characteristics. For example, some details are more closely aligned in one framework over another, one framework provides more of a roadmap for program development while another offers factors to think about, but each has special components that can guide evaluation. In conducting evaluations, we can use one framework or borrow components from more than one framework to make our equity lens clear for our work.

An **evaluation equity framework** provides guidance for conducting evaluations focused on or incorporating equity. The evaluation frameworks focus on understanding and applying the concept of equity first before there is focus on the technical aspects of the evaluation. This type of framework promotes a certain mind-set that is required to comprehend first and then apply the framework.

Evaluators have built these frameworks working in multiple disciplines and with diverse populations representing a variety of demographic characteristics. Applying a consistent, standard approach to your work and offering a standard set of concepts and variables to consider as you conduct your program evaluation can benefit current and future work (Office of Management and Budget, 2018). Frameworks support systematic inquiry that is critical in the work we do as evaluators. Some of these frameworks are based on theory while others represent a consistent way of thinking and are based on concepts just shy of formalized theory (Partelow, 2023).

The first step in applying an equity framework to evaluation is to understand where and how equity fits into the program being evaluated. Was the program designed with equity in mind? If not, the evaluator needs to take special considerations in determining how the program can be evaluated with an equity perspective. An increased understanding can happen through asking the right questions, collecting the right data, and analyzing the data as required, if there are sufficient data. For example, being asked to evaluate a behavioral health **evidence-based intervention** designed with special attention to the racial and cultural differences between participants is different from being asked to evaluate an intervention that was not designed to account for any participant racial or cultural differences but at the same time was implemented in a racially diverse community. In either case, equitable results for all participants are possible but may require more effort when evaluating the "nontailored" intervention if differences are thought to exist between the racial and cultural groups. The additional effort may come from the need to spend more time researching and understanding the intervention to determine how to infuse equity in the evaluation. The evaluation will require more on how to explore and analyze the data and disseminate the findings when acknowledging all participants. Post hoc exploration of data with equity in mind is not too late.

Whether equity is built into the program or is considered after-the-fact at the evaluation stage, the evaluator can integrate it into the evaluation design and consider a few things. For example, you will want to understand how management works equity into their processes at the organizational level and ultimately its programming. Did they ensure that their programs are tailored for specific population subgroups that the organization serves and not offering a one-size-fits-all approach for their target populations? While we hope to get to a place where organizations routinely integrate equity into their planning and processes, we want to also ensure it is included in the program evaluation. You may want to include collaborators in meaningful positions to give them a voice in designing the evaluation. Collaborators such as persons with lived experiences can play a meaningful role in the evaluation design. Their input can be valuable and help to provide that equity lens that is so critical. Some collaborators may be able to provide perspectives from the participants' viewpoints on how a program works and the best approaches for designing effective data collection methodologies for a particular population. While evaluators can define methodological approaches, individuals with a closer knowledge of the population and a strong focus on equity may be able to improve upon evaluators' methods.

Box 6.2 highlights three frameworks that focus strategies for engaging an equity perspective within the evaluation process. They provide for structured thinking about programs and how and where equity may have been integrated into the program's design.

BOX 6.2. Examples of Evaluation Equity Frameworks

The CDC Framework

The CDC's framework (Practical Strategies for Culturally Competent Evaluation) identifies practical strategies evaluators should apply when conducting culturally competent evaluation. Specifically, their guide presents six steps for conducting culturally competent evaluations. These steps help the evaluator and others conducting the evaluation to ground themselves in understanding what the program is and how cultural issues play a role in its implementation.

1. **Engage interest holders**—While it may seem easy to engage collaborators and partners, the CDC cautions evaluators that it may not be. It is often important for the evaluator to engage in self-reflection before recruiting the right partners. First, evaluators need to be open to bringing on collaborators who will add value to the evaluation whether they have the same philosophical positions as the evaluators or not. If indeed they do have different positions, this diversity can lead to a better evaluation. Diverse discussions often lead to better products (Chamorro-Premuzic, 2017; Phillips, 2017; Miller, 2023). These discussions can also lead one to strengthening their positions and thoughts on equity or open doors to new ways of thinking about equity. In any event, diverse interactions require self-reflection. Similarly, it is important for the evaluator to understand how the partner views themself and what they may bring to the evaluation as well as what others may bring to the evaluation. In these types of discussions where there may be differences of perspectives, the evaluator should lay the ground rules of participation for partners and create safe spaces for discussions where everyone involved feels comfortable to express their opinions. There may be occasions where people express long-held opinions that may not be consistent with an equity approach or biases toward another group. Everyone should discuss and address the ideas for the betterment of the evaluation.

2. **Describe the program**—Evaluators need to create an accurate description of the program, including using both current and historical information. Information gathered from program participants can ensure that the program descriptions resonate with them as characterizing the true nature of the program.

3. **Focus the evaluation design**—The evaluation design should also be reflective of how partners see that program. Partners, people with interests in the program topic, target populations, and/or communities being served have a unique view of the program that is different from the evaluator's view. The multiple views should be reflected in the design. The evaluation questions and design should be consistent with the program intent and utility of the potential results.

4. **Gather credible evidence**—The components of the data collection activities should all be reflective of gathering information to address program participants and partners. Data collection instruments should be appropriate for the participating target groups and have the ability to analyze and report data as needed to address partners' needs.

5. **Justify conclusions**—Data interpretation and reporting should also be consistent with partners' needs and should maximize the potential for using the results to improve equitable program outcomes.

6. **Ensure the use of evaluation findings and share lessons learned**—Results and recommendations should also be directed to participant and partner needs, and be disseminated in culturally appropriate ways.

The CDC encourages evaluators to use this guide in conjunction with the Framework for Program Evaluation in Public Health. This is an integrative approach to marrying traditional evaluation strategies with strategies that are equity focused. While these six steps are helpful in thinking through the process of how to conduct the evaluation to ensure equity is incorporated, evaluators must be careful in how they are implemented. It all starts with the evaluators' self-reflections and self-awareness.

The Equitable Evaluation Framework

The Equitable Evaluation Initiative has created a framework to consider when conducting evaluations. It is based on three principles: (1) the work that is done should be for a purpose and be "in service" of equity—all that is done should support equity, (2) evaluation work should be "designed and implemented" with acceptable values—those that support equity, and (3) these types of evaluations should "answer critical questions" of today—the historical and structural issues that have led us to where we are today as a nation focusing on equity.

While this framework lays out principles to follow, it does not provide a 'how to' for conducting an evaluation. The essence of the principles is to set a framework for how to think about designs and conduct the evaluation to achieve an equitable approach and equitable outcomes. Key questions include Will the work be useful from an equity perspective?, Does it address values that are relevant to the program and target population?, and Is the evaluation responsive to current issues and needs we have as a nation?

The Center for Culturally Responsive Evaluation and Assessment (CREA) Framework

CRE and assessment is another philosophical approach to conducting program evaluation. It is not just a model or framework but a way of thinking about how to conduct an evaluation. At its core, CRE looks to include culture in all aspects of evaluation and indicates that there is no "culture-free" evaluation. Culture should be embedded in each evaluation. Each and every aspect of evaluation is subject to CRE analysis and interpretation from the evaluation preparation to the dissemination of results.

The CRE framework includes nine steps that should be followed when implementing CRE (Hood et al., 2015; Frierson et al., 2002):

1. **Prepare for the evaluation**—When beginning an evaluation, evaluators need to do a fair amount of research to learn about the culture of who and what is being evaluated. They also need to learn the language of the community and how they view diversity.

2. **Engage interest holders**—Evaluators need to identify the interest holders. Interest holders are the ones who can inform the evaluators, provide useful information and context for the evaluation, and support data analysis and interpretation.

3. **Identify evaluation purpose(s)**—It is clear that evaluators need to understand the purpose of the evaluation, understand the dynamics under which it is being done, and be clear on how it may benefit the community and if social justice will prevail.

4. **Frame the right questions**—It is important to ask the right questions. And there should be input from the interest holders as well as the evaluators. The questions should not be generated and reviewed by the evaluators alone. Once the questions are generated, a serious discussion must be held to determine the data needed to answer the questions sufficiently.

5. **Design the evaluation**—The evaluation design must complement the objectives of the evaluation. There is nothing special noted in CRE about the evaluation design. It calls for an appropriate design to answer the questions using either experimental or quasi-experimental designs, and collecting both qualitative and quantitative data, as appropriate.

6. **Select and adapt instrumentation**—It is important, though not required, to use instruments that have validity and reliability. It is also useful to use instruments that have been tested on the population of focus for the evaluation. While many instruments have not been tested on a variety of populations, the instruments may need to be adapted to be considered culturally sensitive for the target population.

7. **Collect the data**—Data collection methods should be considered especially when qualitative data are collected. When collecting qualitative data, consideration should be given to the characteristics of the data collector, to account for any possible interaction between the respondent and the collector.

8. **Analyze the data**—It is key for the evaluators to think through how the data were collected when analyzing them. And it is important for the evaluator to involve, in the sense of making the data, those who are familiar with the culture and context to more accurately analyze the data. Engaging others, besides the evaluators, in the analysis process ensures that all perspectives, especially cultural perspectives, are included in the interpretations.

9. **Disseminate and use the results**—Using these CRE steps increases the chance that the evaluation will be used and the results will be disseminated. Having the evaluator engage in these steps makes sure that culture is infused in the evaluation from all perspectives. Finally, the evaluator also needs to consider how the information will be disseminated and how it can be used early on in the process to increase the probability that dissemination and utilization will happen.

What to Consider When Conducting Equity-Focused Program Evaluations

As with any evaluation, challenges may arise before, during, and after you select a framework and also while conducting the evaluation. For example, you may find limitations in the framework you select for the evaluation. The framework may not be flexible enough to include components that you think are important to your evaluation or it may not work if key elements of the framework are not possible. With a framework centered around understanding how an intervention works for specific population subgroups and making sure that the data are appropriate to conduct analyses for those subgroups, it is key to have the right data elements for the analysis. These data may not be available for the evaluation. Conducting the evaluation without the appropriate data will limit what can be said about the results. Another example of a "not-so-good" fit is when the framework calls for including interested parties in the evaluation design and you are not able to include them for reasons beyond your control. For example, if you are unable to identify or reach out to the appropriate interested parties or those you ask decline your invitation to join an advisory group, then you may need to proceed without them. In this situation your evaluation will not be meeting the recommended criteria of the framework, which is to include interested parties in the evaluation as advisors. In these cases, you may need to proceed without them and if needed, indicate in a final evaluation report why you were unable to include interested parties as a part of the evaluation team.

What Is the Evaluator's Responsibility?

A critical first step in any evaluation is for evaluators to assess their understanding of the evaluation and its objectives—that is, what you think about what's being evaluated, who the participants are, and the nature of the program. While we, as evaluators, have had discussions about value-free evaluation, ideas brought up in these discussions about values are really important here. Evaluators who come to an equity-focused evaluation with biases, either acknowledged or not, will not be able to conduct an unbiased equity-focused evaluation. The following is a short list of factors to consider as you approach the evaluation to support the appropriate inclusion of equity as a valid component of the work.

First, Know Yourself and Acknowledge Your Level of Self-Awareness

What are your beliefs, values, and what is your objectivity? How do you, the evaluator, address your potential biases and limitations? Can you be objective in your approach? Will you be sufficiently confident to do this work in a field where no one has conducted an equity-focused evaluation? How do you need to prepare to appropriately integrate an equity perspective in the evaluation? Having an equity focus in your evaluation may challenge you and require you to expand your thinking personally, professionally, and technically. There are a few basic steps required to address these questions: Be honest with yourself and acknowledge what you believe; engage others in conversation to share your thoughts, refine what you think, and maybe learn something from someone else who has been engaged in similar thinking; and do a little research to boost your level of self-awareness.

Are you being personally aware: Are you, the evaluator, being thoughtful and sensitive to the individuals involved and issues of interest? Who are you and what experiences have you had, as a person and as an evaluator, that will help shape the tone of the evaluation? As the evaluator, can you be sensitive in your approach to the populations with whom you will work? You also need to assess how well you can work with those individuals who may serve on the evaluation team. What is your personal reaction to statements supporting cultural stereotypes? What is your personal reaction, your honest reaction, to the following stereotypical statements: Asians are strong in math and science; Black students' performance is substandard to White students; and girls' performance is substandard to boys in math? We know that sensitivity is key and important to the evaluation. Evaluators should not support racial and cultural stereotypes of the populations they are working with—either knowingly or unknowingly, intentions rule. This is where it can be helpful to have carefully composed advisory groups or people with lived experiences involved in the process to help you become aware of the issues associated with your line of thinking and help you avoid any inappropriate statements or behaviors.

Acknowledge What You Know about the Populations of Interest

Are you knowledgeable about the target populations of interest to the evaluation? Is this book knowledge or based on real-world experience? Is it from the context you are working in or another context (this can include time as well as geographic context)? It is key to understand the nuances that exist when studying racial and cultural issues and characteristics and how they can be contextually based as well.

When research questions address demographic characteristics, such as race/ethnicity and Hispanic origin or sexual orientation or gender identity, they are sometimes discussed by evaluators without understanding much about the groups or who they are. People often group diverse ethnic groups together without understanding the difference that culture plays in these groups and how they may differ from one another. For an equitable evaluation, the heterogeneity that may exist within each of the ethnic groups must be acknowledged. It is important that the results address subpopulations for the results to be accepted and utilized by those included in the evaluation. For example, blanket statements are often made about Black people without acknowledgment of the many different groups and cultures that exist. Many subgroups are encompassed within those who identify as Black or African American due to family origins either within or outside of the United States. And if the family origins are outside of the United States, where the family is from, such as Africa, the Caribbean, or South America, also carries important distinctions about culture and ethnicity. These differences need to be acknowledged and not glossed over as if they do not exist, not only because it is more culturally appropriate but also because the distinctions can offer greater validity to the constructs we use and how we understand what works for whom. I address this later in the chapter when discussing issues associated with having sufficient sample sizes of subgroup populations for certain types of analyses.

Understand the Budget You Have to Work With

Thinking about the funds that are available to conduct the evaluation is a high priority. The level of funding determines what you are able to do in spite of what you may want to do. The budget shapes all aspects of the methodology and, if funds are limited, the evaluation design needs to be creative in order to accomplish what you would like to do but do not have sufficient funding to carry out. These evaluation components need to be addressed and potentially downsized or tailored to fit the budget constraints:

- *Evaluation questions*—Revisit the questions posed for the evaluation to determine whether they are all needed; prioritize them based on the evaluation objectives. Reduce where you can so that the evaluation will be tighter and more streamlined.

- *Data collection*—As evaluators, we always want data and more data. When funds are limited you may need to reduce plans for primary data collection and research secondary data sources that may be available to answer your evaluation questions. If primary data collection is a must, consider less expensive strategies to avoid—for example, on-site in-person data collection. In our current environment where many types of interactions, including research activities, are virtual, make the most of less expensive data collection through the use of the internet and computer technology.

- *Sample and sample size*—While a common desire is to have a large number of respondents, we know that evaluations can sometimes be conducted with fewer respondents. Of course, when required, power analyses should be conducted to determine the appropriate sample size needed to determine program effects. In the end, the goal is to have a sufficient sample to be able to confidently make statements about, for example, program effectiveness. The evaluator needs to determine the importance of how far they will be able to disaggregate the data to address findings of subpopulation groups.

- *Duration of the evaluation*—A longer time period may translate into higher costs. Consider reducing the timeframe of the evaluation to help reduce costs.

- *Advisory groups including persons with lived experiences involved*—While advisors are critical, especially in an equity-focused evaluation, you may need to limit the number you include on your team. Set your objectives and only bring on the experts that are required to do the job.

- *Reports and dissemination activities*—Evaluators can take many approaches to getting the findings and results out to those who need them. As evaluators we can get fancy with how documents are styled and how data are presented. You may need to cut back on the fanciest approach to fit your budget but still produce appealing materials.

The approach is to make sure that you can conduct the evaluation even in the midst of financial restraints. You need to figure out a way to make sure that your resources are sufficient to meet the design requirements. The last resort is to not conduct the evaluation if you believe it cannot adequately address equity. It may be better to cut back your budget than to cut back on including equity in the evaluation.

If You Are Clueless, Seek Proper Guidance

If you feel clueless or that your level of expertise is limited with specific populations or in a specific area, then you may need to seek guidance to conduct your work with more legitimacy and authenticity. This may be done by bringing on equity experts and/or individuals from the populations or areas that you are studying to inform your work as well as expanding your team with others with equity-focused evaluation experience. In addition, this may be done by doing some research to find evaluation reports others have done to get some ideas and by researching the literature on how equity may impact the content of your evaluation. For example, if you are evaluating health programs, there is a wealth of literature on health disparities to help guide your thinking.

What about the Client's Perspective and Others Who Will Participate in the Evaluation in a Significant Role?

Know Your Client

Understand the client's needs for an evaluation. When embarking on this potentially new approach to conducting your evaluation work, it is important to know your client. While an equity lens should be incorporated early and often throughout the development and implementation of all our work, you should know your client's acknowledgment of and priorities on equity (e.g., race, culture, sexual orientation and gender identity, economic class) and articulate approaches accordingly. You should also know whether your client is receptive to the concept of equity and including it in the evaluation. While equity is based on justice and fairness, it may not be acceptable as a theme in the evaluation for your client. Understand their position early on in the process. Acknowledging and understanding their perspectives helps you to determine how to approach the evaluation. This may be an opportunity to request that your client think about equity if they have not done so before and offer this as a "learning moment" for them. As evaluators, this is a part of our responsibility, as outlined in the American Evaluation Association's Guiding Principle E: Common Good and Equity—evaluators strive to contribute to the common good and advancement of an equitable and just society, as a reminder (American Evaluation Association, 2018).

If you encounter some level of resistance to your ideas about including an equity focus in the evaluation, you may want to do a little research on your client's organization to determine how equity has and is currently perceived and addressed. You may also locate evaluations or other work produced by the organization or that the client has participated in that did have this focus to substantiate your approach. If your research does not yield any useful information, then you may consider revisiting with the client why this work is important, how it can benefit program participants, and the impact the organization can have on the field if it is seen as a trailblazer for equity. You may also discuss the importance of the evaluation to others beyond your client—for example, conducting work with an equity focus may be seen in a positive light to funding agencies, including the federal government. Engaging in this work may put you in a stronger position for getting additional work with funding agencies that are also dedicated to equity.

Know the Beneficiaries

Understand who the beneficiaries are and how they can benefit from the evaluation so that their needs can be met through the evaluation results and recommendations. Again, this is a reference to knowing and understanding the populations involved in the evaluation. It is your responsibility as the evaluator to either learn more about the participants and how the evaluation may impact them or involve others who do know something about the participants in some type of an advisory role.

Know Your Partners

Understand who the partners (e.g., board of directors, funders, and community organizations) are and their interests in conducting the evaluation. They may serve as allies in conducting the evaluation and support the inclusion of an equitable approach. You may have different types of partners when conducting an evaluation, those you have selected and others who come with the evaluation as members of the community and other interested parties. In either case, it is important to understand who they are and what their philosophies and interests are in conducting the evaluation. Your partners may turn out to be a diverse group. If this is the case, be prepared for discussions that may be risky when talking about equity but in the end will hopefully be fruitful for an equitable process. Risky conversations include statements that may offend someone in the discussion and potentially turn them off from participating. When it is time to make decisions, overriding others can be challenging and can potentially create tension in the group. If you do have a diverse group of partners and there is a fair amount of disagreement in how to include equity in the evaluation design, then you need to decide whether you move forward based on a consensus of the approach or if you as the evaluator needs to make that decision.

Consider the Benefits of an Advisory Committee and Expert Panel

As noted, you may consider including persons with lived experiences and people who represent the target populations in your evaluation. If you do include them, consider how you will compensate them for their time or provide incentives to them to participate in the work and provide advice. These individuals may serve as advisors or experts who have experience either working with or representing these populations. They may also have experience conducting evaluations that include an equity focus. If any of these individuals are not familiar with the evaluation process, you may need to spend some time supporting their participation. This support may come in many different forms from raising their awareness of the technical aspects of conducting an evaluation and what is acceptable protocol to providing technology to facilitate participation as an advisor. These groups can serve as sounding boards and provide guidance in many aspects of the evaluation design. They may also help to expand the network of experts who may be needed to provide advice on specific aspects of the evaluation. For example, when determining how to recruit participants for the evaluation, persons with lived experiences may provide useful advice on where and how best to recruit participants. In regard to data collection, advisory committee members may be able to review draft data collection instruments even before they are piloted to make recommendations on how to refine the items for accuracy and sensitivity, the length of the instrument, and the flow of the items. When instruments are translated into other languages, advisory committee members may be able to comment on the quality of the translations. They may also be able to provide guidance on the use of incentives and what might be an appropriate incentive for participants.

Engage the Right Representatives to Sit at the Table for Your Evaluation

You will want to engage the appropriate representation in the evaluation. It is important to ensure that you have appropriate representation when identifying your target populations, constructing your partner groups, and identifying members of your evaluation team. While it may be easy to identify people to serve on committees and panels, are they the right people? While deciding to include an advisory committee or panel of experts is important, it is critical to ensure that you select the most appropriate people to serve in these roles. A team of people who are not in agreement with ensuring the conduct of an equitable evaluation may not serve the evaluation well in the short term but having discussions with a diverse group may offer up important topics to consider that can allow people to either confirm their own positions or make a change. In either case it is indeed important to get these perspectives out and this can only be accomplished with the right set of people around the table. As the evaluator, it is important to offer diversity in thinking and experiences to the evaluation team. You may use the "snowball" approach to identifying the right representatives for your evaluation. Once you recruit one person to serve on the committee, you may ask them for recommendations for others who you can reach out to. You may also reach out to colleagues for recommendations. Reaching out to people you know may yield better success at getting the right people to serve. But remember to be open during this process so that you get a diverse set of perspectives at the table.

If you consider people with lived experiences to sit at the table, be prepared to hear and understand their perspectives—they may be different from yours. The purpose of inviting persons with lived experiences to the table is to have them offer ideas and perspectives that only they can bring. Identifying individuals who also bring a knowledge of research and evaluation is a plus. They will bring multiple perspectives to the discussions.

The idea that diversity breeds innovation is talked about in the business world and there can be synergies to it within the field of evaluation (Chamorro-Premuzic, 2017; Miller, 2023). Following this logic, a diverse team of people is more likely to design an evaluation that is less traditional than a group of seasoned, yet more uniformly thinking, members of an evaluation team.

Consider Community-Based Participatory Research

Evaluations that include an equity focus often include a **community-based participatory research (CBPR)** approach. CBPR is based on an equitable approach according to the Kellogg Foundation (2001):

> a collaborative approach to research that equitably involves all partners in the research process and recognizes the unique strengths that each brings. CBPR begins with a research topic of importance to the community with the aim of combining knowledge and action for social change to improve community health and eliminate health disparities. (p. 2)

This is one of the most commonly used definitions and comes from the Foundation's Community Health Scholars Program (Kellogg, 2001).

The CBPR approach incorporates input from members of the community who are under study, serve as partners, are prominent members of the community who have a vested interest in the evaluation results, and gives them a significant role in shaping the evaluation (Wallerstein et al., 2018). Again, because this approach may lead to including *persons with lived experiences* and those closely aligned with evaluation participants and beneficiaries, be prepared to hear and understand their perspectives—they may not be the same as yours.

A popular component now of CBPR is engaging youth. There is **youth participatory action research** that is being used to ensure that the ideas and perspectives of youth are included in the evaluation design discussions. It focuses on authentic and useful engagement of youth and helps to broaden understanding of "expertise" to encompass multiple ways of learning (Teixeira et al., 2021). As an example, you could involve youth who transitioned from the foster care system to participate in an evaluation of child welfare policies and practices in a local county. Who better than youth who have been involved in the child welfare system to participate in work to improve system policies, programs, and practices? Since youth are less familiar with research and evaluation, they are supported through their participation to provide as much useful information as possible to improve their ability to contribute to the evaluation.

Will a New and Different Approach Impact the Quality and "Acceptance" of My Work or Jeopardize My Work in Any Way?

Quality and acceptance should only be negatively affected if you conduct an evaluation that is not technically sound. One of the first things to realize is that including equity in your evaluation means that you can continue to conduct technically sound evaluations of high quality and in fact, may heighten the quality with a deeper understanding of the population and program context. You will continue to design your evaluation based on your research questions and use methods that are consistent with the design. What may be different is the types of questions you ask, what outcomes you select and how they are measured, how data are collected and analyzed, and who is on your evaluation team to make these types of decisions.

Will This Approach to Evaluation Be More Expensive?

This is a good question. Unfortunately, the answer is not straightforward: The answer is maybe. Conducting an evaluation with an equity focus may not be more costly. It all depends on your design, who the participants are, if you collect additional data (more than you would have without an equity focus), if the analysis plan is more extensive, and who you involve on your evaluation team. If you have interested partners or people with lived experiences who either require compensation or you would like to compensate, then yes, you may incur additional expenses. Involving additional partners and perspectives also may take more process and planning time. The evaluation may take additional time for your evaluation team to do more preparation work to be ready to think through methodological issues, such as crafting the research questions and all aspects of data collection and forming study groups if required.

If you find that your budget for the program evaluation is limited, there are a few things for you to consider. First, determine what is important for the evaluation, prioritize those items, and determine what must be done to conduct the evaluation with an equity perspective. Using your list of "essential evaluation elements," you can reach out to the funder to negotiate for additional funding, explaining the need and justification for implementing an equity approach in the evaluation. You may also consider redistributing funds within the existing budget by shifting how the funds are allocated. For example, if site visits are included in the budget, be purposeful in how the sites are selected. You may visit sites that require using less travel funds, such as those that are local to the evaluation team site visitors. The savings from the site visits could be redistributed to paying for the time of individuals with lived expertise, for example.

What Are Some Potential Technical Issues or Challenges to Consider in Incorporating Equity in Your Evaluation Design?

A number of issues require the evaluator's attention in the design of the evaluation. The authenticity of the approach is essential for a quality and useful product.

Formulating the Evaluation Design

For effectiveness evaluations, experimental or quasi-experimental designs are considered the gold standard of research and are still in the mix for many evaluators. Will you be able to generate comparison groups that make sense based on the preferred approach of building equity into the design? Indeed, you may be able to. Especially with the right group of advisors and persons with lived experiences, you may be able to generate comparison groups that fit your design.

A mixed methods approach to conducting the evaluation should certainly be considered (see Azzam & Jones, Chapter 18, this volume). While quantitative data can provide required information to determine whether some outcomes have been met, the role of qualitative data should not be overlooked. Collecting qualitative data can complement the quantitative data that are collected to explore the answer to evaluation questions. This mixed methods strategy of triangulation is useful for a better understanding of the data collected (Creswell & Plano, 2007). Depending on your objectives and questions, qualitative data could be considered "co-equal" with quantitative data. It can certainly provide context, which is critical to better understand the target populations, their culture, environment, and experiences in the programs. Whether the qualitative data comes from open-ended items in a survey, interviews, or focus groups, these data often provide insights into the evaluation questions otherwise not captured with numbers. Due to the nuances and perspectives that qualitative data provide, a data strategy is to combine the two approaches. This can be tremendous for providing a better understanding of results and crafting solid recommendations.

Formulating the Evaluation Questions

Consideration should be given to who the target populations are and what their role is in the evaluation. The evaluation questions should be relevant for the groups being evaluated so that when the data are analyzed they can provide the types of answers needed to understand outcomes and potentially improve programs (Barroga & Matanguihan, 2022). When evaluating an evidenced-based program designed to improve chronic health conditions in a diverse community, the evaluator will want to understand how the program impacts each of the cultural and ethnic groups that participated. The program may have worked for one group but not another due to cultural differences. This is important to know and could be included as an evaluation question to determine whether there were differences in outcomes based on cultural group.

Data Collection Methodologies

Attention should be paid to the data collection methodologies employed. These methods should be based on pertinent characteristics of the potential respondents. The types of either primary and/or secondary data collection should be appropriate for the target populations. Consideration should be given to how they are able to participate, and the methods should be in alignment with what they find acceptable. For example, conducting a self-administered survey that will take an hour to complete with participants who may be under time constraints due to inflexible work schedules when completing the survey may not be appropriate and yield low response rates. Asking youth who live in rural areas where cell phone coverage is sometimes not dependable to participate in a telephone survey may also yield low response rates.

Knowing the respondents' capabilities to respond to data collection requests is central to higher response rates. For example, these situations may warrant alternate data collection strategies or accommodations to collect the data when respondents do not speak or their English is limited, or do not have a mailing address or access to a computer. Often these accommodations are straightforward to implement. In another example, if one method of data collection is focus groups on the topic of how gender roles and identities influence the decision-making process and family dynamics and the respondents are youth and their families, you may not get a true picture of what the youth think when the data strategy is to collect data from the family simultaneously. Consideration should be given to conducting separate groups for the youth and family members to understand what participants really think without being influenced by other family members. This is a straightforward change though it may require additional funds to make this accommodation.

In another example, when conducting an evaluation with a transient population that is often homeless, it is inappropriate to use a mail survey to collect data or conduct in-person home interviews; and if they are asked to complete an online survey, the data collector should make a laptop computer available to the respondents. While these examples are obvious situations, others may not be; the key is to be in tune with the target population and understand how they can best provide the data you need to conduct the evaluation. Data collection methods, the types of questions posed, the way they are asked, and the available response options all need to be carefully thought through.

Another component of the data collection methods is for the data collection tools to have the appropriate items and response options required to address the questions. When asking questions of women who live in a male-dominated society about roles, responsibilities, and decision making, questions should be crafted to permit respondents to select an appropriate response option that is consistent with their culture. Surveys and other data collection tools that have been normed in the United States may not work the best when administered to respondents who may live in the United States but are from and practice other cultures. While national health surveys may ask about medical decision-making behaviors, the norms for these behaviors in another culture may be quite different (Moyer, 2023). The decision-making authority is different among cultural groups. While for some in the United States, women make their own decisions; in other cultures they generally do not but defer these decisions to more senior members of their family. Therefore, when conducting an evaluation that explores health care and medical compliance, it may be insufficient to include only the patients but also expand to others who participate in the decision making.

Adequate Sample Sizes

When conducting evaluations where the target populations may be small to begin with and then grow smaller as data are disaggregated for analysis to answer the evaluation questions, you may have a challenge that needs to be addressed. Know in advance that this may be an issue and begin early on to make the most of your design, maximize your sampling plan, and define some analytic strategies to address sample size. For example, you may need to collect your sample over a longer period of time to get a sufficient number or you may need to expand the geographical area of your recruitment. Each of these strategies may yield larger numbers to support stratification and disaggregating the data to what is "appropriate" for the evaluation. (See Harbatkin et al., Chapter 16, this volume, for more information on planning quantitative evaluations.)

Analytic Strategies

When your samples sizes are questionable, then your analytic strategies are limited, and some may be called into question. You may not have sufficient data to conduct the types of analyses needed to answer the evaluation questions. In addition, the analytic strategies play a role in outcomes and how they are perceived. It is essential to think about this upfront. In these cases, you may need to adjust your analysis plans and apply analyses that work with the limitations you have. You may need to apply a mixed methods approach, which may give you data for some of your questions even if less precise or generalizable to support your questions and identify the need for further exploration.

Reporting and Dissemination

Often, evaluation reports are submitted to the client and evaluators do not know what happens with the information. On the other hand, sometimes they are reviewed and analyzed, and recommendations are implemented. The idea is to deliver a report with findings and recommendations that will be used. Patton (2008) describes this as **utilization-focused evaluation**. Part of this approach is to be inclusive in the entire evaluation process to ensure that those interested parties will get results that they can use. Similarly, by applying an equity approach to the evaluation, the findings likely will be more useful than without it, will be seen as more authentic, and consequently may have a greater probability of being used. Targeting the right audiences and venues for distribution of the evaluation report is key for getting the information to those who need and will most likely implement the findings. Having a dissemination plan for sharing the evaluation report with the intended audiences should be thought about carefully. (See O'Neil, Chapter 25, for more information on communication strategies that are relevant to evaluators.)

PLANNING THE EVALUATION

How Do You Prepare for Implementing the Evaluation with an Equity Focus?

Select the Most Appropriate Framework for the Evaluation

We know that there is no one model that fits every evaluation. When selecting the framework for the evaluation, it is especially important to the evaluation goals to conduct a type of "goodness-of-fit" test. You want to make sure that the model you select works well for your evaluation goals, is consistent with how you define equity, and is consistent with your approach to evaluation. And, that the model has the potential to frame the results in an effective manner, one that is consistent with the direction you are looking to achieve.

Consider these factors and include them in your decision-making process:

1. *Evaluation goals: technical and conceptual*—Are the goals consistent with the framework you selected? If engaging in an evaluation to assess the effectiveness of a teaching curriculum for multiple target populations, yet the model is unidimensional and does not consider multiple populations, it may not be the model for your evaluation.
2. *Design characteristics*—You must determine whether you can meet the characteristics of the framework requirements. Are you able to include the target populations, are you permitted to ask the right questions, and can you get enough data to answer your questions to fulfill the requirements?
3. *Cost*—If the framework requires more data and more detailed data than you are able to afford, then it might not be the one for your evaluation this time around. You may be limited to data that have already been collected.

Plan to Include Equity in Your Evaluation

By now, it is clear that an equity perspective in your evaluation likely may make it more comprehensive and useful. Inclusion of the equity perspective may improve the probability that the results and recommendations will be accepted and applied. As you start planning the evaluation, consider these steps:

- *Step 1: Start thinking early about how equity can be a fundamental component in your evaluation.* Evaluators should think about equity in the very beginning of the evaluation so that it can be woven throughout the process. This thinking should occur as soon as you know that there will be an evaluation. Whether you are an internal or external evaluator, start the thought process early so that you can be comprehensive in how you will think about and design the evaluation, prime your team to be on board with your thinking, and identify any required resources you may need to help your team in the process. This is a step that is often not thought of until much later in the process, if at all.

- *Step 2: Include equity in your initial meeting agenda and subsequent agendas when discussing all aspects of the evaluation design.* Potentially, the most significant change needed for evaluators who have yet to integrate an equity, inclusive and/or a justice perspective in their evaluations, is to think about equity. It is a simple step but one that is often not achieved even though the intention is there. And when you are not accustomed to including these thoughts in your conversations as you begin your work, it is easy to overlook. Remember this should not be an afterthought. One way to make this change, if needed, is to always consider including equity in each meeting agenda. It may be appropriate to include or may not be a desire of the client but if it is included in early conversations about the evaluation, then at least it is considered and not overlooked.

- *Step 3: Identify your working definition of equity, inclusivity, and justice!* In order to think about equity, you need to understand what it is. Make sure you have a definition to guide you and your thinking. Make sure you have a definition to guide your team members' thinking too.

- *Step 4: Broaden the conversation, get input, and do your homework.* Search the literature, presentations, guidance documents, grey literature, and other publications to assist in shaping your thoughts and the evaluation design. Publications on the topic may be available as resources as you formulate your evaluation design. Also, a number of evaluations have been conducted with an equity focus. Take a look at them and see how they were designed, implemented, and reported. There may be colleagues that you can reach out to or organizations you can contact who can serve as advisors and offer experiences that can help you shape the evaluation.

- *Step 5: Conduct a gap analysis to determine where you need additional support.* After you do your research and identify information that can support your work, take a look at what experiences you have, who you have on your team, and where the gaps are. From this analysis you may further refine your team by including others with not only the technical skills needed but familiarity with the target populations included in the evaluation. These team members could include evaluators with the types of experiences you are looking for, persons with lived experiences who can prove useful to the evaluation design discussions, and a partner organization that brings the skill sets and knowledge you need of the program and the community.

Remember that there is no "one-size-fits-all" approach to including equity in your evaluation. Each client is different, each program is different, target populations are different, and consequently, each evaluation is different. The key to achieving equity in your evaluations is to think about it early and often, seek the support you may need, and conduct a technically solid evaluation that can determine the merits of a program *for all participants*.

REFERENCES

American Evaluation Association. (2018). Preface to evaluators' ethical guiding principles. Available at *www.eval.org/Portals/0/AEA_289398-18_GuidingPrinciples_Brochure_2.pdf*

Annie E. Casey Foundation. (2023). *Equity and inclusion*. Author.

Armstrong, K. (2012). Methods in comparative effectiveness research. *Journal of Clinical Oncology, 30*(34), 4208–4214.

Barroga, E., & Matanguihan, G. J. (2022). A practical guide to writing quantitative and qualitative research questions and hypotheses in scholarly articles. *Journal of Korean Medical Science, 37*(16), e121.

Centers for Medicare and Medicaid Services. (2023). *CMS framework for health equity*. Available at *www.cms.gov/priorities/health-equity/minority-health/equity-programs/framework*

Chamorro-Premuzic, T. (2017, July 28). Does diversity actually increase creativity? *Harvard Business Review*. Available at *https://hbr.org/2017/06/does-diversity-actually-increase-creativity*

Cook, T. D., & Campbell, D. T. (1979). *Quasi-experimentation: Design and analysis issues for field settings*. Houghton Mifflin.

Creswell, J. W., & Plano, C. V. L. (2007). *Designing and conducting mixed methods research*. Sage.

Dean-Coffey, J. (2018). What's race got to do with it? Equity and philanthropic evaluation practice. *American Journal of Evaluation 39*(4), 527–542.

Feng, A., & Schwabish, J. (2021). Are your data visualizations racist? *Stanford Social Innovation Review*. Available at *https://ssir.org/articles/entry/are_your_data_visualizations_racist*

Frierson, H. T., Hood, S., & Hughes, G. B. (2002). A guide to conducting culturally responsive evaluations. In J. Frechtling (Ed.), *The 2002 user-friendly handbook for project evaluation* (pp. 63–73). National Science Foundation.

Hood, S., Hopson, R., & Kirkhart, K. (2015). Culturally responsive evaluation. In K. E. Newcomer, H. P. Hatry, & J. S. Wholey (Eds.), *Handbook of practical program evaluation* (4th ed., pp. 281–317). Jossey-Bass.

Inouye, T. E., Yu, H. C., & Adefuin, J. (2005). *Commissioning a multicultural evaluation: A foundation resource guide*. Partners for Advancing Health Equity.

Kellogg Foundation. (2001). *Stories of impact community health scholars program*. Author.

Kellogg Foundation. (2021). *New series of how-to guides for evaluators advancing racial equity*. Author.

Kellogg Foundation. (2023). *Diversity, equity and inclusion*. Author.

Kresge Foundation. (2023). *Diversity, equity, and inclusion*. Author.

Masters, G. (2018). *What is "equity" in education?* Available at *www.teachermagazine.com/au_en/articles/what-is-equity-in-education*

Merriam-Webster. (n.d.). Equity. In *Merriam-Webster.com dictionary*. Retrieved November 30, 2024, from *www.merriam-webster.com/dictionary/equity*

Miller, J. (2023, August 16). The power of diversity and inclusion: Driving innovation and success. *Forbes*.

Moyer, K. (2023). *How patients' culture influences health care*. Rendia. Available at *https://rendia.com/resources/insights/culture*

National Equity Project. (2022). Educational equity definition. Available at *www.nationalequityproject.org/education-equity-definition*

Office of Management and Budget. (2018). Program Evaluation Standards OMB M-20-12, Phase 4 implementation of the foundations for Evidence Based Policymaking Act of 2018: Program Evaluation Standards and Practices. Author.

Ogden, T. (2010, August 30). Lies, damned lies, statistics, and data visualization. *Stanford Social Innovation Review*. Available at *https://ssir.org/articles/entry/lies_damned_lies_statistics_and_data_visualization#*

Partelow, S. (2023). What is a framework? Understanding their purpose, value, development and use. *Journal of Environmental Studies and Sciences, 13*, 510–519.

Patton, M. Q. (2008). *Utilization-focused evaluation* (4th ed.). SAGE.

Phillips, K. W. (2017, September 18). How diversity makes us smarter. *Greater Good Magazine*. Available at *https://greatergood.berkeley.edu/article/item/how_diversity_makes_us_smarter*

Robert Wood Johnson Foundation. (2017). *Visualizing health equity: Diverse people, challenges, and solutions infographic*. Author.

Robert Wood Johnson Foundation. (2022). *Health equity: Everyone counts*. Author.

Robert Wood Johnson Foundation. (2023a). *Our guiding principles*. Author.

Robert Wood Johnson Foundation. (2023b). *Why focus on health equity and social determinants of health?* Author.

Rossi, P. H., Lipsey, M. W., & Freeman, H. E. (2004). *Evaluation: A systematic approach* (7th ed.). SAGE.

Rudiger, A. (2022). *Advancing racial equity: A framework for federal agencies*. Local and Regional Government Alliance on Race and Equity.

Schwabish, J., & Feng, A. (2021). *Do no harm guide: Applying equity awareness in data visualization*. Urban Institute.

Scriven, M. (1991). *Evaluation thesaurus* (4th ed.). SAGE.

Shadish, W. R., & Luellen, J. K. (2005). History of evaluation. In S. Mathison (Ed.), *Encyclopedia of evaluation* (pp. 183–186). Sage.

Shonhe, L. (2017). A literature review of information dissemination techniques in the 21st century era. *Library Philosophy and Practice*.

Sox, H. C., & Goodman, S. N. (2012). The methods of comparative effectiveness research. *Annual Review of Public Health, 33*, 425–445.

Stern, A., Guckenburg, S., Persson, H., & Petrosino, A. (2019). *Reflections on applying principles of equitable evaluation*. WestEd.

Teixeira, S., Augsberger, A., Richards-Schuster, K., & Sprague Martinez, L. (2021). Participatory research approaches with youth: Ethics, engagement, and meaningful action. *American Journal of Community Psychology, 68*(1–2), 142–153.

Tufte, E. (1983). *The visual display of quantitative information*. Graphics Press.

U.S. Centers for Disease Control and Prevention. (2014). *Practical strategies for culturally competent evaluation*. U.S. Department of Health and Human Services.

U.S. Centers for Disease Control and Prevention. (2023). A practitioner's guide for advancing health equity: Community strategies for preventing chronic disease: Section 1. Addressing health equity in evaluation efforts Available at *cdc.gov*

Wallerstein, N., Duran, B., Oetzel, J., & Minkler, M. (2018). *Community based participatory research for health: Advancing social and health equity*. Jossey-Bass.

White House. (2021, January 20). *Executive order on advancing racial equity and support for underserved communities through the federal government*. Author.

Chapter 7

Ethical Challenges

Michael Morris

CHAPTER OVERVIEW

The distinctive complexity of ethical challenges in evaluation arises in large part from the multiple-interest holder nature of the endeavor and its implications for programmatic decisions affecting human welfare. Against this background it is useful to conceptualize ethical challenges in terms of the stage of the evaluation where a particular conflict is likely to manifest itself: entry/contracting, design, data collection, data analysis, reporting, or utilization of findings. Overall, being pressured to misrepresent findings during reporting appears to be the ethical conflict most frequently encountered by evaluators. Systematic data are scarce on how interest holders other than evaluators view ethical issues in evaluation projects. Major sources of ethical guidance for evaluators in the United States include the American Evaluation Association (AEA) Guiding Principles for Evaluators and the Program Evaluation Standards. Strategies for preventing and responding to ethical conflicts in evaluation include psychological contracting, minimizing personal defensiveness, consulting with colleagues, journaling, self-reflection, and appreciating the relevance of moral courage.

Although the core questions that drive an evaluation can vary—Does Program A make a difference?; Has Program B been faithfully implemented?; Do the monetary benefits generated by Program C exceed its costs?—there are certain questions that are relevant to *every* evaluation. One of the most crucial is the subject of this chapter: What can the evaluator do to ensure that the evaluation is carried out in an ethical fashion?

After introducing the concept of ethical practice within the context of evaluation, the chapter explores the major ethical challenges that evaluators report they encounter in their work. This is followed by an overview of professional resources that provide ethical guidelines to evaluators. The chapter's final section presents recommendations for planning and conducting evaluations in a way that facilitates the prevention of, and effective response to, ethical difficulties.

Simply put, **ethics** deal with "what is good and bad and with moral duty and obligation" (Merriam-Webster, n.d.). The focus here is on *behavior*—in colloquial terms, "doing the right thing" as opposed to doing the wrong thing. Research that engages human participants raises familiar ethical issues, such as informed consent, confidentiality/privacy, risk of harm, deception, and incentives for involvement—issues that **institutional review boards (IRBs)** typically focus on. These concerns, as well as others, can become especially challenging in evaluation, given that evaluation is a multiple-interest holder endeavor that has the potential to affect decision making concerning programs that are linked to a myriad of vested interests. Even small-scale evaluations, carried out on a local level, can evolve into affairs of intimidating complexity. Although there are values, principles, and standards that one can look to for guidance, it is not always self-evident how they might be best applied in a given set of circumstances. Indeed, evaluators must sometimes grapple with what philosophers call "ethical dilemmas" (O'Neill & Hern, 1991), where two or more valued principles come into conflict (e.g., honoring confidentiality vs. serving the common good).

Against this background, it is not surprising that most evaluators indicate that they have faced ethical conflicts (Morris, 2015), and that the more experience one has, the more likely it is that such an encounter has occurred (Morris & Clark, 2013; Morris & Cohn, 1993). The next section explores the specific types of ethical challenges that are reported most frequently by evaluators (Morris, 2015).

NAVIGATING THE TERRAIN OF ETHICAL CHALLENGES IN EVALUATION: A STAGE-BASED JOURNEY

Most evaluations proceed through a series of stages encompassing the following:

- Entry/contracting
- Designing the evaluation
- Data collection
- Data analysis and interpretation
- Reporting the results
- Utilization of findings

These stages can overlap in practice, but in conceptual terms they are fairly distinct. What ethical challenges are most likely to emerge during each phase, according to evaluators?

Entry/Contracting

The entry/contracting stage is when, ideally, the evaluator and key interest holders develop a shared understanding of what the core focus and purpose of the evaluation will be. In other words, what are the major questions that the evaluation will attempt to answer, why are those questions important, and what decisions are likely to be influenced by the answers obtained?

A major ethical challenge that can arise during this phase is when the evaluator believes that a primary interest holder has already decided what the findings "should be" and/or intends to use the findings in an inappropriate fashion (e.g., to support a course of action that has previously been decided upon). In this situation, evaluators see themselves being presented with a subtle—or not-so-subtle—message that amounts to "If your findings don't confirm my expectations, there will be trouble—not just for the program but for you as well." For instance, an interest holder who has publicly committed to expanding a program is not likely to be pleased with evaluation results that cast doubt on the program's effectiveness.

Conflicts of interest are another problem that can occur during the entry/contracting stage. These come about when "a primary interest (e.g., validity of research) is unduly influenced by a secondary interest (e.g., financial gain, academic success, community leadership)" (Ross et al., 2010b, p. 42). For example, an evaluator anticipates that their spouse's consulting firm might be awarded a lucrative contract by a local school district if the evaluator produces a glowing report on a program offered by that district. Conflicts of interest can abound in multiple-interest holder environments, and while the mere *existence* of incompatible loyalties is not proof of unethical behavior, the ways in which evaluators respond to these conflicts can vary in their ethicality.

A third type of ethical challenge that can take place during entry/contracting is when the primary client for the study does not want certain evaluation questions to be addressed, despite their substantive relevance. For instance, the client may not wish to gather data from program dropouts, even though the experience of this group could shed significant light on the quality of service implementation, which is claimed to be a major focus of the evaluation.

Additional ethical difficulties involve the participation of interest holders in the entry/contracting phase itself. Legitimate interest holders may be omitted from the planning process, especially if they possess little power as a result of being marginalized on dimensions such as education, income, race/ethnicity, sexual orientation, or disability. Even if all key interest holder groups participate meaningfully during the entry/contracting stage, problems can arise when interest holders' goals and expectations for the evaluation are in conflict. How should the evaluator handle fundamental disagreements that appear to be irreconcilable? Whose perspectives should be privileged? Should the views of interest holders funding the evaluation be accorded first priority by the evaluator?

Designing the Evaluation

The critical task of developing the detailed methodology for the evaluation takes place during this stage. A well-designed evaluation, if implemented properly, should produce the data needed to answer the major questions driving the evaluation. Unfortunately, for a variety of reasons, evaluators can find themselves being pressured to use designs that fall short of this goal.

For example, interest holders may lobby vigorously for a design that emphasizes measures of client *satisfaction* with services, even though the espoused objective of the evaluation is to demonstrate a programmatic *impact* on the problem targeted by the intervention. Thus, parents may be more invested in how much their children enjoy an after-school educational program, rather than in the effect the program has on the students' grades or other indicators of learning. Of course, this issue could emerge during the entry/contracting stage, when the focus of the evaluation is being determined. If so, it should be addressed then.

In certain cases, the resources available for the evaluation (including time) might be insufficient to support a meaningful examination of the program and its effects. For instance, there could be severe limitations on the evaluator's ability to employ comparison or control groups to assess program efficacy. Complicating these dynamics even further is research by Azzam (2010), which suggests that evaluators may be more likely to alter their proposed design when recommendations for change come from interest holders with the greatest amount of power and influence over the logistics of the evaluation. Unfortunately, power and influence are not necessarily synonymous with substantive design expertise.

Realistically, evaluators are not in a position to dismiss or ignore the views of those who are funding the evaluation, but they *are* responsible for making these interest holders, as well as others, aware of the consequences of those views for the quality of the evaluation. Doing so lessens the chances that the evaluator will face the ethically compromising prospect of conducting a fatally flawed evaluation, one that is not valid for its stated purposes.

Data Collection

The problems encountered during data collection are the ones that people most intuitively associate with the ethics of applied research. Foremost among these are situations where the rights and dignity of those providing data are threatened or violated.

Informed consent is a key area where evaluators have consistently reported difficulties. Research indicates that program staff can overestimate the extent to which service recipients comprehend the evaluation details that are provided to them (Walker et al., 2008). In participatory-oriented evaluations involving multiple interest holders, the logistics of obtaining informed consent at individual, group, and community levels can be daunting (Ross et al., 2010a). And in some cases, the temptation to use passive consent—which can maximize participation rates—rather than active consent might be very strong, even though the latter is seen as ethically preferable by most evaluators (Morris & Jacobs, 2000).

Protecting the confidentiality and/or anonymity that may have been promised to evaluation participants is another data collection challenge reported by evaluators. In some cases evaluators experience direct pressure from interest holders to reveal the identities of confidential data sources. Increasingly, however, problems emerge when comprehensive, electronic databases maintained by local, state, or federal agencies are used by researchers to establish and monitor rosters of evaluation participants. The vulnerability of these databases to both inadvertent and deliberate sharing of identifiable information can put large numbers of individuals at risk (Marquart, 2005).

Finally, during data collection evaluators occasionally become aware of behavior in the program setting that is illegal, unethical, or dangerous. For instance, the evaluator may strongly suspect that sexual harassment or misappropriation of agency funds is occurring. What are the ethical obligations of evaluators in such circumstances? Although evaluators are not typically considered "mandated reporters" in a legal sense, the absence of a legal duty to report wrongdoing does not necessarily answer the question of what the most ethical course of action is to take, especially when competing ethical principles are involved.

Data Analysis and Interpretation

During this stage the evaluator examines the data in an effort to address the questions framing the evaluation, explore possible side effects, and draw conclusions about what it all means. A significant challenge here is being cognizant of the ways in which one's values and opinions can influence this process. Evaluators are often concerned that their personal views might skew their analysis and "sensemaking" of the data. For instance, an evaluator who greatly admires the frontline staff of a program serving persons who are homeless and mentally disabled might worry that this high regard could motivate them to search more thoroughly for positive findings than would otherwise be the case. Conversely, a researcher who doubts the validity of the logic model underlying a substance abuse prevention program might be inclined to exaggerate the importance of incidental negative results in a pattern of outcomes that is largely supportive of the intervention.

Another challenge that can manifest itself during data analysis is one that typically has its roots in the planning stage. Specifically, it is when methodological decisions made during planning focus attention on certain types of findings at the expense of others. For example, an evaluation of the work requirements in a welfare program might target in great detail the intervention's impact on employment rates and hours worked, while neglecting side effects, both positive and negative, of the program on the quality of parents' interactions with their children. Or research on a school-based intervention designed to increase standardized achievement test scores might overlook the degree to which these programs reduce the amount of classroom time devoted to other worthwhile educational endeavors.

Reporting the Results

Research suggests that this is the phase where evaluators are most likely to confront ethical difficulties. Specifically, many practitioners report that they have been pressured by a key interest holder, usually the evaluation client, to misrepresent findings. Indeed, Morris and Clark (2013) found that 42% of their random sample of AEA members indicated that they had experienced such pressure. Of this subgroup, 70% said that they had been pressured on more than one occasion in their career. By far, misrepresentation pressure appears to be the ethical conflict most frequently reported by evaluators (Morris & Cohn, 1993; see also Pleger et al., 2017).

In most cases this pressure takes the form of being asked to make findings look more positive, or less negative, than the evaluator believes is warranted. Occasionally an interest holder may request a more *negative* report than the evaluator thinks is justified. Sometimes the interest holder is seeking a small change ("Can you soften the wording a bit?"), and other times a much more substantive one ("Don't include that finding"), but the common denominator is the evaluator's belief that the requested change is not supported by the data.

Confidentiality challenges can also occur during this stage. For example, an interest holder may want the evaluator to reveal the source of a quote that appears in a draft of the final report. On other occasions the problem is not interest holder pressure but the evaluator's concern that specific individuals could be identified from the way in which results are presented. This threat of inadvertent identification is especially likely in small-scale evaluations with a modest number of participants providing data. In these circumstances, evaluators must be careful when using demographic and other characteristics to organize findings, in order to avoid generating subgroups that could provide clues to how specific individuals responded or performed.

Utilization of Findings

The utilization phase is when key interest holders make decisions based on the evaluation and take action to implement those decisions. Of course, in some cases they may conclude that no changes need to be made in the program.

Of all the stages in an evaluation, this is the one where the evaluator has the least direct influence; primary responsibility rests with the interest holders who commissioned the evaluation, not the evaluator. That being said, professional standards indicate that there is a role for evaluators here. For instance, the Program Evaluation Standard Concern for Consequences and Influence (U8) states that "evaluations should promote responsible and adaptive use while guarding against unintended negative consequences and misuse" (Yarbrough et al., 2011, p. 65). From the very beginning of a project, the evaluator should be interacting with interest holders in a fashion that facilitates the effective, meaningful use of the research.

Not surprisingly, the most frequent challenge reported by evaluators in this domain is when evaluation findings are suppressed or ignored by key interest holders. Here we have the proverbial situation of a final report "gathering dust" on an administrator's shelf. Of course, this outcome is likely to be seen as most *ethically* problematic when the evaluator believes that the study's results, if widely shared, would have a significant impact on the way the program is viewed by others with a vested interest in it.

There are also instances where evaluators perceive interest holders as misrepresenting the evaluation's results when communicating with others. This misrepresentation can be deliberate or unintentional. Examples of the former can include making changes to the actual report, or preparing written summaries that do not accurately convey key aspects of the findings. Misrepresentation that is based in interest holder misunderstanding is a more benign occurrence than intentional distortion but the evaluator's ethical burden of bringing the matter to the attention of relevant interest holders remains.

A related problem arises when interest holders apply the findings of a program evaluation to a second program that differs in significant ways from the first one. In many of these cases it is likely that the evaluator and interest holders differ in the criteria they employ to judge how similar the two programs must be in order to justify grouping them together for analytical purposes using the evaluation.

Disagreements over the ownership/sharing of the evaluation's final report and/or raw data can also wreak havoc after the study is completed. Does the evaluator have the right to present the study's findings at a professional conference? What about publishing in a scholarly journal? In theory, issues such as these should have been discussed and resolved during the entry/contracting stage but sometimes they are not, and on other occasions verbal agreements that are not put in writing are the subject of conflicting memories.

Finally, there are instances when evaluators believe that their work has been used by interest holders to punish individuals (e.g., terminating the director of a program that has received a less-than-stellar evaluation). Program evaluations are not reviews of individual job performance and should not be used as such. In practice, however, the line distinguishing the two can get blurred, particularly when the program in question is small and there are few staff responsible for running it.

Evaluators also report that *they* have occasionally been the ones targeted for punishment, in a kill-the-messenger fashion, by interest holders displeased with an evaluation report. Internal evaluators may fear for their job security in these episodes, while external evaluators are likely to worry about negative word of mouth influencing their ability to secure future clients.

Implications

Most of what we know about ethical challenges in evaluation comes from self-reports provided by evaluators. Given that research on attribution processes indicates that most individuals have a tendency to externalize the sources of the problems they encounter (e.g., Kelley, 1973), it is likely that the preceding section understates, to an unknown degree, ethical problems that are rooted in the behavior of evaluators themselves or in the dynamics of evaluation–interest holder interaction. For example, a survey of philanthropic foundation officers suggests that, in many cases, what evaluators view as misrepresentation pressure, foundation officers regard as good-faith disagreement over how findings could be most accurately presented (Morris, 2007; see also Perrin, 2019). This finding is supported by data indicating that most evaluators who report misrepresentation pressure do *not* necessarily believe that the interest holders involved were acting out of an intent to deceive readers of the evaluation report (Morris & Clark, 2013). Clearly, a comprehensive understanding of ethical challenges in evaluation requires a great deal more research incorporating the perspectives of interest holders who work with evaluators.

SOURCES OF PROFESSIONAL GUIDANCE

For evaluators in the United States, the two major published sources of ethical guidance are the Guiding Principles for Evaluators (AEA, 2018) and the Program Evaluation Standards (Yarbrough et al., 2011). IRBs can also be of great help in designing an ethical evaluation, although interacting with IRBs can be a challenging endeavor in its own right.

The Guiding Principles were developed by AEA in 1994 and are periodically revised; the latest revision was in 2018 (AEA, 2018). Each of the five principles consists of a core statement followed by several substatements that provide elaboration.

Systematic Inquiry

This principle states that "evaluators conduct data-based inquiries that are thorough, methodical, and contextually relevant" (AEA, 2018, A). Evaluators have an ethical responsibility to apply sound methodological approaches to the evaluation's core questions, and to explore with interest holders the strengths and limitations of those approaches within the context of the evaluation setting and the resources available for the research. There may be occasions when these resources, or other logistical problems, do not permit the most-preferred methodology to be employed. In these instances, there need to be candid conversations about the implications of those limitations for the conclusions that can be drawn from the evaluation. For instance, an evaluator may need to make it clear that a design lacking a comparison or control group can place severe constraints on one's ability to judge the impact of a particular intervention.

These conversations should generate among all key interest holders a thorough understanding of *what* the evaluation is attempting to accomplish, *how* the evaluation will attempt to accomplish it, and *why* the approaches taken in the evaluation make sense. Throughout this process, evaluators must communicate, to the best of their ability, the various factors (e.g., values, assumptions, theories) that will contribute to their interpretation of the evaluation's findings. Doing this allows interest holders to consider, in an explicit fashion, the extent to which alternative perspectives might lead to different conclusions. What is being underscored here is that the *systematic inquiry* principle focuses on more than just the *evaluator's* confidence in the methodological approaches being employed; an ethical evaluation engages all key interest holders in exploring design issues and their significance.

Competence

The *competence* principle requires that "evaluators provide skilled professional services to stakeholders" (AEA, 2018, B). In order to put this straightforward assertion into practice, several issues need to be attended to. First, there must be a good match between the type of evaluation being conducted and the skills possessed by the evaluator or evaluation team. As the contents of this volume demonstrate, evaluation is a multifaceted field, and it is virtually certain that any given evaluator will have expertise in some areas but not others. One can have extensive knowledge of implementation evaluation but only an introductory-level familiarity with cost–benefit analysis. In addition, certain overall approaches to evaluation imply the possession of skills that would not be needed, at least to the same degree, by those who were not followers of that approach. For instance, evaluators who embrace a participatory/collaborative orientation should have extensive training in group facilitation and conflict resolution (Morris, 2021).

Evaluators cannot assume that interest holders will know what questions to ask to determine whether a particular researcher is the right fit for the technical demands of a specific project. Many interest holders probably view evaluators the way a lot of people look at automobile mechanics: "No matter what type of car I drive, a good mechanic should be able to diagnose the problem and fix it." That is an inaccurate perception of mechanics, and the same applies to evaluators. The burden is on evaluators to make sure that interest holders grasp what types of projects are relevant to their expertise.

In cases where the match between project and expertise is not ideal, the evaluator should clearly communicate what the limitations of the evaluation are likely to be if it went forward, as well as "make every effort to supplement missing or weak competencies directly or through the assistance of others" (AEA, 2018, B2). Accordingly, it is not surprising that the competence principle stresses the importance of continuing education for evaluators.

Finally, the competence principle acknowledges the importance of being responsive to the *cultural* context of the evaluation setting. This topic is explored in depth by Stewart Donaldson (see Chapter 27, this volume), so it will not be discussed further here, except to note that attention to cultural concerns is not presented in the Guiding Principles as something that it is simply nice or desirable to do, but as an endeavor that evaluators are ethically required to engage in. It is not optional.

Integrity

According to the *integrity* principle, "evaluators behave with honesty and transparency in order to ensure the integrity of the evaluation" (AEA, 2018, C). While the first two Guiding Principles emphasize the substantive expertise of the evaluator, integrity focuses primarily on the evaluator's *character* as displayed by their interactions with interest holders.

Several domains are pertinent here. One is the evaluator's responsibility for communicating with interest holders in a way that maximizes their understanding of all aspects of the evaluation, including plans for the project, the implementation of those plans (including any changes and their rationales), and the findings that are produced. It is here where the obligation to report honestly is most explicit, with the evaluator having a mandate to "accurately and transparently represent evaluation procedures, data, and findings" (AEA, 2018, C5). Moreover, if evaluators believe that the integrity of the evaluation is threatened, they must take steps to address that threat, including seeking advice from colleagues and even disengaging themselves from the project if necessary.

Conflicts of interest are also relevant to the integrity principle. They must be identified and responded to in some fashion. In certain instances a conflict could be so potentially damaging to the credibility of the evaluation that the evaluator might need to withdraw from it (e.g., evaluating a program administered by a close friend). In this context it is important to note that the *appearance* of a conflict of interest can be just as problematic for an evaluation's credibility as a genuine conflict. If interest holders believe that the integrity of a project has been compromised, their trust of the evaluation's findings and conclusions will be severely undermined, and indeed, their participation in the evaluation could be influenced in ways that produce a self-fulfilling prophecy of justified skepticism.

The integrity principle is perhaps most ambitious when it urges evaluators to "assess and make explicit the stakeholders', clients', and evaluators' values, perspectives, and interests concerning the conduct and outcome of the evaluation" (AEA, 2018, C4). Although at first glance (and second, and third . . .) this task may seem overwhelming, it is best seen as a process that unfolds over the course of the evaluation. Practitioners should be skilled at engaging in the sorts of inquiry that seek not only interest holders' opinions and preferences regarding the evaluation but also the fundamental assumptions and orientations underlying those positions. Doing so increases the likelihood that areas of overlapping intentions and "common ground" among interest holders will be identified, establishing a framework for collaborative effort in which honesty and transparency become a shared responsibility.

For example, certain interest holders may assign greater credibility to quantitative indicators of program effectiveness than qualitative ones, while other interest holders might hold the opposite view. Both groups, however, are presumably motivated by a desire to find the best possible evidence of beneficial outcomes, a motivation that the evaluator can tap into when working with them to develop a multifaceted approach to conceptualizing the evaluation's methodology.

Respect for People

The principle of *respect for people* states that "evaluators honor the dignity, well-being, and self-worth of individuals and acknowledge the influence of culture within and across groups" (AEA, 2018, D). When conceptualized narrowly, respect for people addresses the domains that have traditionally been associated with the protection of human subjects in medical research—for instance, preventing/minimizing harm, informed consent, confidentiality, and incentives for participation. Evaluators should be familiar with, and abide by, professional norms in these areas.

A potentially relevant source of guidance here is the IRB, which can be concisely described as follows:

> [IRBs] are responsible for reviewing plans for research before any data are collected; monitoring research as it is being conducted, usually on an annual basis; and reviewing the results of research to assure that it is compliant with federal policy on the protection of human subjects. The principal role of IRBs is to make sure that research or evaluation is done in such a way that the rights and well-being of participants are protected. (Cooksy, 2005, p. 354)

An evaluation that is supported by federal funding may require an IRB review (in some cases, by more than one IRB). The key factor here is whether the evaluation is considered to be *research*. Research is defined as systematic investigation intended to develop or contribute to generalizable knowledge that will be disseminated beyond the setting in which it is conducted. Evaluations occupy a gray area in this regard. They clearly represent systematic investigations but they vary in the extent to which they are designed to produce generalizable knowledge that is disseminated. Many do not, but even small-scale evaluations within local agencies can result in the sharing of findings at professional conferences, which is a form of dissemination.

Excellent discussions of the research/evaluation distinction can be found on university websites devoted to IRB matters (e.g., Oregon State University, 2020; University of Southern California, n.d.b; University of Washington, 2020). Also, the Office for Human Research Protections of the U.S. Department of Health and Human Services (n.d.) provides detailed commentary, with examples, of the conditions under which an organization's quality-improvement activities, a domain closely tied to program evaluation, would not require IRB approval.

It is important to note that there is a distinction between not having to obtain IRB approval *at all* versus having a study classified by an IRB as "exempt." Exempt studies must pose no greater than minimal risk to participants *and* fall into one or more of six categories (e.g., research on "normal" educational practices; benign behavioral interventions involving adults; surveys and observation of public behavior). Exempt studies require the evaluator to interact with the IRB in order to confirm the project's exempt status (University of Southern California, n.d.a).

Overall, the safest course of action for uncertain evaluators in these matters is to seek advice from trusted colleagues with IRB experience or a representative of an actual IRB. Although an evaluator might not be required to obtain IRB approval for a particular study, making voluntary use of the IRB process can strengthen the evaluation's ability to ensure the welfare of participants. One caveat, however, is that IRBs can vary widely in how they interpret their charge to protect research participants. The result is that some IRBs have been criticized for passing judgment on aspects of the proposed research that are beyond their jurisdiction (Speiglman & Spear, 2009). Given this concern, evaluators should be cautious when choosing among several IRB candidates (assuming they have a choice), getting input from researchers who have previously worked with the IRBs in question.

One consequence of the multiple-interest holder nature of evaluation is that the "human subjects" focus of IRBs, which emphasizes service/intervention recipients, can be too limiting for the purposes of exploring the ethical implications of the respect for people principle. In order for interest holders to be respected they must first be identified, and this principle explicitly states that the perspectives of interest holders who "are not usually included or oppositional" (AEA, 2018, D1) need to be taken into consideration. For example, low-income parents of children participating in a school-based intervention could be a difficult group to engage in an evaluation of that program. As a result, an evaluator might be reluctant to invest the time and energy necessary to achieve an effective level of engagement. The respect for people principle reminds us that following the path of least resistance in such situations is ethically suspect.

These interest holder dynamics can become even more complicated when, in accordance with this principle, one attempts to address cultural influences. Lakes et al. (2012), for example, found that White, Latina, and Asian American groups differed in the orientations they brought to the informed consent process on dimensions such as perceived risks/benefits, participant burden, and the information needed to make a participation decision. These results suggest that evaluators must be prepared to develop multiple, nuanced approaches when working with various groups to achieve consent that is truly "informed."

The theme of maximizing benefits while minimizing risk is also prominent in the respect for people principle. Although most evaluations are unlikely to pose the clear-cut health risks frequently associated with medical research, there are other sorts of harm (e.g., data collection procedures that are burdensome, generate emotional discomfort, or put staff at risk if poor program performance is revealed). Evaluators need to be sensitive to these possibilities and address them straightforwardly.

The benefits of an evaluation to participants can perhaps be most easily seen in formative evaluations where the focus is on improving program implementation. More challenging are impact studies that employ comparison or control groups whose members, at least in the short run, will not experience the positive outcomes produced by an effective intervention or program. At a minimum, these participants should be made aware of other relevant resources and services they are eligible for. And evaluators should not underestimate the appeal that altruistic motivation can have for some individuals. Participating in an evaluation that one believes is contributing to the greater good can provide significant intrinsic gratification, especially if the evaluator is skilled at emphasizing that dimension of the study. Indeed, this observation, when applied to evaluators themselves, brings into focus the final Guiding Principle.

Common Good and Equity

According to the fifth Guiding Principle, "evaluators strive to contribute to the common good and advancement of an equitable and just society" (AEA, 2018, E). In aspirational terms, this is the loftiest of the Guiding Principles, focusing as it does on the evaluator's responsibility to society as a whole.

In practice, what does this mean? For one thing, evaluators should be mindful of the ways in which the interests and priorities of the most visible interest holders in a given evaluation relate to the broader public interest. Consider the previously mentioned example of a school intervention that narrowly targets students' standardized achievement test scores. Would an evaluation that only examined these test results be responsive to the *common good and equity* principle? What if the intervention consumed so much classroom time that other, presumably important, educational activities associated with public education were undermined? Would an ethical evaluator insist that the scope of the evaluation be expanded?

The common good and equity principle, by itself, does not provide definitive answers to these questions. However, the principle would almost certainly call for the evaluator to reflect on those issues when deciding how to proceed. In doing so the evaluator would need to explore the relevance of their own personal values regarding the common good, equity, and social justice (see Morris, 2009).

The elaborations of this principle emphasize the need to take action when "stakeholder interests conflict with the goals of a democratic, equitable, and just society" (AEA, 2018, E2), to "address the evaluation's potential risks of exacerbating historic disadvantage or inequity" (E3), and to "mitigate the bias and potential power imbalances that can occur as a result of the evaluation's context [including] self-assess[ing] one's own privilege and positioning within that context" (E5). There is a clear theme here, one closely aligned with Schwandt's (2002) claim that evaluation is "first and foremost a . . . moral–political and interpretive practice, not a technical endeavor" (p. 196).

Consider, for example, the case of public flogging. In 2011, sociologist Peter Moskos authored *In Defense of Flogging*, in which he proposed giving individuals convicted of a crime the choice of receiving corporal punishment rather than going to prison. Imagine that a state has passed legislation authorizing this option, and that you have been asked to evaluate the impact of this policy on such variables as crime rates, incarceration rates, and prison costs. Would you accept this evaluation offer, or would you see the project as not embodying the goals of a "democratic, equitable, and just society"?

Thinking about evaluation in this fashion, one that extends ethical considerations beyond the restricted parameters traditionally associated with respect for human subjects, is likely to be an unsettling, and perhaps even threatening, experience for many evaluators. What cannot be denied, however, is that attention to these matters is growing in the field, and their relevance has been institutionalized in an ethical principle that all evaluators are expected to adhere to. At a minimum, evaluators need to familiarize themselves with the work of prominent theorists in this domain (e.g., Donaldson & Picciotto, 2016; House & Howe, 1999; Schwandt, 2018; Schwandt & Gates, 2021).

The Program Evaluation Standards

The Program Evaluation Standards are a book-length set of 30 standards that "when implemented will lead to greater evaluation quality" (Yarbrough et al., 2011, p. 292). The standards address virtually all of the areas targeted by the Guiding Principles, but in much greater detail. The presentation of each standard is followed by an extended discussion of its underlying rationale, recommendations for implementing the standard, hazards associated with the standard, and a relevant case scenario for analysis.

The standards are organized into five groups: utility, feasibility, propriety, accuracy, and evaluation accountability. The eight utility standards are concerned with the "extent to which program stakeholders find evaluation processes and products valuable in meeting their needs" (Yarbrough et al., 2011, p. 4), and their goal is to "increase the likelihood that the evaluation will have positive consequences and substantive influence" (p. 8). Although most of these standards (e.g., *evaluator credibility*, *attention to stakeholders*, *explicit values*) deal with issues that are addressed by the Guiding Principles, presenting them within a utilization framework is distinctive. The message here is that in order to be of high quality, an evaluation must be useful, a stance that has long been championed by Patton (2008) and is explored in depth by Alkin and Vo (see Chapter 8, this volume).

The feasibility standards focus on the "extent to which resources and other factors allow an evaluation to be conducted in a satisfactory manner" (Yarbrough et al., 2011, p. 288). Of the four standards in this group, three pertain to matters that are primarily logistical in nature (*project management*, *practical procedures*, and *resource use*). The fourth, *contextual viability*, states that "evaluations should recognize, monitor, and balance the cultural and political interests and needs of individuals and groups" (Yarbrough et al., 2011, p. 93). This standard brings to mind novelist Kurt Vonnegut's (1952) observation in *Player Piano*: "if it weren't for the people . . . always getting tied up in the machinery . . . the world would be an engineer's paradise" (p. 59). Interest holders tangled up in the machinery is a given in evaluation, and evaluators who attempt to avoid this challenging reality do so at their peril, and the peril of the evaluation for which they are responsible, ethically and otherwise. Evaluators whose work is characterized by an interest holder-involvement philosophy (see Fetterman et al., Chapter 10, this volume) are likely to be particularly sensitive to the demands of these contextual dynamics, especially in terms of showing respect for the diverse values and priorities of multiple interest holders while actually attempting to get the evaluation done. These evaluators take a relationship-based approach to their practice, one that emphasizes notions of both procedural and responsive justice in order to ensure that typically marginalized interest holders are fully engaged participants (see Bromley et al., 2017).

The eight propriety standards address the "extent to which the evaluation has been conducted in a manner that evidences uncompromising adherence to the highest principles and ideals (including professional ethics, civil law, moral code, and contractual agreements)" (Yarbrough et al., 2011, p. 291). This group of standards emphasizes the ethical domains addressed by the integrity and respect for people Guiding Principles. In addition, the crucial role of formal agreements in evaluation is directly acknowledged by a standard stating that "evaluation agreements should be negotiated to make obligations explicit and take into account the needs, expectations, and cultural contexts of clients and other stakeholders" (Yarbrough et al., 2011, p. 119).

Formal agreements represent binding contracts, and it can be tempting to view the process of developing them as a tedious exercise that one should simply endure and "get through" as quickly as possible. This would be a serious mistake, given that the entry/contracting phase represents an opportunity to explore a variety of ethical issues relevant to the evaluation. Formal agreements that reflect this consideration are likely to prove extremely valuable as the evaluation unfolds.

The accuracy standards are concerned with the "extent to which an evaluation is truthful or valid in the scope and detail of what is communicated about a context, program, project, or any of their components" (Yarbrough et al., 2011, p. 283), especially communications that support judgments of quality. These standards most directly overlap the systematic inquiry and integrity Guiding Principles and apply the notion of accuracy to aspects of the evaluation that go beyond findings and conclusions to domains such as theoretical frameworks, analyses, and program contexts.

Throughout the accuracy standards attention is paid to the possibility that different interest holders might conceptualize any given evaluation component in different, even conflicting, ways. Using a previous example, certain interest holders might view client satisfaction with services as evidence of program impact, while others, including the evaluator, might not. Drawing "accurate" conclusions about the performance of the program would require the evaluator to make explicit the reasoning processes underlying the disparate interpretations, examining the justifications that might exist for favoring one interpretation over the others. It would be nice if "the facts spoke for themselves" in evaluation, but in many cases they do not.

Finally, the three evaluation accountability standards recommend that all aspects of an evaluation be fully documented, and that this documentation be used by the evaluator and external experts to assess the quality of the evaluation, with special attention paid to the evaluation's adherence to the Program Evaluation Standards. Adapting the accountability standards to the focus of this chapter, a wise evaluator would, at a minimum, monitor throughout the evaluation the steps that are taken to ensure ethical practice, including reviewing the adequacy of any actions that were taken in response to ethical problems.

With the exception of the propriety standards, the Program Evaluation Standards are not presented as a document that is designed to provide explicitly ethical guidelines to evaluators. That being said, one can certainly make the case that conducting high-quality evaluations is an evaluator's ethical responsibility, and it has been noted that, conceptually, the Guiding Principles and the Program Evaluation Standards traverse a common territory for the most part. The standards are an extremely valuable resource that should be regularly consulted by all evaluators who are committed to ethical practice.

PREVENTING AND RESPONDING TO CHALLENGES: STRATEGIES FOR THE PROFESSIONAL, ETHICAL EVALUATOR

Putting a familiar observation in polite terms, "challenges happen," no matter how conscientious an evaluator might be in trying to prevent them. That reality certainly should not dissuade evaluators from attempting to forestall ethical conflicts, or from developing strategies to handle them effectively once they occur. This section presents a number of concrete suggestions for how evaluators can strengthen their ethical practice.

Take Advantage of the Entry/Contracting Stage

Establishing in this phase a foundation for discussing ethical issues is probably the single most important action that an evaluator can take to ensure the ethical "health" of the project. This involves doing several things:

- Consider the sorts of ethical challenges that are likely to arise in the evaluation and share your concerns with key interest holders. Seek feedback on how they view these issues, and how they might be handled. For example, if a summative evaluation is taking place in a highly politicized, high-profile environment, pressures to misrepresent findings are a distinct possibility. What are interest holders' opinions about what could be done to prevent this from happening? What expectations should there be regarding criteria for modifying drafts of final reports?

- Educate interest holders about the professional guidelines and standards that you need to be responsive to as an evaluator. The Guiding Principles are concise enough to be included as an addendum to your research proposal or the evaluation contract itself. However, simply giving people a copy of the Guiding Principles is not enough. You should highlight and interpret the parts of the document that hold the most relevance for the upcoming evaluation. A complex impact evaluation, for instance, can raise systematic inquiry issues that require attention to technical considerations (e.g., control groups, randomization) that interest holders might not understand or approve of. You have a responsibility to go beyond stating methodological requirements to helping interest holders grasp the ethical justifications for those requirements.

- Make sure that interest holders have an opportunity to bring up any ethical concerns that *they* might have regarding the project. However, keep in mind that interest holders might not conceptualize ethical matters in the same way, or using the same language, that you do. Thus, rather than asking, "What ethical concerns do you have?" it probably makes more sense to pose a more general query, such as "What sorts of worries, concerns, or questions do you have about this evaluation?" This will bring to the surface both ethical and nonethical issues, both of which deserve to be explored.

Do not be surprised if interest holders, at least initially, are somewhat uncomfortable with the ethical conversation you are introducing into the entry/contracting process. They may have limited experience with such discussions. What you are engaging them in is what consultants call **psychological contracting** (e.g., Block, 2011; Boss, 1985), a process in which individuals share concerns about a relationship they are about to embark upon. It is your job to help interest holders see the importance and value of such an exchange. A challenging conversation during the entry/contracting stage can help prevent a much more difficult one later in the evaluation.

When Challenges Arise, Minimize Your Defensiveness

As previously noted, most of us are not prone to seeing our own actions as the cause of the conflicts we experience. This tendency can interfere with constructive problem solving when responding to ethical challenges that occur during an evaluation. For example, Pleger and Hadorn (2018) found that interest holder behavior that evaluators might view as misrepresentation pressure can often result from a sincere attempt on the former's part to produce a more accurate depiction of the program being evaluated. They conclude that "the notion of the 'evil' client and the 'good' evaluator is . . . too simplistic" (p. 471) and stress the need for enhanced communication between the two parties that can result in influence attempts that facilitate the betterment of, and support for, the evaluation (see also Pleger & Sager, 2018).

A crucial implication of this line of analysis is that making negative assumptions about interest holder motivation is likely to lead to interaction cycles that exacerbate rather than resolve them. Searching for constructive intent is a more productive path, especially when combined with a humility that acknowledges the possibility that one's own actions have contributed to the ethical difficulties being faced. Adopting such an orientation can introduce the possibility that an ethical challenge will actually provide an opportunity to *enhance* the quality of the evaluation, not just maintain it. Perrin (2019), for instance, in his detailed listing of recommendations for managing interest holder pressure to alter final reports, encourages evaluators to "welcome comments, even critical ones" (p. 365), on the report.

Consult with Your Colleagues

No matter what the ethical challenge is that you're dealing with, the odds are good that other evaluators have encountered it at some point in their career. Seek their input, either from your own personal network or from professional sources like the EVALTALK listserv. Colleagues may be able to help you frame the challenge in a way that you had not previously considered, and/or identify courses of action (and their side effects) that you had overlooked.

For example, internal evaluators are often embedded in interlocking organizational hierarchies that render them vulnerable to retribution if powerful interest holders are displeased with what is reported about their favored programs. "Killing (or at least *wounding*) the messenger" scenarios can pose serious ethical challenges to evaluators who wish to display integrity while also retaining their job. In these circumstances an evaluator would do well to seek mentoring from experienced internal evaluators they respect who work in similar settings. How have they dealt with these pressures?

Ultimately, of course, collegial input and advice can only take you so far. No two situations are exactly alike, your colleagues have their own biases (conscious or unconscious) that might affect their counsel, and you are the one who is responsible for the decisions you make. That being said, there are few resources more valuable than a seasoned, wise evaluation colleague when one is facing an ethical conundrum.

Keep an Ethics Journal

Documentation of the real-time unfolding of an evaluation project is the foundation of the evaluation accountability standards, and is clearly relevant to the ethical domain. The salience of technical and political considerations during the early stages of an evaluation can make it easy to overlook important ethical concerns, establishing a pattern that can become self-sustaining. This can lead to incremental wrongdoing, where little-noticed, minor ethical compromises grow over time into more serious problems that call for major remedial attention.

Journaling about ethical matters throughout an evaluation forces the sort of self-reflection that makes this phenomenon less likely. The documentation involved need not be unduly laborious. The key is to briefly note the proactive steps you are taking to ensure ethical practice, as well as highlight any developments, however subtle, that give you ethical pause. The very fact that you are recording these developments increases the chances that you will feel obligated to address them, just as one must address other issues (e.g., methodological, political, analytical) to produce a credible evaluation.

Know Thyself

Your actions as an evaluator are not just influenced by the field's professional guidelines and standards; the personal values you have developed over a lifetime also play a crucial role. The more self-aware you are in this regard, the more readily you can mobilize your personal resources to analyze ethical questions and reach decisions about how to deal with them (Newman & Brown, 1996). Consider a situation where your primary client is resistant to involving low-status interest holders in planning the evaluation. If you strongly value collaboration and equality, you may well see this as an ethical challenge that requires you to take a firm stand in favor of inclusion. Another evaluator—one who is comfortable operating out of a more conventional "expert" mode—might not take such a position.

Personal values can also help you tackle ethical dilemmas when professional principles do not offer clear guidance because they are in conflict or are simply too general (see Mabry, 1999). In an impact evaluation, to what extent should one continue to advocate for a methodologically powerful design that certain interest holders oppose in principle due to its use of a comparison group that will not receive the intervention? Should you opt for a less-strong design that will gain wider acceptance? Simultaneously maximizing systematic inquiry, respect for people, and common good and equity might not be possible in such a circumstance. To what degree should knowledge building in the name of the public interest be accorded more importance than honoring the preferences of particular interest holders? Ultimately, you will probably need to draw upon your personal prioritization of the values involved here, in conjunction with examining the specifics of the situation, when deciding how to proceed.

Sometimes, You Need Courage

To be sure, figuring out what one should do when confronted with an ethical challenge can be a difficult task. In many cases, however, the tougher task is actually putting into practice the behavior you have decided is ethically required. This occurs when the behavior in question would put you *at risk*. In these instances you are being called upon to display **moral courage**. Morally courageous actions embody two characteristics: they stem from a commitment to ethical principles, and they are willingly engaged in by individuals who understand that they are putting themselves at risk of harm by behaving in this fashion (Kidder, 2005).

There are occasions when living up to one's principles, professional or otherwise, could threaten the job security of an internal evaluator, or the chances of an external evaluator being awarded future contracts. Of course, there is always the possibility of being unfairly bad-mouthed by influential, vindictive interest holders, regardless of one's internal or external status.

What should you do if a powerful interest holder orders you to misrepresent a key finding? Violate confidentiality? Implement a flawed informed-consent policy? Remain silent when other interest holders provide misleading summaries of the evaluation to the public? What if your good-faith attempts to reach agreements with interest holders on these matters have not been persuasive? And retribution is virtually certain if you do not comply? Box 7.1 provides such an example.

As the saying goes, sometimes the only reason for doing the right thing is that it is the right thing to do. You can look to courageous role models for inspiration, seek out supportive colleagues and build alliances, and reflect upon your most cherished values, but in the end you need the courage to translate those values into action: "I'm sorry, but I just can't do that. What I must do is this, and here are the reasons why."

The chapters in this handbook are devoted to the distinctive characteristics of theory and practice in evaluation. With respect to ethical challenges, however, sometimes it all comes down to making the sorts of fundamental choices that define us more as a person than as an evaluator: Do I do what I believe is right, even at my own peril? Professional principles and personal values can bring you to that point of decision, but they cannot walk you through the door.

Additional Resources

EVALTALK listserv. Available at *www.eval.org/Community/EvalTalk*

Mertens, D. M., & Ginsberg, P. E. (Eds.). (2009). *The handbook of social research ethics*. SAGE.

Morris, M. (Ed.). (2008). *Evaluation ethics for best practice: Cases and commentaries*. Guilford Press.

REFERENCES

American Evaluation Association. (2018). *Guiding principles for evaluators*. Retrieved December 18, 2022, from *www.eval.org/About/Guiding-Principles*

Azzam, T. (2010). Evaluator responsiveness to stakeholders. *American Journal of Evaluation, 31*, 45–65.

Block, P. (2011). *Flawless consulting* (3rd ed.). Jossey-Bass.

Boss, R. W. (1985). The psychological contract: A key to effective organization development consultation. *Consultation, 4*, 284–304.

Bromley, E., Mikesell, L., & Khodyakov, D. (2017). Ethics and science in the participatory era: A vignette-based Delphi study. *Journal of Empirical Research on Human Research Ethics, 12*, 295–309.

Cooksy, L. J. (2005). The complexity of the IRB process: Some of the things you wanted to know about IRBs but were afraid to ask. *American Journal of Evaluation, 26*, 352–361.

Donaldson, S. I., & Picciotto, R. (Eds.). (2016). *Evaluation for an equitable society*. Information Age.

House, E. R., & Howe, K. R. (1999). *Values in evaluation and social research*. Sage.

Kelley, H. H. (1973). The process of causal attribution. *American Psychologist, 28*, 107–128.

Kidder, R. M. (2005). *Moral courage*. Morrow.

Lakes, K. D., Vaughan, E., Jones, M., Burke, W., Baker, D., & Swanson, J. M. (2012). Diverse perceptions of the informed consent process: Implications for the recruitment and participation of diverse communities in the National Children's Study. *American Journal of Community Psychology, 49*, 215–232.

BOX 7.1. Reverse Bait and Switch?

A couple of months ago, you delivered the final report of an impact evaluation focused on an innovative community reintegration program for offenders released from prison. Overall, the results were quite positive. For example, the recidivism rate among participants was significantly below that of the comparison group, and the employment rate was higher.

This morning, the governor announced that the program would be introduced into 10 communities throughout the state, and cited, without mentioning your name, the supportive results of your external evaluation of the program. So far, so good.

What is not so good is what you learn when you talk to your contacts at the state's Department of Correction (DOC), which will be funding the dissemination effort. To put it mildly, the disseminated program will be a watered-down version of the program you evaluated. Several key components of the intervention you studied have been seriously weakened or diluted. Although it would not be accurate to say that the program has been totally "gutted," you believe that it is disingenuous to claim that the two versions of the program are the same, and that is exactly what the governor has done. In its diluted form, it's hard for you to imagine that the program will be effective. Distressed, you share your concerns with one of your DOC contacts. Her response:

> "Listen, it's an election year, and the state budget is a mess. The governor needs to do something to show that he cares about reintegrating offenders but there's no way he can fund the full-fledged program, so he's done some trimming. OK, maybe it's a bit more than just trimming. But at least a version of the program will be out there, and perhaps more funds can be allocated for it down the road. Heck, I wouldn't be surprised if they wanted you to evaluate the statewide implementation. They respect your work. All things considered, this situation is a net positive. We're practicing the 'art of the possible' here."

Your friend's comments leave you conflicted. On the one hand, they have used your research to justify a severely compromised program that, in your opinion, is likely to be ineffective. That ineffectiveness could *lower* support for reintegration efforts, not strengthen them. On the other hand, you did your job, and you did it well. You produced and delivered a high-quality evaluation report to your client, the local office of the DOC. This matter has now moved on to the next level. How far do your responsibilities extend? And your friend could be right. Implementing a "Reintegration Lite" program could build support for later efforts. It's also possible that even a diluted intervention could have a positive impact. Yes, this is politics, and it smells bad, but something good could emerge. Being a purist in these circumstances might not be warranted.

But it still smells bad.

What, if anything, should you do?

Issues to Consider

Let's take a brief look at this case from the perspective of the Guiding Principles. The systematic inquiry principle requires evaluators to "make clear the limitations of the evaluation and its results" (AEA, 2018, A4). An obvious limitation here is that your evaluation pertains to the program you actually studied, not the diluted version that is about to be implemented. With respect to the competence principle, if the (unacknowledged) watered-down version of the program fails to have a beneficial impact, it could cast unjustified doubt, in the eyes of the public or other key interest holders, on the competence displayed in your evaluation of the original program.

Where integrity is concerned, it is clear that you believe "honesty and transparency" have been compromised during the utilization phase of the evaluation, making you feel personally uncomfortable, even though it is the governor and the DOC that are engaging in the sleight-of-hand maneuver, not you. But does remaining silent make you an accomplice?

There is no indication that the evaluation itself has failed to uphold the principle of respect for people, but one could argue that the common good and equity principle is now endangered. This principle calls for evaluators to "recognize and balance the interests of the client, other stakeholders, and the common good while also protecting the integrity of the evaluation" (AEA, 2018, E1). The common good is not served if the public is led to believe that Program B is a faithful replication of Program A, when it is not. At the very least, the interests of the released offenders participating in a weak Program B would not seem to be receiving equitable consideration.

The preceding analysis suggests that action on your part might be ethically warranted at this point. Should you ask for a formal meeting with representatives of the DOC? What would you hope to achieve in such a meeting? Would it be enough to have them commit to greater transparency in communicating the nature of the disseminated program to the public? If you were not satisfied with the outcome of this meeting, would you consider contacting a local news reporter in order to tell your side of the story? How risky a step might that be for you professionally? Does the magnitude of the issue require taking such a risk? At what point do you say, "Ethically, I've done all that I could . . . or should . . . in this case"?

Mabry, L. (1999). Circumstantial ethics. *American Journal of Evaluation, 20*, 199–212.

Marquart, J. M. (2005, October). *Ethical issues in state-level evaluation settings.* Paper presented at the meeting of the American Evaluation Association, Toronto, Ontario, Canada.

Merriam-Webster. (n.d.). *Ethics.* Retrieved December 18, 2022, from *www.merriam-webster.com/dictionary/ethic*

Morris, M. (2007). Foundation officers, evaluation, and ethical problems: A pilot investigation. *Evaluation and Program Planning, 30*, 410–415.

Morris, M. (2009). The fifth guiding principle: Beacon, banality, or Pandora's box? *American Journal of Evaluation, 30*, 220–224.

Morris, M. (2015). Research on evaluation ethics: Reflections and an agenda. *New Directions for Evaluation, 148*, 31–42.

Morris, M. (2021). Ethical considerations. In R. P. Kilmer & J. R. Cook (Eds.), *The practice of evaluation: Partnership approaches for community change* (pp. 81–102). Sage.

Morris, M., & Clark, B. (2013). You want me to do what? Evaluators and the pressure to misrepresent findings. *American Journal of Evaluation, 34*, 57–70.

Morris, M., & Cohn, R. (1993). Program evaluators and ethical challenges: A national survey. *Evaluation Review, 17*, 621–642.

Morris, M., & Jacobs, L. (2000). You got a problem with that? Exploring evaluators' disagreements about ethics. *Evaluation Review, 24*, 384–406.

Moskos, P. (2011). *In defense of flogging.* Basic Books.

Newman, D. L., & Brown, R. D. (1996). *Applied ethics for program evaluation.* SAGE.

O'Neill, P., & Hern, R. (1991). A systems approach to ethical problems. *Ethics and Behavior, 1*, 129–143.

Oregon State University. (2020). *Human research protection program and institutional review board.* Retrieved December 18, 2022, from *https://research.oregonstate.edu/irb*

Patton, M. Q. (2008). *Utilization-focused evaluation* (4th ed.). SAGE.

Perrin, B. (2019). How to manage pressure to change reports: Should evaluators be above criticism? *American Journal of Evaluation, 40*, 354–375.

Pleger, L. E., & Hadorn, S. (2018). The big bad wolf's view: The evaluation clients' perspectives on independence of evaluations. *Evaluation, 24*, 456–474.

Pleger, L. E., & Sager, F. (2018). Betterment, undermining, support and distortion: A heuristic model for the analysis of pressure on evaluators. *Evaluation and Program Planning, 69*, 166–172.

Pleger, L., Sager, F., Morris, M., Meyer, W., & Stockmann, R. (2017). Are some countries more prone to pressure evaluators than others? Comparing findings from the United States, United Kingdom, Germany, and Switzerland. *American Journal of Evaluation, 38*, 315–328.

Ross, L. F., Loup, A., Nelson, R. M., Botkin, J. R., Kost, R., Smith, G. R., Jr., & Gehlert, S. (2010a). The challenges of collaboration for academic and community partners in a research partnership: Points to consider. *Journal of Empirical Research on Human Research Ethics, 5*, 19–31.

Ross, L. F., Loup, A., Nelson, R. M., Botkin, J. R., Kost, R., Smith, G. R., Jr., & Gehlert, S. (2010b). Nine key functions for a human subjects protection program for community-engaged research: Points to consider. *Journal of Empirical Research on Human Research Ethics, 5*, 33–47.

Schwandt, T. A. (2002). *Evaluation practice reconsidered.* Lang.

Schwandt, T. A. (2018). Acting together in determining value: A professional ethical responsibility of evaluators. *Evaluation, 24*, 306–317.

Schwandt, T. A., & Gates, E. F. (2021). *Evaluating and valuing in social research.* SAGE.

Speiglman, R., & Spear, P. (2009). The role of institutional review boards: Ethics: Now you see them, now you don't. In D. M. Mertens & P. E. Ginsberg (Eds.), *The handbook of social research ethics* (pp. 121–134). SAGE.

University of Southern California. (n.d.-a). *Exempt.* Retrieved December 18, 2022, from *https://oprs.usc.edu/irb-review/types-of-irb-review/exempt*

University of Southern California. (n.d.-b). *IRB review.* Retrieved December 18, 2022, from *https://oprs.usc.edu/irb-review*

University of Washington. (2020). *Do I need IRB review?* Retrieved December 18, 2022, from *www.washington.edu/research/hsd/do-i-need-irb-review/is-your-project-considered-research*

U.S. Department of Health and Human Services. (n.d.). *Quality improvement activities FAQs.* Retrieved December 18, 2022, from *www.hhs.gov/ohrp/regulations-and-policy/guidance/faq/quality-improvement-activities/index.html*

Vonnegut, K., Jr. (1952). *Player piano.* Charles Scribner's Sons.

Walker, R., Hoggart, L., & Hamilton, G. (2008). Random assignment and informed consent: A case study of multiple perspectives. *American Journal of Evaluation, 29*, 156–174.

Yarbrough, D. B., Shulha, L. M., Hopson, R. K., & Caruthers, F. A. (2011). *The program evaluation standards: A guide for evaluators and evaluation users.* SAGE.

Chapter 8

Fostering Evaluation Use

Marvin C. Alkin
Anne T. Vo

CHAPTER OVERVIEW

Literature pertaining to research on evaluation use indicates that specific evaluator behaviors and the consequent actions of those impacted by the evaluator foster evaluation use. In this chapter we present a set of guidelines for fostering evaluation use. These guidelines are derived from our analysis of evaluation use literature. Using Miller's (2010) standards for examining evaluation as a framework, we document our definition of use and develop a set of well-defined guidelines that are use oriented and, specifically, context bound. These are stated as specific observable actions of the evaluator.

This chapter deals with the topic of fostering evaluation use. Evaluation use might occur quite by accident or unrelated to the actions of the evaluator. However, we firmly believe that most evaluation use derives from the specific actions of the evaluator and the consequent actions of those impacted by the evaluator. Thus, the focus we take is on the actions of the evaluator in fostering evaluation use.

Now, let us consider the question "Why all the fuss?" Why is evaluation use important? We maintain that evaluation use is at the heart of evaluation; it is the reason for performing evaluation. Classic definitions of evaluation affirm the importance of use. Scriven (1991) makes the distinction between "merit" (denoting that the entity performs well on some or all aspects of what it intended to do) and "worth," which refers to whether the entity does well in terms of the characteristics that are valued within *that particular context* and to *these particular interest holders*. Worth is usefulness and implies the importance of future use. Emily Gates and Tom Schwandt (see Chapter 5, this volume) delve more fully into the role of valuing in evaluation.

The relevance of evaluation use is further affirmed by many other leading scholars. Carol Weiss (1977), whose initial writings on evaluation use spurred the decades of research that ensued makes the case well:

> The basic rationale for evaluation is that it provides information for action. Its primary justification is that it contributes to the rationalization of decision-making. [U]nless it gains a hearing when program decisions are made, it fails in its major purpose. (p. 318)

To be clear, use occurs when interest holders consider evaluative information (i.e., findings about a program or insights gained through participating in an evaluation) in the course of making decisions or altering attitudes. We elaborate on this later in the chapter.

PURSUING THE GOAL OF FOSTERING EVALUATION USE

So, how does an evaluator pursue the objective of fostering evaluation use? What are the guidelines? One source might be the various prescriptive theories that purportedly provide a framework for conducting evaluation. Many of these theories are presented in the book *Evaluation Roots* (Alkin, 2013). Scholars on the "use branch" of the evaluation theory tree presented in that book affirm (or at least Alkin & Christie [2005] contend so) that evaluation use is the goal of their various theoretical frameworks. Clearly then, employing one of these use branch theoretical frameworks might be a start to fostering evaluation use. Utilization-focused evaluation, for example, aims to attain use by prioritizing the information needs of primary intended users—that is, those who are in decision-making positions (Patton, 2008). In contrast, participatory evaluation focuses on engaging interest holders as partners throughout the evaluation process; their firsthand experience in evaluation offers opportunities for determining how use can take place as the investigation unfolds (Cousins & Earl, 1992; Cousins & Whitmore, 1998). Evaluative approaches that take capacity building as the focus prioritize interest holder learning and the installment of organizational infrastructure to support evaluation use (Volkov & King, 2007; Preskill & Boyle, 2008). Tom Archibald and colleagues (see Chapter 3, this volume) provide more detail on evaluation capacity building, specifically the role of evaluative thinking in evaluation capacity building.

Theorists on other branches of the evaluation theory tree have also expressed concern for attaining evaluation use—although perhaps not as their primary goal. Theorists and theories that appear on the "methods branch," for instance, prioritize methodological rigor and accuracy of results in the hopes that technically sound evaluations will more likely be used (Chen, 2005; Mark et al., 2000; Boruch, 1997). Many of the theorists that appear on the "valuing branch" seek inclusion of diverse interest holder perspectives as a means of promoting equitable access to opportunities for underrepresented communities. The hope is that not only will use occur but the resulting decisions will be more equitable and just (House & Howe, 1999; Greene, 2005; Mertens, 2009).

Using a theory from a branch of the theory tree is a start but only if it is specific enough in describing proposed evaluator actions, and if they are adhered to well. That is not always the case. In their analysis of a well-known evaluation theory, Miller and Campbell (2006) identified three areas of critique of current evaluation theories: conceptual ambiguity, lack of unanimity in practice, and limited documented evidence of success (p. 298). Specifically, they noted that while the theory was inspired by various other evaluative approaches, "it is not adequately differentiated from [them]" and "its lack of specificity regarding its theorized mechanisms of change" makes implementing the approach with precision an obstacle in practice (pp. 298–299).

Further, we maintain that in many cases attempting to follow a particular theoretical framework may be insufficient for actually fostering evaluation use. As noted, some of these theories may have other secondary goals that could, in minor ways, deflect from a primary emphasis on use. Most importantly, we believe that most theories do not adequately portray sufficient elements of what is actually required for fostering evaluation use. We come to this view by having been greatly influenced by the writings of Robin Miller (2010)—particularly her article entitled "Developing Standards for Empirical Examinations of Evaluation Theory." Miller maintains that "The evaluation profession must gain a better understanding of the requirements needed to concretize, measure, and test the effects of evaluation frameworks and procedures empirically" (p. 396). Toward this end, she outlined five criteria by which prescriptive theories of evaluation can be judged: operational specificity, range of application, feasibility in practice, discernible impact, and reproducibility.

Most, if not all, theories do not live up to the standards that Miller (2010) developed. What she calls the "theoretical signature" of most models are not sufficiently detailed so that a potential user can properly implement the theory in the manner that the theorist intended or in the way that theorists themselves might have done so. Here too there is a dilemma—many theories as written may not conform to or be detailed enough to describe what a theorist really does when they evaluate. Take, for example, Alkin and Christie's (2005) effort to study the alignment between theory and practice by inviting a representative from each branch of the evaluation theory tree to evaluate a fictitious educational program: the Bunche–Da Vinci Learning Partnership Academy. In doing so, each theorist was encouraged to indicate if, how, and the ways in which they would engage interest holders; evaluation methods to be used; and any assumptions they had to make along the way (e.g., about timeline, budget, intended use). In this exercise theorists say what they would do in evaluating the program but it may not be precisely what they have said they would do in their prior writings.

NECESSARY ELEMENTS FOR AN EVALUATION USE THEORY

In examining the writings of theorists, what must we look for to determine whether it is an adequate prescriptive theory—and in our case, one for facilitating evaluation use? We have taken Miller's (2010) standards and converted them into four major elements that must be precisely defined: (1) the goal, (2) the area of applicability, (3) the type of evaluation, and (4) the specific observable actions that can be seen in implementing the theory.

The *goal* of a theory to be employed (or of one's own formulated working theory) must be clearly defined and well understood. For our purpose, and for that of this chapter, the goal is *use*. However, use may be viewed in multiple ways and it is important that we specify precisely what we mean by use.

Another area derived from Miller's formulation is *the area of applicability*. This refers primarily to the program's scale. Does the theoretical formulation refer to small-scale or large-scale programs? We think of small scale as local or limited state programs and large scale as programs of greater size, typically federally funded. Consider the differences in what might be entailed to foster evaluation use in each of these instances. Both Patton and Weiss referred to this in the early literature of our field as a "paradigms debate." For example, we noted in their debate the differences in frames of reference that influenced perceptions toward and understandings of the extent to which evaluation utilization occurs (Alkin, 1990). Weiss's work, at the time, was grounded in policy evaluation that took place at the highest levels of government—a context in which evidence of utilization was seldom directly observable—and, instead, required the evaluator to rely on partnerships with unlikely interest holders, including policy aides, special commissions and panels, the media, and interest groups. Patton, whose work offered a different sense of appreciation for the intimacy of contexts in which an evaluator practices, offered suggestions that can be realistically implemented on a scale that is more narrowly defined. He emphasized, for example, the importance of being situationally responsive, reflective, and an advocate for evaluation. Weiss's approach takes into account the real chasm that exists between evaluators and decision makers in the policy arena, whereas Patton's approach assumes direct evaluator access to interest holders as primary intended users of evaluation results. This "paradigms debate" reflected in the literature underscores the importance of the program context and of depicting with great specificity the size of the program for which the theoretical approach is most applicable.

The third area to be considered in the development of a theoretical signature is the *type of evaluation* being performed. There are differences in actions that must be taken related to whether the program is undergoing formative, summary formative, or summative evaluation. Formative evaluation is conducted to "provide an indication of how things are going," whereas summative evaluation offers "information designed to serve [major, end of program or end of cycle] decisions" and summary formative evaluation is a hybrid process involving a formative period that, at some point, is brought to a discrete conclusion (Alkin & Vo, 2018, pp. 12–13). What observable steps, actions, or activities might we expect in each of these instances? In the most simplified sense, we could anticipate great probing and investigation in the conduct of formative evaluation, more observation and summarization during a summative evaluation, and some combination of both in the case of a summary formative evaluation. Evaluation, however, is anything but simple. Clearly, a precise set of guidelines and observable actions differ by evaluation type and reflect the inherent messiness often brought about by contextual differences.

Finally, for the theoretical signature to be complete, some *observable actions* would need to be formulated. These are the specific actions that must be performed relevant to that particular program. As Miller (2010) states, "A recognizable signature is necessary to support the claim that any particular theory adds value to practice" (p. 392)—that is, these elements must be readily recognizable when observed in action. Generally stated evaluator actions are insufficient. Actual statements that the evaluator might make and specific actions taken are necessary for inclusion.

ADEQUACY OF THEORIES

As noted, extant evaluation use theories might qualify as clear choices for fostering evaluation use. However, most theories are deficient in specificity related to the areas that Miller (2010) indicated. The precise definition of use is usually lacking. It is highly unlikely that the theory under consideration is applicable for both small-scale local programs and large national programs. Many theories are broad sweeping and do not specify an area of applicability for the theory. Likewise, they do not specify the type of evaluation for which the theorist's approach is most appropriate—that is, does the theorist's approach have equal applicability for both formative and summative evaluations? Finally, the specificity of observable actions is generally lacking. While examples exist, they are generally not stated as statements an evaluator could make during the evaluation or discrete actions that could be definitively observed.

Miller (2010) also mentions another criterion as part of her standards, one that we have not mentioned—namely, discernible impact. In essence, this criterion seeks to examine evidence of "whether the use of a particular theory actually leads to the impacts that are expected and desired. . . ." (p. 395). All existing theories are weak on this criterion because there simply is not sufficient evidence of impact—in this case, of "use"—from implementing particular theoretic models.

We present a package of evaluator actions and consequent observable actions for fostering evaluation use. While we note that they have not yet demonstrated discernible impact, the individual evaluator actions that we discuss are derived from the research conducted on evaluation use. In essence, the factors that have been established through the body of research form the basis for evaluator actions and subsequent observable actions.

DESIGNING GUIDELINES FOR FOSTERING EVALUATION USE

In the previous sections we have discussed the necessary elements for a comprehensive evaluation use theory. We examine each of these to create our mini-theory (or guidelines) for fostering evaluation use. The first of these is a specific definition of use. We lean on a paper by Alkin and King (2017), where a Guttman scale mapping sentence was described, as an aid in defining a specific use model. We begin by defining some of the elements of that model.

First, what is the nature of the evaluation information that might ultimately be used? Obviously, findings of one type or another, whether quantitative or qualitative, are one kind of information for potential use. Other types are the various views, attitudes, and perceptions acquired by interest holders as a consequence of participating in the evaluation.

Second, who are the potential users? Or, more directly, who are the individuals who might employ the information for a useful purpose? This category consists of interested primary interest holders, other local interest holders, or external users.

Third, in what way might the information be used? Was the information a dominant factor in the use that occurred? Or was it one of multiple influences on use or was it one of multiple cumulative influences?

Fourth, what aspect of the program was addressed in the use? Was it the total program, any of its components, the role of individuals in any way associated with the organization, or the values and understandings of individuals in any way associated with the organization?

Fifth, what was the use purpose? It could be making decisions about any of the aspects discussed in the previous paragraph—either at the end or during the program implementation. It could have the purpose of establishing or altering attitudes. The purpose might be substantiating previous decisions or actions. Further, the purpose might be building an individual's or an organization's evaluation capacity.

This generic definition of evaluation use has within it a number of elements, which provide a variety of possible kinds of use. This definition is quite inclusive and does not offer sufficient specificity for theory development.

Starting with this generic definition, we are obligated to define use in a more specific way. In the second cluster, we conceive of an evaluation as oriented toward "this program at this time." Thus, we *exclude* evaluations that deal with "external users" (i.e., those who are external to the project or its constituencies because we view issues of use as specific to a particular program and context rather than the building of a research knowledge base). We also exclude in the third cluster, the idea of "multiple cumulative influences" (specifically if it implies influence of findings over an extended period of time). Further, in the last cluster we exclude "substantiating previous decisions or actions" (if there was no openness by users to potential change being made). Thus, in this chapter, our definition of use is:

> *The making of decisions, establishment or altering of attitudes, or building of an individual or organization's evaluation capacity by an interested primary user or other local users through information acquired as findings and/or a consequence of participating in the evaluation. Importantly, the evaluation information must serve as a dominant (or one of multiple) influence(s) related to the program being evaluated, any of its components, the role of individuals in any way associated with the organization, and/or the views and understandings of individuals in any way associated with the organization.*

We rely on this refined definition of evaluation use as the basis for our theoretical formulation and subsequent prescriptions for fostering use.

Next, we indicated that the proposed guidelines must define an "area of applicability." For our purposes, we have defined that area as small- and medium-scale programs. For "type of evaluation," we focus on formative and summary formative evaluations. We consider the issue of "observable actions" later in this chapter.

RESEARCH ON EVALUATION USE AND CONSEQUENT EVALUATOR ACTIONS

We now go about the task of developing our guidelines for fostering evaluation use in a sequence of activities:

1. Examine the research on evaluation use.
2. From that research specify evaluator actions that correspond to fulfilling what the research dictates; these are the specific elements required for fostering evaluation use.
3. Provide some examples of observable actions or dialogue for each evaluator action that would provide evidence that the action had been attended to.

The research on evaluation use is quite extensive with much of it having taken place from 1980 to 2004. The studies that were conducted focused on an examination of particular factors that tend to be associated with use occurring. What does this research tell us? These studies employed a variety of research techniques and investigators examined evaluation practice in many kinds of program contexts. The research is nicely summarized in various compendia that sought to aggregate this body of work and compile perceptions about factors affecting evaluation use (Leviton & Hughes, 1981; Alkin, 1985; Cousins & Leithwood, 1986; Shulha & Cousins, 1997; Johnson et al., 2009). A summary of the derivation of factors from this literature is found in Alkin and Vo (2018, pp. 314–316).

We have examined the research in each of these compendia and the way in which factors were placed into larger categories. Further, we noted the extent to which factors were present across the various research syntheses (Alkin & Vo, 2018). These factor summaries were aggregated into a cohesive framework consisting of four main categories: the *evaluatOR* category, the *user* category, the *organizational/cultural/*

social context category, and the *evaluatION* category.

The fourth category, the evaluation, refers to the evaluation itself. It includes particular aspects of the evaluation that have relevance to facilitating evaluation use, including:

- Attaining technical quality (appropriate to the situation).
- Doing work that has relevance (meets information needs).
- Understanding the relationships of findings to existing and competing information.
- Proposing work that has high communication quality and appropriateness.
- Preparing work in a timely manner.
- Structuring options that are easily understood and show directions for potential use.

We focus on the particular actions of the evaluator that lead to a high level of use. Thus, we focus on the first three categories, which would lead to the fulfillment of the fourth category and the attainment of a high-quality use-oriented evaluation.

The factors within the first three of these categories are presented in Table 8.1. Each of the items listed in the first column were the elements specifically identified in the research literature. Each employs one (or more) specific "evaluator actions" as noted in the second column.

We briefly comment on some of these research use factors. The first of these is the evaluator category. These are factors that are directly related to the evaluator's professional identity and their competencies, beliefs, and value positions on various evaluation-related issues. In our approach to fostering evaluation use, by far

TABLE 8.1. Evaluation Use Research Factors and Relevant Evaluator Actions

Research factors	Evaluator actions
A) Evaluator Factors 　* Evaluator commitment to use 　* Evaluator technical competence 　* Evaluator credibility 　* Individual/organizational/personal context	A1) Evaluator personally and intensely commits to attaining evaluation use. A2) Evaluator assesses her own technical competencies and determines areas in need of further development A3) Evaluator engages in actions that build greater credibility A4) Evaluator works on relationship building A5) Evaluator works towards developing further understanding of the individual and organizational contexts and assesses her own values in relationship to the various contexts
B) User Factors 　* User commitment to use 　* Initial attitude toward evaluation 　* User influence capability 　* Evaluator/user relationship	B1) Evaluator works on developing in interest holders a positive attitude toward evaluation and a commitment to evaluation use B2) Evaluator identifies those who have or might have influence capability and helps interest holders to understand the role they might play in decision making B3) Evaluator actively involves users in all major phases of the evaluation B4) Evaluator engages in ongoing communication
C) Organizational/Cultural/Social Context Factors 　• Preexisting evaluation policy and legal boundaries 　　* Written evaluation requirements 　　* Other contractual obligations 　　* Organizational evaluation policy 　　* Fiscal constraints 　• Organizational and programmatic arrangements 　　* Development stage of the program 　　* Type of evaluator 　• Interorganizational elements 　　* Interest in evaluation from higher organizational level 　　* Relationship to the broader program 　　* Relationship to related programs in the organization	1) Evaluator seeks to understand evaluation policy and legal boundaries and ensures that these are considered in the evaluation 2) Evaluator accommodates the evaluation to the stage of the program and type of evaluation 3) Evaluator seeks to understand the interests and values of those at other organizational levels and use that information to enhance the evaluation

Note. Asterisks (*) indicate research factors drawn from a major compilation of evaluation use research (see Alkin & Vo 2018, pp. 309–310).

the most important element is the evaluator's personal commitment to use. By this we refer to the way in which the evaluator in their actions and interactions demonstrates that attaining use is a very high personal priority. Moreover, it must be a priority of such importance that the evaluator seeks to infuse it into users' thinking. Another evaluator factor, within this category, is of great importance. The evaluators' credibility is an essential part of the evaluation being viewed as credible and thus worthy of use. It is important to note that credibility on the part of the evaluator, while partially attained at the outset, may be enhanced through the evaluator's actions.

The user category describes actions that the evaluator must take in relationship to actual and potential users. The evaluator's personal commitment to use is reflected in their attempt to gain interest holders' attention to this priority. It is attained by actively teaching interest holders to be users. This involves, at minimum, a willingness on the part of evaluators to involve users in the conduct of the evaluation. Involvement is a continuous endeavor that involves specific teaching activities as well as attention to relationship building. Another area within the evaluator user category is influence capability. This refers to the potential role that users might have in making decisions about program change or their ability to modify attitudes about the program. For a user's commitment to use to have impact, the interest holder user must have the capability, directly or indirectly, to influence actions or attitudes. Many interest holders are capable of having influence. The evaluator must seek to determine this potential influence and enhance it where possible.

In the third category, we note that programs exist within their larger organizations and within communities. This we refer to as the organizational/cultural/social set of factors. This consists of the individual context, the organizational context, and the community context. Each of these and their constituent parts, as well as their rules and expectations, exert influence on an evaluation. Discovery of these factors is not enough. Attention to these factors by the evaluator as reflected in their actions is essential. That is why context awareness is repeated (further reflected) in the first set of evaluator factors.

FROM RESEARCH TO EVALUATOR ACTION/OBSERVABLE ACTION

The specific evaluator actions that the evaluator must engage in to foster evaluation use are found in the second column of Table 8.1. We have considered the evaluation research-based factors and converted them to descriptions of evaluator actions that summarizes that research. We anticipate that pursuing the evaluator actions described above and instantiating them through examples of behaviors provided will lead to the conduct of a credible and useful evaluation that meets empirical standards defined in the research literature—namely, that a credible and relevant evaluation will be produced. To achieve credibility, the evaluation process and outcomes must demonstrate high technical quality that is appropriate to the situation. For an evaluation to be relevant, it must examine questions that are of genuine concern to users, the measures for determining success are considered appropriate by users, and the valuing process must be user engaged.

In the following, we list each evaluator action including a general description of what the action means. It is important to note that particular evaluator actions may be ongoing and occur at various points throughout the conduct of the evaluation.

These evaluator actions alone, however, may be best understood by more detailed examples. Miller (2010) reminds us that actions are best understood when amplified by a sampling of particular *observable* behaviors or statements that the evaluator might make in promoting that action. They must be directly observable in a particular evaluation situation. Thus, we consider what the evaluator could specifically be observed doing or saying, so that there is verification that the action has taken place. We refer to these as *observable actions*. The examples that we provide following each description of evaluator actions are consistent with our goal definition and are most applicable to small-scale formative or summary formative evaluation. Many of these may not be unique to our approach—they could, for example, be considered a part of other approaches but perhaps to a lesser extent. Other observable actions that we devise might be adopted here more fully than in other theories. However, there are several elements that are particularly unique to our approach:

A1. Evaluator Personally and Intensely Commits to Attaining Evaluation Use

Committing to the attainment of evaluation use is inherently a value position. Such a commitment is typically made in advance of the commissioned evaluation. However, because it is a professional value—one that has been shaped and articulated through prior training—it is also essential for evaluators to reaffirm this value throughout the evaluation.

The evaluator's awareness of their positionality and motivation for engaging in evaluation is not simply important, it is what gives the evaluator's practice an identity. Attainment of use is but one value position an evaluator could take. There are many others, including ensuring diverse representation of interest holder value perspectives or achieving methodological rigor (see Alkin, 2013). For us, these are important and may be viewed as subsidiary but evaluation use must remain the priority. The evaluator benefits greatly from having a strong sense of professional self and values along with personal standards for gauging the evaluation's success and the success of one's own practice.

Note that a declaration—whether internal or public—to the attainment of evaluation use has the potential to be understood as a form of advocacy—that is, advocacy for use of evaluation processes and findings. We do not reject this possibility. Rather, in our view, this is what gives evaluation meaning and value. It is imperative that evaluators be clear on their own stances on this issue and the conditions under which adoption of this position would be acceptable.

Sample Observable Actions

• The evaluator introduces self to interest holders as committed to use and points out that evaluation has little value unless it is used.

• The evaluator comments on and emphasizes use in meetings with interest holders.

• The evaluator takes on the role of being a teacher (or facilitator) of evaluation use. This involves asking questions about potential use during the evaluation, such as "How could we apply what we are learning from this evaluation or the way the program is being run?" or "What are you learning from the evaluation and is it changing your perspective in any way?"

• The evaluator also seeks to help interest holders understand use alternatives at various summary points in the evaluation. At that time the evaluator may be seen teaching or facilitating interest holders to engage in an analysis of use alternatives.

A2. Evaluator Assesses their Own Technical Competencies and Determines Areas in Need of Further Development

Evaluations that are conducted today are informed by similar logic and procedures that were used perhaps 10, or even 20, years ago. What has continued to evolve, however, are the principles, tools, and values that have emerged as part of the evaluator's toolkit. The evaluative contexts and questions that interest holders are required to address have also have grown in complexity as well. As such, it is beneficial for the evaluator to position themselves as a reflective, lifelong learner. As we have noted elsewhere, the evaluator is always a learner first (Alkin & Vo, 2018, p. 306). Adopting this perspective also means that the evaluator takes on questions of whether they have the necessary technical, methodological, theoretic, and cultural know-how to conduct the desired evaluation even before agreeing to actually do it. Likewise, it is reasonable to anticipate, in a multiyear contract for instance, that interest holders might inquire about evaluation approaches or methods that are different from what was originally agreed upon. It is important for the evaluator to remain regularly apprised of developments in the field and continuously upgrade their skills.

Sample Observable Actions

• The evaluator assesses the evaluator actions required in the conduct of the evaluation and the requisite technical skills. The evaluator assesses their own technical capabilities and either develops missing requisite skills or provides appropriate technical assistance.

• The evaluator, in determining the areas that need further development, engages in self-reflection, whether on paper or internally, after each evaluation and is able to concisely acknowledge their strengths and weaknesses as an evaluator when asked.

- The evaluator also seeks input about their evaluation competencies by asking interest holders the questions, "How could that have gone/been better?" and "What is something I am doing well and something that I can improve?"

- When the evaluation is unusually complex, the evaluator, at completion, discusses the methodologies employed with another experienced evaluator.

- The evaluator stays aware of technical advances in evaluation and seeks out continuing professional development opportunities as appropriate.

A3. Evaluator Engages in Actions That Build Greater Credibility

Evaluation, unlike many other practice-centered disciplines (e.g., medicine, education, and law), is not a clearly understood field. It is challenging, in turn, to judge an evaluator's credibility because certifications that are analogous to a medical license or a teaching credential do not exist on a broad scale yet. The "Credentialed Evaluator" designation from the Canadian Evaluation Society is perhaps the only exception at present (Buchanan, 2015; Love, 2015). This is problematic to the extent that the evaluator's "credibility" is the part of the evaluation that is subsequently judged as trustworthy and thus usable. While professionalization questions are being considered throughout the United States and around the globe, two documents serve as beacons for guiding evaluation practice: the American Evaluation Association Guiding Principles for Evaluators (2018, pp. 320–321) and the Joint Commission Program Evaluation Standards (Yarbrough et al., 2011). It is important to note that credibility on the part of the evaluator, while partially attained at the outset, is mostly acquired through the evaluator's actions. And situating one's practice within the guidelines outlined in these documents helps frame those actions in an understandable, credible manner.

Sample Observable Actions

- The evaluator reflects on and is honest with themselves and others about their areas of expertise and limitations. The evaluator shares what they know while also not being afraid of saying, "I don't know" and seeks out resources (e.g., professional development opportunities) to address gaps in knowledge and skills.

- The evaluator engages interest holders as thought partners by offering them a menu of possible routes to pursue in an evaluation while facilitating their consideration of the advantages and disadvantages of each rather than approaching them with hubris. For example, the evaluator could state, "Well, let's think about that possibility for a moment. What has to be true for that to work? What are the possible challenges and how can we address them?"

- The evaluator obtains and updates existing programmatic events. They obtain a schedule of program activities and regularly ask program staff, "What's new in the program?" and "Are there special events planned that I might observe?" The evaluator attends as many events as possible.

- The evaluator has a unifying characteristic of integrity and of commitment to doing what they say they will do and communicating clearly and consistently about the evaluation's progress while acknowledging support received and challenges encountered along the way.

- The evaluator demonstrates professional credibility by producing work in a timely manner.

- The evaluator dresses in a professional manner but adapts behavior reflective of the local context. One of the authors tells his students, "When in doubt, dress Macy's."

A4. Evaluator Works on Relationship Building

Evaluation is inherently a social and political activity (Weiss, 1993). For it to have meaning and drive change, we must pay attention to the social environment in which it is unfolding. An understanding of who the interest holders are, what is important to them and why, along with the organization and environment in which they are situated helps evaluators build constructive relationships that support the end goal of use.

The occurrence of evaluation use benefits from, but is not solely contingent on, the quality of professional relationships established and maintained during the project's life cycle. Instead, those relationships have the potential to influence the evaluation's feasibility and the extent to which interest holders value related efforts—that is, they can inform interest holders' perceptions of the evaluation and whether they choose to approach it as a punitive or as a formative experience. Further, interest holder relationships can influence the quality of communication—how messages are relayed, heard, and interpreted—which, in turn, moderates potential fear and anxiety that is associated with evaluation activities. Thus, while use relies on a combination of complex factors, establishing positive relationships with interest holders can buffer the sense of threat that surrounds the evaluative process. Connecting with interest holders as people rather than clients alone by relating their experiences with your own and vice versa is an advantageous approach to consider.

Sample Observable Actions

• The evaluator situates themselves as a learner and asks questions that offer a window into interest holders' social histories by making inquiries, such as "How did you become involved with this program?" and "What motivated you to pursue work in this area?"

• The evaluator shows interest in and seeks to learn about interest holders' experiences with the program in general. The evaluator asks questions like "What is your favorite part of this program?" and "What has been most rewarding and challenging about your work with the program? Why do you think that's the case?"

• The evaluator also tries to understand interest holders' prior experiences with evaluation. Questions such as the following tend to be helpful: "Were you involved in the process when the program was last evaluated? What was that like?" and "What do you hope will be different about your experience this time?"

• The evaluator seeks to demonstrate that interest holders are valued by acknowledging interest holder input through phrases like "That was a great question" or "Thank you for bringing that perspective."

• The evaluator accepts and offers feedback graciously. The evaluator responds quickly and kindly to any communications or questions.

• The evaluator establishes avenues for bidirectional communication with interest holders throughout the evaluation by exchanging contact information with them.

A5. Evaluator Works toward Developing Further Understanding of the Individual and Organizational Contexts and Assesses their Own Values in Relationship to the Various Contexts

One important part of organizational context is the organizational structure—the way the organization operates and the levels of responsibility contained therein. Another important aspect involves gaining clarity of the organizational values. An organization's values serve as guideposts for how it conducts business. Examples include integrity, generosity, transparency, excellence, inclusion, learning, sustainability, innovation, and social impact. Individual interest holder values are also a part of the organizational context. They may include ideas such as these, but they could also be expanded upon to reflect the importance placed on faith, family, and community. These organizational and individual values at times support each other while at other times compete with each other.

An evaluator's values likewise include some combination of these personal and professional dimensions. As we noted earlier, and it is worth repeating here, it is imperative that evaluators firmly understand their own personal and professional value positions because these views inherently shape their practice. One of the moments in which this influence is perhaps most observable is when an evaluator's values brush up against the value positions of interest holders and the organizations they aim to serve. While perfect alignment of individual, interest holder, and organizational values is not a requisite for a successful evaluation, understanding where there may be differences will be helpful in fostering respectful and constructive social interactions.

Sample Observable Actions

• The evaluator observes and keeps a field guide of notes about the program's organizational processes, including how decisions are made, by whom, and when, throughout the evaluation.

- The evaluator interviews all primary user interest holders to better understand their values and also snowball interviews various other relevant interest holders. Along the way, the evaluator seeks information that supports or disconfirms alignment between their own values and those of interest holders' and the organization's, among interest holders, and between interest holders and that of the organization's.

- The evaluator systematically examines their own personal values and convictions before beginning an evaluation so that they are aware of how these personal contexts might influence their observations and questions. Further, the evaluator seeks to understand interest holder cultural background and values and also seeks to understand differences from their own positions.

- The evaluator reads local newspapers to stay abreast of community-specific issues that may affect the program and the evaluation.

- The evaluator discusses the need to understand the community, engages in a "neighborhood walk," and invites interest holders to participate as well to better understand the community.

B1. Evaluator Works on Developing in Interest Holders a Positive Attitude toward Evaluation and a Commitment to Evaluation Use

Evaluation has not typically been an activity that most organizations pursue willingly. Rather, many evaluations are compulsory. They are completed in response to requirements that have been mandated by some other entity, such as a funding agency (i.e., federal government, charity, private investor) or an accrediting body (e.g., Western Association of Schools and Colleges, Liaison Committee on Medical Education). There are many interest holders. Some might not take kindly to evaluation. Some have reported fearing it. Indeed, evaluation anxiety is a reported phenomenon in the literature (Donaldson et al., 2002). Still, it is possible to begin addressing this angst. One approach involves actively teaching interest holders to be users, empowering them to own the evaluative process. This involves, at minimum, a willingness on the part of evaluators to involve users at various points throughout the evaluation. Involvement is a continuous endeavor that requires specific teaching activities that call attention to the importance of use. These intentions and activities encourage interest holders to not only consider how to learn from the evaluation process and use evaluation findings but it also offers them a means to demystify and find value in evaluation.

Sample Observable Actions

- The evaluator seeks to become more aware of the past evaluations conducted and what type of attitude this might have developed in the program's interest holders. They ask questions like "How did you feel after the evaluation?" or "How did the evaluators engage you with their work?" Such questions are used by the evaluator to begin conversations about how they conduct evaluations and why they do/do not do things differently than other evaluators.

- The evaluator demonstrates excitement when talking about how the evaluation can benefit the program and discusses why it is a waste of resources and time if the evaluation is viewed only as a required exercise. This involves asking questions like "Why are we doing this evaluation?"; "What use might be made of it?"; "Would program changes be possible?"; "What do you think you might learn about your program?"; and "What do you hope/think you might learn about evaluation?"

- The evaluator seeks to engage interest holders in priority-setting activities. These "reality testing" opportunities offer interest holders and evaluators opportunities to discuss the relevance of evaluation questions and data collection measures. Questions that are used to structure these discussions include the following: "Why is this question important?"; "Might the answer to that question provide support for program changes or for modified attitudes?"; and "Would you be satisfied if this measure (i.e., an exam, a survey, an interview, etc.) provides relevant evidence related to the question that you have asked?"

- The evaluator aims to understand and manage expectations throughout the evaluation so that potential surprises are kept to a minimum and do not detract from the use mission. This can be accomplished by asking questions, such as "What about this process has been rewarding/positive/surprising/frustrating/challenging for you?"; "Moving forward, what could be different?" or "Were the preliminary evaluation results in line with what your experiences suggest?" and "What had you expected to see instead? Why might that have been the case?"

• The evaluator asks, after initial program results are reported, "What are your next steps now that the evaluation has reached this summary stage?" and "What do you think can be done differently to improve the program?"

B2. Evaluator Identifies Those Who Have or Might Have Influence Capability and Helps These Interest Holders to Understand the Role They Might Play in Decision Making

An evaluation's context is complex. Interest holders are an important element of that landscape. As has been described elsewhere (Alkin & Vo, 2018), being able to identify primary interest holders and to understand their perspectives and inclinations, along with the sources and motivations for these views, is a significant aspect of constructive evaluation practice. Because evaluators encounter and interact with diverse individuals throughout the evaluation, it is important to differentiate between interest holders who are intended users (i.e., individuals at all levels who are able to make decisions about the program), influencers (i.e., those whose views and positions may indirectly affect final decisions), and general audiences (i.e., those who will receive information about the evaluation and its findings and be affected but may not be able to act on this information). Doing so enhances the likelihood of instrumental use, but also broadens the sphere of the evaluation's potential to influence decision making during and after the study is completed. The process of identifying interest holders with influence capabilities lies greatly in the evaluator's own abilities to understand who interest holders are, what informs their views, what their motivators are, and what compels them to act. Prioritizing the task of getting to know interest holders beyond their identities as evaluation clients is a key element of supporting use. Evaluators may also take an active role in helping interest holders to modify and increase their influence capability.

Sample Observable Actions

• The evaluator interviews program participants and community members to understand who benefits from a positive or negative evaluation of the program and how. They ask various interest holders, "Who are the people who have a stake in the outcomes of the evaluation?" and "How are they already positioned to affect changes in this program?"

• The evaluator creates an inventory of primary potential users and possible uses of evaluation findings by each interest holder. This mapping of the interests and influences of interest holders is frequently referred to by the evaluator and used to determine overlapping areas of interest among interest holders. In particular, the evaluator uses it to determine how individuals' interests and roles within the program can be combined to incite evaluation use.

• The evaluator seeks to work with individual interest holders/users who will (or might) have the ability to influence decisions within the program and/or the organization of which they are a part. The evaluator asks such questions as "What does 'evaluation use' mean to your program?"; "What role might you have in influencing program changes of any type during or at the summary stages of evaluation?"; and "How might that role be enhanced?"

• The evaluator asks potential evaluation users, "How might this evaluation add to your personal understanding of the program or of evaluation in general?"

B3. Evaluator Actively Involves Users in All Major Phases of the Evaluation

Interest holder engagement is a heavily studied issue that is of long-standing interest for evaluators as they may be involved in various activities throughout the evaluation, including identification and refining of guiding questions, facilitating access to study sites, piloting data collection instruments, data analysis, interpretation of results, and setting parameters for evaluation use. The research literature further unpacks related topics on interest holder engagement, such as how to identify interest holders to include in the evaluation process; once identified, how to select and invite these individuals; ways in which to define the breadth and depth of their involvement; and how to determine the potential consequences of their engagement on the evaluation's trajectory (Taut & Alkin, 2010). These issues highlight the technical importance of the practice of actively involving interest holders as a means of fostering use. However, it is critical to ensure that such involvement is authentic and additive not only for the evaluation but for the interest holder as well. Evaluators, thus, should explicitly consider interest holders' interests to determine which evaluation phases and specific activities would benefit most from collaboration and support from a broader group. These assessments and decisions take place throughout the evaluation upon careful observation by the evaluator and thoughtful discussions with interest holders.

Sample Observable Actions

- The evaluator refers to the work to be done as "our evaluation," and points out that interest holder knowledge and participation are essential for success.

- The evaluator engages interest holders in logic modeling with the evaluator questioning input/output/use/outcome use relationships. The evaluator may posit potential outputs and outcomes (positive and negative) and ask interest holders to talk about possible use.

- The evaluator involves interest holders in defining questions and the relevance of measures.

- The evaluator's approach is particularly defined by a priori valuing by interest holders (in *our* particular approach). The evaluator asks, "If I told you at the end, or some other summary point of the evaluation, that the level of accomplishment for this particular question was X, would you conclude that was an indication of success?"; "What if it was Y?"; "What would you consider to be an appropriate level/standard for the program to be deemed successful?"; and "If the measure of success is qualitative (or, cannot be quantified), help me to describe the characteristics and general description of 'success.'"

- The evaluator develops simulations for interest holders to practice using data to inform decision making.

- The evaluator develops working groups, learning communities, or data inquiry groups to explore results and interpret them in context.

B4. Evaluator Engages in Ongoing Communication

Clear communication is critical in a well-conducted, successful evaluation. Unlike a few other evaluation activities, such as question definition or data analysis, which occur at discrete stages during an evaluation, communication takes place throughout the project's life cycle. Evaluators might find different modes of communication—meetings (in-person or virtual), phone calls, e-mails, and so on—especially effective, depending on the particulars of the evaluation context and the stage or phase of the evaluation (Alkin et al., 2006). Understanding interest holders' preferred mode of communication and expectations for updates is an important issue that the evaluator needs to firmly grasp early in the project. Doing so supports the evaluator's position as a collaborative professional and, perhaps more important, creates opportunities for evaluators to share tentative findings, which can be helpful in priming interest holders to think about how to use such results throughout the process.

Sample Observable Actions

- The evaluator indicates their availability to talk about the program and its evaluation and encourages interest holders to contact them when they have questions or as issues arise. The evaluator might ask, "What would be the most convenient way for us to communicate about the evaluation and its progress?"

- The evaluator works with interest holders to develop a timeline for formal and informal discussions about the evaluation's progress.

- The evaluator actively seeks and listens to interest holder input about what works best for them.

- The evaluator communicates in a clear and professional manner. The evaluator formats and frames complicated issues in easily understood language or appropriate data visualizations.

- The evaluator regularly clarifies and reminds interest holders of the status of the evaluation process and the progress that has or has not been made.

C1. Evaluator Seeks to Understand Evaluation Policy and Legal Bounds and Ensures That These Are Considered in the Evaluation

Evaluations are bounded by a number of program external factors. These tend to be policy related in nature, which constrain and enable what an evaluator can feasibly pursue and accomplish in an evaluation. The implication for practice is determining what processes and workflows must be developed, reviewed, and approved and from whom such approvals must be sought to ensure the evaluation's successful implementation. A common scenario that evaluators encounter, for instance, involves securing approval from an organization's ethics review board (or institutional review board) in addition to their own institutional review board, to conduct the study, particularly if it involves underage youth or other vulnerable populations. In the context of an educational program evaluation, an evaluator might be faced with the need to work within the confines of a school district's existing data access and security policies along with Family Educational Rights and Privacy Act (1974) regulations. Or if working in the health care sector and with patients' medical records, then stipulations of the Health Insurance Portability and Accountability Act (2004) will certainly be a factor. While many policies are driven by federal regulations, there may be other locally implemented policies—official and otherwise—that the evaluator will need to uncover and learn. Many of these may be written into the contract. Explicit and implicit rules will quickly complicate the evaluation landscape and push the evaluator to consider the trade-offs that must be made to ensure that interest holders' questions can be addressed in a timely fashion. These insights help the evaluator locate the evaluation within a social and political landscape and shepherd it in a manner that supports the attainment of use.

Sample Observable Actions

- The evaluator clarifies the fiscal and reporting constraints imposed by the organization on the evaluation to be conducted and uses this to guide their initial proposal and future work. The evaluator refers back to these understandings frequently to do time-cognizant work for the program being evaluated.

- The evaluator checks and double checks all evaluation requirements and contractual obligations to be certain that they are being met. The evaluator seeks to operate within these evaluation bounds.

- The evaluator seeks to understand organizational policy that might impact the evaluation. For example, the evaluator might ask, "Who is the contact person for arranging site observations?" Or the evaluator might provide a list of the various intended evaluation procedures and ask about approvals and organizational lessons related to each.

- The evaluator keeps on hand organizational charts, the contract, and summaries of what has been learned about the approaches and refers to them as needed.

C2. Evaluator Accommodates the Evaluation to the Stage of the Program and Type of Evaluation

The usefulness of an evaluation's process and its findings are contingent on whether they match the program's developmental stage and fit the needs of the organization that commissioned the study. A program that is still in the process of being designed or one that has been implemented for less than 2 years, for example, should not be held to the same standards as one that has been offered for more than 5 years. In the same vein, the evaluation's purpose should also be taken into consideration as this will inform the type of evaluation that should be conducted. For instance, a summative evaluation—one whose results are intended to inform "go/no-go" or "fund/defund" types of decisions—should not be conducted on programs that have not been given the opportunity to deliver on its stated objectives. Formative or summary-formative evaluations may be more fitting if the emphasis is on iterative and incremental improvement. We focus on formative and summary formative evaluation. But even within these categories there may be great variation in what is needed and what is to be accomplished based on age and development of the program.

Pinning down where the program is in its developmental cycle and how the commissioning organization hopes to use the evaluation early on is helpful in charting the study's course. This also helps the evaluator begin guiding interest holders in considering and recognizing which evaluation actions are most appropriate. Certainly, an important component of these discussions also includes setting interest holders' expectations about the evaluation's scale, scope, and what can be accomplished in light of the resources that have been allowed.

Sample Observable Actions

- The evaluator, at the start of the evaluation process, tries to pin down where the program is in its development cycle. They will note that some adjustments may need to be made along the way—as in different ways of collecting data but not drastically changing the scope and focus of the evaluation.

- The evaluator keeps in mind what the goals of the program are in relation to how long they have been established. By understanding how long certain inputs have been available and whether the activities have been clearly implemented by program management, the evaluator makes decisions on what evaluation questions would provide the most helpful feedback for the stage of the program being evaluated.

- The evaluator demonstrates an understanding of the program's history and development by asking such questions as "How did the program come about?"; "What needs is the evaluation intended to address?"; and "How have its goals and objectives evolved, if at all, and why?"

- The evaluator considers the evaluation budget so that they do not overpromise and underdeliver.

- The evaluator focuses evaluation questions on and uses study designs that are appropriate for the program's stage. Doing so requires the evaluator to understand the program's scale: "Has the program been piloted?"; "What was learned from that experience?"; "How many sites is the program currently offered in? How has that changed over time?"; and "How many participants have completed, are currently engaged in, or have prematurely left the program?"

- The evaluator needs to understand interest holders' views toward various types of evidence, such as those generated from a case study compared to a study using observational or experimental designs. Questions such as the following shed light on these perspectives: "Was an evaluation conducted on this program in the past? How was it received and why?"

- The evaluator asks, "Given what we have discussed, what must be true about the current evaluation for it to be useful and used?"; "Has the program reached the stage where this question is answerable?"; and "Is it premature to ask this evaluation question?"

C3. Evaluator Seeks to Understand the Interests and Values of Those at Other Organizational Levels and Uses That Information to Enhance the Evaluation

We have emphasized the importance of context throughout this chapter and revisit the element here; this time, focusing chiefly on the program's organizational context and, specifically, how it is situated within the broader environment. The assumption here is that the program is neither a start-up nor a stand-alone operation. Rather, it is part of a larger and more established organization, such as a school, school district, nonprofit organization, state department, and so forth. Each of these types of entities has its own culture and operational systems and is organized differently. For instance, some may be hierarchical while others are "flatter." Some organizations, likewise, may have highly established and fluid processes by which business is conducted while others have processes that are being developed or refined. It is important for evaluators to understand these structures and systems because it will help to clarify the program's relationship to other programs and processes that can be found in the same ecosystem. This understanding will, in the same vein, help evaluators to paint a more complete picture of ways in which the program, its implementation, and the accompanying evaluation complements or competes with existing priorities within the program and the larger organization. The implication of this broader view into the program is the evaluator's ability to accurately locate what motivated the evaluation, and interest holders' interest in it along with anticipated use(s) of the evaluation across the organization.

Sample Observable Actions

- The evaluator obtains an organization chart for the program and the larger organization of which it is a part.

- The evaluator interviews individuals at various levels in the organization to discern their views. Questions the evaluator could ask in these discussions include "How does this program fit with the organization's mission?"; "What is its relationship to other programs within the organization?"; "What makes it unique or similar to other programs the organization offers?"; and "How do you anticipate the program and the organization benefiting from this evaluation?"

- The evaluator asks questions like "Who does the head of this program report to?"; "What is your understanding of how they perceive the program?"; "Have you had any indication of concerns that they or other organization administrators feel about the program?"; and "Have there been any expressions of satisfaction or displays of disaffection about the program from members of the governing board?

Summary Comment

We have presented a prescriptive approach to fostering evaluation use. Precision in theory construction demands that a theory has a unique and defined focus. Our guidelines are designed to be particularly appropriate for small- and medium-scale formative and summary formative evaluations that are focused on a specific definition of evaluation use as an objective. The 12 evaluator actions are written with that context in mind. The observable actions provide examples of what might be seen or heard when the evaluation actions are implemented.

FOSTERING EVALUATION USE FOR OTHER CONTEXTS

The evaluator actions that we have presented and the attendant observable actions provide an approach to fostering evaluation use that we maintain is feasible. This may fit the reader's particular evaluation need if they are similar to what we have selected: goal, area of applicability, and evaluation type. Even then, they might need to be somewhat modified based upon the unique program and organizational context encountered.

The research factors that form the basis for this theory were derived from a variety of settings and very likely are generally applicable to large-scale and/or summative evaluations. What may be different in the effort to be responsive to other settings is the ways in which our defined evaluator actions are eventually translated into different observable actions. Different settings require different approaches. An evaluation purpose of summative evaluation rather than formative imposes different demands on the evaluator. Size of program also affects the observable actions that might be applicable (e.g., closeness to interest holders and possibilities or participation and the nature of interactions).

For example, in small-scale summative evaluations, a judgment of whether the program will continue is made at the end of the evaluation. The procedure for small-scale summative evaluations may be like small-scale formative evaluations. However, the focus is on the success of the program at meeting intended outcomes, rather than identifying areas for program improvement. In these contexts, evaluators must identify measures that will accurately capture program impact. Additionally, evaluators must focus more directly on gathering credible evidence of the program's ability to meet intended outcomes and its success.

Similarly, large-scale summative evaluations will result in a judgment about whether the program will continue. Large-scale summative evaluations can occur at the national level with large government agencies. In these contexts, interpersonal communication is more limited. Furthermore, these evaluations can be highly political and involve a variety of interested parties.

Readers considering an evaluation—any combination of small or large scale, formative or summative—should consider whether the observable actions that we have advocated are applicable. Then they may use the evaluator actions proposed and modify or create new observable actions.

USING "FOSTERING EVALUATION USE"

A few words are in order as to how you, the reader, might most beneficially use the fostering evaluation use framework that has been presented. This work might guide an evaluation practitioner as they conduct their work. Another use of this chapter is to teach students how to better attain use in their forthcoming work. Finally, this chapter might provide the stimulus and insights into potential future research that would enhance use.

Use by Evaluation Practitioners

We urge practitioners to read and understand what we mean by the *evaluator actions*. Consider whether these actions seem appropriate in the context of evaluations you conduct. Generally, they are applicable to most settings. Then turn to the *observable actions*. Are you currently doing them? Do they make sense to you and are they compatible with how you do things, your personality, and so on? Try gradually introducing them into your evaluation practice.

Further, we note that the guidelines described in this chapter only partially reflect how to do an evaluation. They only address a limited number of additional things to attend to and particular attitudes and ways of thinking. That is to say: This is only a *partial* prescriptive theory focusing on further things to attend to in seeking to foster evaluation use. The evaluator still must gain an understanding of the program, the theory of action, program-relevant questions, instruments, appropriate designs, appropriate analyses, valuing of findings, communication to interest holders, and so on. Many of these may follow naturally from the evaluator actions and specific observable actions that we have noted. These further essential elements of an evaluation are spelled out in many leading evaluation textbooks and covered in many of the chapters in this handbook.

Doing Research on Use

Factors leading to the development of evaluator actions have been identified in the research literature. However, we do not have knowledge of the specific impact of each of the research factors. Further, research might be conducted on the evaluator actions themselves. Are the translations from research factors to evaluator actions totally appropriate? Perhaps investigations of individual, or a small collection of, intentionally implemented evaluator actions could begin to shed light on ways in which they contribute to the fostering of evaluation use. Likewise, case studies of evaluator practice in various sectors and contexts could further understandings about the prevalence, form, and applicability of these suggested actions to further solidify them. Building the knowledge base on descriptive practice in these ways would directly address Miller's (2010) call for more explicitly articulated evaluation theories.

Teaching Use to New Learners

"Fostering evaluation use" is not a prescription that is to be filled—it is a *mind-set, worldview,* and *value orientation*. Attaining evaluation use demands a desire to do so. This is the most important thing to teach students, and we situate this frame of mind in our discussion of context-sensitive evaluation (Alkin & Vo, 2018)—that is, we emphasize the importance of talking about it. Showing its relevance. Promoting it as a worthy goal—indeed, it is the ultimate goal in conducting an evaluation given the definitions of evaluation noted earlier in this chapter. Fellow evaluation educators could have students read and understand these actions and observable actions. Discuss them. Finally, provide in-class or training opportunities to role-play these observable actions within evaluation simulations.

REFERENCES

Alkin, M. C. (1985). *A guide for evaluation decision makers*. SAGE.

Alkin, M. C. (1990). *Debates on evaluation*. SAGE.

Alkin, M. C. (2013). *Evaluation roots* (2nd ed.). SAGE.

Alkin, M. C., & Christie, C. A. (Eds.). (2005). Theorists' models in action. *New Directions for Evaluation, 106*.

Alkin, M. C., Christie, C. A., & Rose, M. (2006). Communicating evaluation. In I. Shaw, J. Greene, & M. Marks (Eds.), *Sage handbook of evaluation* (pp. 384–403). SAGE.

Alkin, M. C., & King, J. (2017). Definitions of evaluation use and misuse, evaluation influence, and factors affecting use. *American Journal of Evaluation, 38*(3), 434–450.

Alkin, M. C., & Vo, A. T. (2018). *Evaluation essentials: From A to Z* (2nd ed.). Guilford Press.

American Evaluation Association. (2018). Guiding principles for evaluators. Available at *www.eval.org/About/Guiding-Principles*

Boruch, R. (1997). *Randomized experiments for planning and evaluation*. SAGE.

Buchanan, H. (2015). A made-in-Canada credential: Developing an evaluation professional designation. *Canadian Journal of Program Evaluation, 29*(3), 33–53.

Chen, H. (2005). *Practical program evaluation: Assessing and improving planning, implementation, and effectiveness.* SAGE.

Cousins, J., & Earl, L. (1992). The case for participatory evaluation. *Educational Evaluation and Policy Analysis, 14*(4), 397–418.

Cousins, J., & Whitmore, E. (1998). Framing participatory evaluation. In E. Whitmore (Ed.), *New directions for evaluation: Vol. 80. Understanding and practicing participatory evaluation* (pp. 5–23). Jossey-Bass.

Cousins, J. B., & Leithwood, K. A. (1986). Current empirical research on evaluation utilization. *Review of Educational Research, 56*, 331–364.

Donaldson, S. I., Gooler, L. E., & Scriven, M. (2002). Strategies for managing evaluation anxiety: Toward a psychology of program evaluation. *American Journal of Evaluation, 23*(3), 261–273.

Family Educational Rights and Privacy Act of 1974, 20 U.S.C. § 1232g (1974).

Greene, J. C. (2005). Evaluators as the stewards of the public good. In S. Hood, R. Hopson, & H. Frierson (Eds.), *The role of culture and cultural context: A mandate for inclusion, the discovery of truth, and understanding in evaluative theory and practice* (pp. 7–20). Information Age.

Health Insurance Portability and Accountability Act (HIPAA). (2004). U.S. Department of Labor, Employee Benefits Security Administration.

House, E., & Howe, K. (1999). *Values in evaluation and social research.* SAGE.

Johnson, K., Greenseid, L. O., Toal, S. A., King, J. A., Lawrenz, F., & Volkov, B. (2009). Research on evaluation use: A review of the empirical literature from 1986 to 2005. *American Journal of Evaluation, 30*, 337–410.

Leviton, L. C., & Hughes, E. F. (1981). Research on the utilization of evaluations: A review and synthesis. *Evaluation Review, 5*, 525–548.

Love, A. (2015). Building the foundation for the CES professional designation program. *Canadian Journal of Program Evaluation, 29*(3), 1–20.

Mark, M. M., Henry, G. T., & Julnes, G. (2000). *Evaluation: An integrated framework for understanding, guiding, and improving policies and programs.* Jossey-Bass.

Mertens, D. M. (2009). *Transformative research and evaluation.* Guilford Press.

Miller, R. L. (2010). Developing standards for empirical examinations of evaluation theory. *American Journal of Evaluation, 31*(3), 390–399.

Miller, R. L., & Campbell, R. (2006). Taking stock of empowerment evaluation: An empirical review. *American Journal of Evaluation, 27*(3), 296–319.

Patton, M. Q. (2008). *Utilization-focused evaluation* (4th ed.). SAGE.

Preskill, H., & Boyle, S. (2008). A multidisplinary model of evaluation capacity building. *American Journal of Evaluation, 29*(4), 443–459.

Scriven, M. (1991). *Evaluation thesaurus* (3rd ed.). Edgepress.

Shulha, L. M., & Cousins, J. B. (1997). Evaluation use: Theory, research, and practice since 1986. *Evaluation Practice, 18*, 195–208.

Taut, S., & Alkin, M. (2010). The role of stakeholders in educational evaluation. In B. McGraw, P. Peterson, & E. Baker (Eds.), *International encyclopedia of education* (pp. 629–635). Elsevier.

Volkov, B. B., & King, J. A. (2007). *Checklist for building organizational evaluation capacity.* University of Minnesota Press.

Weiss, C. H. (1977). *Using social research in public policy making.* Lexington Books.

Weiss, C. H. (1993). Where politics and evaluation research meet. *American Journal of Evaluation, 14*(1), 93–106.

Yarbrough, D. B., Shulha, L. M., Hopson, R. K., & Caruthers, F. A. (2011). *The program evaluation standards: A guide for evaluators and evaluation users* (3rd ed.). SAGE.

Chapter 9

Illuminating Evaluation's Kaleidoscope
Beautiful, Diverse, Ever-Changing Manifestations

Michael Quinn Patton

CHAPTER OVERVIEW

This chapter examines and illuminates diverse perspectives on and dimensions of the field of evaluation: (1) using applied social science methods, (2) evaluation's development as a profession, (3) evaluation's status as a discipline and (4) transdiscipline, (5) evaluation as science, (6) evaluation as technology, (7) artistic/creative aspects of evaluation, and (8) evaluation practice. The image of an evaluation kaleidoscope is meant to convey the variations that emerge when combining these dimensions in diverse evaluation contexts and inquiries. Depicting evaluation as a kaleidoscope of diverse and many-splendored perspectives and contributions invites assessment of each element and their interrelationships.

EVALUATION AS KALEIDOSCOPE

A kaleidoscope, made up of mirrors and colored materials that reflect light, produces changing patterns when the tube is rotated thereby creating emergent patterns through the interactions of its constituent elements. Kaleidoscopic light patterns were discovered in 1816 by Scottish inventor David Brewster. He was studying the properties of light and noticed that reflected objects at the end of two mirrors created beautiful patterns. He turned this knowledge into an invention he named combing three Greek words meaning beautiful form watcher: *kalos*, meaning beautiful; *eodos*, meaning shape; and *scopeo*, to look at. This chapter looks at beautifully diverse forms of evaluation.

Jean King's chapter (see Chapter 2, this volume) on evaluator competencies highlights the diverse skills evaluators need. This chapter builds on that work by examining the dimensions of the field of evaluation more broadly. Figure 9.1 displays these kaleidoscopic elements. Imagine an evaluation kaleidoscope that turns to adapt the combination of elements and relative dominance of each one to the context in which evaluation is both receiving and reflecting *light*—illuminating evidence, findings, conclusions, judgments, and options for future action.

The thrust of this analysis of the beautifully diverse and ever-changing manifestations of *what evaluation is* will be to more fully illuminate the evaluation kaleidoscope. The result, I hope, is to ensure that evaluators can turn the

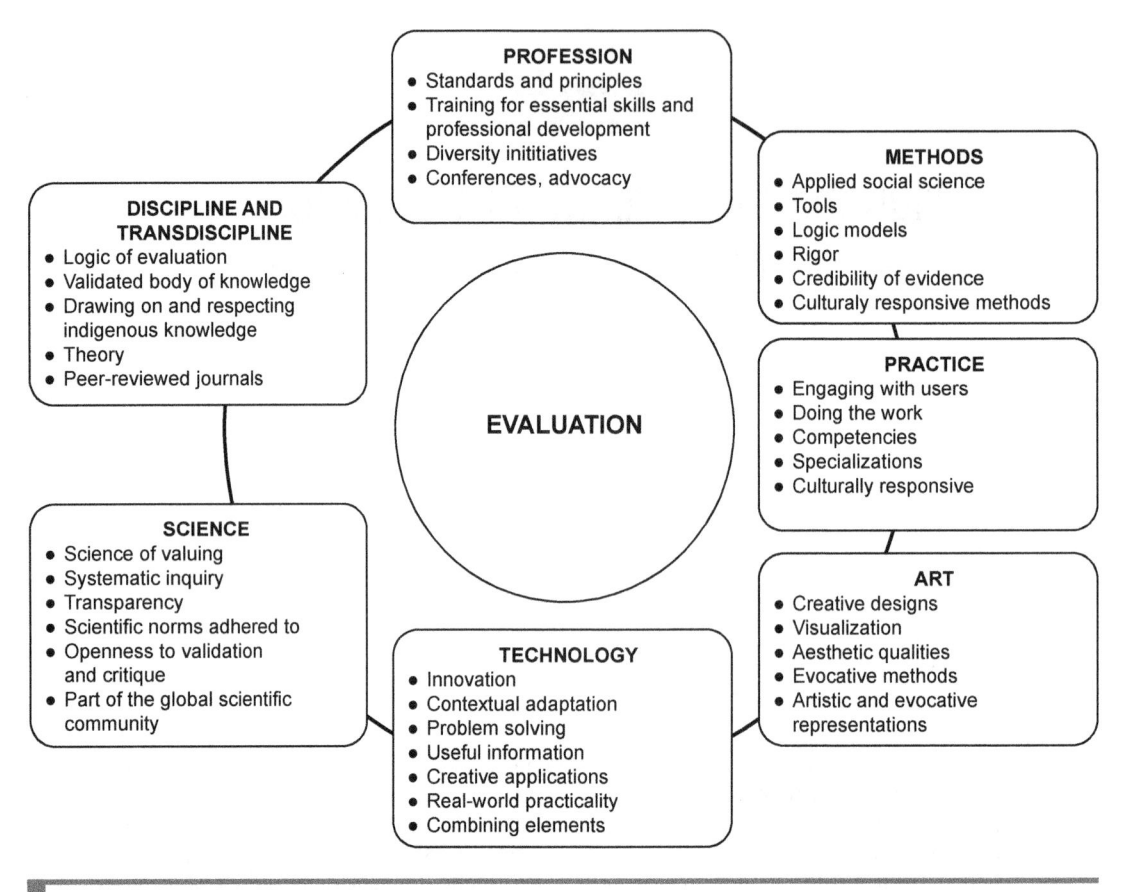

FIGURE 9.1. The evaluation identity kaleidoscope.

PROFESSION
- Standards and principles
- Training for essential skills and professional development
- Diversity inititiatives
- Conferences, advocacy

METHODS
- Applied social science
- Tools
- Logic models
- Rigor
- Credibility of evidence
- Culturaly responsive methods

DISCIPLINE AND TRANSDISCIPLINE
- Logic of evaluation
- Validated body of knowledge
- Drawing on and respecting indigenous knowledge
- Theory
- Peer-reviewed journals

PRACTICE
- Engaging with users
- Doing the work
- Competencies
- Specializations
- Culturally responsive

EVALUATION

SCIENCE
- Science of valuing
- Systematic inquiry
- Transparency
- Scientific norms adhered to
- Openness to validation and critique
- Part of the global scientific community

ART
- Creative designs
- Visualization
- Aesthetic qualities
- Evocative methods
- Artistic and evocative representations

TECHNOLOGY
- Innovation
- Contextual adaptation
- Problem solving
- Useful information
- Creative applications
- Real-world practicality
- Combining elements

kaleidoscope to match diverse evaluation situations, contexts, uses, users, and related complexities. We begin with evaluation as methods.

EVALUATION AS APPLIED SOCIAL SCIENCE METHODS

Rossi et al. (1979), in the first widely used evaluation methods textbook, *Evaluation: A Systematic Approach*, defined evaluation research as the systematic application of social science research procedures in assessing social intervention programs. The book, now in its eighth edition (Rossi et al., 2019), positions evaluation as applying social science methods. Rigorous methods, in this positioning, define evaluation quality.

In their classic review of *Foundations of Program Evaluation*, Shadish et al. (1991) observed that "as a specialty, evaluation is most like methodological specialties—ethnography, psychometrics, experimental design, or survey research" (p. 31) and

> The most widely used textbooks and sourcebooks in program evaluation deal primarily with methods. . . . The popularity of methodological books is no surprise, given that program evaluation is a pragmatic activity. Evaluation practitioners need to act and need tools to use in their daily work. Methods texts are their essential references. (p. 34)

Methodological Debates

Early in the development of evaluation, the relative merits of quantitative versus qualitative methods were debated. That debate gave way to a recognition that all methods have strengths and weaknesses, and that mixed and multiple methods are stronger than singular methods. A central argument for mixing methods comes from "Critical Multiplism" (Shadish, 1993), which argues that any single method is biased and that only by thinking critically about the strengths and weaknesses of various methods, and using multiple methods to overcome single-methods biases, can rigorous results be achieved. Over time, valuing multiple and mixed methods countered arguments about the inherent superiority of a particular method. The challenge has become choosing methods appropriate to answer priority evaluation questions with available resources to meet timelines for use.

Being practical and flexible allows one to eschew methodological orthodoxy in favor of *methodological appropriateness* as the primary criterion for judging methodological quality, recognizing that different methods are appropriate for different situations. Situational responsiveness means designing a study that is appropriate for a specific inquiry situation or interest. A wide range of possibilities exist when selecting methods. The point is to do what makes sense and report fully on what was done, why it was done, and what the implications are for making evaluative judgments.

But debate about what constitutes rigorous methods continues. The qualitative–quantitative debate has morphed into the gold-standard debate. For example, the What Works Network rates rigor and quality from low to high according to a hierarchy of evidence that places randomized controlled trials (RCTs) or a synthesis of multiple RCTs at the top of the hierarchy, followed by quasi-experimental designs, cohort studies, case-control studies, cross-sectional surveys, and case reports. What Works has 10 centers in the United Kingdom applying this hierarchy in different policy areas with over £200 (over $262) billion in funding (Marett, 2018).

While experimental evaluations are part of the evaluation toolkit, to assert an absolute hierarchy of methodological rigor ignores the need for different methods at different stages of program development and in different contexts. Rather than celebrated as the "gold standard," RCTs can be viewed as one among many options where methodological appropriateness is the standard. This means choosing the right design for the inquiry questions, nature and type of intervention, existing knowledge, available resources, the intended uses of the results, and other relevant factors. This is but a glimpse into the issues that arise in emphasizing evaluation as application of social science methods. Is evaluation a branch of social science, a specialization within applied social science? Turning the kaleidoscope, an alternative emphasis is to view evaluation as a profession.

EVALUATION AS A PROFESSION

Professional Identity

When I was president of the American Evaluation Association (AEA) in 1988, the application to join the AEA asked for primary area of specialization: education, health, psychology, sociology, economics, criminal justice, and so forth. . . . Evaluation was not among the options listed. We changed the application so that members of the AEA could identify their primary area of specialization as *evaluation*. How we identify ourselves, both individually and collectively, affects how we present ourselves to others and how they see us. We've long debated the status of evaluation: Profession? Discipline? Both? Neither? Let's consider these alternative ways of positioning evaluation. For evaluation old-timers, this will be a walk down memory lane. For youngsters, it will give you a glimpse of the history of ideas you are heir to as an evaluator.

Evaluation as a Profession

The shift from positioning evaluation as applied social science to emphasize the professional nature of evaluation was influenced, in part, by a distinction between conclusion-oriented versus decision-oriented research (Cronbach & Suppes, 1969), the former focused on informing professional judgment and the latter emphasizing research methods. The distinction proved too absolute but it did focus attention on evaluation's service purpose. Evaluators provide services to decision makers, program staff, funders, policymakers, and other interest holders. As service providers, evaluators play a professional role. Evaluation pioneer Ernie House examined evaluation's emergent professional status in 1993 and asked:

> What shape has evaluation taken as a profession? Legitimation of professional authority involves three claims: that the knowledge and

competence of the professional have been validated by a community of peers, that this consensually validated knowledge rests on scientific or scholarly grounds, and that professional judgment and advice are oriented toward important social values. In other words, a modern profession rests on collegial, cognitive, and moral authority. Evaluation has established itself as a profession in ways similar to those of the other professions—through university training, professional associations and journals, and official recognition. (p. ix)

House has long been concerned about the actual and potential co-optation of evaluation professionals in the service of funders and authorities, thus his advocacy of deliberative democratic evaluation (House & Howe, 2000). He has insisted on the importance of putting ethics at the center of the evaluation profession and emphasized our responsibility, as professionals, to serve the public interest and social justice. His own stance in this regard is a call for evaluators to engage professionally in societal issues of the day, especially racial inequality and the increasing gap between rich and poor (House, 2017; see also Morris, Chapter 7, this volume).

Skepticism about evaluation's professional status centers primarily on the lack of a credentialing process. Anyone can hang out an evaluation shingle and declare themselves an evaluator. What kind of profession is that? Or so goes the critique. The response is caveat emptor. Of course, it is altogether appropriate for evaluation, as a profession, to aspire to improvement and advancement. The work led by Jean King (2007) on essential competencies, and presented in King (see Chapter 2, this volume), is an example of such advancement and resulted in AEA membership endorsing the essential competencies (and in this handbook), but certification is nowhere in sight in the United States. Canada, New Zealand, and Japan have been leaders in developing evaluation competency frameworks and voluntary certification. The United Nations Evaluation Group has competencies for both evaluators and commissioners of evaluation. These frameworks specify competencies in (1) methods, (2) professional practice, (3) interpersonal skills, (4) project management, and (5) context sensitivity (see King, Chapter 2, this volume).

The AEA endorsed cultural competence in evaluation in 2011. The AEA statement explains:

To draw valid conclusions, the evaluation must consider important contributors to human behavior, including those related to culture, personal habit, situational limitations, assimilation and acculturation, or the effect of the evaluand. Without attention to the complexity and multiple determinants of behavior, evaluations can arrive at flawed findings with potentially devastating consequences. (p. 2)

Bob Picciotto (2011), former director of the Independent Evaluation Group of the World Bank, drew on the sociological literature on professions to examine the intersection between evaluation and professionalism, identify the extent to which evaluation fulfills the main attributes of professionalism, and apply logical models of professionalism to the practice of independent and self-evaluation. He concluded that without meeting "the imperative of occupational self-management" evaluation "is highly vulnerable to capture by vested interests" (p. 165):

Evaluation is not a profession today but it could be in process of becoming one. Much remains to be done to trigger the latent energies of evaluators, promote their expertise, protect the integrity of their practice and forge effective alliances with well-wishers in government, the private sector and the civil society. It will take strong and shrewd leadership within the evaluation associations to strike the right balance between autonomy and responsiveness, quality and inclusion, influence and accountability. (p. 179)

In a wide-ranging chapter examining evaluation professionalization for the book *The Future of Evaluation* (Stockman & Meyer, 2016). Wolfgang Meyer (2016) judges professionalization by the criteria of having standardized training programs for developing professional expertise, offering a "homogeneous bundle of well-weighted general and specific competences which [sic] give the participants a relevant, unique and applicable profile," professional identity and language, and "expert autonomy in a difficult expert–client relationship." Using these criteria, Meyer concludes that the state of evaluation professionalization "is poor." With particular attention to university-based training programs, he judges evaluation professionalization to be in a state of "stagnation" (p. 109).

On the other hand, the existence of over 130 voluntary organizations for professional evaluation at the national and regional levels around the world, and emergence of the International Organization for Cooperation in Evaluation, demonstrates the global reach of the profession with estimates of more than 50,000 practicing evaluation professionals worldwide. The quality of professional training and practice will, and should, be a matter of ongoing concern but the trajectory of the profession strikes me as impressive.

Thinking of ourselves as professionals, or more specifically, as members of a global professional community, does not seem to come naturally for evaluators. For some years, I have taught a course at The Evaluators' Institute on how to become a consultant. One of the exercises participants undertake is crafting an elevator speech to introduce themselves as an evaluator to a stranger. Having heard hundreds of such presentations, I don't recall any that included being a member of a global evaluation profession, one with standards, principles, journals, conferences, and professional development opportunities. Thus, while we may debate our professional strengths and weaknesses internally, and do so appropriately with an eye toward improvement and advancement, to the outside world, including funders, commissioners of evaluation, users, and the general public, I think it behooves us to present ourselves as a profession—without reservation—a profession that is still developing, improving, and striving for advancement but our professional status is not in doubt, at least in my view.

EVALUATION AS A DISCIPLINE AND TRANSDISCIPLINE

Another turn of the kaleidoscope brings us to evaluation as discipline. Disciplines, given birth by the mother of all disciplines, philosophy, can be distinguished by their core burning questions. For sociology, the burning question is the Hobbesian question of order: What holds society or social groups together and what keeps societal groups from falling apart? Psychology asks why individuals think, feel, and act as they do. Political science asks "What is the nature of power, how is it distributed, and with what consequences?" Economics studies how resources are produced and distributed. Disciplines and subdisciplines reveal layers of questions. Biologists inquire into the nature and variety of life. Botanists ask how plants grow, while agriculturists investigate the production of food, and agronomists narrow their focus still further to field crops (Patton, 2015, pp. 97–98).

To be sure, reducing any complex and multifaceted discipline to a single burning question oversimplifies the focus of that discipline. But what is gained is clarity about what distinguishes one lineage of inquiry from another. It is precisely that clarity I strive for in identifying the burning questions that distinguish major lineages of inquiry such that evaluation can be recognized as a discipline. Evaluation's burning disciplinary question is "What are the factors that contribute to, methods for determining, and criteria for judging interventions' successes and failures?" Interventions are any effort, program, project, initiative, product, policy, organization or community development, or activity aimed at bringing about change. As a professional practitioner, an expert evaluator knows how to conduct an evaluation of a particular intervention in a particular context for a particular purpose. As an evaluation scholar in the *discipline of evaluation*, a knowledgeable evaluator contributes to and has access to a *body of knowledge* about ways of studying and judging interventions and ways of applying knowledge to design and improve interventions, both based on empirically and theoretically validated patterns of successes across interventions and evaluations. It is because evaluation has become a reservoir of knowledge about effectiveness that we are consulted about how to design, plan, and implement new interventions, not just evaluate them once implemented.

In their classic *Foundations of Program Evaluation: Theories of Practice*, Shadish et al. (1991) examined evaluation as a methodological specialty and a profession of practice but it was evaluation theory made coherent by a validated body of knowledge that made evaluation a discipline:

Program evaluators are slowly developing a unique body of knowledge that differentiates evaluation from other specialties while corroborating its standing among them. Evaluation is diverse in many ways, but its potential for intellectual unity is what Scriven calls "the logic of evaluation," which might bridge disciplinary boundaries separating evaluators. (p. 31)

They identified five fundamental issues that are at the core of evaluation's disciplinary body of knowledge:

1. *Social programming*: ways that social programs and policies develop, improve, and change, especially in regard to social problems.
2. *Knowledge construction*: the ways researchers learn about social action.
3. *Valuing*: the ways value can be attached to program descriptions.
4. *Knowledge use*: the way social science information is used to modify programs and policies.
5. *Evaluation practice: the tactics and strategies evaluators following the professional work, given the constraints a face.* (p. 32)

The body of knowledge accumulated around these five conceptual issues constitute evaluation's distinctive theory. Specific approaches to addressing and understanding these issues is what distinguish particular evaluation theories.

More than a decade later, Alkin (2004) created an evaluation theory tree providing both the conceptual framework and image for evaluation's body of knowledge based on attention to evaluation use, evaluation methods, and valuing—the three branches of the theory tree. They subsequently expanded the theory tree with recent and international contributors to evaluation's body of knowledge (Alkin, 2013). The third edition of the book maps theories rather than theorists, an important shift in emphasis from spotlighting people to highlighting ideas and approaches (Alkin & Christie, 2023).

Stufflebeam et al. (2000), Madaus et al. (2012), and Stufflebeam and Coryn (2014) are among many other examples of efforts to document, capture, synthesize, and report evaluation's rapidly evolving body of knowledge represented by diverse viewpoints, models, methods, and approaches. The disciple of evaluation has handbooks (Guttentag & Struening, 1975; Shaw et al., 2006; Kellaghan & Stufflebeam, 2003; Newcomer et al., 2015), an encyclopedia (Mathison, 2005), and peer-reviewed journals (e.g., *American Journal of Evaluation, New Directions for Evaluation, Evaluation, Evaluation Review,* and *Evaluation and Program Planning*). Our disciplinary stature is solid and growing as evidenced in this handbook.

Pioneering evaluation thought leader and philosopher Michael Scriven (2004) posits four criteria to merit disciplinary status:

1. A distinguishable subject matter.
2. Subject-specific methods.
3. Substantial field of application.
4. Production of results that serve substantial social and/or intellectual improvement.

He finds that evaluation meets all of these criteria (p. 186). In Scriven's (1993) masterful and enduring "Hard-Won Lessons in Program Evaluation" treatise, he sings such praises of evaluation as a discipline as to make a shy evaluator blush, to wit:

Evaluation, the ugly frog, turns into a prince when the spell on us is broken. Evaluation is all that distinguishes astronomy from astrology, good explanations from bad ones, good experimental designs—or bridge designs—from inferior ones, good scientists and engineers and technologists from run-of-the-mill ones. It is a discipline that is part of every discipline because it distinguishes the discipline from pretentious jargon, just as one distinguishes good food from garbage. (pp. 47–48)

In this way Scriven (2013) eloquently and forcefully envisions and advocates positioning evaluation as the *alpha transdiscipline*: As a transdiscipline, evaluation sits atop the disciplinary, scholarly, and academic hierarchy with philosophy, logic, and statistics as bodies of knowledge, theory, and methods that are essential for the scholarship and knowledge creation of all other disciplines. Evaluation is the *alpha* transdiscipline because "its domain includes the methodology of the task of validation at any discipline's claim to legitimacy as a discipline: it is the master of credentials" (Scriven, 2013, p. 175).

Here again, as with evaluation's professional status, academics will argue among themselves about whether, and the extent to which, evaluation is a discipline. Arguing about definitions and boundaries is what academics do, and I've had my share of fun so indulging. But to the outside world, when I am talking about evaluation, I proclaim, assert, and celebrate without reservation evaluation's disciplinary status as a theory-based body of knowledge. Our peer-reviewed journals capture, adjudicate, and report that body of knowledge. The nature and depth of our disciplinary status may be a matter for academic debate but the fact that we have a reservoir of disciplinary theory and knowledge should, from my perspective, be part of our public persona and identity to the larger world.

Still, Scriven's argument primarily concerns evaluation's status and function within academia and the scientific community. The case for evaluation as science and evaluators identifying themselves as scientists concerns how we present ourselves to the larger world, how we join with scientific specializations under the common banner of "science," and why we should do so. To that issue, I now turn.

EVALUATION AS SCIENCE

On April 22, 2017, millions marched for science in 600 cities worldwide (*New York Times*, 2017). The AEA was one of 270 partner organizations that supported the March for Science. One of the central issues that emerges in focusing on evaluation methods as the defining characteristic of the field is whether those methods are sufficiently rigorous to be considered worthy of the designation science. Science, in this tradition, is often equated with the scientific method. "When conducting research, scientists use the scientific method to collect measurable, empirical evidence in an experiment related to a hypothesis (often in the form of an if/then statement), the results aiming to support or contradict a theory" (Bradford, 2015, p. 1).

We have long debated whether we are a profession, discipline, or specialization within applied social science. These distinctions matter within academia and contention about evaluation's academic status and professional stature will no doubt continue. But the stakes have changed. Science is under attack. Culturally and politically, the anti-science trends include "alternative facts," "fake news," and a "post-truth" world. In November, 2016, Oxford Dictionaries announced *post-truth* as its international Word of the Year.

> **post-truth** *adjective:* Relating to or denoting circumstances in which objective facts are less influential in shaping public opinion than appeals to emotion and personal belief.

Casper Grathwohl, president of *Oxford Dictionaries*, explained: "Given that usage of the term hasn't shown any signs of slowing down, I wouldn't be surprised if *post-truth* becomes one of the defining words of our time" (Grathwohl, 2016).

While evaluators continue to split hairs and parse terms about how we position ourselves within the ivy walls and debate our professional status in conferences, the current anti-science political climate calls us to unite with others engaged in defending and supporting science, creating a *united front to the larger world*—for example, "I am an evaluation scientist. I do evaluation science. I join with other scientists and supporters of science to defend and support science."

In what follows I consider the case for **evaluation science** (Patton, 2018; Patton & Campbell-Patton, 2022). This requires examining what science is, what evaluation is, and thereby, what evaluation science is, or might be. I also address arguments to the contrary, that evaluation is not science. I then consider how thinking of evaluation as science complements but is different from thinking of evaluation as a profession, discipline, or applied social science.

What Is Science?

> Science is the intellectual and practical activity encompassing the systematic study of the structure and behavior of the physical and natural world through observation and experiment. 2. Science is a systematically organized body of knowledge on a particular subject. (Online dictionary, 2017)

> *Science:* systematized knowledge derived from observation, study, and experimentation carried on in order to determine the nature of principles of what is being studied. (Webster's New World Dictionary, 1982, p. 1275)

The *Random House Unabridged Dictionary* defines science as

> A branch of knowledge or study dealing with a body of facts or truths systematically arranged . . . ; Systematized knowledge in general; knowledge, as of facts or principles; knowledge gained by systematic study; a particular branch of knowledge. (Stein & Urdang, 1966)

In the same citation, a scientist is defined as an expert in science. A scientist, it turns out, is a person who works in and has expert knowledge of a particular field of science, or more generally, any person who studies or works in a scientific field.

Evaluation Science

In considering whether evaluation is science, and whether evaluators are scientists, two distinct levels of social construction are involved. First, individual evaluators decide how to identify themselves within their own contexts and frames of reference. Second, as a community of practitioners and members of a professional evaluation association, we construct and establish shared norms about what it means to be an evaluator. A critical mass of individuals taking a position together creates a shared community perspective, though not everyone will agree with whatever that perspective may be. How we perceive and identify ourselves, at both the individual and collective levels, affects how others view us. Both how we view ourselves, and how others view us, has social, cultural, economic, academic, and political implications. The Thomas theorem applies: What is perceived as real is real in its consequences (Thomas & Thomas, 1928, p. 572).

The core consequence of perceiving and asserting evaluation as science, I am suggesting here, is that it enhances our credibility, responsibility, capability, and effectiveness in supporting the importance of science in our world and brings us together with other scientists to make common cause in supporting and advocating for science. That is a potential political consequence, as is AEA's endorsement of the March for Science on behalf of the evaluation community. There are other consequences we'll explore, like communicating our role more clearly and credibly to those who value science but haven't thought of evaluation as a scientific activity. Viewing evaluation as science may also have consequences for how we are viewed, treated, positioned, and located in academic institutions, government agencies, and by funders and users of evaluation. So, with that introduction of what is at stake, I turn to defining evaluation science.

Earlier, I presented dictionary definitions of science. There are variations on the precise wording in different dictionaries, but the consistent theme is systematic inquiry to understand and explain how some aspect of the world works. Evaluators do that. Indeed, the first AEA Guiding Principle on *systematic inquiry* states "Evaluators conduct systematic, data-based inquiries about what is being evaluated."

The Science Council defines science as "the pursuit and application of knowledge and understanding of the natural and social world following a systematic methodology based on evidence" (*www.sciencecouncil.org/about-us/our-definition-of-science*). Data and evidence are foundations of evaluation practice. Common signs at the March for Science were "Evidence NOT Ideology" and "Data NOT Dogma."

Defining Evaluation Science

Based on common understandings, perceptions, wisdom about, and definitions of science and evaluation, I proffer a working definition of evaluation science:

> *Evaluation science is systematic inquiry into the merit, worth, and significance of whatever is being evaluated by adhering to scientific norms that include employing logic, using transparent methods, subjecting findings to verification, and providing evidence to support reason-based valuing and judgment; evaluation science generates and applies knowledge based on the science of valuing.*

Here's a version of the elevator speech I used during the March for Science:

> *Science is systematic inquiry into how the world works. Evaluation science is systematic inquiry into how, and how well, interventions aimed at changing the world work.*

How does characterizing evaluation as science compare and contrast to other ways of describing evaluation? I review major alternatives before returning to the pros and cons of evaluation as science.

Foundations of Evaluation Science

Stewart Donaldson's (2007) book on program theory-driven evaluation science defined the term as follows:

> *Evaluation science* (instead of evaluation) is intended to underscore the use of rigorous scientific methods (i.e., qualitative, quantitative, and mixed-method designs) to attempt to answer valued evaluation questions. A renewed emphasis in evaluation practice on relying on systematic, scientific methods is especially important for overcoming the profession's negative reputation in some contexts. That is, in some settings, evaluation is criticized for being an unreliable, soft, or second-class type of investigation. The term *evaluation science* signals the emphasis placed on the guiding principle of systematic inquiry (Guiding Principles for Evaluators, 2004) and the critical evaluation standard of accuracy (Joint Committee on Standards for Educational Evaluation, 1994). (p. 11; emphasis in original)

Donaldson's book provides important guidance for the practice of evaluation science, especially highlighting program theory as the centerpiece of such practice. He began deliberately using the terminology "evaluation science" as he encountered evaluation in academic settings being treated as second-class, not really science. Since having taken to referring to what he does as "evaluation science," he reports gaining credibility and greater acceptance among social and behavioral scientists with whom he interacts (Donaldson, 2017). The issue here is our identity as much as our practice.

The Science of Evaluation: A Realist Manifesto by Ray Pawson (2013) offers another window into the practice of evaluation science. He examines whether evaluation has produced a cumulative and authoritative body of knowledge deserving of the designation evaluation science. He provides a detailed blueprint for an evaluation science based on realist principles. Though his primary concern is with making the case for realist evaluation as the primary legitimate and credible approach to evaluation science, his positive experience explaining evaluation inquiry as worthy of scientific designation merits our attention.

Michael Scriven pioneered treating evaluation as the science of valuing (Shadish et al., 1991, p. 74). Scriven (2004) has reflected that "much of my early work in evaluation was devoted to attacking various attempts to . . . marginalize evaluation into the category of decision-support apparatus, *by contrast with* truth-seeking efforts of 'true science' " (p. 188; emphasis in original). For Scriven (2013), evaluation is without question "*scientifically legitimate*. . . . The bottom line . . . is that a competent program evaluator can show that, for example, a program for teaching reading is truly excellent or truly worthless *as a matter of scientific fact*" (p. 171; emphasis in original).

Scriven (1976) does not aspire to have evaluation become more like science, for he has long been scathing in his critique of shoddy reasoning and judgment in much scientific practice. Rather, he challenges science to become more evaluative. Indeed, he is critical of evaluators for failing to recognize evaluation's preeminent scientific status:

> Some leading texts on evaluation describe evaluation as a branch of social science, which is surely not true since the social sciences have no methodology for dealing with evaluative propositions, and are only partially recovered from the days when they put all evaluation in the untouchable class. I would like to see the exact reverse of this relationship come to pass. . . . [Instead of] the view of evaluation fields as being satellites circling social science's sun. I think a more appropriate model is the reverse. (p. 20)

As for scientists' failure to recognize evaluation as science, his eloquence resists summary:

> The status of evaluation in the twentieth century represents one of the most striking paradoxes in the history of thought: An essential—and perhaps the most important—ingredient in all intellectual and practical activity has been explicitly banned or implicitly excluded from discussion or acknowledgment in most of its natural territory.
>
> The psychological, social, and political reasons, as well as the intellectual ones, for this bizarre situation—for this "intellectual treason of

the intellectuals" ... [has come with enormous cost] ... If the status of evaluation as an "untouchable" subject is to be radically changed, there must be a direct attack on the myths responsible for this paradox, and there must also be works that set out the elements of an alternative view of evaluation, a view of it as perhaps the most important and pervasive process in which the human mind is capable. (Scriven, 1991, p. 10)

You can see how Scriven (1993) builds on that judgment to assert evaluation's rightful status as the alpha transdiscipline of all sciences, which means it must, logically, be a science:

What science should be is an evaluative decision, and it is hard to argue that there is a more important kind of decision anywhere in science. This is the decision, or a refinement of it, after all, that we call on many of our peer review panels to make. In particular we ask them to review the scientific *quality* of the proposals in front of them. They are indeed evaluators, and on them and on their peers on editorial boards and appointment committees rest the whole definition and quality of science, and eventually the whole future of science—and of mathematics, and engineering, and technology. . . . Science is at its core as well as in all of its applications an evaluative enterprise.

If science is an evaluative enterprise, then where in the whole of science and scientific training is the training in evaluation? It is not there. (p. 48)

The Ascendance of Scientific Designation as a Source of Legitimacy

Language matters. Evaluation language matters.
—RODNEY HOPSON (2000)

Precedent-setting examples of branding a field as science include policy science (Lasswell, 1970) and action science (Argyris et al., 1985). New fields of inquiry and practice are flourishing—and asserting their legitimacy by taking on the moniker of science:

- Complexity science (Jensen, 2023)
- Cognitive science (*www.cognitivesciencesociety.org*)
- Improvement science (Christie et al., 2017)
- Implementation science (Eccles & Mittman, 2006)
- Translational science (Pardridge, 2003)
- Urban science (Townsend, 2015)
- Management and service science (Management and Service Science, 2017)
- The sciences of learning and instructional design (Lin & Spector, 2017)
- Developmental science (Nelson et al., 2016)
- Community science (Chavis, 2015)
- Big data science (*https://datascience.berkeley.edu/what-is-big-data*)

Viewing evaluation science as the alpha transdiscipline à la Scriven, these could all be considered specializations within evaluation science, and *evaluation science* might well be the umbrella under which they all operate. Let's take a closer look at one such new specialty: *sustainability science*:

Sustainability science has developed from a new research field into a vibrant discipline in its own right, with scientific conferences, journals and scientific societies dedicated to its pursuit. Characterized more by its research purpose than by a common set of methods or objects, sustainability science can be subdivided into the more traditional disciplinary-based science for sustainability and the transdisciplinary science of sustainability. Whereas the former consists of more descriptive, analytical and basic science, the latter is characterized by reflexivity and applicability; on a meta level, the emergence of the latter can be understood as a new step in the evolution of science. (Spangenberg, 2011, p. 275)

With all these emergent self-designated scientific arenas, who decides what field of inquiry is worthy of the designation science? Sustainability science offers one pathway:

Like "agricultural science" and "health science," sustainability science is a field defined by the problems it addresses rather than by the disciplines it employs. In particular, the field seeks to facilitate what the National Research Council has called a "transition toward sustainability," improving society's capacity to use the earth in ways that simultaneously "meet the needs of a much larger but stabilizing human population, . . . sustain the life support systems of the planet, and . . . substantially reduce hunger and poverty." (Clark, 2007, p. 1738)

In early 2005, the National Academy of Sciences approved a new section on sustainability science, which now shares the masthead of the *Proceedings of the National Academy of Sciences* with other long-term residents, such as physics, genetics, and cell biology.

EVALUATION AS TECHNOLOGY

> While evaluation has been practiced for many years, it is only now developing into a discipline. In this way evaluation resembles technology, which existed for thousands of years before there was any substance to the discussion of its nature, its logic, its fundamental differences from science, and the details of its distinctive methods and thought.
> —MICHAEL SCRIVEN (2004, p. 185)

Thus far, we've looked at evaluation as methods (applied social science), a profession, a discipline, a transdiscipline, and as science. Johnny Morell, distinguished recipient of the AEA Paul F. Lazarsfeld Evaluation Theory Award, argues that there is another aspect of evaluation's status that should also be considered—namely, its technological nature. He says that he likes to introduce himself as an engineer. What kind of engineer? Electrical? Civil? Environmental? Chemical? No, none of these. An evaluation engineer (Morell, 2017).

Morell (1979) examines the basic philosophical model of knowledge seeking upon which outcome evaluation is based, how questions are formulated, how variables are chosen, and what decision rules are used to weigh evidence, draw conclusions, and make recommendations. He concludes that the answers to these questions reflect a philosophical model of research that is fundamentally technological in nature:

> There are three main aspects to the argument. . . . First, there are crucial differences between scientific and technological models of knowledge development. Second, these differences have profound implications for the practical value of research. Third, evaluation is far more of a technological than a scientific pursuit. (p. 1)

After systematically comparing science and technology, and the implications of each for evaluation, Morell concludes that because evaluation is a form of inquiry aimed at testing the effectiveness of efforts at solving social problems, evaluation must generate information that is useful to intended users. To do so, evaluation must adapt to ever-changing political, social, and economic constraints.

The scientific model, with its main goals of advancing truth and theory development, is attuned to surmounting those constraints by developing artificial situations that interact as little as possible with the practical world. Although scientists . . . may be interested in helping with practical issues, the logical structure of their work is oriented toward goals that are, at best, irrelevant to the development of innovations that will survive the rigors of wide-scale implementation. Hence the need for conceptualizing evaluation as technology, a system in which the reward structure and the use of resources are intimately attuned to the issues involved in developing and testing practical innovations (Morell, 1979, p. 120).

A parallel perspective emphasizes the technological nature of medicine. In her highly respected *History of Medicine*, Jacalyn Duffin (2010) asserts: "Medicine is not a science; rather, it is an applied technology or an art that makes extensive use of science" (p. 65).

Jane Fields and Tim Sheldon (2017) use a technological lens to communicate about their evaluation of EngrTEAMS, a 5-year, $8 million project funded by the National Science Foundation, designed to increase students' learning of science content, as well as mathematical concepts related to data analysis and measurement. Because the program uses an engineering design-based approach to teacher professional development and curriculum development, they do the same for the evaluation:

> With EngrTEAMS, we recognized early on that the steps in an evaluation cycle are closely aligned to the steps of the engineering design process. . . . Focusing the evaluation design is similar to the planning stage in the engineering design process. Gathering credible evidence, justifying conclusions, and using the lessons learned are similar to the solution phases in the EngrTEAMS design process of trying, testing, and deciding. When we were able to demonstrate that the problem-solving process used in evaluation was similar to that used in their engineering design framework, program staff easily saw the connections and were even more

receptive to the evaluation side of the work. (p. 1)

Morell's (1979) full rationale for viewing evaluation as technology is available online and provides a comprehensive review of the implications of technological versus scientific identity and practice. Interestingly, science and technology are so closely associated in the public mind, and apparently among policymakers, that the American Association for the Advancement of Science (AAAS; 2017) integrates science and technology in its mission statement:

> The AAAS seeks to "advance science, engineering, and innovation throughout the world for the benefit of all people." To fulfill this mission, the AAAS board has set the following broad goals (partial list)
> - Enhance communication among scientists, engineers, and the public.
> - Strengthen support for the science and technology enterprise.
> - Strengthen and diversify the science and technology workforce.
> - Foster education in science and technology for everyone.
> - Increase public engagement with science and technology.

The essence of both science and technology is reality testing. Richard Phillips Feynman, 1965 recipient of the Nobel Prize in Physics, observed that "For a successful technology, reality must take precedence over public relations, for Nature cannot be fooled." This comment was occasioned by his involvement in the presidential commission inquiring into the explosion of the space shuttle *Challenger* following a cold-weather liftoff on January 28, 1986. Professor Feynman's demonstration of reality versus public relations came during the televised hearings on the cause of the *Challenger* disaster:

> Interrupting the ponderous, defensive proceedings, he put a sample of the rubber used for the booster rockets' O-ring seals into a glass of ice water, then clamped the sample and released it; the rubber had lost its resilience. A month later NASA conceded that the joint failure was the most likely cause of the explosion. (Miner & Rawson, 2000, p. 441)

Technology is certainly subject to evaluation, as is evaluation viewed as technology.

EVALUATION AS ART (CRAFT)

Lee J. Cronbach (1982), introduced earlier in this volume as an evaluation pioneer and author of several major books on measurement and evaluation, observed that designing an evaluation is as much art as science: "Developing an evaluation is an exercise of the dramatic imagination" (p. 239). This perspective can help free practitioners and other primary users who are nonresearchers to feel they have something important to contribute. It may also open the evaluator to valuing their contributions and facilitating their "dramatic imaginations."

Another distinguished evaluation pioneer, Bob Stake (1995), has emphasized that qualitative methods and responsive evaluation involve substantial creativity: "Finishing a case study is the consummation of a work of art" (p. 136).

The art of evaluation involves creating a design that is appropriate for a specific situation and particular action or policymaking context. In art there is no single, ideal standard. Beauty is in the eye of the beholder, and the evaluation beholders include decision makers, policymakers, program managers, practitioners, participants, and the general public. Thus, any given design is necessarily an interplay of resources, possibilities, creativity, and personal judgments by the people involved (Patton, 2008, p. 393). The increased emphasis on data visualization is grounded in creative and artistic renderings of findings. *Creative Evaluation* (Patton, 1981) invites attention to the artistic dimensions of evaluation practice.

EVALUATION AS PRACTICE

Scholars of decision making and expertise have found that what distinguishes people with great expertise is not that they have more answers than others but they are more adept at situational recognition and more intentional about their decision-making processes (Klein, 1999). We can, in fact, come to recognize our heuristic tendencies and learn to identify the heuristic processes that determine our impressions, and to make appropriate allowances for the biases to which our thought processes make us liable (Tversky & Kahneman, 1974, pp. 1124–1125). We can do this through ongoing and in-depth reflective practice to become reflective practitioners (Schön, 1983, 1987). We can do this by systematically evaluating our evaluation work, engaging in case learning (Patrizi & Patton, 2005), and deconstructing our design tendencies and methodological decision making. I reiterate the overall point here. Our evaluation practice depends on using some set of theoretical screens and constructs that operate through decision heuristics, cognitive algorithms, paradigm parameters, and contingency-based, satisficing, and bounded rationality shortcuts. The issue is whether and how we become more intentional and deliberative about how we practice. Toward that end, I share the results of my own journey toward such greater intentionality and deliberativeness in my own evaluation situation recognition and decision-making processes.

Utilization Heuristic

Basically, the utilization heuristic for managing situational complexity in **utilization-focused evaluation** is to stay focused on use (Patton & Campbell-Patton, 2022). For every issue that surfaces in evaluation negotiations, for every design decision, for every budget allocation, and for every choice among alternatives, keep asking, "How will this affect use in this situation?" But upon further reflection, I have discovered that I apply the utilization heuristic through six conceptual screens that guide and inform my situation recognition about what to do.

Figure 9.2 presents my practice framework for utilization-focused evaluation. It presents the six conceptual screens that, in combination, as near as I can tell, constitute my practice situation recognition framework: (1) intended users' contingencies, (2) nature of the evaluand, (3) evaluation purpose: findings use options, (4) process options, (5) context and situational contingencies, and (6) evaluator characteristics. I hasten to add that I offer this scheme as an example of what a practice framework might look like and to encourage evaluators to become intentional, explicit, and deliberate about their own practice algorithms and heuristics. I am not suggesting that others adopt the framework in Figure 9.2. It is meant to stimulate reflection and discussion, not pose as a prescriptive framework for adoption. Given limitations of space, I discuss each one only briefly.

Intended Users' Contingencies

Situation analysis starts for me in identifying and engaging the primary intended users of the evaluation: their perspectives, commitment, capacity, interest, and power, all personal factor considerations (Patton, 2012, pp. 61–85; Patton & Campbell-Patton, 2022, Ch. 6).

Nature of the Evaluand

What is being evaluated? A beginning point for situation recognition in contingency theory is the extent to which the evaluand is, or aspires to be, a standardized, high-fidelity, best-practice model versus an innovative, adaptive set of principles that are implemented variously depending on context.

Evaluation Purpose: Findings Use Options

The purpose of an evaluation conditions the use that can be expected of it. Specific inquiry questions flow from intended use. Eleanor Chelimsky (1997, 2006, 2007) pioneered the importance of distinguishing evaluation purposes and the implications of different purposes for how an evaluation is conducted. Accountability evaluations serve a purpose quite different from improvement-oriented evaluations. Knowledge generation has emerged as one of the principal purposes of evaluation. Being clear about an evaluation's purpose is central to evaluating the

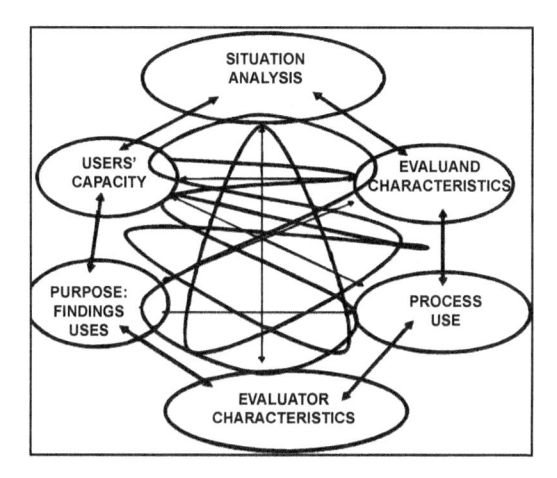

FIGURE 9.2. Reflective practice framework for understanding utilization-focused evaluation practice decision making.

evaluation and the source of our own professional accountability (Patton, 2012, pp. 113–138; 2022a, 2022b). Chelimsky (1983) has posited that the most important kind of accountability in evaluation is use that comes from "designed tracking and follow up of a predetermined use to predetermined user." She calls this a "closed-looped feedback process" in which "the policy maker wants information, asks for it, and is interested in and informed by the response" (p. 160). This perspective solves the problem of defining use, addresses the question of who the evaluation is for, and builds in evaluation accountability since the predetermined use becomes the criterion against which the success of the evaluation can be judged. Such a process has to be planned and evaluated.

Process Options

How an evaluation is conducted varies along many dimensions, including the extent to which the process is completely independent versus highly interactive. Interactive, participatory, collaborative, empowerment, and **developmental evaluations** are heavily relationship based. Evaluators work closely with intended users to build trusting, mutually respectful, and close working relationships (Patton, 2011; Patton, 2012, pp. 140–166; Patton & Campbell-Patton, 2022, Ch. 2). Credibility, and therefore utility, are affected by "the steps we take to make and explain our evaluative decisions, [and] also intellectually, in the effort we put forth to look at all sides and all interest holders of an evaluation" (Chelimsky, 1995, p. 219).

Context and Situational Contingencies

The theme of the 2009 AEA annual conference was "Context and Evaluation." AEA president Debra J. Rog articulated the challenge of taking context seriously:

> Context has multiple layers and is dynamic, changing over time. Increasingly, we are aware of the need to shape our methods and overall approach to the context. Each of the dimensions within the context of an evaluation influences the approaches and methods that are possible, appropriate, and likely to produce actionable evidence.

In understanding context to inform situation analysis, I have found it helpful to distinguish simple, complicated, and complex situations (Patton, 2011, Ch. 4; Patton, 2012, pp. 253–258). Simple, complicated, and complex is not a taxonomy of operationally distinct, mutually exclusive and exhaustive categories. Rather, the distinctions constitute a typological continuum. In working with clients on these distinctions, it is illuminating to engage them in the discussion about what aspects of what they do are relatively simple, relatively complicated, and relatively complex. First, staff do not typically agree about which is which, so that discussion itself is illuminating. And there are clear evaluation implications for aspects of interventions that are simple, complicated, and complex. Different kinds of evaluation designs are called for under different conditions and in varying contexts.

Chelimsky has argued insightfully that the strength of an evaluation is context dependent. The judgment that an evaluation is "strong" can only be made within some context where the kind of strength manifest is appropriate to the situation. The strength of an evaluation has to be judged within the context of the question, the time and cost constraints, the design, the technical adequacy of the data collection and analysis, and the presentation of the findings. A strong study is technically adequate and useful.

Evaluator Characteristics

> Know thyself [γνῶθι σεαυτόν in Greek].
> —Inscription in ancient Temple of Apollo at Delphi

My final practice screen involves thinking about how well my approach would fit with the context, intended users, evaluation findings, process options, and nature of the evaluand. Does the evaluation interest me? Would I learn from it? Would it engage my capacities? I took on a major meta-evaluation of the evaluation of the Paris Declaration primarily because the nature, scope, and challenges would expand my horizons (Patton, 2013). The capacity to reflect on our practice and on the underlying theories that inform our practice—and taking the time to do so—is a critical characteristic on which evaluators vary. The term *reflexivity* has entered the evaluation lexicon as a way of emphasizing the importance of deep introspection, political consciousness, cultural awareness, and ownership of one's perspective. Reflexivity calls on us to think about how we think and inquire into our thinking patterns even as we apply thinking to making sense of the patterns we observe around us. Being reflexive involves self-questioning and self-understanding, including "critical self-reflection on one's bases, theoretical predispositions, preferences, and so forth" (Schwandt, 2007, p. 260). Reflexivity reminds us as evaluators to be attentive to and conscious of the cultural, political, social, linguistic, and economic origins of our own perspective and voice as well as the perspective and voices of those with whom we engage. This is emphasized in the AEA Evaluator Competencies (see King, Chapter 2, this volume). To excel in integrating theory with practice requires astute self-awareness. It turns out that people who excel in all kinds of endeavors share the quality of being self-aware and using that awareness to adapt to whatever presents itself in the course of taking action (Sweeney & Gosfield, 2013).

Evaluation Practice Specializations

Evaluators are an eclectic group working in diverse arenas using a variety of methods drawn from a wide range of disciplines applied to a vast array of efforts aimed at improving the lives of people in places throughout the world. Over the last 50 years, evaluation has become characterized by specialized areas of practice and theory. For example, the AEA has over 50 topical interest groups—subgroups of evaluators with specialized interests and capabilities. Many specializations are sector specific: education, health, criminal justice, human services, social work, arts and culture, environment, business, technology, disaster and emergency assistance, and international development. Some specializations focus on particular evaluation methods: quantitative methods, qualitative methods, mixed methods, social network analysis, experimental designs, performance measurement, systems in evaluation, and data visualization.

Evaluation niches include targeting evaluations for specific populations and institutions: people with disabilities; youth; the poor and disadvantaged; indigenous people; lesbian, gay, bisexual, and transgender people; military and veterans; underrepresented populations; policy-makers and leaders; philanthropic foundations, nonprofits, government programs, and private sector evaluation; and extension services and higher education, including science, technology, engineering, and mathematics programs. Then there are subgroups that have formed around specialized issues facing evaluators: evaluation theories, program design, use and influence of evaluation, multiethnic issues, ethics, needs assessments, translational research, international and cross-cultural evaluation, empowerment, collaboration, theory-driven evaluation, teaching evaluation, organizational learning, capacity building, democracy and governance, evaluating advocacy, and integrating technology into evaluation. In addition to program evaluation, the broader field includes product evaluation, personnel evaluation, policy evaluation, and specializations in evaluating strategy, organizational effectiveness, community change, and sustainability development goals.

In the chapter on evaluation focus options in *Utilization-Focused Evaluation* (Patton, 2008), I identified and discussed 80 different evaluation options, including summative evaluation, formative evaluation, developmental evaluation, participatory evaluation, outcomes evaluation, process evaluation, cost–benefit evaluation, internal evaluation, external evaluation, realist evaluation, quality assurance, responsive evaluation, independent evaluation, real-world evaluation, accountability, monitoring, knowledge-generating evaluation, and utilization-focused evaluation. This broad panorama of evaluation types, approaches, methods, models, and specializations is one set of refracting crystals that gives evaluation its kaleidoscopic complexity (Patton, 2022a, 2022b).

WHAT I SEE WHEN I LOOK THROUGH THE EVALUATION KALEIDOSCOPE

I introduced the evaluation kaleidoscope earlier, in Figure 9.1, to present the elements that define evaluation: using social science methods, development as a profession, status as a discipline, evaluation as science, evaluation as technology, the art of evaluation, and evaluation practice. I invited you to imagine turning the evaluation kaleidoscope to adapt the combination of elements and relative dominance of each one to the context in which you are working. Depicting evaluation as a kaleidoscope of diverse and many-splendored perspectives and contributions invites assessment of each element and their interrelationships. Table 9.1 describes what I see when I look through the evaluation kaleidoscope and turn it circularly from one element to the next. I invite you to make your own assessments.

I opened with the invention of the kaleidoscope by David Brewster. In 1817 he patented his creation, but apparently worded the patent application incorrectly, which made it easy for others to copy without legal recourse. As a result, he saw no financial gain from his invention but could revel in the popularity that ensued. Kaleidoscopes became popular during the Victorian age as an amusement for children and adults. In 1980 a first exhibition of kaleidoscopes helped fuel renewed interest and elevated the making of kaleidoscopes to an art form. Today there are hundreds of great kaleidoscope makers and artists. I daresay there are thousands of evaluators engaged in kaleidoscopic design, creating new patterns of illumination by integrating diverse elements of this many-splendored and multifaceted thing we call evaluation. It's just that most don't know they're *kaleidoscopers*. Now, perhaps, they will.

TABLE 9.1. Looking through the Evaluation Kaleidoscope to the Future

Evaluation perspective	Status assessment and future challenges
1. Evaluation as methods and tools	1. Methods and tools proliferating; the hunger for tools is insatiable; mixed methods have become accepted as legitimate and desirable; methodological appropriateness has replaced the notion of a methods hierarchy (gold standard privileging certain designs over others). Rossi's "good enough" rule prevails: "Choose the best possible design taking into account practicality and feasibility" (Shadish et al., 1991, p. 377).
2. Evaluation as a profession	2. Evaluation's Standards and Principles widely acknowledged and accepted; professional development opportunities expanding nationally and globally; diversity initiatives gaining traction and seeing results; essential skills conceptualization is crystalizing what evaluators need to know and be able to do to be effective. The AEA and other voluntary organizations for professional evaluation becoming increasingly respected and effective. However, the notion of credentialing and certifying evaluators remains controversial and the focus of those who dissent from recognizing evaluation as having achieved full professional status.
3. Evaluation as a disciple	3. Evaluation's body of knowledge, theories of evaluation, and scholarly contributions are increasingly recognized. However, evaluation is viewed largely as a specialty in other disciplines, not as a discipline in its own right. The academic status of evaluation in universities remains fragile and dependent on the whims of deans and department heads.
4. Evaluation as a transdiscipline	4. The logic that evaluation is essential to every other discipline is irrefutable. But few evaluators can articulate why and how evaluation is a discipline, much less a transdiscipline. The hutzpah needed to assert evaluation's alpha transdisciplinary status is largely absent among meek evaluators who are shy about asserting even professional status for evaluation; recognition as the alpha transdiscipline is viewed as hallucinogenic by all but the most visionary.
5. Evaluation as science	5. Rumblings are being heard; the idea remains largely emergent, but as the demonstrable need grows for solidarity in support of science, there is reason to hope evaluators, and the evaluation community, will join in common cause against anti-science and post-truth forces.
6. Evaluation as technology	6. Silicon Valley has yet to call. But they should. We have a lot to offer technologically.
7. Evaluation as art	7. The artistic dimensions of evaluation are evident in creative thinking and adaptive designs, evocative communications, data visualization, artistic representational aesthetics, dramatic imagination, creative syntheses, and creative evaluations (Patton, 1981; Patton, 2015, pp. 687–690).
8. Evaluation as practice	8. Essential competencies having been identified and adopted by the AEA, the challenge ahead is supporting use of the competencies to inform practice.

Additional Resources

Blackburtn, S. (2005). *Truth: A guide.* Oxford University Press.

Cronbach, L. J. (1980). *Toward reform of program evaluation.* Jossey-Bass.

Dangermond, J. (2017). *The science of where.* Available at *www.esri.com/videos/watch?channelid=UC_yE3TatdZKAXvt_TzGJ6mw&playlistid=PLaPDDLTCmy4b4_faC7—TcEP9OMcUXXYU&title=esri-2017-uc-plenary*

Eyben, R., Guijt, I., Roche, C., & Shutt, C. (2015). *The politics of evidence and results in international development: Playing the game to change the rules?* Practical Action.

Goldacre, B. (2009). *Bad science.* Fourth Estate.

Harris, R. F. (2017). *Rigor mortis: How sloppy science creates worthless cures, crushes hope, and wastes billions.* Basic Books.

Koch, R. (2014). *The 80/20 principle and 92 other powerful laws of nature: The science of success.* Brealey.

Lincoln Motor. (2017). The science of seduction of luxury. *New York Times.* Available at *https://paidpost.nytimes.com/lincoln/the-science-and-seduction-of-luxury.html*

Mann, T. (2017). *Secrets from the eating lab: The science of weight loss, the myth of willpower, and why you should never diet again.* HarperCollins.

Matthews, M. (2016). *Bigger leaner stronger: The simple science of building the ultimate male body.* Waterbury.

Nelson, T. (2017, June 28). *Minnesota scientist says EPA pressured her to change congressional testimony.* Minnesota Public Radio. Available at *www.mprnews.org/story/2017/06/28/minnesota-scientist-says-epa-pressured-her-to-change-congressional-testimony*

Offit, P. (2017). Pandora's lab: Seven stories of science gone wrong. *National Geographic.*

Olmstead, M. (2017). *Seeking the unheard voices of science: How science journalists consider diversity when finding sources.* Available at *https://mospace.umsystem.edu/xmlui/bitstream/handle/10355/61082/ProjectReport.pdf?sequence=1*

Partnow, E. (Ed.). (1977). *The quotable woman: An encyclopedia of useful quotations, Vol. 1, 1800–1899.* Pinnacle Books.

Patton, M. Q. (2014). What brain sciences reveal about integrating theory and practice. *American Journal of Evaluation, 35*(2), 237–244.

Peter, L. J. (1977). *Peter's quotations: Ideas for our time.* Bantam Books.

Phillips, D. J. P. (2017). The science of storytelling: Key neurological findings on storytelling. Available at *www.youtube.com/watch?v=NjhdQMa3uA*

Roach, M. (2017). *GRUNT: The curious science of humans at war.* Norton.

Scriven, M. (2003). Differences between evaluation and social science research. *The Evaluation Exchange IX* (4, winter). Harvard Family Research Project.

Simon, H. (1957). *Administrative behavior.* Macmillan.

Simon, H. (1978). On how we decide what to do. *Bell Journal of Economics, 9,* 494–507.

Southqwick, S. M., & Charney, D. S. (2012). *Resilience: The science of mastering life's greatest challenges.* Cambridge University Press.

Time Magazine. (2017a). *The science of exercise: Younger, smarter, stronger.* Author.

Time Magazine. (2017b). *The science of happiness: New discoveries for a more joyful life.* Author.

Tversky, A., & Kahneman, D. (2000). Advances in prospect theory: Cumulative representation of uncertainty. In D. Kahneman & A. Tversky (Eds.), *Choices, values, and frames* (pp. 44–65). Cambridge University Press.

Van Edwards, V. (2017). The science of storytelling. Available at *www.scienceofpeople.com/2017/01/the-science-of-storytelling*

Wattles, W. D. (2009). *The science of getting rich.* Thrifty Books.

Weiss, C. (2002). Less learned: A comment. *American Journal of Evaluation, 23*(2), 229–230.

Wheeling, K. (2017, June 30). EPA creates initiative dedicated to questioning climate science. *Pacific Standard.* Available at *https://psmag.com/environment/scott-pruitts-epa-working-to-undermine-climate-science*

Wootton, D. (2015). *The invention of science: A new history of the scientific revolution.* Harper.

Young, S. D. (2017). *Stick with it: A scientifically proven process for changing your life—for good.* Harper.

REFERENCES

American Association for the Advancement of Science. (2017). *Mission and history.* Available at *www.aaas.org/about/mission-and-history*

American Evaluation Association. (2011). *Public statement on cultural competence in evaluation.* Available at *www.eval.org*

Alkin, M. C. (Ed.). (2004). *Evaluation roots: Tracing theorists' views and influences.* SAGE.

Alkin, M. C. (Ed.). (2013). *Evaluation roots* (2nd ed.). SAGE.

Alkin, M. C., & Christie, C. A. (Eds.). (2023). *Evaluation roots: Theory informing practice (3rd ed.). Guilford Press.

Argyris, C., Putnam, R., & Smith, D. M. (1985). *Action science*. Jossey-Bass.

Bradford, A. (2015). *Science & the scientific method: A definition*. LiveScience. Available at *www.livescience.com/20896-science-scientific-method.html*

Chavis, D. (2015). Community science. Available at *www.communityscience.com*

Chelimsky, E. (1983). Improving the cost effectiveness of evaluation. In M. C. Alkin & L. C. Solomon (Eds.). *The costs of evaluation* (pp. 149–170). SAGE.

Chelimsky, E. (1995). *The political environment of evaluation and what it means for the development of the field*. American Evaluation Association Presidential Address, November, Vancouver, Canada. *Evaluation Practice, 16*(3), 215–225.

Chelimsky, E. (1997). The coming transformations in evaluation. In E. Chelimsky & W. Shadish (Eds.), *Evaluation for the 21st century*. SAGE.

Chelimsky, E. (2006). The purposes of evaluation in a democratic society. In I. F. Shaw, J. C. Greene, & M. M. Mark (Eds.), *The SAGE handbook of evaluation: Policies, programs and practices* (pp. 33–55). SAGE.

Chelimsky, E. (2007). Factors influencing the choice of methods in federal evaluation practice. *New Directions for Program Evaluation, 113*, 13–33.

Christie, C. A., Inkelas, M., & Lemire, S. (Eds.). (2017). Improvement science in evaluation: Methods and uses. *New Directions for Evaluation*, No. 153.

Clark, W. C. (2007). Sustainability science: A room of its own. *Proceedings of the National Academy of Sciences, 104*(6), 1737–1738.

Cronbach, L. J. (1982). *Designing evaluations of educational and social programs*. Jossey-Bass.

Cronbach, L. J., & Suppes, P. (1969). *Research for tomorrow's schools: Disciplined inquiry for education*. Macmillan.

Donaldson, S. I. (2007). *Program theory-driven evaluation science: Strategies and applications*. Erlbaum.

Donaldson, S. I. (2017, June 20). *Evaluation science*. AEA eStudy webinar.

Duffin, J. (2010). *History of medicine* (2nd ed.). University of Toronto Press.

Eccles, M. P., & Mittman, B. S. (2006). Welcome to implementation science. *Implementation Science, 1*(1). Available at *https://implementationscience.biomedcentral.com/articles/10.1186/1748-5908-1-1*

Fields, J., & Sheldon, T. (2017, July 9). *Aligning concepts and language demystifies evaluation* [AEA365 blog]. Available at *http://aea365.org/blog/aligning-concepts-and-language-demystifies-evaluation-by-jane-fields-and-tim-sheldon/?utm_source=feedburner&utm_medium=email&utm_campaign=Feed%3A+aea365+%28AEA365%29*

Grathwohl, C. (2016). "Post-truth" declared word of the year by Oxford Dictionaries. BBC News. *www.bbc.com/news/uk-37995600*

Guttentag, M., & Struening, E. (Eds.). (1975). *Handbook of evaluation research*. SAGE.

Hopson, R. (Ed.). (2000). How and why language matters in evaluation. *New Directions for Evaluation*, No. 86.

House, E. (1993). *Professional evaluation: Social impact and political consequences*. Sage.

House, E. R. (2017). Evaluation and the framing of race. *American Journal of Evaluation, 38*(2), 167–189.

House, E. R., & Howe, K. R. (2000). Deliberative democratic evaluation. *New Directions for Evaluation, 85*, 3–12.

Jensen, H. J. (2023). *Complexity science: The study of emergence*. Cambridge University Press.

Kellaghan, T., & Stufflebeam, D. (Eds.). (2003). *International handbook of educational evaluation*. Springer.

King, J. A. (2007). Developing evaluation capacity through process use. *New Directions for Evaluation, 116*, 45–59.

Klein, G. (1999). *Sources of power: How people make decisions*. MIT Press.

Lasswell, H. D. (1970). *Policy sciences*. Available at *www.policysciences.org*

Lin, L., & Spector, J. M. (Eds.). (2017). *The sciences of learning and instructional design: Constructive articulation between communities*. Routledge.

Madaus, G. F., Scriven, M., & Stufflebeam, D. L. (Eds.). (2012). *Viewpoints on educational and human services evaluation: Vol. 6. Evaluation models*. Springer Science and Business Media.

Management and Service Science. (2017, October 23–25). *Management and service science*. 11th International Conference on Management and Service Science, Guilin, China. Available at *www.engii.org/conference/MASS/?utm_campaign=mass&utm_source=e_cp&utm_medium=conf_mass_d2_20170718_pan_119747*

Marett, G. (2018, December). *Growing the evidence base through evaluation* [ARDT Consultants blog]. Available at *https://artd.com.au/growing-the-evidence-base-through-evaluation/16:225*

Mathison, S. (Ed.). (2005). *Encyclopedia of evaluation*. SAGE.

Meyer, W. (2016). Toward professionalization? The contribution of university-based training programs in pioneer countries. In R. Stockman & W. Meyer (Eds.), *The future of evaluation: Global trends, new challenges, shared perspectives* (pp. 98–112). Palgrave Macmillan.

Miner, M., & Rawson, H. (Eds.). (2000). *The new international dictionary of quotations* (3rd ed.). Signet.

Morell, J. (1979). Evaluation as social technology. Available at *https://evaluationuncertainty.com/evaluation-as-social-technology*

Morell, J. (2017, June 22). *Evaluation science*. AEA eStudy Webinar.

Nelson, C. A., de Haan, M., & Quinn, P. C. (Eds.). (2016). *Developmental science*. Wiley.

Newcomer, K. E., Hatry, H. P., & Wholey, J. S. (Eds.). (2015). *Handbook of practical program evaluation* (5th ed.). Wiley.

Pardridge, W. M. (2003). Translational science: What is it and why is it so important? *Drug Discovery Today, 8*(18), 813–815.

Patrizi, P., & Patton, M. Q. (Eds.). (2010). Evaluating strategy, New Directions for Evaluation, No. 120 (Winter).

Patton, M. Q. (1981). *Creative evaluation*. Sage.

Patton, M. Q. (2008). *Utilization-focused evaluation* (4th ed.). SAGE.

Patton, M. Q. (2011). *Developmental evaluation: Applying complexity concepts to enhance innovation and use*. Guilford Press.

Patton, M. Q. (2012). *Essentials of utilization-focused evaluation* (4th ed.). SAGE.

Patton, M. Q. (2013). Metaevaluation: Evaluating the evaluation of the Paris Declaration. *Canadian Journal of Program Evaluation, 27*(3), 147–171.

Patton, M. Q. (2015). *Qualitative research and evaluation methods* (4th ed.). SAGE.

Patton, M. Q. (2018). Evaluation science. *American Journal of Evaluation, 39*(2), 183–200.

Patton, M. Q. (2022a). *The panorama of evaluation approaches*. YouTube video. Available at *https://youtu.be/GEGtBnkDyBk*

Patton, M. Q. (2022b). *Why so damn many options: The 10 competing values that explain the panoramic evaluation landscape*. YouTube video. Available at *https://youtu.be/YReAFxv_31s*

Patton, M. Q., & Campbell-Patton, C. E. (2022). *Utilization-focused evaluation: Premises and principles* (5th ed.). SAGE.

Pawson, R. (2013). *The science of evaluation: A realist manifesto*. SAGE.

Picciotto, R. (2011). The logic of professionalism. *Evaluation, 17*(2), 165–180.

Rog, D. (2009). *Context and evaluation*. Presidential explanation of the American Evaluation Association annual meeting theme.

Rossi, P. H., Freeman, H. E., & Wright, S. R. (1979). *Evaluation: A systematic approach*. Sage.

Rossi, P. H., Lipsey, M., & Henry, G. (2019). *Evaluation: A systematic approach*. Sage.

Schön, D. (1983). *The reflective practitioner: How professionals think in action*. Basic Books.

Schön, D. A. (1987). *Educating the reflective practitioner*. Jossey-Bass.

Schwandt, T. (2007). *The Sage dictionary of qualitative inquiry* (3rd ed.). SAGE.

Scientists Feeling Under Siege, March Against Trump Policies. (2017, April 22). *New York Times*. Available at *www.nytimes.com/2017/04/22/science/march-for-science.html?emc=edit_nn_20170426&nl=morning-riefing&nlid=44499219&te=1&_r=0*

Scriven, M. (1976). *Reasoning*. McGraw-Hill.

Scriven, M. (1991). *Evaluation thesaurus*. SAGE.

Scriven, M. (1993). Hard-won lessons in program evaluation. *New Directions for Program Evaluation, 58*, 1–57.

Scriven, M. (2004). Reflections. In M. Alkin (Ed.), *Evaluation roots: Tracing theorists' views and influences* (pp. 183–195). SAGE.

Scriven, M. (2013). Conceptual resolutions and evaluation: Past, present, and future. In M. Alkin (Ed.), *Evaluation roots* (2nd ed., pp. 167–179). SAGE.

Shadish, W. (1993). Critical multiplism: A research strategy and its attendant tactics. *New Directions for Program Evaluation, 60*, 13–57.

Shadish, W. R., Cook, T. D., & Leviton, L. C. (1991). *Foundations of program evaluation: Theories of practice*. SAGE.

Shaw, I. F., Greene, J. C., & Mark, M. M. (Eds.). (2006). *The Sage handbook of evaluation: Policies, programs and practice*. SAGE.

Spangenberg, J. H. (2011). Sustainability science: A review, an analysis and some empirical lessons. *Environmental Conservation, 38*(3), 275–287.

Stake, R. E. (1995). *The art of case study research*. Sage.

Stein, J., & Urdang, L. (Eds.). (1966). *The Random House dictionary of the English language* (unabridged ed.). Random House.

Stockmann, R., & Meyer, W. (2016). The future of evaluation: Global trends, new challenges and shared perspectives. In R. Stockmann & W. Meyer (Eds.), *The future of evaluation*. Palgrave Macmillan.

Stufflebeam, D. L., & Coryn, C. L. S. (2014). *Evaluation theory, models, and applications* (2nd ed.). Jossey-Bass/Wiley.

Stufflebeam, D. L., Madaus, G. F., & Kellaghan, T. (Eds.). (2000). *Evaluation models: Viewpoints on educational and human services evaluation*. Kluwer.

Sweeney, C., & Gosfield, J. (2013). *The art of doing: How superachievers do what they do and how they do it so well*. Penguin.

Thomas, W. I., & Thomas, D. S. (1928). *The child in America: Behavior problems and programs*. Knopf.

Townsend, A. (2015). The future of urban science. Available at *www.citiesofdata.org/report-the-future-of-urban-science*

Tversky, A., & Kahneman, D. (1974). Judgment under uncertainty: Heuristics and biases. *Science, 185*(4157), 1124–1125.

Webster's New World Dictionary. (1982). *Science*. Simon & Schuster.

Part III

ANSWERING EVALUATION QUESTIONS
DESIGNS, METHODS, AND ANALYSES

Chapter 10

Collaborative, Participatory, and Empowerment Evaluation

From Community Consultation to Community Control

David M. Fetterman
Liliana Rodríguez-Campos
Ann P. Zukoski

CHAPTER OVERVIEW

Community consultation to control approaches to evaluation engage people and help address pressing social issues. These approaches value community knowledge and local control. They are designed to ensure that the appropriate people are identified, involved, and in many cases, in control of the evaluation. In addition, these approaches contribute to program improvement, build capacity, and produce sound results. Collaborative, participatory, and empowerment evaluations are believed to be more credible than traditional approaches in culturally diverse contexts and communities. They give voice to previously marginalized populations, honoring the knowledge held within communities. They cultivate a sense of ownership, which increases the probability of use and programmatic sustainability.

Community consultation to control approaches to evaluation are designed to ensure that the appropriate people are identified, involved, and in many cases, in control of the evaluation. Community members using this approach, are in a position to inform evaluation design and implementation. The findings and recommendations are credible because they were generated from within the group or community. Ownership increases the probability that community interest holders will use the findings and accept the recommendations. The degree and type of community involvement varies, depending on the approach needed. Community interest holders may include policy decision makers, funders, program staff members, clients, and community members.

There is a continuum of community involvement approaches to evaluation, ranging from primary interest holders being consulted to assuming complete control of the evaluation (with the assistance of a trained evaluator). Community involvement approaches are also committed to varying levels of evaluation capacity building, ranging from enhancing skills to nurturing an evaluative way of thinking. Archibald et al. (see Chapter 3, this volume) provide more information about evaluative thinking. These approaches support sustainability because community interest holders are able to use this capacity long after the formal evaluation has been completed.

Community consultation to control-oriented evaluators enlist or simply support and coach people as they identify a question, problem, or challenge; develop a methodology; implement an evaluation; and interpret, share, or apply evaluation findings and recommendations. Community interest holders may serve on evaluation steering committees, become co-principal investigators, or be responsible for the evaluation (with evaluator guidance). Most approaches help to institutionalize evaluation (e.g., contributing to accreditation task forces, cultivating communities of practice, and launching learning organizations).

COMMUNITY CONSULTATION TO CONTROL APPROACHES

There are many types of community consultation to control approaches to evaluation. A few include collaborative, participatory, and empowerment evaluation. One essential way to highlight the difference between approaches is to focus on the role of the evaluator:

• **Collaborative evaluators** are *in charge* of the evaluation, but they create an ongoing engagement between evaluators, staff members, and participants, contributing to stronger evaluation designs, enhanced data collection and analysis, and results that people understand and use (Rodríguez-Campos et al., 2018; O'Sullivan, 2018). Collaborative evaluation covers the broadest scope of practice, ranging from an evaluator's consultation with the client to full-scale collaboration with specific staff members and participants in every stage of the evaluation (Rodríguez-Campos, 2018; Rodríguez-Campos & O'Sullivan, 2010).

• **Participatory evaluators** *jointly share* control of the evaluation. Participatory evaluations include program staff members and participants, as well as relevant community interest holders, in an evaluation that is jointly designed and implemented by the evaluator and program staff members. Participatory evaluators encourage participants to become actively engaged in defining the evaluation, developing instruments, collecting and analyzing data, and reporting and disseminating results (Guijt, 2014; Shulha, 2010; Zukoski & Bosserman, 2018; Zukoski & Luluquisen, 2002). Typically, "control begins with the evaluator but is divested to program community members over time and with experience" (Cousins et al., 2013, p. 14).

• Empowerment evaluators view *program staff members, program participants, and community members as in control* of the evaluation. However, empowerment evaluators serve as critical friends or coaches to help keep the process on track, rigorous, responsive, and relevant. Empowerment evaluations are not conducted in a vacuum. They are conducted within the conventional constraints and requirements of any organization. Program staff and participants remain accountable to meeting their goals. However, program staff and participants are also in the best position to determine how to meet those external requirements and goals (Fetterman & Wandersman, 2005, 2010, 2018; Fetterman, Kaftarian, et al., 2015).

Community consultation to control approaches have clear distinctions between them, as demonstrated. However, in many respects these approaches have more in common than the differences that distinguish them from one another. For example, community involvement approaches are in alignment with the philanthropic sectors' commitment to community power. They appreciate community knowledge and recognize the need for communities to guide the development of interventions and solutions to their own problems. In addition, each approach has articulated a set of guiding principles that are used to inform evaluation practice.

Substantial underlying similarities can be surfaced with even a cursory review of each of the approaches' principles. For example, explicitly, they share many of the same principles, including involvement, community, staff member, and participant interest holder focus, capacity building, valuing community knowledge, learning, and improvement. In addition, depending on the circumstances and context, they each may share principles of empowerment and social justice. Implicitly, they share the following principles:

trust, ownership, qualifications, empathy/sympathy, and democratic participation.

GUIDING PRINCIPLES IN COMMON

The American Evaluation Association (AEA) Collaborative, Participatory, and Empowerment Evaluation Topical Interest Group generated a list of principles in common,[1] with their corresponding definitions (see Fetterman et al., 2018). This list of guiding principles in common was further refined and prioritized.[2] Principles held in common across approaches (70–92% in agreement) included the following:

- **Capacity building**—enhance the community interest holders' ability to conduct evaluation and to improve program planning and implementation.
- **Improvement**—help people improve program performance; help people build on their successes and reevaluate areas meriting attention.
- **Evaluation use**—helping people use evaluation to inform decision making, program planning and implementation, and strategic planning.
- **Trust**—treating people honestly, fairly, and reliably to build relationships such that people can take risks and depend on each other.
- **Organizational learning**—data should be used to evaluate new practices, inform decision making, and implement program practices; evaluation is used to help organizations learn from their experience (building on successes, learning from mistakes, and making mid-course corrections).
- **Community knowledge**—respect and value community knowledge.
- **Accountability**—focus on outcomes and accountability; did the program or initiative accomplish its objectives.
- **Empathy**—demonstrate sensitivity and understanding, concerning the feelings of others.
- **Evidence-based strategies**—respects and uses the knowledge base of scholars (in conjunction with community knowledge).
- **Sustainability**—focused on helping people continue their work for the long term (beyond initial pilot program or seed money).

Principles held in common at the 45–66% level included social justice, democratic participation, community ownership, competence, empowerment, social support, and self-determination (see also Emerson, 1993, concerning self-reliance). The Black Lives Matter-led racial justice movement generated in large part as a result of George Floyd's death in 2020; high-profile entertainers and athletes openly spouting antisemitic tropes; anti-Asian violence; and the rising hatred directed against the lesbian, gay, bisexual, transgender, queer or questioning, plus community have thrust social justice and related principles deeper into the heart of community consultation to control approaches. *Empowerment Evaluation and Social Justice: Confronting the Culture of Silence* (Fetterman, 2023) reflects the increasing centrality of social justice principles in community, staff member, and program participant interest holder approaches to evaluation.

An additional list of principles and attributes guiding the membership (based on the survey results) includes equity, accessibility, results, cultural competence, integrity, fairness, standards, diversity, open communication, resilience, ethics, transformativeness, transparency, respect, accuracy, collaborativeness, humility, courage, engagement, and humor.

AEA GUIDING PRINCIPLES

The majority of community consultation to control approach evaluators (95%) stated they were also guided by the AEA Guiding Principles. In addition, empowerment evaluation explicitly adheres to the spirit of the Joint Committee on Standards for Educational Evaluation (2011), concerning utility, feasibility, propriety, and accuracy (see Fetterman, 2001, pp. 87–99).

---

[1] The American Evaluation Association's Collaborative, Participatory, and Empowerment Evaluation Topical Interest Group held several conference sessions over a 5-year period, focusing on "features in common." They generated a list of principles associated with each approach, highlighting the most important principles guiding their work.

[2] CPE conducted a survey of its membership based on this list of "most important" guiding principles. This refined the list of principles guiding interest holder involvement approaches.

SHARED METHODS AND SKILLS

In addition to principles, community consultation to control evaluators use many of the same methods in practice. This is in part because the approaches are more about a systematic way of thinking and practicing evaluation than they are about the use of particular methods. For example, they all use qualitative and quantitative methods.

Typical methods used across approaches include literature searches, data collection (e.g., surveys, interviews, observations, storytelling, photo voice, and fieldwork), and analysis. Tools include self-rating exercises, logic models, **dialogue**, document review, and dashboards to monitor performance. Equipment includes flip chart paper, computers, smartphones with cameras, digital recorders, and poster boards to record group exchanges. Qualitative data analysis software includes NVivo, Atlas.ti, MAXQDA, and HyperResearch. Quantitative software includes Excel, SAS, and SPSS. Web-based tools include videoconferencing and email to facilitate communication (e.g., Zoom, Google Meet, Skype, and Gmail). Online surveys are used to take the pulse of the group, program, and community (e.g., SurveyMonkey, Qualtrix, and Google Forms). Collaborative documents, spreadsheets, and slide sharing software are used to encourage participation, build rapport, and enhance quality. Blogging, social media, and infographics/data visualization are used to report on progress, problems, and accomplishments. Artificial intelligence is rapidly being used to generate logic models, theories of change, conduct analyses, and even draft reports.

Facilitation skills are required in all community consultation to control approaches to evaluation, given the diversity of most groups and the vested interests entrenched in program and community dynamics. The ability to work within and across communities is critical. Research and management skills are also an absolute requirement. Cultural sensitivity and competence are needed. A nonjudgmental approach is highly valued. Interpersonal communication skills, verbal and written skills, and a concern and deep respect for other people are also required. Fundamentally, however, one of the most important skills among these approaches is the ability to share and/or relinquish power. Strategies for developing this skill and others are explored in the sections to follow and in the community consultation to control literature (Fetterman & Wandersman, 2018; Fetterman, 2023; Fetterman, Kaftarian, et al., 2015; Rodríguez-Campos, 2005; Rodríguez-Campos & Rincones-Gómez, 2013).

COLLABORATIVE, PARTICIPATORY, AND EMPOWERMENT EVALUATION

A comparison of the major community consultation to control approaches provides an insight into how they are conducted. The comparison also highlights the range and variability of community interest holder approaches used and is aimed at helping evaluators select the most appropriate community consultation to control approach for the task at hand.

Collaborative Evaluation

Collaborative evaluation is practiced in the United States and in countries around the world, such as Brazil, Chile, China, Costa Rica, Ecuador, Korea, Puerto Rico, Saudi Arabia, Spain, and Vietnam. It has been applied to a wide variety of settings, including business, nonprofit, and education (Rodríguez-Campos, 2015). In the last decade, due to an increasing desire for people to have a voice concerning the development and implementation of programs designed to assist them, collaborative evaluation has grown in popularity along with similar approaches, bringing together evaluators, program staff members, and participant interest holders from different disciplines and cultures to exchange knowledge on how collaboration can be used as a strategic tool for fostering and strengthening evaluation practice (Rodríguez-Campos & Rincones-Gómez, 2016). This approach has a growing number of supporters and has benefited immensely from feedback by colleagues (e.g., Arnold, 2006; Bledsoe & Graham, 2005; Cousins et al., 1996; Fetterman & Wandersman, 2007; Gajda, 2004; Gloudemans & Welsh, 2015; Green et al., 1996; Guerere & Hicks, 2015; Martz, 2015; Morabito, 2002; O'Sullivan & Rodríguez-Campos, 2012; Ryan et al., 1998; Scriven, 1994; Stufflebeam & Shrinkfield, 2007; Veale et al., 2001; Yeh, 2000).

Definition

Collaborative evaluation involves a substantial degree of collaboration between evaluators, program staff members, and participant interest holders throughout the evaluation process to the extent that they are willing and capable of being involved (e.g., Cousins et al., 1996; O'Sullivan, 2004; Rodríguez-Campos, 2005; Rodríguez-Campos & Rincones-Gómez, 2013, 2016). Collaborative evaluators are in charge of the evaluation but they create an ongoing engagement between evaluators, staff members, and program participant interest holders, contributing to results that are understood and used. A collaborative evaluation fosters personal, team, and organizational learning (Morabito, 2002).

Advantages

Collaborative evaluation is an approach, based on field experience, that offers access to information, quality of information gathered, opportunities for creative problem solving, and receptivity to findings. This approach distinguishes itself in that it uses a sliding scale for levels of collaboration, as different evaluations experience different levels of collaboration. For instance, the range can be from an evaluator's consultation with a client to a comprehensive collaboration concerning all phases of an evaluation (planning, executing, and reporting). Collaborative evaluation assumes that active, ongoing involvement between evaluators, staff members, and program participant interest holders results in stronger evaluation designs, enhanced data collection and analysis, and results that people understand and use.

Disadvantages

Collaborative evaluations cover a broad scope of practice but are typically conducted with the involvement of smaller groups or populations. In addition, they take more time than traditional evaluations, and less time than participatory or empowerment evaluations. Building trust is critical, as it is in traditional evaluation approaches, but once again, requires additional time not always allotted in traditional approaches. The cost of not allowing the requisite time is poor-quality data, minimal ownership, and reduced effectiveness. Managing expectations can be complex and may shift during the course of an evaluation as **collaboration members (CMs)** become more proficient in their roles. Interest holders may seek more opportunities to build capacity than is available during the course of an evaluation.

Essential Features

Collaborative evaluation's essential features include its conceptual framework, principles, roles, and specific steps. These features provide an insight into the nature of collaborative evaluation. (See Rodríguez-Campos & Rincones-Gómez, 2013; Rodríguez-Campos, 2015, for a more detailed description.)

CONCEPTUAL FRAMEWORK

There are several collaboration frameworks that could be used and adapted. For instance, the **model for collaborative evaluations (MCE)** is a comprehensive framework for guiding collaborative evaluations in a precise, realistic, and useful manner (e.g., Rodríguez-Campos, 2005, 2008, 2015; Rodríguez-Campos & Rincones-Gómez, 2013). This model has a systematic structure and revolves around a set of six interactive components specific to conducting collaborative evaluations, providing a basis for decision making. The MCE helps to establish priorities in order to achieve a supportive evaluation environment, with a special emphasis on collaboration. The MCE has been used in multisite and multiyear evaluations, at the national and international levels, and for both formative and summative purposes.

Figure 10.1 provides the conceptual framework for viewing the MCE components interactively: (1) identify the situation, (2) clarify the expectations, (3) establish a collective commitment, (4) ensure open communication, (5) encourage effective practices, and (6) follow specific guidelines. Additionally, each of the MCE subcomponents, shown as bullet points in the outer circle of the figure, includes a set of steps suggested to support the proper understanding and use of the model. The implementation of the MCE has been very effective, because it is possible to make adjustments during execution as well as to immediately recover from unexpected issues, such as the extent and various levels of collaboration required throughout the evaluation (Rodríguez-Campos, 2005).

Each of the MCE components influences the others and, as a consequence, the overall collaborative evaluation. Even though the MCE could create an expectation of a sequential process, it is a system that incorporates continuous feedback for redefinition and improvement in which changes in one element affect changes in other parts of the model. To accomplish a comprehensive collaborative evaluation, interactive use of the MCE elements on a rotating and remixing basis is recommended. This interactive model establishes a solid basis for auto-analysis and a feedback mechanism to manage the unintended events. However, new insights and associated benefits may be gained by using each of the model components individually as well.

Identify the Situation. The situation is a combination of formal and informal circumstances determined by the relationships that surround and sustain the collaborative evaluation. It sets the foundation for everything that follows in the evaluation. This component of the model also considers issues related to the applicability of a collaborative approach to ensure it is appropriate given the current situation. The evaluation situation represents an early warning signal, highlighting potential constraints and benefits (e.g., funds, staff, materials, and time needed to support the collaboration process) associated with the collaborative evaluation. It can help evaluators better manage the effort and anticipate potential barriers.

This MCE component is divided into the following subcomponents: (1) identify community interest holders; (2) identify logic model

Model for Collaborative Evaluations (MCE)
© 2005, 2013 by Liliana Rodríguez-Campos and Rigoberto Rincones-Gómez. All rights reserved.

- Identify stakeholders
- Identify logic model elements
- Identify potential SWOTs
- Identify the evaluation scope
- Identify critical evaluation activities

- Clarify the role of the evaluator
- Clarify the role of the CMs
- Clarify the evaluation criteria and standards
- Clarify the evaluation process
- Clarify the evaluation budget

- Follow guiding principles for evaluators
- Follow evaluation standards (such as personnel, program, and student evaluation standards)
- Follow the collaboration guiding principles

- Establish a shared evaluation vision
- Establish recommendations for positive actions
- Establish means toward conflict resolution
- Establish decision-making procedures
- Establish reward options

- Encourage appreciation for individual differences
- Encourage fairness and sincerity
- Encourage benchmarking
- Encourage teaching by example
- Encourage flexibility and creativity

- Ensure active participation
- Ensure careful listening
- Ensure the message is clear
- Ensure immediate feedback
- Ensure the need for change is justified

MCE core: Planning → Executing → Reporting
Sections: Identify the situation; Clarify the expectations; Establish a collective commitment; Ensure open communication; Encourage effective practices; Follow specific guidelines

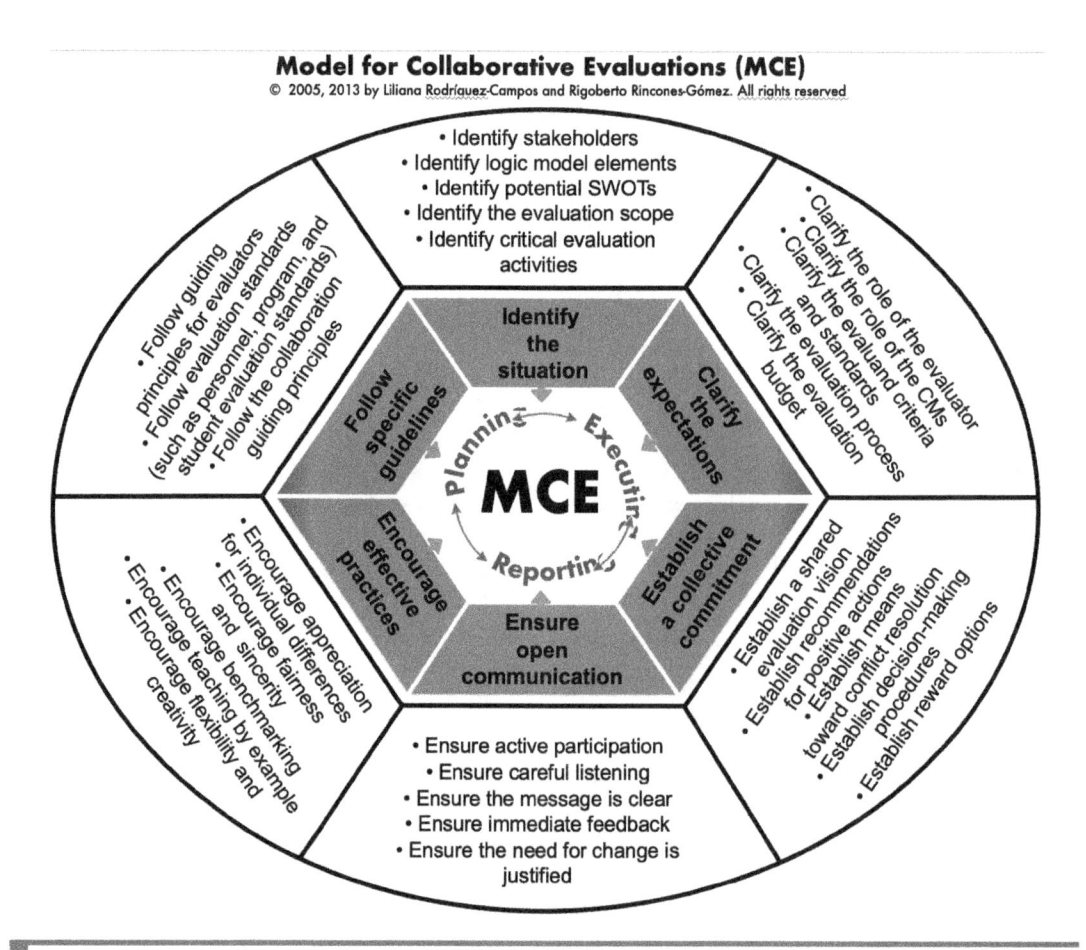

FIGURE 10.1. Model for collaborative evaluations (MCE). From Rodríguez-Campos and Rincones-Gómez (2013). Reprinted with permission from Stanford University Press.

elements; (3) identify potential strengths, weaknesses, opportunities, and threats (**SWOTs**); (4) identify the evaluation scope (e.g., evaluation questions, work breakdown structure); and (5) identify critical evaluation activities.

Clarify the Expectations. An expectation is the anticipation that good (or bad) may come out of the collaborative evaluation. It is the assumption, belief, or idea evaluators have about the evaluation and the people involved. A clear expectation is very important because it influences all the decisions made during the evaluation. By clarifying the expectations, everyone understands which issues must be addressed and what the best ways are to achieve desired results in order to make effective contributions. As a result of clarifying the expectations, it is possible to understand the implications of each evaluation choice made. In addition, a control process can be followed to show whether evaluation activities are being carried out as planned.

This MCE component is divided into the following subcomponents: (1) clarify the role of the evaluator, (2) clarify the role of the collaboration members or CMs, (3) clarify the evaluand criteria and standards, (4) clarify the evaluation process, and (e) clarify the evaluation budget.

Establish a Collective Commitment. A collective commitment is a compromise to jointly meet the evaluation obligations without continuous external authority or supervision. In a collaborative evaluation there is a need for this type of commitment in order to promote a desire to take responsibility and accountability for it. Through a collective commitment, the collaborative evaluator and the CMs gain a sense of ownership of the effects of this process and its commitment to continuous improvement. This increases awareness and the willingness to make adjustments to enhance the quality of the collaborative evaluation. Love and Russon (2000) stated, "evaluation will remain one of the world's best kept secrets unless we build strong coalitions that go beyond our own backyards" (p. 458).

This MCE component is divided into the following subcomponents: (1) establish a shared evaluation vision, (2) establish recommendations for positive actions, (3) establish means toward conflict resolution, (4) establish decision-making procedures, and (5) establish reward options.

Ensure Open Communication. Communication is a process of social interaction (such as speaking, listening, or writing) used to convey information and exchange ideas in order to influence specific actions within the collaborative evaluation. Both formal (evaluation-related) and informal (personal) communication strategies must be planned to reflect the diverse styles of the collaborative evaluator and the CMs (and other community interest holders) within the collaborative evaluation. Effective communication involves understanding others as well as being understood (Gibson et al., 2008). Thus, it is important to foster a group dialogue of openness and exploration that continues among the CMs themselves (even outside of formal meetings).

This MCE component is divided into the following subcomponents: (1) ensure active participation, (2) ensure careful listening, (3) ensure the message is clear, (4) ensure immediate feedback, and (5) ensure the need for change is justified.

Encourage Effective Practices. Effective practices are sound established procedures or systems for producing a desired process and effect within the collaborative evaluation. Among others, this can be accomplished by balancing evaluation resource needs. Also, fostering an atmosphere in which everyone is supportive of everyone else's capabilities increases recognition that each individual provides important input to the evaluation process. As a result, people feel empowered and able to actively interact in the collaborative evaluation activities because (e.g., by focusing on strengths) there is a belief that each contribution makes a difference.

This MCE component is divided into the following subcomponents: (1) encourage appreciation for individual differences, (2) encourage fairness and sincerity, (3) encourage benchmarking, (4) encourage teaching by example, and (5) encourage flexibility and creativity.

Follow Specific Guidelines. Guidelines are principles that direct the design, use, and assessment of the collaborative evaluations, their evaluators, and their CMs. Guidelines provide direction for sound evaluations, although they alone cannot guarantee the quality of any collaborative evaluation. By identifying and addressing where the collaborative evaluation meets the necessary guidelines, the evaluator(s) and the CMs demonstrate a clearer understanding of what the process is about and how it should be carried out. If adopted and internalized, these guidelines may serve as a baseline for the collaborative evaluators and the CMs to use and improve them.

This MCE component is divided into the following subcomponents: (1) follow guiding principles for evaluators, (2) follow evaluation standards (such as program, personnel, and student evaluation standards), and (3) follow the collaboration guiding principles.

The greatest strengths of the MCE are that it gives focus to collaborative evaluations and provides a strong basis for establishing long-term relationships. This model provides information on how to build collaborative relationships within an evaluation, while recognizing that the level of collaboration will vary for each evaluation. It is a tool that helps better understand how to develop priorities and achieve a high level of support within a collaborative evaluation. According to James Sanders (2005, p. iii): "The model, based on the author's experience and extensive reading, serves as a guide for evaluators who believe that making evaluation an integral part of everyday work in programs and organizations is important . . .)." There are also other collaborative evaluation approaches that can be also used and adopted. O'Sullivan (2018), for example, highlights many similarities and differences between the MCE and the collaborative evaluation techniques approach.

PRINCIPLES

Collaborative evaluation is shaped and influenced by the collaboration guiding principles, which are established tenets that guide the professional practice of collaborators (Rodríguez-Campos & Rincones-Gómez, 2013). The principles are implicitly present throughout a collaborative evaluation, helping to blend together the six MCE components. They represent the diversity of perceptions about the primary purpose of collaboration and guide its everyday practice. Hence, they are conceptualized here as general ideals or expectations that need to be considered in collaborative efforts. They include (1) development, (2) empathy, (3) empowerment, (4) involvement, (5) qualification, (6) social support, and (7) trust. They are briefly described below:

1. **Development** is the use of training (such as workshops or seminars) or any other mechanism (e.g., mentoring) to enhance educational learning and self-improvement.

2. **Empathy** is the display of sensitivity, understanding, and a thoughtful response toward the feelings or emotions of others, therefore better managing a positive reaction to your collaborative environment.

3. **Empowerment** is the development of a sense of self-efficacy by delegating authority and removing any possible obstacles (such as inadequate feelings) that might limit the attainment of established goals.

4. **Involvement** is the constructive combination of forces (such as strengths and weaknesses) throughout the collaboration in a way that is feasible and meaningful for everyone. The level of involvement varies among everyone who collaborates in the effort.

5. **Qualification** is the level of knowledge and skills needed to achieve an effective collaboration. It is the preparation for dealing with relevant performance issues that are directly affected by the individual's background.

6. **Social support** is the management of relationships with others in order to establish a sense of belonging and a holistic view of social-related issues. It is the ability to develop productive networks in order to find solutions in a collaborative way.

7. **Trust** is the firm confidence in or reliance on the sincerity, credibility, and reliability of everyone involved in the collaboration. Although a high level of trust must exist for a successful collaboration, trust takes time to build and can be eliminated easily.

Evaluators benefit from guidelines developed by various associations regarding appropriate activities that need to be followed and met. The collaboration guiding principles together with other guidelines (such as the AEA's guiding principles for evaluators) direct the design, use, and assessment of the collaborative evaluations, their evaluators, and their CMs. They provide direction for responsibly conducted evaluations, a clearer understanding of what the process is about, and how it should be carried out.

ROLE

In a collaborative evaluation, there are a set of actions expected from the evaluator(s) and the CMs in terms of what needs to be done. The evaluator accepts responsibility for the overall evaluation and its results, employing defensible criteria to judge the evaluand value. The CMs are specific interest holders (possessing unique characteristics) who work jointly with the evaluator(s) to help with particular tasks in order to achieve the collaborative evaluation vision.

The roles in a collaborative evaluation are multifaceted, and everyone involved is required to have a mix of strong conceptual, technical, and interpersonal skills. Everyone's roles should be clearly defined, without being overly restrictive, to avoid overlap with the evaluator(s) and other CM roles. In addition, roles should be suited to everyone's interests, skills, and availability. (See Rodríguez-Campos & Rincones-Gómez, 2013, for a more detailed description of the roles of the evaluator and CMs.)

STEPS

There are many ways in which to implement a collaborative evaluation. The MCE serves as an iterative checklist that provides consistent step-by-step guidance for the collection of relevant evidence to determine the value of the evaluand. Specifically, each of the MCE subcomponents includes a set of 10 steps suggested to support the proper understanding and use of the model. (See Rodríguez-Campos & Rincones-Gómez, 2013, for a traditional formulation of such a checklist.) For example, the following steps are suggested to identify potential SWOTs, which is a subcomponent of *Identify the Situation* in Figure 10.1:

1. Create a SWOT matrix on a flip chart (poster or other similar option) and have available a variety of color-coded, self-adhesive cards (such as blue for strengths, yellow for weaknesses, green for opportunities, and red for threats).

2. Review relevant data (e.g., historical information on this and other evaluands) to have some examples that could be identified as SWOTs, such as technology and information availability, assigned budget, and time considerations.

3. Divide the participants (including CMs and other interest holders as needed) into four teams representing strengths, weaknesses, opportunities, and threats. Then provide each team with the color adhesives identifying their particular SWOT.

4. Instruct each team to write one specific idea per adhesive, under their specific team SWOT, until they run out of ideas. Then the team leader will read to their members each of the ideas and, with their feedback, eliminate any overlap.

5. Place the color adhesives on the flip chart under the specific team SWOT so the rest of the teams can read them. In the case of the opportunities and threats, only leave those that have at least a 50% chance of occurrence.

6. Solicit participants to each make note of their own new ideas about the SWOTs (to make sure all of the most important ideas are addressed) and share each of those ideas while adding them to the SWOTs matrix as appropriate.

7. Ask for ideas or feedback from other interest holders who may help identify additional realistic SWOTs (such as unintended results or areas that may have been overlooked). Then question every alternative before adding it to the SWOTs matrix.

8. Agree with all of the participants and other specific engaged parties, as feasible, on a definitive SWOTs matrix. This final version of the SWOTs matrix should be clearly aligned with the evaluand vision and mission to understand which issues deserve attention.

9. Design with the participants' emergency procedures (e.g., risk analysis, predefined action steps, or contingency plans) and plan for timely feedback throughout the evaluation to provide early warning signs of specific problems.

10. Gather feedback on a regular basis using a previously agreed-upon system, such as meetings, and summarize it in a written

format (including an updated version of the SWOTs report) so it is available to each CM and other interest holders as appropriate.

The MCE steps have a wide potential applicability for conducting collaborative evaluations because different aspects will have greater relevance in certain cases depending on specific contextual factors. Each set of steps can be visited individually as needed because they are easy to follow and allow for quick guidance. For example, each program evaluated has its own unique group of people, interests, and disagreements. Thus, the steps for the subcomponent *Establish Means Toward Conflict Resolution* could be more relevant in one evaluation than in another. The MCE provides an important learning opportunity on how to conduct collaborative evaluations step-by-step. A more in-depth discussion of the steps is available in various publications (see Rodríguez-Campos, 2005; Rodríguez-Campos & Rincones-Gómez, 2013).

Group Dynamics: Locus of Control

Collaborative evaluators are in charge of the overall evaluation from the first step to the last one. However, they engage community interest holders at various levels throughout the evaluation. Typically, collaborative evaluators begin by meeting with the client and as many relevant members of the community as is feasible. They recruit individual CMs and with their assistance break the larger group into smaller ones. The evaluator may be responsible for data collection and analysis but consults with community members throughout the evaluation to continually improve its quality. Reporting may include CMs but is typically performed by the evaluator.

Participatory Evaluation

Participatory evaluation is a community consultation to control approach in which program planners, staff members, participants, and other community interest holders actively engage with an evaluator to implement an evaluative process. This method is used widely throughout the United States and in international settings to create opportunities to engage diverse groups in evaluation—examples include young people in the United States, social activists in Bangladesh, and indigenous communities in Columbia (Jupp et al., 2010; Guijt & Gaventa, 1998; Sabo Flores, 2007). Participatory evaluation may enhance evaluation use by increasing the depth and range of participation. It builds on participatory action research and participatory research models. Participatory evaluation, much like other similar approaches, has benefited from ongoing critiques designed to help define and distinguish it from other community consultation to control approaches (Daigneault & Jacob, 2009; Fetterman et al., 2014).

Definition

Participatory evaluation is a community consultation to control approach to evaluation that enables evaluators, program staff members, participants, and other community interest holders to design and implement an evaluation together, leading to joint ownership and joint control of the evaluation process and learnings (Cousins & Whitmore, 1998). Decision making and leadership of the process begins with the evaluator and over time is divested to community and related program interest holders (Cousins et al., 2013; Fetterman et al., 2014). Levels of community participation vary widely from nominal to transformative, depending on the purpose of the evaluation (Cornwall, 2008; Guijt, 2014). In addition, participation can occur at any stage of the evaluation process in the design, data collection, analysis, and reporting phases (Guijt, 2014; Shulha, 2000; Zukoski & Luluquisen, 2002; Cousins et al., 2013; Jackson & Kassam, 1998; Upshur & Barretto-Cortez, 1995). Participatory evaluation typically involves "a relatively small number of primary users" (Cousins & Earl, 1992, p. 400). However, Guijt (2014) explains that involvement can include a range of different community interest holders but the emphasis should be on "meaningful participation of programme participants" (p. 4). Participatory evaluation is designed to ensure the evaluation addresses relevant questions that can inform program improvement (Guijt, 2014; Chambers, 2009).

Two Streams

Participatory evaluation, similar to empowerment evaluation (as described below), has two streams: practical and transformative. **Practical participatory evaluation** is focused on use, not empowerment, and specifically on producing evaluation findings that can be used for immediate program improvement. It is rooted in organization learning theory and designed to support program or organizational decision making and problem solving. **Transformative participatory evaluation** draws on principles of emancipation and social justice (Cousins & Chouinard, 2012, pp. 23–25). Transformative participatory evaluation, unlike practical participatory evaluation, is designed to empower and give voice to members of the community with limited access to power or oppressed by dominating groups. The type of participatory evaluation stream is determined by both the evaluator and community members and may overlap in practice.

BOX 10.1. Collaborative Evaluation Illustration: Six-Component Approach— A Collaborative Evaluation of an Aquarium[1]

- Identify the situation
  - Evaluation key interest holders were identified (e.g., client, board members, program's staff members, local school teachers) and meetings scheduled to understand specific needs and who should become a collaboration member (CM).
  - Relevant interest holders (including the client) identified the evaluation scope, based on the available resources (e.g., time required to gather pertinent information).
  - The collaborative evaluation (CE) team, evaluators, and CMs identified the critical evaluation activities and made necessary adjustments to the evaluation plan in order to present the results to the client on time.
- Clarify the expectations
  - The evaluators met with the client and selected key interest holders (e.g., CMs) to clarify roles, responsibilities, and anticipated needs during the evaluation process. It was emphasized that recommendations for improvement were welcomed.
  - The evaluation team clarified the evaluand criteria and standards after the client solidified the evaluation scope, including the evaluation questions.
  - The CE team formally delivered to the client the evaluation plan, after it was clear that all of the CMs involved in the process agreed with the evaluation. Appropriate adjustments to the plan were made based on feedback received.
- Establish a collective commitment
  - Meetings were held with each CM to decide on a preliminary vision statement. Then, besides a shared evaluation vision, the CE team created recommendations for positive actions, means toward conflict resolution, decision-making procedures, and reward options throughout the collaborative effort.
  - The collective commitment established early in the evaluation helped to foster a positive working relationship among the CE team, so issues were solved in a straightforward and proactive way.
- Ensure open communication
  - The CE team engaged in dialogue on a regular basis, among themselves and relevant interest holders (e.g., to discuss concerns, needs, and results). When not on-site, the primary mode of communication was by email and phone.
  - The CE team ensured immediate feedback in a timely fashion. This feedback was useful to both understand and validate the need to adjust during the evaluation. These adjustments were beneficial and neither caused a delay or inconvenience.
- Encourage effective practices
  - The CE team encouraged appreciation for individual differences throughout the evaluation (e.g., fostering the collaboration of diverse interest holders).
  - Flexibility was encouraged by adapting to several changes in the logistics of the program and dependence on scheduling information for program participants.
  - The CMs provided expertise in the program's operations and proactively recognized benchmarks with potential issues that were encountered throughout the evaluation.
- Follow specific guidelines
  - Everybody involved in the CE received training on the Guiding Principles for Evaluators, the Evaluation Standards, and the Collaboration Guiding Principles. Although those alone cannot guarantee the quality of evaluations, they are helpful in providing sound direction.

[1]Rodríguez-Campos et al. (2018).

Advantages

Based on experience, there are many advantages associated with the use of participatory evaluation, including:

- *Identification of locally relevant questions*—Participatory approaches allow community members, program staff members, and participants to determine the most important evaluation questions to address that will most directly impact and improve the programs and systems that serve their communities.
- *Improving program performance*—Participatory evaluation supports reflection about program progress and generates knowledge to support continual improvement. It can support corrective action and midcourse improvements during program implementation. The main goal is for findings to drive action and change.
- *Engaging community interest holders*—Participating in an evaluation from start to finish supports community ownership and commitment to accomplishing program goals and outcomes.
- *Building capacity*—Through the process, participants learn and strengthen their own evaluation skills. It can result in new knowledge and increased understanding of the program context. This can build a group's capacity to identify action steps and advocate for policy changes, as well as create systems for ongoing evaluation and improvement.
- *Developing leaders and teams*—The process of collaborative inquiry can create new opportunities for teamwork and leadership.
- *Sustaining organizational learning and growth*—Participatory evaluation creates a learning process that can be applied to other programs and projects. The techniques and skills acquired through the evaluative process can support organizations in their efforts to use data to improve program performance. (See Sette, 2016, for additional advantages to using this approach.)

Disadvantages

Participatory evaluation requires lengthy discussions over each significant component of the evaluation. It is a more time-consuming process than traditional evaluation approaches in large part because decision making is shared. Participatory evaluators work closely with community members, program staff members, and participants to help build evaluation capacity. However, helping those members learn how to conduct interviews and surveys takes more time than conducting non-capacity-building evaluations. Reaching consensus can be contentious and add time to the evaluation timeline. In addition to the length of time required, the degree of participation (for evaluator and staff or community member) is more substantial than a traditional evaluation. These time commitments have direct and indirect costs implications, including community members' compensated and not compensated time.

Essential Features

Participatory evaluation is grounded in organizational learning theory and based on principles of engagement. The participatory evaluation process is implemented through a series of specific steps, and calls for a unique role for the evaluator. (See Cousins & Chouinard, 2012; Cousins & Earl, 1992, 1995; Guijt, 2014; Guijt & Gaventa, 1998; Sette, 2016; Zukoski & Luluquisen, 2002, for more detailed descriptions of participatory evaluation.)

CONCEPTUAL FRAMEWORK

Participatory evaluation is based in part on an organizational learning theoretical framework (Argyris & Schön, 1978). Organizational learning theory proposes that organizations improve performance by continually examining and learning from their own behavior (see Fetterman, 2009, 2012; Fetterman et al., 2010; Liker, 2004; Van der Weile et al., 2000). Organizational learning involves the integration of new ideas and constructs into existing mental maps and cognitive structures. This process of integration is a result of linkage mechanisms (Huberman, 1987; Mathisen, 1990), such as communication and collaborative group activity. According to Hedberg (1981), it "can only take place in the language of the learners, and on their terms" (p. 5).

Participatory evaluation enhances communication about relevant organizational concerns, creates an environment that enables people to think critically and creatively about how things are done, and generates new and ideally more effective ways of operating.

CONDITIONS

There are a number of conditions that have been identified from decades of field experience that must be met to conduct a participatory evaluation effectively and authentically. Cousins and Earl (1992) include the following organizational requirements:

- Evaluation must be valued by the organization.
- Time and resources are required.
- Organizations need to be committed to organizational learning (to improve performance).
- Primary users must be motivated to participate in evaluation activities.
- Organization members are capable of learning how to conduct an evaluation (even though they typically begin with insufficient research experience).

In addition to having the time to devote to a labor-intensive participatory approach and the resources to conduct a participatory evaluation, evaluators need to have a diverse set of skills, including:

- Training and expertise, including technical skills, as well as conflict negotiation and group facilitation skills.
- Ability to function as an "evaluator as teacher"; evaluators must be capable of training practice-based staff in the skills of systematic inquiry.
- Appropriate interpersonal and communication skills.
- Motivation to participate.
- Tolerance for imperfection.

These conditions and attributes increase the probability that the participatory evaluation will yield valuable information and be a productive experience for all community interest holders.

PRINCIPLES

Although participatory evaluation principles have not been formally stated or ratified, the literature consistently cites a set of core principles that range from cultivating ownership to supporting learning, reflection, and action. These include:

1. **Participant focus and ownership**—Participatory evaluation seeks to create structures and processes to engage and create ownership among all key community interest holders. The process seeks to honor the perspectives, voices, and knowledge of those most impacted, including program participants or recipients who are often voiceless in the evaluation process (Institute of Development Studies, 1998; Canadian International Development Agency, 2001).
2. **Negotiation and balance of power**—Participants commit to work together to decide on the evaluation approach. There is a balance of power among team members and the evaluator to determine each step of the evaluation process.
3. **Learning**—Participants learn together about what is working in a program and what is not, and together determine what actions are needed to improve program outcomes.
4. **Flexibility**—The evaluation approach will change based on resources, needs, and the skills of participants (Guijt & Gaventa, 1998).
5. **Focus on action planning**—The main purpose of participatory evaluation is to identify points of action to improve program implementation.

ROLES

In the participatory evaluation process the trained evaluator leads the process but shares control with participants over time (Cousins, Whitmore, & Shulha, 2014). According to Cousins and Earl (1992):

> In the participatory model the evaluator is the coordinator of the project with responsibility for technical support, training, and quality control, but conducting the study is a joint responsibility.... The evaluator's role may evolve into a posture of support and consultation as time elapses and local skills are developed and refined. (p. 400)

Similar to other community consultation to control approaches, the evaluator serves as a facilitator, coach, negotiator, and capacity builder, ensuring the process moves forward and comes to completion.

Participants can play a variety of roles and be engaged at different levels of decision making and involvement in the process (Sabo Flores, 2007). Participants may contribute to identifying relevant questions, planning the design, selecting appropriate measures and data collection methods, gathering and analyzing data, reaching consensus about findings, and disseminating results.

STEPS

There are many approaches to conducting a participatory evaluation. A five-step model is presented below (see Figure 10.2):

Step 1. Decide to Use a Participatory Evaluation Process. Conducting participatory evaluation requires additional time, resources, and commitment to fully engage community interest holders throughout all the steps. Considerations should include:

- What purpose will community participation serve to support the evaluation? Is a participatory evaluation appropriate (Guijt, 2014)?
- Are your potential team members interested? Do you have a group of people who express interest and enthusiasm?
- Does your funder support a participatory evaluation approach? Not all funders will support participatory evaluation because it may be an unfamiliar or nontraditional approach, and it may be more time and resource intensive than desired.
- Do you have an adequate timeline? Participatory evaluation is generally a lengthier process than other evaluation approaches because it requires more time for engagement, decision making, and building consensus.
- Does your group have the potential to work well together? Does your group have the necessary skills and trust to do challenging work and resolve conflicts?

It is not necessary to have all of these factors in place to move forward. However, enthusiasm for the project among the group members, funder support, adequate time, and the potential for participants to build mutual trust are important building blocks for a successful participatory evaluation process. In addition, authoritarian, dictatorial, and abusive environments, where there is a significant lack of trust, are not conducive to participatory evaluation.

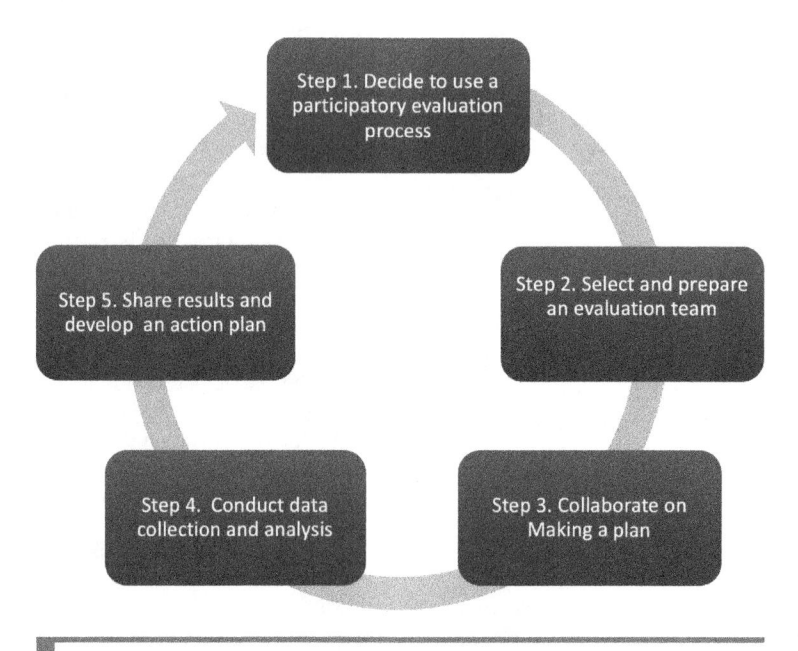

FIGURE 10.2. Participatory evaluation steps.

Step 2. Select and Prepare an Evaluation Team. Participatory evaluation requires participation from a broad range of people. Community interest holders may include program recipients, program staff, organizational leadership, and funders. It is important to include those with different roles, knowledge, and power within the program context, including people who are most affected by the program. While asking for broad representation is a good place to start, it may be appropriate to establish a smaller working group with representatives of different community groups to enable the process to move forward in a timely manner.

All members of the evaluation team or work group should be oriented to align the goals of the group and ensure a shared understanding of the evaluation process. Together the group should be determined to participate in the decision-making process and establish a mechanism for handling power differentials and potential conflict. Groups need to be aware of existing power dynamics and work to actively counter them. An appreciation for the dynamics related to differences in power among those with diverse cultural, language, and socioeconomic backgrounds is imperative. The role of an evaluator is to coach the group through the formation process, and to continue to facilitate, educate, and train the group throughout the evaluation process.

Establishing clear roles is critical to the participatory evaluation process. The UNICEF Methodological Brief on Participatory Approaches provides a set of questions that can guide decisions about what roles community interest holders should play in each step of the evaluation, from framing the questions to supporting use of evaluation findings (Guijt, 2014; UNICEF, 2005).

Step 3. Collaborate on Making a Plan. Collectively, the group—with direction from the evaluator—will:

- Define the evaluation priorities.
- Identify evaluation questions.
- Select indicators that the group views as important for documenting change or demonstrating evidence of progress.
- Agree on appropriate ways to collect the information and create plans for data collection, analysis, interpretation, and the development of an action plan.

Step 4. Conduct Data Collection and Analysis. Determining a data collection methodology that builds on team strengths and maximizes team participation requires thought and consideration (Guijt & Gaventa, 1998; Zukoski & Luluquisen, 2002). Participatory evaluation can include both quantitative and qualitative approaches and may or may not directly involve evaluation team members in data collection activities.

Rapid appraisal techniques have been often used to actively engage program participants in international settings (Chambers, 2009; UNICEF, 2005). These methods are simpler, quicker, and less costly than other data collection methods. When engaging participants in data collection, evaluators should select methods that are both rigorous and easy to use. These methods should be appealing to participants and take relatively short amounts of time to accomplish (Canadian International Development Agency, 2001). The role of participants should be acknowledged and compensated when appropriate.

Step 5. Share Results and Develop an Action Plan. Following the gathering of data, the group should work to collectively develop a shared understanding of the evaluation results. The group should develop recommendations based on evaluation findings and create an action plan to begin program improvement (Zukoski & Luluquisen, 2002).

Group Dynamics: Locus of Control

Participatory evaluation uses many of the tools of traditional evaluation. However, the locus of control for the evaluation is shared by the evaluator and program or community members. Typically, the evaluator asks program staff and/or community members to work together to design the evaluation, conduct it, and report on progress and findings. One member of the group may become a co-principal evaluator or a lead task force member. Together they discuss the pros and cons of specific evaluation designs and data collection techniques. They also exchange views about how to meaningfully interpret the data and responsibly report on findings and recommendations. The evaluator helps to build community interest holder capacity to define the scope of the evaluation, collect and analyze data, and share results. In addition, the evaluator attempts to shift as much control toward the community interest holder as possible during the course of the evaluation. Reporting may be shared. The goal is for the participants to do the bulk of the dissemination, as well as performed by the evaluator.

Empowerment Evaluation

Empowerment evaluation is practiced throughout the United States and in over 18 countries, ranging from Australia to Israel and Japan to South Africa. It has been applied to a wide variety of settings, including Google (Fetterman & Ravitz, 2018), Hewlett-Packard's $15 Million Digital Village Initiative (Fetterman, 2013a), Stanford University's School of Medicine (Fetterman, 2009; Fetterman et al., 2010), Arkansas's tobacco prevention programs (Fetterman,

---

BOX 10.2. Participatory Evaluation Illustration: Five-Step Process—A Participatory Evaluation of a Community Health Improvement Initiative

- Goal
  - Conduct a meaningful participatory evaluation of the Healthy Communities Partnership, a 3-year initiative designed to improve the health of residents in 13 communities throughout Minnesota and western Wisconsin. The initiative funded local health systems to partner with community organizations to implement strategies to strengthen the health systems role within the local community wellness infrastructure and to improve community health outcomes.
- Step 1. Decide if a participatory approach is appropriate
  - As part of the bidding process for the evaluation contract, the evaluation lead pitched the idea of a participatory approach emphasizing that this method allows for interest holders to co-design the evaluation and share in the process of discovery as they assess a program's impact. The evaluation lead outlined the pros and cons, the time needed, and the resource commitment. The funder chose this approach, launching the project.
- Step 2. Select and prepare an evaluation team
  - The evaluation lead created two teams. An advisory group, made up of the foundation's executive director and key staff, provided broad oversight. A program advisory group with members from 13 communities guided the design, data collection, and findings interpretation.
  - At a grant kickoff meeting, the evaluation lead provided an overview of the process, roles, and expectations. There was time to explain how this process differs, answer questions, and explain what to expect next.
- Step 3. Collaborate on creating an evaluation plan
  - Following the kickoff, the evaluation lead invited program leads and community partners to a three-quarter-day meeting to answer key questions. Using a world café approach, participants rotated between tables answering, "What would success look like for you?"; "What is the most important thing you want to learn from the program?"; and "What methods fit and are feasible (e.g., social network analysis, ripple-effect mapping, focus groups)?" From this work, the evaluation lead developed a plan, sharing and responding to feedback.
- Step 4. Conduct data collection and analysis
  - Program staff actively participated in data collection, analysis, and interpretation.
  - The group chose to conduct ripple-effect mapping and social network analysis at the initiative's midpoint and end stages. Staff collaborated with the evaluation lead to design the questions, convene community mapping sessions, share network surveys with partners, help with analysis, and finalize ripple-effect maps and network diagrams.
- Step 5. Share results and develop an action plan
  - Participatory approaches embrace ongoing sharing and reflection throughout the evaluation.
  - Grantees convened to review baseline results of ripple-effect mapping and social network analysis findings and again a year and a half later. Together, the groups actively discussed what they were seeing in the data and what could be learned. Each session included exercises to explore what should happen next to strengthen the wellness infrastructure in their communities and what the ongoing impact of strategies implemented was and where to go next.

Delaney, et al., 2015), Native American reservations (Fetterman, 2013a), NASA/Jet Propulsion Laboratory's prototype Mars Rover (Fetterman & Bowman, 2002), food banks throughout the United States, villages in India, and townships and squatter settlements in South Africa.

The approach celebrated its 21st anniversary with a panel of luminaries at the AEA (e.g., Alkin, Donaldson, Patton, and Scriven). They presented both compliments and critiques. The most common observation was empowerment evaluators' ability to listen, engage in the discourse, and improve practice (see Donaldson et al., 2010; Donaldson, 2017; Patton, 2017; Scriven, 2017). Empowerment evaluation's development and refinement has greatly benefited from decades of discourse (Alkin, 2017; Datta, 2016; Cousins, 2005; Fetterman, 1997, 2005b; Fetterman & Wandersman, 2007; Fetterman, Wandersman, et al., 2015; Miller & Campbell, 2006; Patton, 1997a, 2015; Scriven, 2005; Wandersman & Snell-Johns, 2005).

Definition

Empowerment evaluation is the use of evaluation concepts, techniques, and findings to foster improvement and self-determination (Fetterman, 1994). They are conducted by community and program staff members, as well as program participants, with the assistance of a professional evaluator. It is an approach that "aims to increase the likelihood that programs will achieve results by increasing the capacity of program staff members and participants to plan, implement, and evaluate their own programs" (Wandersman et al., 2005, p. 28). Empowerment evaluation can be conducted by small groups, as well as large-scale comprehensive (place-based) community change initiatives. It is mainstreamed as part of the planning and management of the program/organization. In essence, empowerment evaluation is a tool to help people produce desired outcomes and reach their goals.

Two Streams

Empowerment evaluation in practice, similar to participatory evaluation, is typically applied along two streams. The first is practical and the second transformative. **Practical empowerment evaluation** is similar to formative evaluation. It is designed to enhance program performance and productivity. It is still controlled by program staff, participants, and community members. However, the focus is on practical problem solving, as well as programmatic improvements and outcomes.

Transformative empowerment evaluation (Fetterman, 2015, 2017) highlights the psychological, social, and political power of liberation. People learn how to take greater control of their own lives and the resources around them. The focus in transformative empowerment evaluation is on liberation from predetermined, conventional roles and organizational structures or "ways of doing things." In addition, empowerment is a more explicit and apparent goal.

Advantages

There are a number of advantages to using empowerment evaluation. Community and staff members, as well as participants, are engaged and build evaluation capacity. They also learn to think evaluatively. In addition, they become more self-determined and produce sustainable outcomes (see Fetterman, 2005a, 2013a; Fetterman, Delaney, et al., 2015). Additional advantages include community members, staff members, and program participants to:

- Produce better-quality data collection, analysis, and reporting (relevant and locally meaningful).
- Use evaluation findings and recommendation (knowledge utilization as a function of ownership).
- Assume programmatic and evaluative leadership roles and responsibilities, often otherwise denied them in society.
- Address social justice issues.

Disadvantages

Empowerment evaluations can take longer than traditional evaluations because, as with all community consultation to control approaches, building evaluation capacity (both skills and a way of thinking) takes time. In addition, everyone is socialized in their own culture, making it difficult and at times stressful to "break away" from existing prescribed roles. Empowerment evaluators must learn to "let go" of as much control as possible but still not abdicate their responsibility to guide a rigorous and useful evaluation. Program staff, community members, and participants must readjust their view of evaluation, perception of their roles in relation to evaluators, and continue to take responsibility for an evaluation (even when scheduling and budgetary considerations make it challenging). Donors also need to rethink their roles, providing insights and guidance based on their vast investment in social program experience. This is in contrast with the traditional pattern of funding projects at the beginning of a project and returning at the completion of the effort without participating in the entire process.

Essential Features

Empowerment evaluation's essential features, based on over two decades of case examples, include a conceptual framework guided by empowerment and **process use** theory as well as theories of use and action. Additional features include the role of the critical friend, 10 principles, and specific steps (3-step and 10-step approaches). Combined, these features provide an insight into the dynamic and synergistic nature of empowerment evaluation (see Fetterman, Kaftarian, et al., 2015, for a more detailed description of empowerment evaluation).

CONCEPTUAL FRAMEWORK

Empowerment theory is about gaining control, obtaining resources, and understanding one's social environment. Empowerment theory processes contribute to specific outcomes. Linking the processes to outcomes helps draw meta-level causal relationships or at least a chain of reasoning. This enables community members, staff, and program participants to determine the logic behind their actions.

Process use represents much of the rationale or logic underlying empowerment evaluation in practice, because it cultivates ownership by placing the approach in community, staff members', and participants' hands. The more that people are engaged in conducting their own evaluations, the more likely they are to believe in them, because the evaluation findings are theirs. This makes them more likely to make decisions and take actions based on their evaluation data. This way of thinking is at the heart of process use.

A by-product of conducting an empowerment evaluation is that people learn to think evaluatively. Thinking evaluatively is a product of guided immersion. This occurs when people conduct their own evaluation with the assistance of an empowerment evaluator. Teaching people to think evaluatively is like teaching them to fish. It can last a lifetime and is what evaluative sustainability is all about: internalizing evaluation (individually and institutionally). A broader discussion of evaluative thinking is described in Archibald et al. (Chapter 3, this volume).

Once the groundwork is laid with empowerment and process use theories, conceptual mechanisms become more meaningful. Theories that enable comparisons between use and action are essential. For example, a *theory of action* is usually the espoused operating theory about how a program or organization works. It is a useful tool, generally based on program personnel views. The theory of action is often compared with the **theory of use**. *Theory of use* is the actual program reality, the observable behavior of community interest holders (see Argyris & Schön, 1978; Patton, 1997b). People engaged in empowerment evaluations create a theory of action at one stage and test it against the existing theory of use during a later stage. It helps people determine consistencies and inconsistencies in organizational and community behavior. A group can identify where and when it is not "walking its talk." This dialectic in which theories of action and use are routinely juxtaposed in daily practice creates a culture of learning and evaluation.

PRINCIPLES

Empowerment evaluation principles provide a sense of direction and purposefulness throughout an evaluation. Empowerment evaluation is guided by 10 specific principles (Fetterman & Wandersman, 2005). They include:

1. **Improvement**—empowerment evaluation is designed to help people improve program performance; it is designed to help people build on their successes and re-evaluate areas meriting attention.

2. **Community ownership**—empowerment evaluation values and facilitates community control; use and sustainability are dependent on a sense of ownership.
3. **Inclusion**—empowerment evaluation invites involvement, participation, and diversity; contributions come from all levels and walks of life.
4. **Democratic participation**—participation and decision making should be open and fair.
5. **Social justice**—evaluation can and should be used to address social inequities in society.
6. **Community knowledge**—empowerment evaluation respects and values community knowledge.
7. **Evidence-based strategies**—empowerment evaluation respects and uses the knowledge base of scholars (in conjunction with community knowledge).
8. **Capacity building**—empowerment evaluation is designed to enhance interest holders' ability to conduct evaluation and to improve program planning and implementation.
9. **Organizational learning**—data should be used to evaluate new practices, inform decision making, and implement program practices; empowerment evaluation is used to help organizations learn from their experience (building on successes, learning from mistakes, and making midcourse corrections).
10. **Accountability**—empowerment evaluation is focused on outcomes and accountability; empowerment evaluations function within the context of existing policies, standards, and measures of accountability; did the program or initiative accomplish its objectives? (pp. 1–2, 27–72)

Empowerment evaluation principles help evaluators and community members make decisions that are in alignment with the larger purpose or empowerment evaluation goals associated with capacity building and self-determination.

ROLE

A **critical friend** is one of the most important roles played in an empowerment evaluation (see Fetterman, 2009; Fetterman et al., 2010). A critical friend is an evaluator who facilitates the process and steps of empowerment evaluation. They believe in the purpose of the program but provide constructive feedback designed to promote improvement. A critical friend helps raise many of the difficult questions and, as appropriate, tells the hard truths in a diplomatic fashion. They help ensure that the evaluation remains organized, rigorous, and honest.

The role of the critical friend merits attention because it is like a fulcrum in terms of fundamental relationships. Applied improperly it can be like a wedge-inhibiting movement and change; applied correctly, this role can be used to leverage and maximize the potential of a group. The empowerment evaluator can differ from many traditional evaluators. Instead of being the "expert" and completely independent, separate, and detached from the people they work with, so as not to get "contaminated" or "biased," the empowerment evaluator works closely with and alongside program staff members and participants. Empowerment evaluators are not in charge. The people they work with are in charge of the direction and execution of the evaluation.

Empowerment evaluators are critical friends or coaches. They believe in the merits of a particular type of program but they pose the difficult questions. Some people ask how can an empowerment evaluator be objective and critical if they are friends and in favor of a type of program? The answer is simple: An empowerment evaluator is critical and objective because they want the program to work (or work better). They may be in favor of a general type of program but do not assume a position about a specific program without data.

Empowerment evaluators are trained evaluators with considerable expertise. They provide it as needed to keep the evaluation systematic, rigorous, and on track. They are able to function in this capacity by advising, rather than directing or controlling an evaluation. They provide a structure or set of steps to conduct an evaluation. They recommend, rather than require, specific activities and tools. They listen and rely on the group's knowledge and understanding of their local situation. The critical friend is much like a financial advisor or personal health trainer. Instead of judging and making pronouncements about successes or failure, compliance or noncompliance, the empowerment evaluator serves the group or community in an attempt to help them maximize their potential and unleash their creative and productive energy for a common good. Important attributes of a critical friend include (1) creating an environment conducive to dialogue and discussion, (2) providing or requesting data to inform decision making, (3) facilitating rather than leading, (4) being open to ideas and inclusive, and (5) willing to learn (see Fetterman, 2009; Fetterman et al., 2010).

Empowerment evaluators help cultivate a culture of evidence by asking people why they believe what they believe. They are asked for evidence or documentation at every stage, so that it becomes normal and expected to have data to support one's opinions and views. Activities can range from poor communication with evidence of overlapping meetings and no agendas to excellent funding with evidence of stable funding streams and generous budgets.

STEPS

There are many ways in which to facilitate an empowerment evaluation. In fact, empowerment evaluation has accumulated a warehouse of useful tools. The three-step (Fetterman, 2001) and 10-step **Getting-to-Outcomes** (Chinman et al., 2004) approaches to empowerment evaluation are the most popular tools in the collection.

Three-Step Approach. The three-step approach includes helping a group (1) establish their mission, (2) take stock of their current status, and (3) plan for the future. The popularity of this particular approach is in part a result of its simplicity, effectiveness, and transparency.

- **Mission.** The group comes to a consensus concerning their mission or values. This gives them a shared vision of what's important to them and where they want to go. The empowerment evaluator facilitates this process by asking participants to generate statements that reflect their mission. These phrases are recorded on a poster sheet of paper (and may be projected using an LCD projector depending on the technology available). These phrases are used to draft a mission statement, crafted by a member of the group and the empowerment evaluator (e.g., see Figure 10.3). The draft is circulated among the group. They are asked to "approve" it and/or suggest specific changes in wording as needed. A consensus about the mission statement helps the group think clearly about their self-assessment and plans for the future. It anchors the group in common values.

- **Taking stock.** After coming to a consensus about the mission, the group evaluates their efforts (within the context of a set of shared values). First, the empowerment evaluator helps members of the group generate a list of the most important activities required to accomplish organizational or programmatic goals. The empowerment evaluator gives each participant five dot stickers, and asks the participants to place them by the activities they think are the most important to accomplish programmatic and organizational goals (and thus the most important to evaluate as a group from that point on). Their use of the dots can range from putting one sticker on five different activities to putting all five on one activity if they are concerned that activity will not get enough votes. The top 10 items with the most dots represent the results of the prioritization part of taking stock (see Figure 10.4). The 10 activities represent the heart of Part 2 of taking stock: rating (see Figure 10.5).

Mission

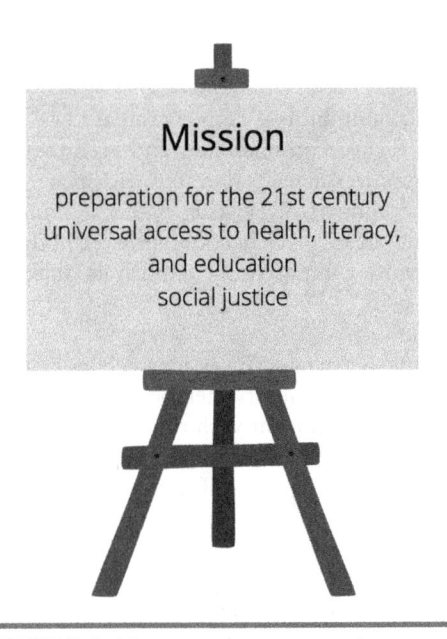

preparation for the 21st century
universal access to health, literacy,
and education
social justice

FIGURE 10.3. Mission statement example.

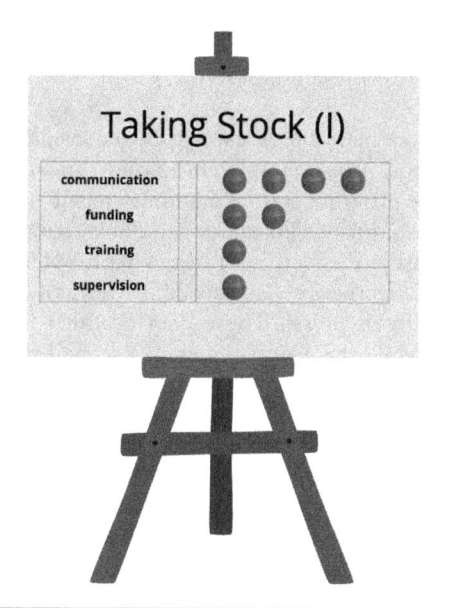

FIGURE 10.4. Taking stock I: Prioritization.

The empowerment evaluator asks participants in the group to rate how well they are doing concerning each of the activities selected, using a 1 (*low*) to 10 (*high*) scale. The columns are averaged horizontally and vertically. Vertically, the group can see who is typically optimistic and/or pessimistic. This helps the group calibrate or evaluate the ratings and opinions of each individual member and helps the group establish norms. Horizontally, the averages provide the group with a consolidated view of how well (or poorly) things are going. The empowerment evaluator facilitates a discussion and dialogue about the ratings, asking members of the community why they gave a certain activity a 3 or 7.

The *dialogue* about the ratings is one of the most important parts of the process. In addition to clarifying issues, evidence is used to support viewpoints and "sacred cows" are surfaced and examined during dialogue. Moreover, the process of specifying the reason or evidence for a rating provides the group with a more efficient and focused manner of identifying what needs to be done next, during the planning for the future step of the process. Instead of generating an unwieldy list of strategies and solutions that may or may not be relevant to the issues at hand, the group can focus its energies on the specific concerns and reasons for a low rating that were raised in the dialogue or exchange.

- **Planning for the future.** Many evaluations conclude at the taking stock phase. However, taking stock is a baseline and a launching off point for the rest of the empowerment evaluation. After rating and discussing programmatic activities, it is important to do something about the findings. It is time to plan for the future (see Figure 10.6). This step involves generating goals, strategies, and credible evidence (to determine whether the strategies are being implemented and whether they are effective). The goals are directly related to the activities selected in the taking stock step. For example, if communication was selected, rated, and discussed, then communication (or improving communication) should be one of the goals. The strategies emerge from the taking stock discussion as well, as noted earlier. For example, if communication received a low rating and one of the reasons was because the group never had agendas for their meetings, then preparing agendas might become a recommended strategy in the planning for the future exercise.

Monitoring the Strategies. Many programs, projects, and evaluations fail at this stage for lack of individual and group accountability. Individuals who spoke eloquently and/or emo-

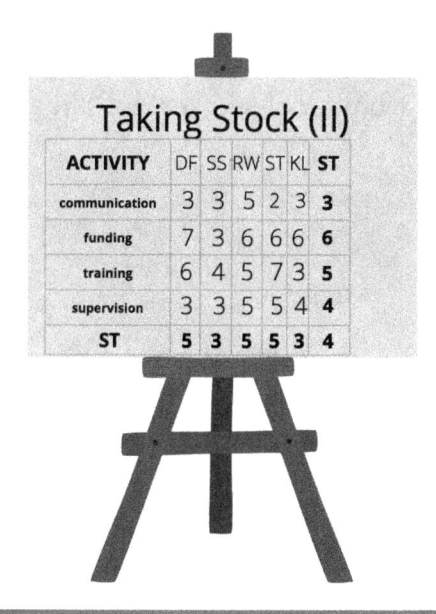

FIGURE 10.5. Taking stock II: Rating and dialogue.

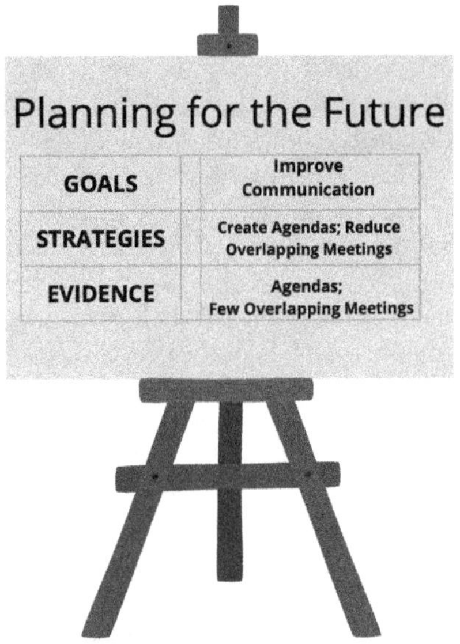

FIGURE 10.6. Planning for the future.

tionally about a certain topic should be asked to volunteer to lead specific task forces to respond to identified problems or concerns. They do not have to complete the task by themselves. However, they are responsible for taking the lead in a circumscribed area (a specific goal) and reporting the status of the effort periodically at ongoing management meetings. Similarly, the group should make a commitment to reviewing the status of these new strategies as a group (and be willing to make midcourse corrections if they are not working). Conventional and innovative evaluation tools are used to monitor the strategies. An **evaluation dashboard** (see Figure 10.7) is a particularly useful tool to monitor change or progress over time. It consists of **baselines**, milestones, goals, and actual performance. For example, a minority tobacco prevention program empowerment evaluation in Arkansas has established:

1. Baselines (the number of people using tobacco in their community).
2. Goals (the number of people they plan to help stop using tobacco by the end of the year).
3. Milestones (the number of people they expect to help stop using tobacco each month or quarter).
4. Actual performance (the actual number of people they help to stop smoking at each interval throughout the year).

These metrics are used to help a community monitor program implementation efforts and enable program staff, community members, and participants to make midcourse corrections and substitute ineffective strategies with potentially more effective ones as needed (Fetterman & Fetterman, in press). These data are also invaluable when the group conducts a second taking-stock exercise (3–6 months later) to determine whether they are making progress toward their desired goals and objectives. Additional metrics, such as an evaluation dashboard, enable community members to compare, for example, their baseline assessments with their milestones or expected points of progress, as well as their goals and actual performance.

In addition, empowerment evaluations are using many other tools, including photo journaling, online surveys, virtual conferencing formats, blogs, shared web documents and sites, infographics and data visualization (Fetterman, 2013b), artificial intelligence, and creative youth self-assessments (Sabo, 2007). (The steps, dialogue, and monitoring can be facilitated online as well, using Zoom, Google Sheets, and Google Forms; see Empowerment Evaluation blog at *eevaluation.blogspot.com*.)

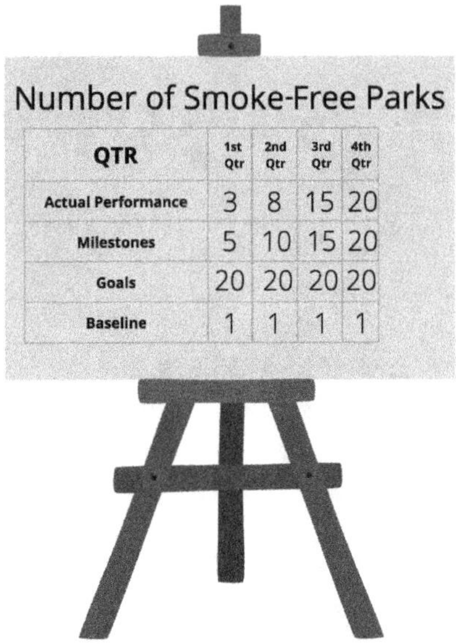

FIGURE 10.7. Monitoring: Evaluation dashboard.

> **BOX 10.3.** Empowerment Evaluation Illustration: Three-Step Approach—USAID-Funded Initiative to Eliminate Tuberculosis in India
>
> - Mission
>   - Assembled national, state, district, and local community members committed to eliminating tuberculosis (TB) in India online using Zoom and Google Sheets.
>   - Participants posted statements about their views of the mission in Google Sheets (e.g., eradicating TB, improving TB care, removing TB stigma).
>   - Empowerment evaluator facilitated a discussion about the statements.
>   - This step helped create a consensus about the mission and prepared participants for Step 2—taking stock.
> - Taking stock (Part 1: prioritization)
>   - Participants listed many of the critical activities they were engaged in to accomplish the mission (e.g., providing rights-based training, serving as TB advocates, changing health care policies, influencing health care providers, providing nutrition support for TB impacted, sensitizing elected officials).
>   - Participants were given five "votes" to select the most important activities on the list to evaluate as a group at that time.
> - Taking stock (Part 2: rating and dialogue)
>   - A list of the top 10 activities (activities receiving the most "votes") were placed on a new Google Sheet.
>   - Members of the group rated how well they thought they were doing in each activity using a 1 (*low*) to 10 (*high*) scale.
>   - The empowerment evaluator or "critical friend" facilitated the discussion about the ratings (e.g., engagement of members was rated high and using social media to promote TB awareness was rated low). The reason for the low social media rating was because they were not posting in social media. The evidence (not posting) was used to guide the development of Step 3—planning for the future.
> - Planning for the future
>   - Members of the group established new goals (e.g., increase the use of social media to increase TB awareness).
>   - Strategies included posting on LinkedIn, Facebook, Twitter, blogs, and web pages.
>   - Evidence included actual postings, comments and responses to postings, number of responses, and so on.
> - Evaluation dashboard
>   - Participants created a dashboard to monitor their "plans for the future" on a quarterly basis (e.g., goal of 24 social media postings per year and milestones of 6 per quarter; goal of 625 TB rights-based trainings per year and approximately 156 trainings per quarter).

Group Dynamics: Locus of Control

Empowerment evaluation is similar to other forms of evaluation, except that it turns it on its head. Instead of the evaluator being in charge, the group or community is in charge. Typically, the evaluator serves as the critical friend or coach and facilitates the three-step process, including mission, taking stock, and planning for the future. However, the group "fills in the blanks" concerning the content for each of these steps. Designated members of the group are responsible for keeping their "task force" moving forward (e.g., implementing plans for the future or new interventions and keeping track of the group's progress). The designated leaders report on any problems or progress at regularly scheduled meetings. Ideally, the meetings are normally scheduled management meetings, rather than special evaluation meetings. This allows the evaluation to become institutionalized and part of the planning and management of the group or agency (instead of a secondary and potentially parasitic activity that drains resources from program activities). The group reports to themselves, the community, and the donor (with the assistance and guidance of the empowerment evaluator).

CONCLUSION

Community consultation to control approaches to evaluation are powerful responses to pressing social issues. These approaches value community knowledge and local control. In addition, they contribute to program improvement, building capacity, and producing sound results (Fetterman et al., 2018). Collaborative, participatory, and empowerment evaluations are often more credible than traditional approaches in culturally diverse contexts and communities. They give voice to previously marginalized populations. They cultivate a sense of ownership, which increases the probability of use and programmatic sustainability.

Community consultation to control approaches to evaluation are conducted worldwide. There are distinctive differences among approaches, particularly concerning the role of the evaluator. While acknowledging the differences between approaches, there are many similarities, as discussed earlier. They share many principles, values, methods, and skills. Although each approach can and often should be applied by themselves, the field is prepared for a new era of community consultation to control approaches to evaluation experimentation. One promising path is combining approaches in the same initiative, depending on the circumstances, purpose, funding, need, and context.

Community consultation to control approaches are a part of the evaluation landscape. They are democratic, inclusive, and transparent in style and substance. The principles and practices presented in this discussion are woven into the fabric of collaborative, participatory, and empowerment evaluation approaches, producing a rich tapestry of evaluation practice. Community consultation to control approaches to evaluation represent a tremendous force for social well-being and equity.

REFERENCES

Alkin, M. (2017). When is a theory a theory? A case example. *Evaluation and Program Planning, 63*, 141–142.

Argyris, C., & Schön, D. A. (1978). *Organizational learning: A theory of action perspective.* Addison-Wesley.

Arnold, M. E. (2006). Developing evaluation capacity in extension 4-H field faculty: A framework for success. *American Journal of Evaluation, 27*, 257–269.

Bledsoe, K. L., & Graham, J. A. (2005). The use of multiple evaluation approaches in program evaluation. *American Journal of Evaluation, 26*, 302–319.

Canadian International Development Agency. (2001). How to perform evaluations: Participatory evaluations. *Performance Review Branch Guides, 3.* Available at *www.acdi-cida.gc.ca/INET/IMAGES.NSF/vLUImages/Performancereview4/$file/participatory_Evl.pdf*

Chambers, R. (2009). Making the poor count: Using participatory options for impact evaluation. In R. Chambers, D. Karlan, M. Ravallion, & P. Rogers (Eds.), *Designing impact evaluations: Different perspectives.* International Initiative for Impact Evaluation. Available at *www.3ieimpact.org/admin/pdfs_papers/50.pdf*

Chinman, M., Imm, P., & Wandersman, A. (2004). Getting to outcomes: Promoting accountability through methods and tools for planning, implementation, and evaluation. RAND. Available at *www.rand.org/pubs/technical_reports/TR101*

Cornwall, A. (2008). Unpacking "participation": Models, meanings and practices. *Community Development Journal, 43*(3), 269–283.

Cousins, J. B. (2005). Will the real empowerment evaluation please stand up? A critical friend perspective. In D. M. Fetterman & A. Wandersman (Eds.), *Empowerment evaluation principles in practice* (pp. 183–208). Guilford Press.

Cousins, J. B., & Chouinard, J. A. (2012). *Participatory evaluation up close: An integration of research based knowledge.* Information Age.

Cousins, J. B., Donohue, J. J., & Bloom, G. A. (1996). Collaborative evaluation in North America: Evaluators' self-reported opinions, practices, and consequences. *Evaluation Practice, 17*(3), 207–226.

Cousins, J. B., & Earl, L. (1992). The case for participatory evaluation. *Educational Evaluation and Policy Analysis, 14*(4), 397–418.

Cousins, J. B., & Earl, L. (1995). *Participatory evaluation in education: Studies in evaluation use and organizational learning.* Falmer.

Cousins, J. B., & Whitmore, E. (1998). Framing participatory evaluation. In E. Whitmore (Ed.), *Understanding and practicing participatory evaluation* (pp. 3–23). Jossey-Bass.

Cousins, J. B., Whitmore, E., & Shulha, L. (2013). Arguments for a common set of principles for collaborative inquiry in evaluation. *American Journal of Evaluation, 34*(1), 7–22.

Daigneault, P., & Jacob, S. (2009). Toward accurate measurement of participation: Rethinking the conceptualization and operation of participatory evaluation. *American Journal of Evaluation, 30*(3), 330–348.

Datta, L. (2016). Book review. In D. M. Fetterman, S. J. Kaftarian, & A. Wandersman. (Eds.). (2015). *Empowerment evaluation: Knowledge and tools for self-assessment, evaluation capacity building, and accountability* (2nd ed., pp. 1–5). Sage.

Donaldson, S. (2017). Empowerment evaluation: An approach that has literally altered the landscape of evaluation. *Evaluation and Program Planning, 63*, 136–137.

Donaldson, S., Patton, M. Q., Fetterman, D. M., & Scriven, M. (2010). The Claremont debates: The promise and pitfalls of utilization-focused and empowerment evaluation. *Journal of Multidisciplinary Evaluation, 6*(13), 15–57.

Emerson, R. W. (1993). *Self-reliance and other essays.* American Renaissance.

Fetterman, D., Rodríguez-Campos, L., Wandersman, A., & O'Sullivan, R. G. (2014). Collaborative, participatory, and empowerment evaluation: Building a strong conceptual foundation for stakeholder involvement approaches to evaluation (a response to Cousins, Whitmore, and Shulha, 2013). *American Journal of Evaluation, 35*(1), 144–148.

Fetterman, D. M. (1994). Empowerment evaluation. *Evaluation Practice, 15*(1), 1–15.

Fetterman, D. M. (1997). Empowerment evaluation: A response to Patton and Scriven. *Evaluation Practice, 15*(1), 1–15.

Fetterman, D. M. (2001). *Foundations of empowerment evaluation*. Sage.

Fetterman, D. M. (2005a). Empowerment evaluation: From the digital divide to academic distress. In D. M. Fetterman & A. Wandersman (Eds.), *Empowerment evaluation: Principles in practice* (pp. 92–122). Guilford Press.

Fetterman, D. M. (2005b). In response to Drs. Patton and Scriven. *American Journal of Evaluation, 26*(3), 418–420.

Fetterman, D. M. (2009). Empowerment evaluation at the Stanford University School of Medicine: Using a critical friend to improve the clerkship experience. *Ensaio,17*(63), 197–204.

Fetterman, D. M. (2012). Empowerment evaluation and accreditation case examples: California Institute of Integral Studies and Stanford University. In C. Secolsky & D. B. Denison (Eds.), *Handbook on measurement, assessment, and evaluation in higher education* (pp. 90–99). Routledge.

Fetterman, D. M. (2013a). *Empowerment evaluation in the digital villages: Hewlett-Packard's $15 million race toward social justice*. Stanford University Press.

Fetterman, D. M. (2013b). *Infographics, data visualizations, and evaluation: Helping evaluators help themselves*. American Evaluation Association. Available at https://higherlogicdownload.s3.amazonaws.com/EVAL/Fetterman%20Infographics%20AEA2013.pdf?AWSAccessKeyId=AKIAJH5D4I4FWRALBOUA&Expires=1391047396&Signature=oqMldk4%2BwtENx1XugaEhrYiDtLg%3D

Fetterman, D. M. (2015). Empowerment evaluation and action research: A convergence of values, principles, and purpose. In H. Bradbury (Ed.), *The Sage handbook of action research* (pp. 83–89). Sage.

Fetterman, D. M. (2017). Transformative empowerment evaluation and Freireian pedagogy: Alignment with an emancipatory tradition. In M. Q. Patton (Ed.), *Pedagogy of evaluation: Contributions of Paulo Freire to global evaluation thinking and practice* (pp. 111–126). Wiley.

Fetterman, D. M. (2023). *Empowerment evaluation and social justice: Confronting the culture of silence*. Guilford Press.

Fetterman, D. M., & Bowman, C. (2002). Experiential education and empowerment evaluation: Mars Rover educational program case example. *Journal of Experiential Education, 25*(2), 286–295.

Fetterman, D. M., Deitz, J., & Gesundheit, N. (2010). Empowerment evaluation: A collaborative approach to evaluating and transforming a medical school curriculum. *Academic Medicine, 85*(5), 813–820.

Fetterman, D. M., Delaney, L., Triana-Tremain, B., & Evans-Lee, M. (2015). Empowerment evaluation and evaluation capacity building in a 10-year tobacco prevention initiative. In D. M. Fetterman, S. J. Kaftarian, & A. Wandersman (Eds.), *Empowerment evaluation: Knowledge and tools for self-assessment, evaluation capacity building, and accountability* (pp. 295–314). Sage.

Fetterman, D. M., & Fetterman, D. M., II (in press). *Artificial intelligence, healthcare, and evaluation: Altering the landscape*.

Fetterman, D. M., Kaftarian, S., & Wandersman, A. (2015). *Empowerment evaluation: Knowledge and tools for self-assessment, evaluation capacity building, and accountability*. Sage.

Fetterman, D. M., & Ravitz, J. (2018). A Google-enhanced empowerment evaluation approach in a graduate school program. In D. M. Fetterman, L. Rodríguez-Campós, A. P. Zukoski, & Contributors (Eds.), *Collaborative, participatory, and empowerment evaluation: Stakeholder involvement approaches* (pp. 105–117). Guilford Press.

Fetterman, D. M., Rodríguez-Campós, L., Zukoski, A. P., & Contributors (2018). *Collaborative, participatory, and empowerment evaluation: Stakeholder involvement approaches*. Guilford Press.

Fetterman, D. M., & Wandersman, A. (Eds.). (2005). *Empowerment evaluation principles in practice*. Guilford Press.

Fetterman, D. M., & Wandersman, A. (2007). Empowerment evaluation: Yesterday, today, and tomorrow. *American Journal of Evaluation, 28*, 179–198. Retrieved January 6, 2014, from *aje.sagepub.com*

Fetterman, D. M., & Wandersman, A. (2010, November). *Empowerment evaluation essentials: Highlighting the essential features of empowerment evaluation*. Paper presented at the American Evaluation Association Conference, San Antonio, Texas.

Fetterman, D. M., & Wandersman, A. (2018). Essentials of empowerment evaluation. In D. M. Fetterman, L. Rodríguez-Campós, A. P. Zukoski, & Contributors (Eds.), *Collaborative, participatory, and empowerment evaluation: Stakeholder involvement approaches* (pp. 74–89). Guilford Press.

Fetterman, D. M., Wandersman, A., & Kaftarian, S. (2015). Empowerment evaluation is a systematic way of thinking: A response to Michael Patton empowerment evaluation: Knowledge and tools for self-assessment, evaluation capacity building, and accountability. *Evaluation and Program Planning, 52*(2015), 10–14.

Gajda, R. (2004). Utilizing collaboration theory to evaluate strategic alliances. *American Journal of Evaluation, 25*, 65–77.

Gibson, J. L., Ivancevich, J. M., & Donnelly, J. H. (2008). *Organizations: Behavior, structure, processes* (13th ed.). McGraw-Hill.

Gloudemans, J., & Welsh, J. (2015). The model for collaborative evaluations in the education sector. In L. Rodríguez-Campos (Ed.), *Collaborative evaluations in practice: Insights from business, nonprofit, and education sectors* (pp. 119–130). Information Age.

Green, B. L., Mulvey, L., Fisher, H. A., & Woratschek, F. (1996). Integrating program and evaluation values: A family support approach to program evaluation. *American Journal of Evaluation, 17*, 261–272.

Guerere, C., & Hicks, T. (2015). The model for collaborative evaluations in the nonprofit sector. In L. Rodríguez-Campos (Ed.), *Collaborative evaluations in practice: Insights from business, nonprofit, and education sectors* (pp. 59–66). Information Age.

Guijt, I. (2014). *Participatory approaches, methodological briefs: Impact evaluation 5*. UNICEF Office of Research.

Guijt, I., & Gaventa, J. (1998). *Participatory monitoring and evaluation: Learning from change* [IDS policy briefing]. University of Sussex. Available at www.ids.ac.uk/files/dmfile/PB12.pdf

Hedberg, B. (1981). How organizations learn and unlearn. In P. C. Nystrom & W. H. Starbuck (Eds.), *Handbook of organizational design: Vol. 1. Adapting organizations to their environments* (pp. 1–27). Oxford University Press.

Huberman, M. (1987). Steps toward an integrated model of research utilization. *Knowledge, 8*(4), 586–611.

Institute of Development Studies. (1998). Participatory monitoring and evaluation: Learning from change, *12*, 1–6.

Jackson, E. T., & Kassam, Y. (1998). *Knowledge shared*. Kumarian Press.

Joint Committee on Standards for Educational Evaluation. (2011). *The program evaluation standards: A guide for evaluators and evaluation users*. Sage.

Jupp, D., Ali, S. I., & Barahona, C. (2010). Measuring empowerment? Ask them, quantifying qualitative outcomes from people's own analysis. *Sida, 9*.

Liker, J. K. (2021). *The Toyota way: 14 management principles from the world's greatest manufacturer*. McGraw Hill.

Love, A. J., & Russon, C. (2000). Building a worldwide evaluation community: Past, present, and future. *Evaluation and Program Planning, 23*, 449–459.

Martz, W. (2015). The model for collaborative evaluations in the business sector. In L. Rodríguez-Campos (Ed.), *Collaborative evaluations in practice: Insights from business, nonprofit, and education sectors* (pp. 3–10). Information Age.

Mathisen, W. (1990). The problem solving community: A valuable alternative to disciplinary community? *Knowledge: Creation, Diffusion, and Utilization, 11*, 410–427.

Miller, R., & Campbell, R. (2006). Taking stock of empowerment evaluation: An empirical review. *American Journal of Evaluation, 27*(3), 296–319.

Morabito, S. M. (2002). Evaluator roles and strategies for expanding evaluation process influence. *American Journal of Evaluation, 23*, 321–330.

O'Sullivan, R. G. (2004). *Practicing evaluation: A collaborative approach*. Sage.

O'Sullivan, R. G. (2018). Collaborative evaluation of a multisite, multipurpose, multiyear early childhood quality care initiative. In D. M. Fetterman, L. Rodríguez-Campós, A. Zukoski, & Contributors. (2018). *Collaborative, participatory, and empowerment evaluation: Stakeholder involvement approaches* (pp. 31–47). Guilford Press.

O'Sullivan, R. G., & Rodriguez-Campos, L. (Eds.). (2012). *Evaluation and program planning: Collaborative evaluation* [Special issue], *35*.

Patton, M. Q. (1997a). Toward distinguishing empowerment evaluation and placing it in a larger context. *Evaluation Practice, 15*(3), 311–320. Available at www.davidfetterman.com/pattonbkreview1997.pdf

Patton, M. Q. (1997b). *Utilization-focused evaluation: The new century text* (3rd ed.). Sage.

Patton, M. Q. (2015). Book review. In D. M. Fetterman, S. J. Kaftarian, & A. Wandersman (Eds.), *Empowerment evaluation: Knowledge and tools for self-assessment, evaluation capacity building, and accountability* (2nd ed., pp. 15–18). Sage.

Patton, M. Q. (2017). Empowerment evaluation: Exemplary is its openness to dialogue, reflective practice, and process use. *Evaluation and Program Planning, 63*, 139–140.

Rodríguez-Campos, L. (2005). *Collaborative evaluations: A step-by-step model for the evaluator*. Llumina Press.

Rodríguez-Campos, L. (2015). *Collaborative evaluations in practice: Insights from business, nonprofit, and education sectors*. Information Age.

Rodríguez-Campos, L. (2018). Essentials of collaborative evaluation. In D. M. Fetterman, L. Rodríguez-Campos, A. P. Zukoski, & Contributors (Eds.), *Collaborative, participatory, and empowerment evaluation: Stakeholder involvement approaches* (pp. 10–20). Guilford Press.

Rodríguez-Campos, L., & O'Sullivan, R. (2010, November). *Collaborative evaluation essentials: Highlighting the essential features of collaborative evaluation*. Paper presented at the American Evaluation Association Conference, San Antonio, Texas.

Rodríguez-Campos, L., & Rincones-Gómez, R.

(2008). *Evaluaciones colaborativas; Un modelo paso a paso para el evaluador* [Collaborative evaluations: A step-by-step model for the evaluator]. Llumina Press.

Rodríguez-Campos, L., & Rincones-Gómez, R. (2013). *Collaborative evaluations: Step-by-step* (2nd ed.). Stanford University Press.

Rodríguez-Campos, L., & Rincones-Gómez, R. (2016). Collaborative evaluations. In B. B. Frey (Ed.), *The Sage encyclopedia of educational research, measurement, and evaluation* (Vol. 1, pp. 327–329). Sage.

Rodríguez-Campos, L., Rincones-Gómez, R., & Roker, R. (2018). A collaborative evaluation of an aquarium [Marine Life Program]. In D. M. Fetterman, L. Rodríguez-Campos, A. P. Zukoski, & Contributors (Eds.), *Collaborative, participatory, and empowerment evaluation: Stakeholder involvement approaches* (pp. 21–30). Guilford Press.

Ryan, K., Greene, J., Lincoln, Y., Mathison, S., & Mertens, D. M. (1998). Advantages and challenges of using inclusive evaluation approaches in evaluation practice. *American Journal of Evaluation, 19*, 101–122.

Sabo Flores, S. (2007). *Youth participatory evaluation: Strategies for engaging young people in evaluation.* Jossey-Bass.

Sanders, J. (2005). Foreword. In L. Rodríguez-Campos (Ed.), *Collaborative evaluations: A step-by-step model for the evaluator* (p. iii). Llumina Press.

Scriven, M. (1994). The final synthesis. *Evaluation Practice, 15*, 367–382.

Scriven, M. (2005). Review of empowerment evaluation principles in practice. *American Journal of Evaluation, 26*, 415–417.

Scriven, M. (2017). Empowerment evaluation 21 years later: There is much to admire about empowerment evaluation. *Evaluation and Program Planning, 63*, 138.

Sette, C. (2016). "Participatory evaluation" [web page]. BetterEvaluation. Available at *http://betterevaluation.org/plan/approach/participatory_evaluation*

Shulha, L. (2010, November). *Participatory evaluation essentials: Highlighting the essential features of participatory evaluation.* Paper presented at the American Evaluation Association Conference, San Antonio, Texas.

Shulha, L. M. (2000). Evaluative inquiry in university-school professional learning partnerships. *New Directions for Evaluation, 88*, 39–53.

Stufflebeam, D. L., & Shinkfield, A. J. (2007). *Evaluation theory, models, and applications.* Wiley.

UNICEF. (2005). Useful tools for engaging young people in participatory evaluation. Available at *www.artemis-services.com/downloads/tools-for-participatory-evaluation.pdf*

Upshur, C. C., & Barretto-Cortez, E. (1995). What is participatory evaluation (PE)? What are its roots? *Evaluation Exchange, 1*(3–4). Available at *www.hfrp.org/evaluation/the-evaluation-exchange/issue-archive/participatory-evaluation/what-is-participatory-evaluation-pe-what-are-its-roots*

Van der Weile, T., Brown, A., Millen, R., & Whelan, D. (2000). Improvement in organizational performance and self-assessment practices by selected American firms. *Quality Management Journal, 7*(4), 8–22.

Veale, J., Morley, R., & Erickson, C. (2001). *Practical evaluation for collaborative services: Goals, processes, tools, and reporting systems for school-based programs.* Corwin Press.

Wandersman, A., & Snell-Johns, J. (2005). Empowerment evaluation: Clarity, dialogue, and growth. *American Journal of Evaluation, 26*(3), 421–428.

Wandersman, A., Snell-Johns, J., Lentz, B. E., Fetterman, D. M., Keener, D. C., Livet, M., Imm, P. S., & Flaspohler, P. (2005). The principles of empowerment evaluation. In D. M. Fetterman & A. Wandersman (Eds.), *Empowerment evaluation principles in practice.* Guilford Press.

Yeh, S. S. (2000). Improving educational and social programs: A planned variation cross-validation model. *American Journal of Evaluation, 21*, 171–184.

Zukoski, A., & Bosserman, C. (2018). Essentials of participatory evaluation. In D. M. Fetterman, L. Rodríguez-Campós, A. P. Zukoski, & Contributors (Eds.), *Collaborative, participatory, and empowerment evaluation: Stakeholder involvement approaches* (pp. 48–56). Guilford Press.

Zukoski, A., & Luluquisen, M. (2002). Participatory evaluation: What is it? Why do it? What are the challenges? *Community-Based Public Health Policy and Practice, 5*, 1–6. Available at *http://depts.washington.edu/ccph/pdf_files/Evaluation.pdf*

Chapter 11

Making the Most of Evaluations
Strategies for Assessing Program Evaluability and Evaluation Feasibility

Debra J. Rog

CHAPTER OVERVIEW

Evaluability assessment (EA) is a key tool that evaluators have at their disposal but too often is left unused. EA offers an opportunity to determine whether a program is ready for an evaluation, and if not, what can be done to improve its readiness. EA is one of the few systematic tools used for evaluation planning, helping ground the evaluation in the reality of the program, ensuring it is focused on the right questions, engaging interested parties in the process, and ensuring that the appropriate design is implemented at the right time in the program process. EA helps to focus evaluation on programs that are designed and implemented with plausibility to achieve their outcomes, and consequently, can provide for wiser investment and use of evaluation funding. In addition, beyond being used as a tool for assessing a program's readiness for evaluation, EA can be used to help develop programs, select sites to use in multisite evaluations, provide quick information on a program, and other purposes. Going through the process of EA itself fosters evaluative thinking among those involved in a program, and an evaluator adopting an evaluability perspective in the design phase of an outcome evaluation may be better informed to focus the evaluation on those features of a program with the greatest plausibility of achieving the outcomes.

Evaluations, especially those focused on outcomes and assessing long-term impact, can be expensive enterprises. Too often, though, an evaluation is not able to yield actionable findings about a program or findings commensurate with the program expenditures made, either because the program is not sufficiently in place to achieve its results, lacks a clear logic of what it intends to achieve, or lacks agreement among key interested parties on what the intended outcomes are or how they should be measured. Each of these situations prevents a fair test of a program's merit and typically does not yield outcome results that are as worthwhile as they might have been if greater attention had been placed on improving the program's readiness.

In other situations, an evaluation is conducted without adequate planning and the program context cannot support implementation of the desired evaluation design. For example, evaluators planning to employ experimental models may encounter resistance to random assignment among the organizations involved; evaluations designed to examine the longitudinal effects of a program may find that the administrative data needed on key outcomes do not exist over time; and in yet another example, evaluations that aim to include data through multiple methods may find limited access to some of the data needed.

Evaluability assessment (EA) was designed to avoid these situations by examining both **program evaluability** and **design feasibility** before an evaluation is initiated (Wholey, 1979; Rutman, 1980). Information on evaluability and feasibility should trigger actions to improve the conditions for evaluation, including strengthening the program design or management, improving the data available or their accessibility, or, at a minimum, question whether conducting an evaluation is a wise expenditure of resources at this time. This chapter introduces and outlines the EA method, describing how it can be used to assess a program's readiness for evaluation, and determine the types of evaluation designs and methods most appropriate and feasible to implement. The chapter begins with a brief overview of the history and background of the method, followed by the types of situations that warrant an EA, and the steps to implementing the method. An example of EA closes out the chapter.

HISTORY AND BACKGROUND OF EA

What Was the Impetus for EA?

EA was created by Joseph Wholey and colleagues at the Urban Institute in the late 1970s (Nay & Kay, 1982; Schmidt et al., 1982; Wholey, 1979; Wholey et al., 1971) to examine the extent to which a program is ready for an evaluation, the changes that are needed to increase its readiness, and the type of evaluation approach most suitable to judge the program's performance (Schmidt et al., 1982). It was developed at a time when the relatively young field of evaluation was experiencing a growth spurt, with the federal government commissioning evaluations in numerous areas. Despite the increasing popularity and use of evaluation, however, researchers noted that few evaluations were having the influence evaluators desired.

Though the absence of **instrumental use** of evaluation results could be due to factors outside the control of the evaluator (such as the closing of a policy window and few opportunities to apply the results), much of the lack of use was attributed to the tendency of evaluations to yield null or negative results (e.g., Schmidt et al., 1982). Nonpositive results occurred for a number of reasons, including the program being evaluated was either not fully implemented or did not even exist; the program goals being evaluated were often "grant goals," reflecting aspirations rather than real goals and typically written in nonoperational terms; or the program lacked an internal logic or theory linking the activities being implemented and the outcomes that were desired (see Frechtling, Chapter 20, this volume, on logic models). Moreover, decision makers at times were not in agreement with which outcomes should be evaluated and had different perspectives on what the program was intended to achieve.

What Was the Focus for EA?

EA assesses the underlying logic of a program or policy, including its goals and objectives, the resources available to implement the program, its proposed activities, and its desired outcomes, as well as the linkages among these different elements. Box 11.1 outlines what EA assesses in a program to determine its evaluability as well as the feasibility of a subsequent evaluation effort. The technique assesses the program as designed as well as implemented, and determines whether, as implemented, it is plausible to expect the program to achieve its desired outcomes. If the program does not have an underlying logic or is not ready to be evaluated, EA outlines what could be done to improve the program's readiness. If it is judged to be ready, the focus then shifts to determining which evaluation design might be most appropriate and feasible.

What Purposes Was EA Designed to Fill?

EA was developed to prevent the waste of resources on premature or inappropriate evaluation; build consensus among decision makers, especially on the desired outcomes; guide decisions on whether and when an evaluation should be implemented; and help design an evaluation appropriate to decision makers' needs

> **BOX 11.1. The Focus of EA**
>
> - Determines if the program has:
>   - Goals and objectives that are clearly specified, measurable, realistic.
>   - Resources that are sufficient to support program activities.
>   - Activities that are well-defined, measurable, implemented consistently across program sites/locations.
>   - Outcomes that are clearly specified, measurable, realistic, comprehensive, agreed upon.
>   - Linkages among goals/objectives that are plausible given research/theory, basic common sense, timeframe, resources, context.
> - Determines if the subsequent evaluation effort:
>   - Is feasible to implement as recommended.
>   - Has data that are available and accessible to support the evaluation.
>   - Has intended users and specific intended uses for the resulting evaluation.

and intended uses. EA is one of the few systematic tools used for evaluation planning, helping ground the evaluation in the reality of the program, ensuring it is focused on the right questions, engaging interested parties in the process, and ensuring that the appropriate design is implemented at the right time in the program process. As described more fully below, however, the purposes for EA have expanded over the years to include selecting sites for multisite evaluations, providing quick turnaround information on a program, and other uses.

Where Has the History of EA's Use Been?

After its initial development, EA was used extensively in the mid-1970s and early 1980s in the federal government, especially by the Department of Health, Education, and Welfare (what is now the Department of Health and Human Services [HHS]), as well as in Canada (Rog, 1985). Wholey's position as deputy Assistant Secretary for Planning and Evaluation was an impetus for using EA as a tool to use to set aside money for evaluation. Few EAs were followed by evaluations, whether they were deemed evaluable or not; in some respects, decision makers used EA information in place of evaluation information (Rog, 1985).

After Wholey's departure from the federal government, however, the use of EA in the government and HHS in particular declined significantly. Among the factors conjectured for its decline include the lack of a strong internal advocate for the technique, a lack of clarity about the methodology and its outcomes (Smith, 1989), and perhaps a penchant for moving to conducting evaluation directly rather than invest in pre-evaluation activity (Trevisan & Walser, 2015). The use of EA reemerged in the mid-1990s and especially increased in the 2000s in both the public and private sectors as a method for learning about interventions quickly as well as how best to approach evaluation (Rog, 2005; Trevisan, 2007; Trevisan & Walster, 2015). In the federal government, the Government and Performance and Results Act (GPRA) of 1993 created a renewed role for EA and evaluation more broadly, requiring that all federal agencies engage in strategic planning and performance management. Agencies were required to set goals, and measure and report results. GPRA was followed by the Program Assessment Rating Tool, instituted in 2002 by the Office of Management and Budget and introduced in the fiscal year 2004 federal budget to assess the effectiveness of all federal programs. For programs such as the Mental Health Block Grant (Mulkern, 2005) that had been in operation for 20 years and had evolved and shifted over that period of time, an EA was a natural first step before embarking on a large-scale evaluation.

Since the early 2000s, EA has experienced a steady growth in use, with a tripling of documented studies between 2008 and 2018 in 14 counties, with its greatest use in North America (Lam & Skinner, 2021). Despite EA's cyclical growth since its inception, it is now a recognized tool for evaluation practice within a range of settings and for a variety of purposes.

WHEN TO CONDUCT AN EA

Ideally, an EA is conducted before there is investment in any type of evaluative activity, especially an **outcome evaluation** or an **impact evaluation**. When an EA is conducted early in a program's life, perhaps even before the program is fully developed, it can serve as a guide to designing the program, ensuring that the program design has goals and outcomes that are realistic and measurable and an internal logic with clear linkages between the planned activities and desired outcomes. Implemented during a program's life, an EA can help guide corrections in the program operations as well as inform the design of the evaluation. In some instances, an EA is conducted for a program that had an evaluation in the past but has shifted or evolved considerably and there is now renewed interest in having another evaluation of the program.

EA can be applied to a wide range of **evaluands**, including single programs or projects, entire portfolios of programs, policies and legislation, processes, and funding streams. In my own work, I have been involved in nearly 100 EAs, both for foundations and the federal government, spanning childhood obesity prevention programs, community networks aimed at enhancing community responses to prevent adverse childhood experiences and foster resilience, supportive housing for families with multiple service needs, medical respite programs, medical legal partnerships, the processing of sexual assault kits, pharmacy interventions, programs serving youth transitioning from foster care, and others. Most of the EAs followed the standard methodology; in a few EA efforts, as noted in sections to follow, we adapted the methodology for specific purposes not originally outlined for EA.

As noted throughout this chapter, EAs are supported by a variety of funders and through a range of funding vehicles and arrangements. The federal government often issues requests for proposals (RFPs) for EAs, either as the sole focus of the work or as a component of a larger government contract. For example, for a project funded through the National Institute of Justice, we conducted EAs of sites receiving funding for processing sexual assault kits within a larger scope of work that also included conducting a subset of process evaluations and developing an evaluation design. Foundations also may issue broad RFPs, may invite a small number of evaluators to compete, or select evaluators noncompetitively if they have experience or background working with the foundation and its programs.

STEPS IN EA

The literature varies somewhat in the number of steps involved in an EA (see Trevisan & Walser, 2015; Lam & Skinner, 2021), though the same activities are generally covered across whatever number of steps are outlined. In this chapter, I outline six main steps I generally follow in conducting an EA. They include:

1. Clarifying the purpose and scope of the EA.
2. Involving interested parties and intended users in the EA process and any potential follow-up evaluation.
3. Documenting the program design/clarifying the program's intent.
4. Documenting the program as implemented and assessing data availability and capacity.
5. Analyzing the **plausibility** of the program to determine its evaluability.
6. Developing options for program design and management, data collection, and evaluation, including collecting information on intended uses for the information.

Step 1. Clarifying the Purpose and Scope of the EA

Purpose

As noted, EA was originally developed to determine readiness for evaluation and that continues to be the major purpose for which it is used. It also can be conducted to provide data for other early design decisions. For example, in programs with many sites, evaluators can use EA (or a modified implementation of the method) to select sites to include in a multisite evaluation (see Box 11.2). A focus on evaluability can direct selection to those sites that can provide the strongest test of the program (i.e., sites that have the strongest theory and implementation) and are most ready for an evaluation (e.g., have data available).

Evaluators can also use EA to collect rapid program information in a systematic manner, either to provide feedback to program sponsors and/or technical assistance providers on what a program is doing and how it aligns with expectations, or to provide information to guide an evaluation that is already decided upon, even if

> **BOX 11.2. Example of EAs Used for Site Selection**
>
> We conducted EAs to select sites for a multisite evaluation on medical respite care for individuals who are chronically homeless. Over 60 medical respite care interventions had emerged across the country to provide individuals with posthospital services for recuperation and recovery. Programs varied widely, from dedicated rooms in shelters to large clinical facilities. With criteria developed from an expert panel, we first identified the subset of medical respite programs that had specific program elements deemed critical for a potentially effective medical respite program. With those 12 programs, we conducted abbreviated EAs (i.e., data collected all by document review and a small number of key informant telephone interviews) to assess if how they were operating aligned with their initial design, if they had data of sufficient quality we could use to understand the population served, and if they had linkages with local hospitals to ensure that a retrospective evaluation was feasible. From the 12 EAs completed, four programs met the criteria for being included in the evaluation.

there is variability among program sites in evaluability. Box 11.3 provides an example of EA's use for rapid information.

Evaluators can initiate EA at the program design stage, helping program developers create a program that has a strong logic and agreed-upon outcomes that are realistic and measurable. When substitute evaluators use EA to design a program, the focus is on applying the concept of evaluability and strengthening the plausibility of the design to achieve the outcomes while it is being developed. Much of the focus is determining what evidence or theory exists to assume these concepts will lead to the outcomes, what needs to be done to ensure that the concepts can be translated into activities that can be implemented with integrity to the concepts, and what data need to be available to assess fidelity to the implementation and the achievement of outcomes. Box 11.4 provides an example of using evaluability principles and processes in intervention development.

Scope

In addition to purpose, evaluators need to clarify the scope of the EA, including what sites are included, what program components are included, whether an assessment of the organization is included in addition to the program, and whether an assessment of the context is included. For example, in a program with multiple sites, it is important for evaluators to clarify if the EA is for the entire program, a representative selection of sites, or specifically selected sites. At times, as the example in Box 11.2 illustrates, funders are interested in evaluating the potential of a program, focusing on a subset of sites with the strongest implementation of a program.

Other questions of scope include whether an EA is being focused on an entire program model or certain components or objectives, especially in very complex initiatives that have many purposes, strategies, activities, and so on (e.g., in a complex mental health treatment program, the interest may be in the peer component of the program).

Similarly, it is important for evaluators to clarify whether the EA is to include an understanding of the organization that operates the program as well as the initiatives themselves, and whether there is to be a focus on the context and possible comparison sites. Expanding the scope of EA to include the organization along with the program can be helpful to understand other resources that may be available to the program being studied; it may help in both assessing its evaluability as well as helping inform how the program can be strengthened if it is not evaluable. For example, several years ago, I conducted an evaluability assessment of an initiative that focused on improving the avail-

> **BOX 11.3. EA for Rapid Program Information**
>
> For a large foundation, we held a contract to conduct EAs of individual projects that had been funded under a broader program announcement. Program officers typically requested EAs to help them learn more about a project and guide their decision whether it was worth continuing to fund. They wanted relatively fast, independent information on how the program was operating and whether it had plausibility of achieving its outcomes. In some instances, the EAs led to additional activities (e.g., strengthening the project's data infrastructure and capacity to participate in future evaluations; conducting process evaluations to provide more in-depth understanding of the project).

BOX 11.4. Using an Evaluability Perspective in Designing an Intervention

With funding from a foundation, we worked as consultants with educators and behavioral psychologists to develop a life-skills professional development intervention for third-grade elementary school teachers. The intervention aimed to integrate reasoning, resilience, and responsibility into teaching to improve student achievement and classroom management. Lessons were developed to infuse these skills into the existing curriculum, with an emphasis on mathematics. The centerpiece of this program was a problem-solving model that encouraged students to reason well, be resilient in the face of challenges, and take responsibility for their learning.

We worked through numerous work sessions with the program development team, determining how best to translate what was tested in more controlled basic research settings into evaluable teacher training programs that can integrate these skills into third-grade curricula. We worked to ensure that the training was well-defined and explicitly included the three key skills, and identified how we could measure that they were evident in the training and in the classroom activities. We outlined what resources were needed to ensure that the training could be implemented to incorporate the key criteria and that teachers had the resources to include the training consistently in their teaching (e.g., what technical assistance and booster training might be needed). We then worked with the intervention development team to determine what short-term outcomes were expected at the teacher and student levels and how they could best be measured. The intervention was aimed at determining the extent to which training teachers in reasoning, responsibility, and resilience increased the knowledge, attitudes, beliefs, and behavioral practices of teachers on these concepts; enhanced teacher self-efficacy and other teacher outcomes; and enhanced students' self-efficacy and other skills and attitudes that optimize their academic functioning. The development of a logic model helped guide the development of an intervention, the implementation and outcome measurement, and the pilot evaluation. The process aimed to ensure that the goals and objectives of the project were linked to how the intervention was articulated and the outcomes also linked to the activities and were clearly specified and validly measured.

---

ability and display of healthier food for children in urban corner stores (having more prominence than less healthy foods) with the aim of preventing childhood obesity. Understanding the broader organization that was implementing the program, including the additional resources it had to help engage corner stores in its efforts (e.g., helping to see funding for refrigeration) and the internal resources it had for evaluation, influenced our assessment of the feasibility of conducting a more rigorous future evaluation.

Including a focus on context and other possible comparison sites in an EA is especially important if the EA is to include a specific evaluation design component or is likely to be followed by an evaluation. EAs do not generally include developing an evaluation design unless it is specifically asked for by the funder, either outlined in an RFP or other funding agreements. When the EA is funded without specification of an evaluation design the focus is typically on assessing a program's readiness for an outcome evaluation. The scope may include describing the feasibility of implementing different evaluation designs. Most EAs do not include funding for implementing the subsequent evaluation but could be followed by a separate project (either through competitive or not competitive funding, depending on the funder).

A variant on EA that affects both its purpose and scope is the **systematic screening and assessment (SSA)** method (Leviton et al., 2010). SSA is a strategy aimed at identifying innovations in a particular substantive area (e.g., childhood obesity prevention, youth transitioning from foster care) that are important to learn more about, have the potential to be effective, and may be appropriate for evaluation. SSA incorporates EA as a key step, following the solicitation and screening of nominated innovations. Identified innovations within a particular intervention area that appear to have the promise of being effective are the focus of EAs. Once the EAs are completed, experts review the EA reports and identify those innovations that are most promising and ready for evaluation—evaluations are then conducted.

The Centers for Disease Control and Prevention (CDC) has funded both EAs and SSAs since 2008, and more recently has created a more streamlined approach that incorporates elements of SSA, entitled the **enhanced evaluability assessment (EEA**; Losby et al., 2015). CDC developed this approach to reduce the time that SSA and the subsequent evaluation takes (averaging 42 months in CDC's experience, with 12 months for the SSA and 30 months for the effectiveness evaluation). EEA replaces the broad nomination process to identify promising programs with nominations by in-house staff, reducing the time needed to collect program nominations and have them reviewed by an external panel. Identified programs are contacted and information is collected to create a comprehensive description of each program aligned with EA criteria, including the development of a logic model. A list of potential programs are assessed using a set of criteria (i.e., potential impact, health effect size, reach, feasibility, sustainability, transferability, and data capacity). Prospective programs are contacted and assessed for their suitability for an effectiveness evaluation. EEA includes an abbreviated approach to EA to decrease the data collection time, relying on telephone calls and documents and not including onsite data collection. An internal, rather than external, panel selects sites for evaluation and sites are selected that have existing data that can shorten the timeframe of the evaluation.

Step 2. Involving Interested Parties and Intended Users

One of the key elements in Wholey's EA approach is involving interested parties in the EA process. Wholey, primarily developing EA for a federal audience in mind, spoke of two key groups with different levels of involvement: a work group and a policy group. The work group typically involved federal managers working on the program who collaborated with the external EA team in organizing and conducting the EA. The policy group, comprising high-level officials, was briefed on the EA at key points in the process and guided decisions about the overall design and use of the EA.

As EA has expanded to a range of institutions, both public and private, the development of work and policy groups has not been a central feature of the approach. Rather, sponsors of the EA and others may be involved in varying ways, depending on the culture and desires of the program organization. In some instances, the program sponsors and/or director may want a great deal of involvement in the process, taking part in each stage (e.g., helping develop logic models, attending site visits, participating in the analysis of plausibility and evaluability), whereas in others, the program sponsors and/or director may prefer to be briefed at key junctures in the process or just at the end of the process to review the findings and their implications for program redevelopment or subsequent evaluation.

Therefore, at the beginning of the EA, the evaluator should determine the needs and expectations of key interested parties with respect to the decision-making, data collection, and analysis steps of the EA; the type of feedback appropriate for the different sets of parties and at what points in the process; and any particular considerations in conducting the EA (such as whether it is important for the evaluators to sign a **nondisclosure agreement** to collect data on the program, especially with private funders). Budget-affected items, such as the nature and timing of feedback, should be considered in the development of the project's cost proposal but other aspects of involvement of invested parties can be discussed in the EA kickoff meeting with the funder.

In many cases, it will not be considered appropriate for all those with an interest in the program to be involved in the steps they expect, especially data collection. Having a program sponsor or staff person in some interviews or focus groups may influence how people answer questions, providing answers they think the program staff want to hear or even at times deferring to them for the "right" response, and in turn, defeating the purpose of the EA. For example, one of the key purposes of the EA is to assess whether everyone involved in the program has the same understanding of its purpose and goals, as differences can create differences in how the activities are conducted and, consequently, their plausibility of achieving the desired outcomes. So setting expectations for program sponsors and staff for their EA participation from the outset and describing the rationale for them is important to facilitating a smooth process.

Step 3. Documenting the Program Design

Reviewing Program Documents

Data collection begins during the proposal process and initial kickoff meeting. Through the proposal process the EA team begins to learn about the program, reviewing documents provided by the funder, and continues with initial discussions about why they funded the program, what they hope it achieves, and other questions that provide a foundation of understanding of the program. The EA team then continues building an understanding of the program by holding introductory conversations with the program director or other leadership to introduce the EA as well as to obtain any basic information on the program. The EA team explains the purpose of the EA (if not already known) and the steps in the process. The EA team asked the program director to provide an overview of the program, including a brief history and current status, and to identify key documents to review, individuals to interview in the next stage, and any key activities to observe in the next stage. This first conversation helps the EA team broaden its data collection efforts.

Program documents are the major source of information to address the questions noted above. These documents include authorizing legislation (for government programs), grant applications, brochures, websites, annual reports, previous evaluation reports, and financial reports, among others. At times, a program may already have a logic model that can provide a starting point for the model used in the EA.

Research literature can also be reviewed at this stage, especially if the program is grounded in an evidence base (e.g., examining research studies on childhood obesity prevention to understand exercise programs aimed at preventing childhood obesity). The literature can inform what theory or conceptualization may underlie the program, and what is known about this program or similar interventions. Among the issues a literature review can address are: what factors influence outcomes; what measures have been used for outcomes; and what research has been conducted that helps inform the assessment of plausibility of various aspects of the program.

Developing a Model of the Program as Designed

This first modeling step in the EA process involves documenting the program design or the program as intended. In this step, the EA team often relies almost exclusively on program documents, abstracting information on the program's design and other relevant information that can inform the development of a **program logic model**, as well as questions to drive interviews with program personnel (in the next stage).

Many evaluators may not be familiar with EA but most are typically familiar with logic models, which were first introduced by EA. A logic model is a visual representation of the underlying logic or theory of a program. It displays a blueprint of how the goals, resources, and activities are aligned and link with the desired outcomes of a program. Logic models were first introduced to evaluators through EA but have transcended the method to be a technique used on its own and often recommended as a first step in most evaluations. RFPs for evaluations typically ask to see a logic model, for example, and evaluation texts often have a section on developing logic models as a first step in guiding an evaluation. Frechtling (see Chapter 20, this volume) reviews the steps in developing a logic model and strategies that can be used in different program situations. Other good resources include Frechtling (2007), W. K. Kellogg Foundation (2004), Knowlton and Phillips (2012), and McLaughlin and Jordan (2015).

To gather data to inform the development of a model, it is advisable for the EA team to develop a protocol or set of questions to guide the document abstraction. The questions can be basic and even somewhat generic in this step, aligning with the features of an evaluable program:

• What are the stated goals and objectives of the program? This can include legislative goals, grant goals, and other stated objectives.

• What resources are available to the program? What are the inputs? Inputs are not limited to funding but can include in-kind supports, partnerships, key tools, and other types of resources that can support the program.

• What is the target population for the program? Is the program reaching and serving the population it intends to serve and in the numbers expected? Although this element is not always explicitly outlined in an EA, it can be a critical piece of information to understand for both the evaluability of the program and the feasibility of conducting an evaluation. As noted later, serving a population different from the one the program intended can have implications for the extent to which program activities are appropriate and/or outcomes are plausible. For example, if a program aims to serve families that need employment assistance but are serving families that do not have child care and cannot yet take advantage of the assistance, the program may either need to include child care resources or recruit families able to participate in the employment assistance. In addition, if the program is not serving as many individuals as it had originally expected, it may not have a service population large enough to support a quantitative outcome evaluation.

- What are the program activities? Activities are the services or elements of a program (e.g., mental health services, educational programming). Some complex initiatives may have many activities, arranged under sets of activities or strategies. In addition, in programs with many sites that do not follow the same model, each program strategy or component may have portfolios of possible activities. For example, in a program funding community collaboratives to prevent community violence, all collaboratives incorporated strategies to organize and mobilize their communities but the specific activities implemented differed across the communities.

- What are the expected outputs of the program? Outputs are what is expected to be produced by a program, not its effects. Outputs can be counts, such as the number of materials produced, the number of training sessions conducted, the number of individuals trained, and so forth. Outputs are what are expected from the inputs. If you receive X amount of funding and other resources, these are the outputs that are expected to be produced. If the outputs are fewer or different than expected, the program may need to adjust expectations for what can be achieved. For example, in an educational program, if fewer training sessions are conducted due to funding cuts, fewer teachers are likely trained, which in turn limits the number of schools and classrooms involved in the program, and, in turn, reduces the number of students taught by trained teachers than originally anticipated.

- What are the desired short-term and longer-term outcomes? Outcomes are what is expected because of the program: changes that result.

In our teacher training program example, we would document the desired chain of outcomes that the program intends to catalyze. The program may intend to increase teachers' knowledge in a certain instructional practice, which in turn is expected to affect changes in how they teach, which in turn are aimed at improving student learning.

- What is the context in which the program is being implemented? In what ways is the context expected to affect the implementation and outcomes of the program? Context is typically considered the setting in which a program takes place (e.g., the school context in which training is taking place) but it can also consider a broader community context as well as the temporal context of the program. For example, in assessing the implementation and outcomes of programs aimed at improving access to and retention in housing, an EA should consider the extent to which housing is available, such as analyzing data on housing stock and vacancy rates, as well as assessing whether other changes occurred during the time of the program that could have affected the program (e.g., changes in the employment environment that affect a program's ability to maintain a workforce to keep the program operating).

At this stage, the logic model depicts the data collected through the document review and other preliminary data collection activities. At a minimum, the logic model should display the key program's goals and objectives, the resources and other program inputs, intended program strategies and activities, and intended outcomes, and the linkages among these elements. The linkages among the elements are what inform the underlying logic, detailing, for example, which resources are supporting which activities, how activities are expected to lead to short-term outcomes, and how short-term outcomes are expected to link to longer-term outcomes. Logic models are developed using an "if–then" logic—for example, "if" a particular activity occurs, "then" it is expected that a particular outcome or outcomes will occur. The assessment, as described below, not only assesses whether this linkage occurs in the program reality but whether the activity is plausibly related to this outcome, given what we know through research and common sense, and given its implementation. Figure 11.1 presents a logic model developed through an evaluabilty assessment of a coalition to address adverse childhood experiences and foster resilience (*https://marc.healthfederation.org/tools/MARC-network-evaluation-toolkit*).

Other elements that may be desirable to have in the logic model include the rationale and conceptual underpinnings of the program, strategies and program components (which may organize the specific activities), the target population or populations for the activities, and the overall context and factors within it that can affect both the different program elements and their outcomes, such as those noted in the housing program example above.

Depending on the complexity of a program or initiative, evaluators may choose to develop one or multiple models. Models can be at different levels of detail, with some very broad to provide the overall logic of an initiative and other more specific models detailing the theory underlying each program component. For example, in a program for youth that has intensive case management, a community drop-in, employment training, employment recruitment, substance abuse support, mental health counseling, and financial training, the evaluator may want to develop an overall model of how youth flow through the program and receive one or more of these different components and then detailed models of the individual program components that have their own outcomes.

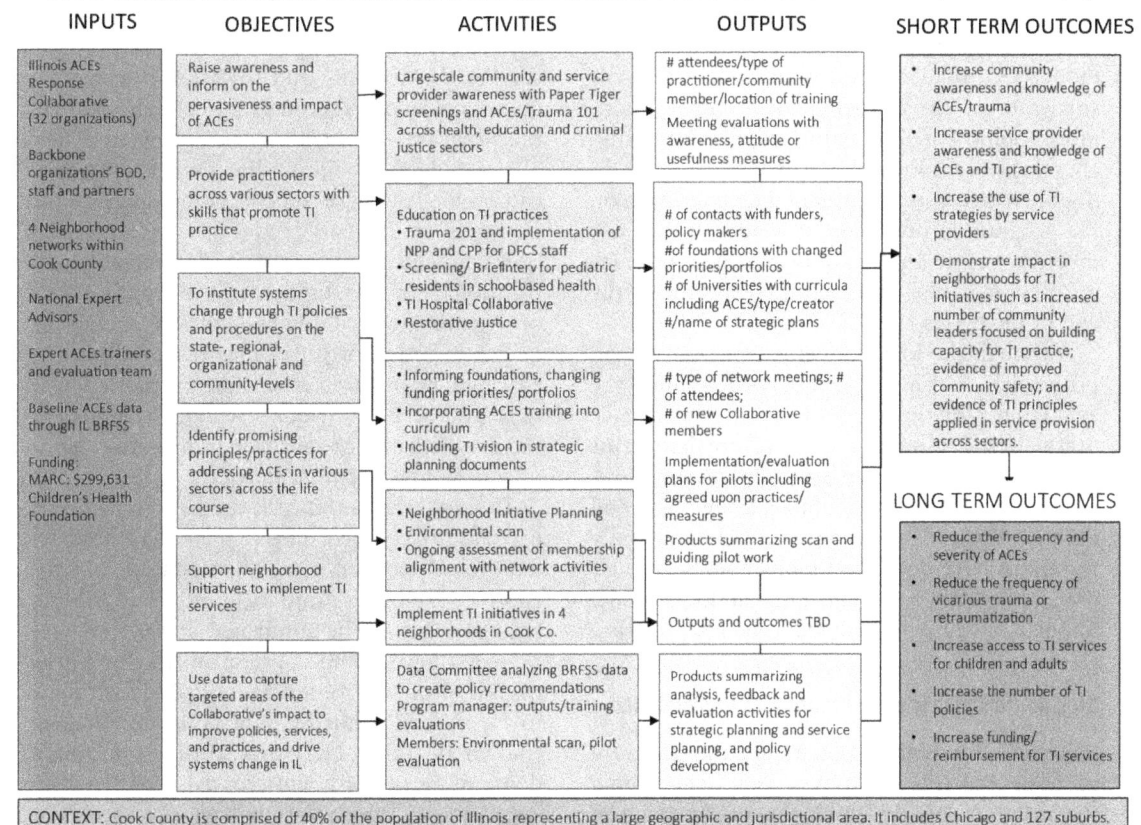

FIGURE 11.1. Logic model for a coalition to address adverse childhood experiences (ACEs) and foster resilience. Reprinted with permission from AEC's Response Collaborative at Health and Medicine Policy Research Group. TI refers to trauma-informed.

Developing program logic models can often be conducted by members of the EA team, drawing upon document information. Others with an interest in the program may also be involved in developing the first model of the program as intended. The process of logic model development can seem overwhelming at its outset, especially for very complex initiatives. To make the process manageable, the EA team might consider first working with all those involved to generate lists of the different program elements (e.g., the goals, activities, and outcomes). Then the EA team can begin to develop the model, recognizing that the process is dynamic and will be shaped and reshaped. To accommodate the process, the EA team can use either physical or electronic Post-it notes, dry erase boards, or other mediums to provide a flexible method for drawing the model, easily making changes in its structure and linkages as more information is received.

A variety of software programs are available for producing the final logic models. Logic models can be developed with basic Microsoft software, such as Word and PowerPoint, or with more sophisticated tools for graphics and flowcharting. As the logic model at this stage will no doubt change with additional data collection on the program in operation, it is advisable to not invest in a large amount of resources to produce a "pretty" model until the final model (at the end of the EA) is ready.

Although the logic model is being developed primarily as an analytic tool to determine the evaluability of the program, it often can have other uses. Programs that have not had prior logic models often find them useful in communicating about the program in a succinct way and even in managing the program. Although many programs have developed logic models on their own, others have not and find the logic model to be a useful by-product from the EA process.

Step 4. Documenting the Program as Implemented

Once the EA team understands the program as designed, the EA moves into determining the program reality—how the program operates on the ground. Documenting the program as implemented typically involves an in-person visit to the program site or sites to interview key program staff and others involved or with an interest in the program, observe relevant activities, and review any data that may be pertinent to review on-site. Abbreviated EAs rely on more limited numbers of telephone interviews and data reviews, and some EAs, especially during COVID-19, relied on virtual meetings in lieu of in-person visits.

Preparing for a Visit

The EA team needs to conduct several activities to prepare for the visit, usually a month or more prior to the time of the visit. The preliminary logic model and accompanying details provides a blueprint to follow for the visit. A call with the project director or key staff contacts prior to a visit provides the EA team an opportunity to learn about the current operation of the program in enough detail to begin to scope out the details of the visit, including people to interview and on what topics, activities to observe, and any data to review. If the program has multiple sites, the EA team should try to encompass in the EA the diversity and variation in type and operation among the sites that is likely to affect the program's evaluability. Interviewees generally include the program director and staff who can provide detail on specific components of the program, individuals in the broader organization who can provide information on the organizational context, funders of the program and/or organizations, individuals in any partnering or participating organizations (especially those that may be involved in specific program activities), and other individuals who have a stake in the program and can provide information on its operation and potential impact.

To guide the initial call, the EA team should use a draft protocol like that used to abstract data from documents, ideally updated with the specifics from the draft logic model that highlight elements to be confirmed as well as elaborated. I have found it useful in developing an overall protocol and data collection strategy to create a domain or data collection matrix (shown in Table 11.1) that outlines the main domains of the protocol crossed with the data sources from which data will be obtained. The matrix provides an opportunity to see where triangulation occurs among the data sources, where there may be gaps, and where there may be more redundancy than needed.

TABLE 11.1. Data Collection Matrix

	Project director	Project staff	Partners	Other interest holders	Documents	Database	Observations
Impetus	X				X		
Goals and objectives	X	X	X	X	X		
Resources	X		X		X		
Activities	X	X	X	X	X	X	X
Outcomes	X	X	X	X	X	X	
Interest holders	X			X			
Future plans	X		X				
Changes in program and rationale	X		X				
Organizational overview	X			X			
Context	X		X	X			
Data and measurement	X	X			X	X	
Past evaluations	X				X		

Scheduling the Visit

Ideally, a site visit is scheduled at least 1 month before it is to occur. The EA team should schedule the visit in concert with the key program staff and at a time that does not conflict with any major events for the program, vacations, or other events that could make people in the context less likely to be available. At times, the visit might be scheduled with another event if it provides an opportunity to either view an activity that offers an important lens on the program (such as a training) or connect with several people efficiently within a window of time (such as a local conference or meeting if people are willing to carve out a bit of their time to meet with you).

The length of the site visit can vary depending on the size and complexity of the program and the number of proposed interviewees. A typical visit, in one general geographic area, takes 2–3 days with approximately five to seven interviews and observations per day (generally the observations or program tours are limited to one to two per visit). Some interviews can be group interviews or focus groups, such as interviews with staff that work in the same or similar areas as well as with beneficiaries of a program. Although interviews are often scheduled for 1-hour slots, the time slots can vary in length depending on the extent of information needed from a respondent. With individuals who have a limited or focused involvement with a program, the interview can be scheduled for 30–45 minutes. With the project director and key staff, the interviews may take more than an hour. It is generally advisable not to schedule more than 2 hours at a time due to diminishing returns from possible fatigue and interruptions. If more time is needed, the EA team can schedule additional interviews with these key staff during the visit or on telephone or video calls after the visit. With a project director, it is often desirable for the EA team to schedule a second meeting at the end of the visit (or shortly after it) to clarify specific topics or ask questions that arise from speaking with others.

Scheduling visits takes strong organizational and communication skills. It involves not only knowing how much time is needed for each person but which interviews are better to schedule earlier in the visit to set a foundation of information for the rest of the interviews, which interviews make sense to schedule in adjacent timeframes to minimize travel time, which interviews include tours or observations, and how much time is needed between interviews to allow for travel. Different times of the day may have different traffic patterns that need to be considered; parking also may be difficult to find or needs to be arranged. In addition, time may need to be allocated for the EA team to go through building security or other processes. The EA team can ask each of these questions in either email or telephone contacts prior to the visit to ensure that sufficient time is scheduled for the process time as well as the interview time. Box 11.5 provides some scheduling tips.

In some instances, it may make sense to have people come to the program site to be interviewed, especially if there is a meeting room the EA team can use. Program directors might even suggest this, especially in communities that are difficult to navigate or where interviewees are very spread out. For many interviewees, their individual office locations do not offer anything substantive to the visit and thus meeting in one location does not detract from the visit.

In scheduling the visits, the EA team should develop an agenda that has all of the information the site visit team needs:

- The name and title of the individuals being interviewed.
- The interviewee's involvement in the program.
- Where the interview will take place—address, room number.
- Whether there is security or other processing to go through and what is needed to go through these processes (e.g., identification).
- What parking is available and at what cost.
- How much time is needed between visits.
- The interviewee's cell phone as well as any other contact information (e.g., name and number of an administrative support person or other staff to contact).

BOX 11.5. Scheduling Tip

The EA scheduler should ask interviewees for all times they are available during the visit to allow for maximum flexibility in scheduling. Doodle polls or other calendar scheduling software (Calendly) might facilitate this activity. Having all times available allows the scheduler to try to put the key interviews early, to schedule geographically when possible, and to provide time for processing. Ask interviewees to hold the times until they receive an email with the set meeting. It is therefore important that the scheduling be done efficiently so that these held times can be released.

In many visits, we also print or have electronically the directions between different interview locations. Although this can be considered "old school" and not needed with current GPS capabilities on cell phones, we have experienced enough difficulties with adequate cell service in rural and other remote areas to continue the hard-copy practice for these situations.

To facilitate scheduling, we often ask program directors to make an initial outreach to their colleagues, or at a minimum, we copy them on the introductory scheduling emails. To facilitate these contacts, we provide the program director with a brief description of the evaluability assessment process, including why it is being done, who is supporting it, and what it entails. In addition, we provide some detail on the scope and nature of the questions to be asked to the interviewee as well as the amount of time needed for the interview. We also at times have called it something other than evaluability assessment (e.g., brief assessment, program assessment) if we felt the term was off-putting and detracted from the process.

Conducting the Visit

Once the data sources are identified, the EA team develops specific interview guides for the key informants. We typically develop a small number of guides for different types of interviews (program staff, activity leads, onsite data/evaluation staff, etc.), with probes included for specific activities, organizations, and so on. In some EAs, we have used one complete protocol that guides all interviews, supplemented by a matrix that identifies the key domains and questions of interest for each interviewee. The protocol includes all of the information that is already known through the documents and highlights questions to supplement or confirm the document information. If answered, the questions in the protocol would provide a full set of information needed to judge the evaluability of the program.

The EA team conducts the interviews in a semistructured manner. The interview provides the information that is needed but the specific questions may vary by respondent. Some respondents start talking and cover many of the questions in their initial response. The interviewer should check to see whether the interviewee has more to add on a topic, but often an interviewee covers several topics in a response to the question "tell me how you are involved in this program." The topics to be covered expand on those addressed in the design documentation phase, addressing many of the same topics but with a focus on implementation. This includes:

- What do different groups of individuals view as the goals and objectives of the program?
- What resources does the program have? For example, what funding has been made available? Are all staff in place as proposed (e.g., have there been any issues with finding or keeping the right people, hiring freezes)? What are the types of partnerships in place? Are they in place as intended? Have there been any changes in level of involvement and level of support expected? Are there other inputs that were planned but not in place? Other inputs in place that were not planned?
- Who is served through the program? Is the program reaching and serving the population it intends to serve and in the numbers expected? What factors account for who is served and the number being served? Do different activities serve different populations? Why?
- What program activities are implemented? What is the level of staffing, intensity of activities, and alignment with original intentions? What factors account for the level of implementation? What challenges, if any, are affecting program implementation?
- What do interviewees expect (based on implementation and resources used thus far) will be the outputs of the program? What accounts for differences in what they expect based on what was initially intended?
- What outcomes are expected? What measures are considered appropriate for those outcomes?
- What is the current context (e.g., economic, political) in which the program is being implemented? How is it affecting the implementation and outcomes of the program? For example, is there a change in the context that has changed the type of individuals who are served by the program (e.g., changes in insurance coverage for health programs)?

Once a visit is underway, additional questions may emerge and can modify the protocol. Modifications may happen as additional activities or other program elements emerge that are not depicted in the draft logic model, as well as if other aspects of the program or the overall context are not clear or need elaboration.

Observations of activities are generally less formal than in bona fide implementation studies (see Powell et al., Chapter 12, this volume) but they provide texture to understanding specific program elements, such as how various activities are conducted, the nature of the setting, and other aspects of the program operation.

Step 5. Collecting Preliminary Data on the Feasibility of Conducting an Evaluation of the Program

As part of the data collection process, the EA team collects preliminary information on key elements of the data and evaluation capacity of the program as well as prospects for conducting an outcome evaluation, if the program is deemed evaluable. During the EA, the EA team is guided by preliminary questions that need to be addressed (either directly or indirectly) through interviews with data staff, reviews of any data collected, and/or reviews of documents that report the data. These questions include:

- What data are available to measure the implementation of the various aspects of the program? Does the program have data on individual-level participation in the program and its specific activities? What data do they collect on outputs and outcomes? Have they collected data from the time the program began? Have there been changes in the data over time that may affect their quality? Are the data accessible by others outside the program and in what timeframe? If there is more than one dataset, can they be merged at the person level?
- Are any data available on program participants before they entered or participated in the program (i.e., a baseline set of measures)?
- What is the program staff's evaluation capacity and receptivity to evaluation? Has the program been evaluated in the past, either internally or externally? Is there capacity in

the program to support an evaluation (i.e., Do they have their own evaluation staff? Are there individuals in the program who support data collection and reporting)?

- What prospects exist in the program setting for conducting a randomized study of the program? Is the demand for the program greater than the program's capacity? Are there formal wait lists for the program? Are there mechanisms in the inflow into the program that would be conducive for randomizing some individuals into the program and others into a services-as-usual condition or some alternative program?
- If randomization might be unlikely, what are the prospects for conducting a quasi-experimental design? Are there alternative programs that serve comparable populations and offer an important contrast in what is being received? Are there databases of comparable individuals not participating in the program from which a comparison group might be constructed?

Step 6. Analyzing the Data and Determining Evaluability

To facilitate analysis, the EA team can organize the data by domain and data source. Depending on the number of data sources, the evaluator may want to use a qualitative software program (such as NVivo, DeDoose, among others) to help organize and manage the data for analysis. Of course, the team can also use Microsoft Excel or nonelectronic means to organize and analyze the data; a software program can provide more efficient cuts in the data by source than other strategies and help the team to arrive more quickly to an analytic summary of the findings on each domain or area of evaluability.

The domains of information the EA team collects map over the key areas of the logic model (noted above), assessing the goals and objectives, the resources, activities, outputs, outcomes, and importantly, the linkages among the different elements of the program to determine whether it is plausible to expect that the activities as implemented are likely to result in the achievement of the outcomes. Table 11.2 outlines the analytic criteria EA uses to determine whether each condition is met for the program to be ready for an evaluation. These criteria include:

- Whether the *goals and objectives* of the program are clearly specified (ideally in writing but also can be articulated by key program staff) and are realistic to achieve, given the nature of the program activities, the resources provided, and the duration of the program. Some program goals are written by developers to sway funders (e.g., eradicate community violence) and are more visionary than providing specific guidance for program operation. Finally, it is important that all key decision makers share the same

TABLE 11.2. Summary of Evaluability Components for the Program

Program coherence		
Goals/objectives	Clearly specified	●
	Realistic to achieve	●
	Shared by interest holders	●
Resources	Sufficient	◉
	Available	◉
	Sustainable	◉
Target population	Well specified	●
	Appropriate	●
Components/strategies	Well-defined	●
	Measurable	●
Implementation	Well-defined	○
	Able to be done with fidelity	○
Outcomes	Clearly specified	◉
	Measurable	◉
	Comprehensive	●
	Agreed upon	◉
Linkages between components and outcomes	Plausible	●
Availability of data		◉
Evaluation capacity		◉
Users and uses for the evaluation		●

Note. Ratings are illustrative. ● Generally meets standards for evaluability. ◉ Questionably meets standards for evaluability. ○ Generally does *not* meet standards for evaluability.

goals and objectives for the program. If there are differences at this level, there will undoubtedly be lack of agreement among them on what the outcomes are and how they are measured. If decision makers do not agree on what the program is aimed at achieving, it may be difficult for an evaluation to produce results that will be convincing or pertinent to all decision makers.

• Whether the *resources* are available and sufficient to implement the program as intended and are sustainable. Sufficient and available resources relate to the program's ability to implement activities in the intensity, frequency, and quality needed to achieve the outcomes. Resources are not limited to funding but also can include the qualifications of the staff providing the services, partnerships, community support, and the suitability of the facilities. Sustainable resources do not relate directly to a program's evaluability but are for the EA team to consider as to whether an evaluation should be conducted if the program does not have the resources to continue over time.

• Whether the *population* that the program aims to serve is well specified and appropriate for the intervention. In some instances, a program may be aimed at serving a vulnerable group but ends up serving people who are higher functioning because the individuals with vulnerabilities may be harder to recruit. The EA can reveal this lack of population alignment and question whether the program as implemented aligns with the goals and objectives. In addition, although numbers served is not always noted as a criterion for evaluation, a program that serves few people may have difficulty achieving desired impacts and the evaluation may not be able to quantitatively assess outcomes. Having small sample sizes in the program may make it difficult for an evaluation to have sufficient **statistical power** to detect program effects through quantitative impact studies (see Harbatkin et al., Chapter 16, this volume) and may limit the evaluation options available (see Kazdin, 2020, for applicability of single-case designs).

• Whether the *program components/strategies/activities* implemented are well-defined and measurable. In multisite programs, especially if the sites are supposed to be implementing the same program model, an additional criterion is whether they are implemented consistently across program sites/locations.

• Whether the *outcomes* are clearly specified, measurable, realistic, comprehensive, and agreed upon. The outcomes should be the corollary to the goals and objectives but outlined in much more specific ways that can be operationalized and measured. The outcomes need to be stated in realistic terms based on the scope of the project, the timeframe of the study, and the resources provided. A key aspect of the evaluability of programs is that the outcomes need to be comprehensive in two ways: (1) they need to represent the key areas of change that are expected to result from the program; and equally importantly, (2) they need to delineate the chaining that is expected, from short-term changes to intermediate to longer-term changes. Frequently, programs have articulated the long-term outcomes desired for a program (such as reducing substance use, improving educational achievement, and improving employment) but lack the initial outcomes that the program intends to achieve that are expected to then bring about these longer-term effects. This chaining of outcomes is an important aspect of logic models that is often missing and, ironically, is among the most important aspects of evaluability as well as for understanding the essence of the program logic. A program aimed at preventing childhood obesity, for example, would need to articulate how it is either reducing access to and consumption of calories or increasing activity to burn calories, two essential elements for preventing childhood obesity based on the research evidence base (Kumanyika et al., 2010). Finally, for a program to be fully evaluable, the outcomes, especially as operationalized, should be those that program decision makers agree are appropriate for the program and upon which a subsequent evaluation should be established.

• Whether it is *plausible to expect that the outcomes can result from the activities in place.* Are the linkages between the activities and the outcomes plausible given basic common sense? Based on what we know from research or theory? Based on the timeframe outlined for the outcomes? Based on the intensity of the activities (e.g., dosage) and the resources provided? Based on the population reach of the program? Based on the context in which the program is operating? The EA is not designed to judge whether a program is effective but whether it is logical to expect that it *could* be effective given what it has set to accomplish and its current implementation.

Some criteria are more fundamental to evaluability than others and some can be remediated. For example, the lack of plausibility to achieve the outcomes given the nature and intensity of the activities in place is a major detriment to evaluability. It does not make sense to evaluate a program against outcomes that are deemed implausible to result from the activities. As noted in the section to follow, recommendations from the EA can address how the program can strengthen the alignment between the program activities and the outcomes. The activities can be refined to increase the plausibility of achieving the outcomes or the outcomes might be adjusted to be more realistic to be achieved by the program. The question is whether the program has the resources and desire to improve its activities or whether the revised outcomes are in line with what decision makers and others believe is a wise investment in the program.

Other evaluability criteria may be even easier to remedy. Increasing the measurability of the outcomes, for example, may involve the EA team working with the program developers/operators to refine the outcomes they are addressing and developing processes for obtaining agreement on the measures they believe are most accurate for measuring the outcomes of their program efforts.

The final determination of evaluability (whether an evaluation is ready for evaluation) is typically a balanced assessment of the criteria and the extent to which any departures from evaluability can be remedied or strengthened. In my experience, few programs that have been through an EA are flawless; most can benefit from some refinement of their program design or measurement before undergoing an evaluation. In some instances, however, the changes a program may need to become evaluable may be quite significant and require considerable resources before undergoing an evaluation.

Whether a program is ready for evaluation, however, is not the only determination of evaluability. Other conditions for determining whether conducting an outcome evaluation makes sense include:

- If the evaluation designs needed are feasible.
- If needed data are available.
- If there is capacity within the program to support it.
- If there are users with specific intended uses for the evaluation.

Taking the last bullet first, if the EA finds that a subsequent evaluation does not have an audience, it is unclear whether the effort should continue. Typically, if there is a funder for the evaluation, it is likely that the same funder has an interest in using the results from the evaluation. However, if it is a third-party funder, and the decisions for the program are in the control of others who are seemingly uninterested in the evaluation, the EA team's recommendation may be to reconsider whether the timing is right for the evaluation.

The feasibility assessment builds on the data collected through the EA (such as if randomization could be possible) and helps inform the development of evaluation options below. Similarly, the extent to which data and evaluation capacity exist also inform options for improving the program's data and evaluation capacity.

DEVELOPING EA FOLLOW-UP OPTIONS

Once an EA is completed, a final section of the report is typically devoted to providing a set of recommendations, often in the form of options for follow-on activities. These options fall into four general categories:

- Evaluation options
- Program design options
- Program management
- Measurement/data options

Evaluation Options

The EA can provide detailed information to guide follow-on evaluation options. Even if there are departures from evaluability based on the data collected, the EA team might still offer evaluation options once other recommendations for improving the program's evaluability are implemented. In some instances, portions of a program might be more evaluable than others and might be the more appropriate focus for an evaluation.

Based on the information collected, the EA report can outline the questions that decision makers have that an evaluation can address and alternative designs that can address them. The report should present the alternative designs within the context of the information needs of the intended users, the bases of comparison available, the timeframe available, whether data are readily available or would need to be collected, the size of the participant pool, the scope of the program, and the capacity and willingness of the program to participate in and/or support an evaluation. In some instances, the best design alternative for an evaluation may be a process or implementation study that can provide more detailed program data before embarking on an outcome evaluation.

Program Design and Management Options

The EA will likely inform modifications needed to the program design or to the management of the program to strengthen the underlying logic of the program and its plausibility of achieving desired outcomes. Program design options may include adding new activities or revising goals, objectives, and intended outcomes. For example, if the goals were not judged to be realistic given the program resources and activities, the EA team may need to recommend that the goals be modified to make them more realistic yet still meet user needs. In other instances, the EA team may recommend that the program be strengthened to make the goals more in reach. The program design options are aimed at improving the alignment between the program as implemented with the expected outcomes so that the outcomes are realistic and plausible.

Some problems with the lack of evaluability may stem from management problems, such as challenges in reaching and engaging the intended population into the program, engaging partners in the work as designed, and ensuring that the implementation of the program across different sites is consistent. The EA report may suggest options for addressing these problems by improving the program management, such as implementing new communication processes, oversight activities, specific program guidelines, and training and supervision.

Measurement/Data Options

The EA may propose options for strengthening the data and measures that would be needed to conduct an evaluation of the desired outcomes. In one EA of a child-serving program we conducted, for example, the program focused on organizational changes that were believed to have outcomes for both staff and the children and families served. Although staff outcomes were well specified, the family and child outcomes were subsumed under a broad category of well-being, with little specificity as to the nature of the changes that were expected and the mechanisms that would bring these changes about. We proposed a set of working meetings that the EA team could facilitate with the program decision makers to discuss what well-being meant to them, the measures that would operationalize these aspects of well-being, and how they believed the program created those changes.

Our EAs generally result in multiple options, within and across the four different types of options. Even in situations where the program is evaluable, some options for tightening the program and its measurement, for example, may be advantageous to implement before embarking on the evaluation.

COMMUNICATING THE EA FINDINGS

An EA is intended as a pre-evaluation activity, aimed at ensuring that an evaluation is not being conducted prematurely or without the full support and engagement of key parties. EA's aims and methodology are reasonably straightforward; therefore, the EA team's feedback to the sponsors can be succinct and focused. Although the EA team typically develops reports, especially if the sponsor is interested in obtaining a detailed understanding of the program, they can also present findings from an EA in short summaries and presentations, with the logic models and charts of evaluability serving as the focus of the findings and the display of options providing recommendations for next steps. Box 11.6 offers a sample EA report outline.

Depending on the purpose of the EA, its outcomes, and the recommendations provided, several next steps are possible. In many instances, the findings from an EA can provide sufficient information for the funder, especially if the purpose is to provide rapid feedback or if the program is not ready for evaluation. In other instances, an evaluation is already slated to occur, regardless of the EA outcomes, and the EA is used as a guide to develop the evaluation plan. Depending on the EA outcome, a sponsor could consider a sequential purchase of information, such as providing resources to strengthen the program and support some evaluation and data capacity building, followed by a commissioning of an evaluation design and subsequent evaluation.

THE EVALUABILITY ADVANTAGE

I learned about EA in graduate school, and was engaged in an EA while finishing my PhD. I was attracted to its simplicity and commonsense appeal and by its roots in providing government sponsors and other program sponsors with a tool that could help them use their resources more wisely. During the period of time when I was in graduate school, much of the nascent evaluation literature was focused on evaluation utilization and trying to understand how we could improve the instrumental use of evaluation findings. The hope that EA brought to evaluators was that by providing early information on whether evaluation was worth doing, evaluators could direct evaluation resources to those situations where the test of outcomes made the most sense and where evaluation information could be most beneficial.

Unfortunately, it has taken many years for EA to become a more standard practice in government and beyond. As I found in my dissertation (Rog, 1985), EA's early expansive use in what is now known as the U.S. Department of Health and Human Services was short-lived. Joe Wholey's leadership as deputy assistant secretary for planning and evaluation in the HHS during the Carter administration was the catalyst for getting it funded but the efforts waned after he left. As noted earlier, however, in the last 20 years EA has become a much more recognized, accepted, and supported tool in many government agencies, philanthropies, and nongovernmental organizations in the United States and globally. Vaessen (2017), in a post for the Independent Evaluation Group of the World Bank Group (WBG), observes:

> Over the last ten years or so, there has been a renewed interest in the international development community (e.g., DFID, ILO, IADB, WBG)[1] for

---

BOX 11.6. Sample EA Report Table of Contents

Introduction	1
Evaluability Assessment Methodology	2
Figure 1. Evaluability Assessment Process	3
Figure 2. Elements of Evaluability	4
Overview of the Program and Its Development	4
Description and Analysis of the Program	6
Figure 3. Logic Model	8
Assessment of the Program	11
Figure 4. Summary of Evaluability Components for the Program	13
Table 1A: Goals/Objectives	14
Table 1B: Resources	14
Table 1C: Target Population	16
Table 1D: Program Strategies and Activities	17
Table 1E: Implementation	19
Table 1F: Outcomes	2
Table 1G: Linkages between the Components and the Outcomes	22
Table 1H: Evaluation Capacity, Data Availability, Users, and Use for Evaluation Results	23
Recommended Options for Consideration	25
Appendix A: Sources of Information for the Evaluability Assessment	30

---

[1] The DFID (Department for International Development of the United Kingdom; now called the Foreign, Commonwealth and Development Office), ILO (International Labour Organization), IADB (Inter-American Development Bank), and WBG (World Bank Group) are international financial organizations.

BOX 11.7. Example of an EA

A number of years ago, I was asked by a foundation to conduct a number of evaluability assessments in the area of childhood obesity prevention. The effort had several purposes: to learn what we could about these relatively small programs; to see which might be ready for evaluation; and to test whether conducting multiple EAs for relatively a small amount of money could, in a short period of time, "separate the wheat from the chaff" with respect to identifying programs most ready to be evaluated and to contribute knowledge on worthwhile interventions. The programs included both exercise-related programs (e.g., dance programs in schools) and food-related programs (e.g., exposing children to healthy foods).

One of the programs we included was a community garden program. It had been initiated by a small community foundation and had many goals, including helping foster community spirit. As the program was being implemented with youth in a variety of settings, the program developers believed the gardens also could help combat childhood obesity. For this EA as well as others in this area, a two-person team planned and conducted the assessment. We began by reviewing foundation-level documents (e.g., the RFP, individual grant funding documents) to understand what the foundation was hoping to get out of this program. For each childhood obesity prevention effort, the foundation's interest was in environmental solutions to prevention, not programs that exclusively focused on changing beliefs and attitudes but that had program elements that changed children's level of activity or food intake.

We conducted telephone interviews with the foundation sponsors to provide greater understanding of what they wanted through the programs, what they hoped to learn from the EAs, and what decisions the EAs could inform.

With each program, we began by sending a description of what an EA is, why the foundation selected their program, what we would like to learn, and a request for setting up a call and scheduling a future visit. We then conducted a call with each program's director, getting some initial information and requesting more through documents that they could send. We specifically were interested in accessing documents that described their program, including initial grant proposals, progress reports, annual reports, program manuals, and others. We discussed the process moving forward, including the nature of the visit we would like to conduct, the types of people we would like to interview, the types of activities we would like to observe, and the data and data systems we would like to review. A significant part of each program director call was describing the purpose of the EA and distinguishing it from an evaluation.

These initial calls were typically followed by several email connections and at least one additional telephone call. The program director sent documents that we reviewed and then we connected back with them to clarify the different program sites they had and the role of the state public health department in helping with measurement of outcomes. We developed a draft logic model that we reviewed with the program director and deputy program director and sent a draft agenda of what we hoped to cover during the visit, including the program sites and people we would like to interview. A key person from the state was not located in the community so we scheduled a call with them after the visit. They provided additional people and partners to include, such as contacts in the local foundation, and we discussed the array of program sites that would allow us to understand the scope of the program (e.g., they were implementing community gardens with recreation centers, schools, and residential programs). We also sought to identify key events that might be good to observe and could influence the timing of our visit. For example, for another program, a dance initiative in several school systems, we attended a train-the-trainers meeting that was a core element of the initiative. We had already received the detailed training manual but having the opportunity to see the training in action helped us to get an understanding of the dynamism of the program.

We sent the proposed agenda to the program director, with proposed times to meet with individuals in selected organizations and the array of sites we would like to visit. The agenda, typical for an EA, began with a 2-hour meeting with the program director and other program staff to build a foundation of knowledge about the program, followed by meetings with the local foundation, and individuals in the other sites. In particular, we visited the different sites where the program operates, interviewing the individuals involved with the program in each site and in one site conducting a focus group with children involved in the community garden. We complemented the visit with telephone interviews with others who were outside of the region (e.g., the state government representative).

The scope of this program was smaller than most programs for which we conduct EAs and the geographic spread between the sites and interviews was limited, so we were able to conduct the visit in a day and conduct the additional phone interviews in a few hours. For many EAs, we generally take 2–3 days to conduct an EA and may even spend more time in additional visits or extended telephone/video interviews if programs are spread across large geographic areas.

We determined that the program was well implemented and according to design but the plausibility of the program preventing childhood obesity was ques-

> **BOX 11.7.** *(continued)*
>
> tionable. The children involved in the community gardens did not generally eat the food or change their eating by becoming more familiar with healthy food and they did not get more exercise than they would in alternative activities (such as playing in the playground). The community garden did not provide an environmental solution to childhood obesity prevention that the foundation was interested in learning more about.
>
> The EA team provided feedback to the developers and operators of the program to either restructure the garden so that the food supplemented the children's diets and had some opportunity to affect caloric intake or reframe the outcomes of the garden that are more consistent to how they are implemented (i.e., increase knowledge of healthy foods, increase familiarity with them, and acceptance of them).

conducting evaluability assessments, mostly at the project level but also at the level of higher-level programs. Evaluability assessments (if used strategically and not as a requirement) can be an effective medicine for treating the metaphorical disease called "evaluitis" (Frey, 2006), thwarting the "ritualization" of evaluation processes in organizational systems. It can help us ask fundamental questions about the strategic allocation of scarce evaluation resources and strengthen our internal monitoring processes to provide timely and relevant evidence to decision makers and other interest holder groups.

Beyond providing a tool, EA has introduced an evaluability perspective into evaluation. It has taught us to question whether an evaluation "should" be done, at least at this point in a program's life cycle, and to guide evaluation sponsors in targeting evaluation resources more wisely. For evaluators, even if they are not afforded the opportunity to implement an EA before embarking on an evaluation, having an evaluability perspective may help them to design evaluations with eyes wide open. Taking an evaluability perspective can, at a minimum, help an evaluator design evaluations that focus on those program elements that have stronger logic and are plausibly linked to outcomes that are both realistic and measurable.

Additional Resources

Craig, P., & Campbell, M. (2015, June). Evaluability assessment: A systematic approach to deciding whether and how to evaluate programmes and policies. *Working Paper*. What Works Scotland.

Davies, R. (2013). Planning evaluability assessments: A synthesis of the literature with recommendations. *Working Paper*, 40. Department for International Development.

Dunn, E. (2008). *Planning for cost effective evaluation with evaluability assessment*. U.S. Agency for International Development.

Leviton, L. C., Kettel-Khan, L, Rog, D. J., Dawkins, N., & Cotton, D. (2010). Evaluability assessment. *Annual Review of Public Health, 31*, 215–234.

Ogilvie, D., Cummins, S., & Petticrew, M. (2011). Assessing the evaluability of complex public health interventions: Five questions for researchers, funders and policymakers. *Milbank Quarterly, 89*, 206–225.

Peersman, G., Guijt, I., & Pasanen, T. (2015). *Evaluability assessment for impact evaluation. A methods lab publication*. Overseas Development Institute.

Wholey, J. S. (1983). *Evaluation and effective public management*. Little, Brown.

Wholey, J. S. (1987). Evaluability assessment: Developing program theory. In L. Bickman (Ed.), Using program theory in evaluation. *New Directions for Program Evaluation*, No. 33. Jossey-Bass.

Wholey, J. S. (2015). Exploratory evaluation. In K. E. Newcomer, H. P. Hatry, & J. S. Wholey (Eds.), *Handbook of practical program evaluation* (4th ed., pp. 88–107). Jossey-Bass.

REFERENCES

Frechtling, J. (2007). *Logic modeling methods in program evaluation*. Jossey-Bass/Wiley.

Frey, B. S. (2006). *Evaluitis—Eine Neue Krankheit*. Working paper series/Institute for Empirical Research in Economics No. 293, University of Zurich.

Kazdin, A. (2020). *Single-case research designs: Methods for clinical and applied settings* (3rd ed.). Oxford University Press.

Knowlton, L. W., & Phillips, C. C. (2012). *The logic model guidebook: Better strategies for great results*. SAGE.

Kumanyika, S. K., Parker, L., & Sim, L. J. (2010). *Bridging the evidence gap in obesity prevention: A framework to inform decision making*. National Academies Press.

Lam, S., & Skinner, K. (2021). The use of evaluability assessment in improving future evaluations: A scoping review of 10 years of literature (2008–2018). *American Journal of Evaluation, 42*(4), 533–540.

Leviton, L., Kettel Khan, L., & Dawkins, N. (Eds.). (2010). *The systematic screening and assessment method: Finding innovations worth evaluating.* Jossey-Bass.

Losby, J. L., Vaughan, M., Davis, R., & Tucker-Brown, A. (2015). Arriving at results efficiently: Using the enhanced evaluability assessment approach. *Prevention of Chronic Diseases, 24*(12), E224.

McLaughlin, J. A., & Jordan, G. B. (2015). Using logic models. In K. E. Newcomer, H. P. Hatry, & J. S. Wholey (Eds.), *Handbook of practical program evaluation* (4th ed.). Jossey-Bass.

Mulkern, V. (2005, October). *Evaluability assessment of the Mental Health Block Grant Program.* Presented at the Annual Meeting of the American Evaluation Association.

Nay, J., & Kay, P. (1982). *Government oversight and evaluability assessment: It is always more expensive when the carpenter types.* Heath and Company.

Rog, D. J. (1985). *A methodological analysis of evaluability assessment* [Doctoral dissertation, Vanderbilt University, Nashville, TN].

Rog, D. J. (2005, October). Evaluability assessment: Then and now [Paper presentation]. Joint meeting of the Canadian Evaluation Society and the American Evaluation Association, Toronto, ON, Canada.

Rutman, L. (1980). *Planning useful evaluations: Evaluability Assessment.* Sage.

Schmidt, R., Beyuna, L., & Haar, J. (1982). Evaluability assessment: Principles and practice. In G. J. Stahler & W. R. Tash (Eds.), *Innovative approaches to mental health evaluation.* Academic Press.

Smith, M. F. (1989). *Evaluability assessment: A practical approach.* Kluwer Academic.

Thurston, W. E., Graham, J., & Hatfield, J. (2003). Evaluability assessment: A catalyst for program change and improvement. *Evaluation and the Health Professions, 26,* 206–221.

Thurston, W. E., & Hatfield, J. (2003). Evaluability assessment: A catalyst for program change and improvement. *Evaluation and the Health Professions,* 206–221.

Thurston, W. E., & Potvin, L. (2003). Evaluability assessment: A tool for incorporating evaluation in social change programmes. *Evaluation, 9*(4), 453–469.

Trevisan, M. S. (2007). Evaluability assessment from 1986–2006. *American Journal of Evaluation, 28*(3), 290–303.

Trevisan, M. S., & Walser, T. M. (2015). *Evaluability assessment: Improving evaluation quality and use.* SAGE.

Vaessen, J. (2017). *Evaluability and why it is important for evaluators and nonevaluators.* World Bank Group.

W. K. Kellogg Foundation. (2004). *Using logic models to bring together planning, evaluation, and action: Logic model development guide.* Author.

Wholey, J. S. (1979). *Evaluation: Promise and performance.* Urban Institute.

Wholey, J. S., Scanlon, J. W., Duffy, H. G., Fukomoto, J. S., & Vogt, L. M. (1971). *Federal evaluation policy: Analyzing the effects of public programs.* Urban Institute.

Chapter 12

Monitoring Program Implementation

Byron J. Powell
Leonard Bickman
Kimberly Eaton Hoagwood

CHAPTER OVERVIEW

The speed and quality of program implementation are increasingly emphasized in the field of evaluation. The purpose of this chapter is to provide an overview of the frameworks, methods, and designs that can be leveraged to monitor program implementation when conducting an evaluation. It includes approaches that are well suited to address the following key questions:

1. What program is being evaluated and what is its theory of change?
2. What is the extent and quality of program implementation?
3. What are key interest holders' perceptions of the program?
4. Was the program sustained?
5. What are the costs associated with implementing the program?
6. What factors facilitated or impeded program implementation?
7. How can the process of implementation be improved?
8. What designs can be leveraged to evaluate programs and implementation strategies?
9. What can be done to ensure that evaluations include implementation data that are sufficiently detailed to inform future efforts?

Evaluations often conclude that programs do not demonstrate their anticipated effects (Bickman & Heflinger, 1995). Bickman & Heflinger discuss three reasons why this occurs: **program failure, implementation failure,** and **evaluation failure.** Program failure is related to a faulty **program theory**: "the plausible and sensible model of how the program is supposed to work," which can be derived from interest holders' beliefs about important factors, theory, and/or data (Bickman, 1987, p. 5; Bickman & Heflinger, 1995). If the underlying program theory is wrong, then the evaluation may correctly show that the program did not have the intended effect. However, before declaring a program failure, evaluators facing null effects need to first rule out the possibility of implementation and/or evaluation failures, both of which would prevent a valid test of the program theory (Bickman & Heflinger, 1995). Implementation failure occurs when the program was not implemented as intended, and evaluation failure occurs when the data collected and/or the data analysis are not well aligned with the targets for measurement suggested by the program theory (see Rog, Chapter 11, this volume, for more on a related concept: evaluability assessment).

Evaluators play a central role in assessing the effectiveness of programs. They are often tasked with monitoring programs to ensure that they are implemented as intended, and if not, improving implementation by providing feedback about how the program was modified (intentionally or unintentionally), what factors are facilitating or impeding implementation, and how the processes and strategies used to implement the program might be improved. In some cases, evaluators monitor programs as they are being implemented and provide feedback to implementers in real time so that they can work to improve the quality of program delivery. In other cases, they evaluate the extent and quality of implementation after the program is implemented, often within the context of the primary outcomes of interest, so that the evaluation of implementation is primarily aimed at improving future implementations of the program.

The purpose of this chapter is to provide an overview of the frameworks, methods, and designs that can be leveraged to monitor program implementation when conducting an evaluation. This includes an examination of the nine key questions described earlier:

1. What program is being evaluated and what is its theory of change?
2. What is the extent and quality of program implementation?
3. What are key interest holders' perceptions of the program?
4. Was the program sustained?
5. What are the costs associated with implementing the program?
6. What factors facilitated or impeded program implementation?
7. How can the process of implementation be improved?
8. What designs can be leveraged to evaluate programs and implementation strategies?
9. What can be done to ensure that evaluations include implementation data that are sufficiently detailed to inform future efforts?

While the guidance provided herein is intended to be broadly applicable to all evaluations, some of the guidance may be particularly applicable to health, mental health, and social service settings given our expertise in these areas.

WHAT PROGRAM IS BEING EVALUATED AND WHAT IS ITS THEORY OF CHANGE?

One of the first tasks of an evaluator is generate a clear understanding of the program being evaluated. Ideally, program developers will have documented the evidence that supports the program, articulated a clear program theory that describes how the program is supposed to work (Bickman, 1987; Bickman & Heflinger, 1995), and will have described the program in enough detail so that it can be replicated (Hoffman et al., 2014). Unfortunately, programs are often not specified in sufficient detail, a deficit that often includes the poor articulation of program theory that would stipulate how and why a program works. Moreover, the "core components" of programs that, based upon theory or evidence, are essential for the program to have an effect, are rarely differentiated from components that may be adaptable to ensure adequate fit with local contexts (Michie et al., 2009). If elements of the program are not already well articulated, evaluators may need to partner with key interest holders (e.g., program developers, providers, and recipients) prior, during, and/or following the program evaluation to specify the aforementioned elements of the program, including a more robust program theory.

Metz (2016) and Metz and Easterling (2016) describe the development of "practice profiles" as a process for operationalizing programs. The methodology begins with the collection of more information about the program through a review of program documents, a scoping review of the literature, and semistructured interviews with practitioners and community members to identify the program's principles as well as the specific activities that are undertaken to carry them out. Community members, practitioners, leadership, and other key interest holders then engage in a process of developing consensus about program activities and functions. Finally, the program is iterated using a plan, do, study, act cycle (Taylor et al., 2014).

A similar process was recently outlined by Kirk and colleagues (2021), who demonstrated a method for identifying core forms (activities) and functions (purposes) of programs that are underspecified by program developers. They reviewed program materials to determine whether a clear theory of change or description of program forms and functions was already described; interviewed program developers to identify usual care pathways and barriers to the outcome of interest, program theory, program forms, and program functions; and mapped the program functions they identified onto theory from the literature to develop a program theory.

Evaluability assessment, another approach to ensuring that a program is properly specified, is covered in detail by Rog (see Chapter 11, this volume).

Many of the methods used to specify a program involve the depiction of program theory through a logic model (Frechtling, 2007; McLaughlin & Jordan, 1999; W. K. Kellogg Foundation, 2004), first developed in evaluability assessment (see Rog, Chapter 11, this volume). Frechtling (see Chapter 20, this volume) provides helpful guidance for developing logic models that reflect program theory and gives several applied examples. She also describes the components of generic logic models, including inputs (resources brought to a program), activities (actions taken to achieve the program's goals and outcomes), outputs (products of activities, often simple counts on products, participants, and events), outcomes (changes in attitudes, skills, and behavior), and impacts (broader systems-level changes that are expected if the program is successful). It is also helpful to rely upon guidance for reporting programs and interventions. For example, for health-related interventions, the Template for Intervention Description and Replication Checklist was developed to improve published descriptions of interventions (Hoffman et al., 2014). It suggests providing details such as (1) name or phrase that describes the program; (2) rationale, theory, or goal of the elements essential to the program; (3) physical or informational materials used in the program and where they can be accessed; (4) description of procedures, activities, and/or processes used in the program; (5) expertise, background, and specific training given to those delivering the program; (6) modes of delivery (e.g., face-to-face, internet, telephone) and whether it is provided individually or in a group; (7) type(s) of location(s) where the program occurred, including any necessary infrastructure or relevant features; (8) number of sessions, their schedule, duration, intensity, or dose; and (9) whether the program is intended to be personalized, titrated, or adapted, and if so, what, why, when, and how (Hoffman et al., 2014).

Specifying a program is a prerequisite to conducting a valid program evaluation, and lays the foundation for monitoring the extent and quality of program implementation to either prevent or diagnose implementation failure, a topic covered in the following section.

WHAT IS THE EXTENT AND QUALITY OF PROGRAM IMPLEMENTATION?

Evaluators seeking to establish the extent and quality of program implementation can draw upon a number of **implementation outcomes**, which can be defined as "the effects of deliberate and purposive actions to implement new treatments, practices, and services" (Proctor et al., 2011, p. 65). Implementation outcomes serve as indicators of implementation success and proximal indicators of implementation processes (Proctor et al., 2011). Proctor and colleagues proposed eight conceptually distinct implementation outcomes (acceptability, appropriateness, feasibility, adoption, fidelity, penetration, sustainability, and cost), and have provided an in-depth exploration of their conceptual grounding, measurement, and reporting (Lengnick-Hall et al., 2022; Lewis et al., 2015; Lewis, Proctor, et al., 2018; Proctor et al., 2014). This conceptualization stems from the mental health field and has been widely used across health and social service settings (Lengnick-Hall et al., 2021). Relatively recent systematic reviews have identified corresponding measures that have been used in physical health (Khadjesari et al., 2020) and behavioral health care settings (Mettert et al., 2020). While we suspect some version of these outcomes will be quite relevant for a range of purposes, it is possible that additional implementation outcomes will be relevant to evaluations conducted for diverse settings and purposes. Notably, while these implementation outcomes are often used in reference to programs, they can also be used in reference to implementation strategies (described in more detail below). For example, there is increasing emphasis on capturing concepts like fidelity to implementation strategies such as audit and feedback and implementation champions (Akiba et al., 2023; Akiba, Powell, Pence, Muessig, et al., 2022; Akiba, Powell, Pence, Nguyen, et al., 2022). Three implementation outcomes are particularly important for evaluators to measure in assessments of the extent and quality of implementation, as they represent concrete, behavioral manifestations of implementation efforts (Lyon & Bruns, 2019). These include adoption, fidelity, and penetration.

Adoption

Adoption is defined as "the intention, initial decision, or action to try or employ an innovation or evidence-based practice" (Proctor et al., 2011, p. 69). Also referred to as "uptake," adoption could be measured from the perspective of an individual or a setting. For example, we could assess whether a classroom-based intervention to prevent behavior problems has been used by individual teachers within a school or adopted by schools within a larger district. As Proctor et al. (2014) note, adoption can often be measured dichotomously ("adopted" or "not adopted")—however, it is recommended that adoption be combined with measures of fidelity and penetration (described below), as the quality and extent to which an intervention is implemented is likely more important than its initial adoption (Dearing & Kee, 2012). In other words, adoption is necessary, but likely insufficient to attain positive outcomes. To return to the previous example, if a teacher has adopted a classroom-based prevention intervention but frequently forgets to use positive reinforcement or other techniques that are core components of the program, it is unlikely that it will result in positive outcomes for students. Similarly, if only a few teachers in a school district have adopted the program, it is unlikely to have widespread effects at the district level. This highlights the importance of assessing fidelity and penetration.

Fidelity

Fidelity is defined as "the degree to which an intervention was implemented as it was prescribed in the original protocol or as it was intended by the program developers" (Proctor et al., 2011, p. 69). For example, during the COVID-19 pandemic, many individuals wore protective masks but did so in a manner that did not confer the intended protection by wearing it below their nose or mouth. They "adopted" the practice of wearing a mask, but had not done so with fidelity to recommended practices. Fidelity is often considered in relation to "core components" of the intervention, or those that are theoretically and/or empirically shown to be fundamental to programmatic impact (Allen et al., 2018; Kirk et al., 2021). The importance of fidelity is illustrated in the case example described in Box 12.1. For many programs, there may not be an adequate underlying theory or model as it may have simply been someone's notion of what would work with little data or theory behind it. In those cases, the evaluator has to decide if fidelity or any other aspect of implementation should be measured. Measurement in this situation is based on the evaluator's belief that it was important enough to measure and thus provides face validation of that measure. The evaluator may judge (yes, it is a judgment) that the program or any aspect of it may not be sufficiently valid to be worth measuring. On the other hand, if there is adequate time and resources, the evaluator may work with interest holders to carefully specify the elements of the program and the associated program theory through the development of logic models (see Frechtling, Chapter 20, this volume) or other systematic approaches (Kirk et al., 2021; Metz & Easterling, 2016). However, the evaluator should recognize that this is an ad hoc activity that the evaluator and other involved interest holders greatly influenced—thus, it may bias the evaluation of the implementation outcomes. Some programs are so poorly conceptualized that they never should have been funded, implemented, or evaluated but that is beyond the control of the evaluator.

Assessing fidelity is essential in conducting a valid test of a program (Allen et al., 2018; Bickman & Heflinger, 1995). When a program demonstrates positive outcomes, careful measure-

> **BOX 12.1. Case Example: The Importance of Monitoring Fidelity**
>
> When I (Leonard Bickman) was director of the Westinghouse Program Evaluation Institute in the late 1970s, I managed the evaluation component of a technical assistance project for a national program called Crime Prevention Through Environmental Design (CPTED). I was to assist local evaluators in their evaluation of this multidisciplinary approach for reducing crime through environmental design in high schools in South Florida. The strategies used in this project were designed to reduce victimization, deter offenders, and build a sense of community among people. The purpose was to give students and school staff a sense of territorial control of areas and reduce opportunities for crime and fear of crime. CPTED contained several strong principles that included natural surveillance, natural access control, and natural territorial control. The director of our group became a major contributor to this approach (Crowe, 2000).
>
> The project involved several strategies that changed the built environment of the schools. Among them were the following changes to the high school environment. To reduce thefts from cars in the parking lot they built patios for students near the lots and included gates that could be locked. To reduce theft in the locker rooms they painted the lockers different colors by class periods so that teachers could quickly see if students belonged in the correct area. To reduce crimes in the bathrooms they removed the outside doors and placed walls in such position so that there was visual privacy. This is now a common strategy in many public locations, such as airports.
>
> As a consultant I made a site visit to look at the changes that were made. First, I visited with the two local evaluators who worked for the school system. I asked them if they had visited the schools. They said they had not and were surprised that I had asked. They were educational evaluators who were accustomed to conducting an evaluation by randomly assigning students to different conditions and then analyzing the test scores. Other than their semiannual surveys they conducted to assess the effects of the program on self-reported victimization, they had no interest in anything else.
>
> I insisted on visiting the schools to see how the changes were made. Given that these were changes in the environment it was easy to see how the program was implemented. The locker room was my first stop. When I tried to visit, I found the door locked. One of the coaches unlocked it and commented that since they locked the door when the students were out playing there had been no thefts. While that is a CPTED strategy, it was not the one that was supposed to be implemented. They were supposed to paint the lockers different colors based on the class period. I did find that they did the painting, but the three-tiered lockers were painted different colors by height and not by location. Not only was the strategy implemented incorrectly but if thefts did drop it would have been misattributed to the painting and not simply locking the doors.
>
> The patios were more or less in place near the parking lots but a brief observation made it clear that students were not arranging themselves so that natural surveillance was occurring. In an attempt to test this strategy, I asked some of my colleagues to make believe they were trying to break into my car. I was surprised when a group of students approached them—however, it was to tell them that the other parking lot had better cars. The gates that were supposed to close the parking lot were wide open. Further investigation disclosed that the gates were poorly installed and the locks that were meant to lock them no longer fit. The locks with longer shanks were on back order for months so none of those gates could be locked.
>
> Finally, the bathroom strategy was well implemented. The doors were gone, and the walls were built. However, it was not clear to me how this was supposed to reduce crime. The point hit home as we were touring the campus with the principal, the superintendent of schools, and some school board members when a boy and girl holding hands exited one of the bathrooms right in front of us.
>
> This experience left me with an appreciation for documenting implementation. Without solid evidence of fidelity of implementation there is little to connect the program or theory of the program to its purported outcomes. It should never be assumed that programs are delivered the way developers intended.

ment of fidelity allows us to understand whether the effects are related to the quality or extent of implementation. For example, if the program wasn't implemented with fidelity, yet the program still obtained positive outcomes, it may be that the program was modified (intentionally or unintentionally) in ways that preserved its intended effect or that factors unrelated to the program may account for observed outcomes. When programs do not achieve intended outcomes, measuring fidelity helps to determine whether results are attributable to inadequate implementation (i.e., Type III error), theory failure, or some combination (Allen et al., 2018;

Bickman & Heflinger, 1995). There is growing evidence that program fidelity is highly associated with success in achieving change in targeted outcomes among programs with strong, plausible theories (Allen et al., 2018; Durlak & DuPre, 2008).

Conceptualizations of fidelity often include one or more of these five elements: adherence, dose, quality of delivery, participant responsiveness, and program differentiation (Allen et al., 2018). Adherence is the extent to which program objectives are met and is generally measured using checklists detailing core components of an intervention that are completed by evaluators who observe sessions or by interventionists themselves following each session (Dane & Schneider, 1998; Power et al., 2005). Dose is the amount, frequency, and/or duration of the program. Quality of delivery reflects how well an intervention is implemented, including things like interventionist effectiveness, enthusiasm, and preparedness (Power et al., 2005). For example, school social workers may technically *adhere* to the steps of a manualized intervention—however, they may not deliver it with quality if poor preparation results in constant note checking such that they are not able to be fully present with the students or exhibit appropriate levels of empathy. Participant responsiveness reflects the degree to which the target audience is engaged in the program. Finally, program differentiation is defined as the identification of unique program components to distinguish between programs and ensure that the program incorporates best practices while excluding contraindicated or irrelevant elements (Power et al., 2005). Program differentiation is particularly important when comparing different programs or program components. When comparing multiple parent training programs, for example, it would be important to identify the program elements that are common and distinct in order to determine what (if anything) contributes to one program being more effective than another.

There are multiple approaches to assessing and monitoring fidelity, and Allen and colleagues (2018) discuss the pros and cons of various methods. Direct methods include the use of trained observers or independent auditors who assess fidelity using structured checklists or coding procedures. These methods often involve direct observation or review of audio or video recordings. These methods are generally viewed as the gold standard (Lewis, Proctor, et al., 2018; Schoenwald et al., 2011) as independent observers are less prone to biased reporting, and direct observation yields highly accurate and valid data. However, direct methods can be more costly and less feasible, especially in large-scale implementation efforts. Indirect methods include collecting data from implementers (e.g., intervention logs or diaries) or collecting data from intervention participants through exit interviews or surveys. Indirect methods are less costly, time-consuming, and labor-intensive than direct methods. Allen et al. note that collecting data directly from implementers and/or program participants can also yield valuable information about the program. However, concerns about indirect data collection include accuracy of the data related to overreporting and social desirability bias, as well as a greater chance of missing data. Beidas, Maclean, et al. (2016) compared different methods of assessing fidelity to cognitive-behavioral therapy (self-report, chart-simulated recall, and behavioral rehearsal) to the gold standard of direct observation, and found that behavioral rehearsal yielded adherence scores comparable to direct observation whereas both self-report and chart-simulated recall yielded inflated adherence estimates (Becker-Haimes et al., 2022). It is encouraging that more feasible approaches to assessing fidelity (e.g., behavioral rehearsal) are being identified and rigorously assessed—however, in the meantime, evaluators must use their best judgment and strike a balance between rigor and feasibility when deciding the best method to use (Bond & Drake, 2020).

If a program is defined well enough for fidelity to be assessed, it could be assessed and reviewed throughout the course of evaluation. It may be desirable to establish a feedback system so that program implementers can be made aware of any deviations in fidelity and can "course correct" as necessary (Allen et al., 2018; Bickman, 2008). In other cases, frequent feedback on implementations is not likely to be a part of future program implementations, and evaluators may be focused on whether interest holders were able to implement the program with fidelity with the support of other strategies, such as training, supervision, or technical assistance. In these cases, it may be best to wait until the conclusion of the evaluation to analyze fidelity data and provide feedback to implementers.

While fidelity to the core components of interventions is generally prized, there is an increasing recognition that interventions may need to be modified to enhance fit with different populations and contexts, and increase the likelihood that they will be implemented, sustained, or scaled up (Aarons et al., 2012; Baumann et al., 2015; Cabassa & Baumann, 2013; Chambers et al., 2013; Wiltsey Stirman et al., 2013, 2019). Wiltsey Stirman and colleagues (2015) suggest that **modifications** are changes to the content or method of a program that are not specified in the protocol, and that **adaptation** is a form of modification characterized by thoughtful and deliberate alteration to the design or delivery of a program to improve its fit or effectiveness in a given context (i.e., planned adaptation). They also distinguish between fidelity-consistent modifications (e.g., tailoring, changing the length of the program, or adding program-consistent modules) from fidelity-inconsistent modifications (e.g., integration of conceptually inconsistent program strategies, removing elements, loosening structure, drifting from the protocol). There are multiple frameworks that can inform the planned adaptation of programs (Escoffery et al., 2018). Once again, evaluators must have a clear understanding of the program's core components and program theory in order to determine what might be a fidelity-consistent or fidelity-inconsistent modification. Recent guidance by Wiltsey Stirman and colleagues (2019) emphasizes the importance of tracking modifications and reporting:

> (1) when and how in the implementation process the modification was made, (2) whether the modification was planned/proactive (i.e., an adaptation) or unplanned/reactive, (3) who determined that the modification should be made, (4) what is modified, (5) at what level of delivery the modification was made, (6) type or nature of context or content-level modifications, (7) the extent to which the modification is fidelity-consistent, and (8) the reasons for the modification. (p. 4)

Multiple methods could be employed to document adaptations within an evaluation. For example, if audio- or video recordings of the program or intervention are feasible, they could be reviewed to both document fidelity and any modifications. Finley and colleagues (2018) demonstrated the use of "periodic reflections," an ethnographically informed approach in which a member of the implementation evaluation team conducted 30- to 60-minute telephone discussions with implementation team members at monthly or bimonthly intervals to assess adaptations to the intervention and implementation plan. That approach has the advantage of providing close to real-time data on potential adaptations. It is also common to assess program adaptations in interviews and/or focus groups with implementers following the program delivery period (Gertner et al., 2021; National Cancer Institute, 2018), though recall bias can be a problem with this approach. Adhering to the recommendations outlined above by Wiltsey Stirman and colleagues (2019) will ensure that the processes used to modify interventions and the modifications themselves are clearly articulated and will enable evaluations to focus on the relationship between modifications and outcomes of interest. The timing of modifications is also a critical element to consider. If modifications are made during different time points of an evaluation period, whether planned or not, then the construct validity of the program could be compromised. Even if the changes are systematic, which is probably rare, the program is not the same over time and thus is not the same to different participants who experience the program. Yet, it is typical that there will be insufficient statistical power to analyze the outcomes for different time periods, so that average effects of the program will be analyzed, even though that may not be a good representation of what the participants received. There is no simple way to deal with this problem and most evaluations simply ignore this complexity—however, it would be preferable to at least document modifications and be transparent about whether and how it may influence the construct validity of the program.

Penetration

Penetration is defined as "the integration of a practice within a service setting and its subsystems" (Proctor et al., 2011, p. 70). Penetration can be assessed by calculating the number of consumers who receive an intervention divided by the number of consumers who are eligible to receive it, or the number of individuals who deliver a program divided by the number of individuals who would be expected to deliver it. In the latter example, penetration could be meaningfully combined with fidelity to indicate, for instance, the proportion of clinicians in a mental health organization who deliver cognitive-behavioral therapy at an acceptable level of fidelity. While penetration may be relatively straightforward to conceptualize, it can be very challenging to measure as it may change over time and be different for different categories of participants and providers. Moreover, without simultaneously assessing fidelity, we do not know whether providers are delivering the program as intended.

WHAT ARE KEY INTEREST HOLDERS' PERCEPTIONS OF THE PROGRAM?

In addition to assessing the extent and quality of implementation, evaluators should consider assessing key interest holders' perceptions of the program. If the program was not well received, these assessments may suggest ways in which the program or its implementation might be enhanced to make it more palatable, and if it is well received, these assessments may help build the case that the program should be implemented more widely (assuming the effectiveness data are also promising). Three implementation outcomes outlined by Proctor et al. (2011) are particularly pertinent, including acceptability, appropriateness, and feasibility.

Acceptability

Acceptability is the extent to which a given program is agreeable, palatable, or satisfactory to interest holders (Proctor et al., 2011). Thus, it can be measured from the perspective of administrators, payers, providers, consumers, or other relevant interest holders. Ideally, acceptability would be assessed based on interest holders' knowledge of and/or direct experience with a program—thus, it may change as interest holders experience the program across different phases of implementation (e.g., initial acceptability could be low in the exploration phase and then increase as interest holders directly experience the benefits of the intervention). Weiner and colleagues (2017) developed the four-item Acceptability of Intervention Measure, a measure with strong psychometric evidence that can be used to quantitatively assess the acceptability of a program or implementation strategy. This measure and the related measures of appropriateness and feasibility described below could be administered to a range of interest holders at one or more time points after they have enough exposure to the program to have perceptions of its acceptability, appropriateness, or feasibility (see Weiner et al., 2017, Additional File 3, for the full version of these measures). This type of approach could easily be combined with qualitative approaches to conduct a simultaneous mixed methods design in which evaluators seek to determine whether quantitative and qualitative perspectives of acceptability converge (e.g., Hamm et al., 2023; Palinkas et al., 2011).

Appropriateness

Appropriateness is the perceived fit, relevance or compatibility of the program for a given problem, practice setting, provider, or consumer (Lewis, Proctor, et al., 2018; Proctor et al., 2011). Proctor et al. (2011, 2014) emphasize that while appropriateness is conceptually similar to acceptability and the literature reflects overlapping and sometimes inconsistent terms when discussing these constructs, the distinction remains important. A program may be perceived as appropriate but not acceptable and vice versa. For example, exposure is certainly an appropriate (and evidence-based) intervention component for treating anxiety—however, clinicians may find it unacceptable due to the discomfort of "creating distress" (Kendall et al., 2005). The construct "appropriateness" may capture "pushback" to implementation efforts, as when providers feel a new program is a "stretch" from the mission of the health care setting, or is not consistent with their skills, role, or job expectations (Proctor et al., 2011). The conceptual distinction between acceptability and appropriateness was supported in the aforementioned measure development work by Weiner et al.

(2017), which resulted in the development of a four-item measure of appropriateness (the Intervention Appropriateness Measure) with strong psychometric evidence.

Feasibility

Feasibility is the extent to which a program can be successfully used or carried out within a particular setting or population (Proctor et al., 2011). While feasibility is conceptually similar to appropriateness, it is distinct in that a program may be appropriate (i.e., compatible with the setting's mission) but not feasible due to resource requirements or other considerations (Proctor et al., 2014). In the aforementioned measurement study, Weiner et al. (2017) developed a measure with strong psychometric evidence that can be used to assess the feasibility of interventions and implementation strategies (the Feasibility of Intervention Measure).

WAS THE PROGRAM SUSTAINED?

Sustainability is the extent to which a program is maintained or institutionalized within a setting (Proctor et al., 2011). Shelton and colleagues (2018) summarize how sustainability has been conceptualized in the literature, noting:

> In recent years, sustainability outcomes have been conceptualized as (a) continuing or improving health benefits or outcomes for patients/consumers at the individual level; (b) maintaining community-level partnerships or coalitions and community capacity for collaboration; (c) maintaining organizational practices, procedures, and policies started during implementation (institutionalization); and (d) continuing the program activities or core elements of the original intervention. (p. 62)

Increasingly, sustainability is conceptualized as a dynamic process. For many programs, entropy will take hold and efforts may be necessary to bolster fidelity to the program (e.g., through booster sessions that provide more training, supervision)—however, there is also recognition that most programs need to be adapted and will evolve over time in order to fit the needs of the settings and populations they are intended to serve (Chambers et al., 2013; Shelton et al., 2018). Moreover, some programs are actually sustained despite evidence that suggests that they are no longer "best practices," signaling the need to consider "de-implementation" (Prasad & Ioannidis, 2014). For example, postoperative antibiotic use in surgical cases that are low risk for infection is an area with substantial overuse of antibiotics in children, so "antibiotic stewardship programs" and related initiatives are focused on helping clinicians prescribe antibiotics appropriately and de-implement the unnecessary use of antibiotics (Malone et al., 2021). Evaluators should consider the extent to which adaptations of intervention components are acceptable or expected, and whether a given threshold needs to be met in order to consider the intervention sustained (Shelton et al., 2018). Shelton and colleagues also recommend that sustainability be measured at least a year after implementation (and ideally 2 or more years later), and that it should be assessed over multiple time points to capture its potentially dynamic and nonlinear nature. Admittedly, this may more often be a decision made by funders than by evaluators.

WHAT ARE THE COSTS OF IMPLEMENTING THE PROGRAM?

Evaluators may wish to evaluate **implementation costs**, or the costs associated with implementing a program, including costs associated with the particular program, the implementation strategy used, and the location of service delivery (Proctor et al., 2011). Unfortunately, implementation evaluations that assess these costs are rare (Reeves et al., 2019; Roberts et al., 2019; Vale et al., 2007), which hampers decision making with respect to implementation (Powell et al., 2019; Saldana et al., 2014). It is beyond the scope of this chapter to provide an overview of various types of economic evaluation. However, readers are encouraged to see Shand et al. (Chapter 14, this volume) as well as Hoomans and Severans (2014) and Eisman et al. (2020) for a review of various types of economic analyses that apply to evaluating program implementation, and Dopp et al. (2019) for a helpful overview of mixed methods approaches to economic evaluation. Finally, Barnett et al. (2020) provide suggestions for collaborating with economists to improve economic evaluations of implementation efforts.

Relationships between Different Implementation Outcomes and Effectiveness Outcomes

It is likely that implementation outcomes (e.g., acceptability, feasibility, fidelity, penetration, sustainability, and cost) are related to one another in dynamic and complex ways (Lewis, Proctor, et al., 2018). At this stage, it is difficult to say which implementation outcomes are most important, or the extent to which they are predictive of more distal effectiveness outcomes. Further empirical work is needed to model these relationships—however, it is probable that the importance or relationship between outcomes is not a universal but is characteristic of the program, the problem, the sensitivity of the measures, and other context issues. Thus, it is likely to be different for every program and possibly every instance of that program.

WHAT FACTORS FACILITATED OR IMPEDED PROGRAM IMPLEMENTATION?

Evaluators are well positioned to identify barriers and facilitators to program implementation. Depending upon the evaluator's role and the type of evaluation, this could be done prior to, during, or after a program is implemented. Prior to implementation, assessing barriers and facilitators can be a useful way of guiding the selection of implementation strategies and informing the development of an implementation plan. During active implementation, evaluators could simultaneously monitor the extent and quality of implementation (as described above) and collect information about interest holders' experiences of barriers and facilitators to program implementation. This may lead to immediate changes in the approach to implementation (if the evaluation design allows for it) or to iterations in the implementation approach after the evaluation period.

Implementation barriers and facilitators can be assessed through qualitative, quantitative, and mixed methods approaches. Qualitative methods often include semistructured interviews (e.g., Beidas, Stewart, et al., 2016; Powell, Hausmann-Stabile, et al., 2013; Yamey, 2012), focus groups (e.g., Bussières et al., 2012; Forsner et al., 2010), direct observation and other ethnographic approaches (e.g., Bunce et al., 2014; Gertner et al., 2021; Palinkas & Zatzick, 2019), and/or document review (e.g., Aarons et al., 2014). Guidance on the use of qualitative methods within implementation evaluations has been published by a National Institutes of Health work group (National Cancer Institute, 2018). Quantitative approaches typically involve surveys, some of which are atheoretical and developed for a specific project (e.g., Jacobs et al., 2010; Powell, McMillen, et al., 2013) and others that are theory based and assess many of the constructs from frameworks that guide assessments of implementation barriers and facilitators (e.g., Beidas et al., 2015; Cook et al., 2015; Huijg et al., 2014; Powell, Mandell, et al., 2017). Increasingly, mixed methods are used to understand barriers and facilitators, including a range of more traditional mixed methods designs (Palinkas et al., 2011), as well as other inherently mixed methods approaches, such as concept mapping (Kane & Trochim, 2007). These involve qualitative approaches to brainstorming and sorting potential barriers and quantitative approaches to develop conceptually distinct categories of barriers and rating them on importance and modifiability (e.g., Green & Aarons, 2011; Lobb et al., 2013). Azzam and Jones (see Chapter 18, this volume) provide informative and practical information on implementing a mixed methods evaluation. Systems science approaches, such as participatory system dynamics modeling, have been proposed as a means of understanding the complex, dynamic nature of barriers and facilitators (Burke et al., 2015; Hovmand & Gillespie, 2010; Luke et al., 2024; Powell, Beidas, et al., 2017; Zimmerman et al., 2016).

Assessments of barriers and facilitators could be strengthened in a number of ways. First, evaluators should examine the literature for studies of barriers and facilitators, including systematic reviews (e.g., Gravel et al., 2006; Overbeck et al., 2016; Powell et al., 2020), so that future evaluations do not "reinvent the wheel" but extend our understanding in meaningful ways. Second, evaluators should carefully consider whether an entirely inductive approach to assessing barriers and facilitators is necessary, as in many cases, conceptual frameworks (e.g., Aarons et al., 2011; Cane et al., 2012; Damschroder et al., 2009; Flottorp et al., 2013; Michie et al., 2005) provide useful guidance about the types of barriers and facilitators that are likely to be encountered. It may be advisable to adapt an existing framework to suit the needs of a given evaluation rather than taking an atheoretical or completely inductive approach. Third, it is essential that evaluators consider barriers and facilitators from the perspectives of multiple interest holders, and involve anyone who may influence or be influenced by the implementation effort given that perspectives may vary substantially between different types of interest holders (Aarons et al., 2009; Beidas, Stewart, et al., 2016). Fourth, whenever possible, evaluators should assess barriers and facilitators longitudinally. This can potentially differentiate perceived barriers and facilitators that may be based upon inadequate exposure to the program being implemented from those actually experienced, and also affords the opportunity to see how these factors change over the course of implementation. Fifth, evaluators should strive to assess barriers and facilitators as efficiently as possible, using **pragmatic measures**, or those that possess desirable properties that make them more likely to be widely used, such as usefulness (e.g., informs clinical or organizational decision making), compatibility (e.g., fits organizational activities), acceptability (e.g., low cost), and ease of use (e.g., uses accessible language, brief; Glasgow & Riley, 2013; Lewis et al., 2021; Powell, Stanick, et al., 2017; Stanick et al., 2018, 2021). Using pragmatic measures increases the likelihood that interest holders could use the assessment tools to inform improvement after the evaluation has concluded. Finally, efforts to help prioritize identified barriers in systematic ways (based upon empirical data, theory, and/or interest holder preferences) should be central to any effort. Evaluations often yield unwieldy lists of determinants (Krause et al., 2014), and it is difficult to ascertain whether and how they might be meaningfully addressed. An important step in this direction would be to evaluate how different barriers and facilitators interact with each other—that is, rather than simply generating lists of barriers and facilitators, evaluators should model how they influence each other. This can be accomplished by formally modeling relationships between barriers and facilitators (e.g., Williams et al., 2018), using methods that capture the complexity of implementation contexts (e.g., Zimmerman et al., 2016) and using mixed methods approaches that help us to understand the nuances of barriers and facilitators and how they operate (e.g., Aarons et al., 2016).

HOW CAN THE PROCESS OF IMPLEMENTATION BE IMPROVED?

Monitoring the extent and quality of program implementation may reveal problems with the implementation process itself. For example, if intended interest holders are not implementing the program with fidelity, it may suggest that anticipated or unanticipated barriers were not well addressed by the strategies used to implement the program. **Implementation strategies** are the methods or techniques used to improve adoption, implementation, sustainment, and scale-up of programs (Powell et al., 2019; Proctor et al., 2013). A range of strategies have been identified (Powell et al., 2012, 2015; Waltz et al., 2015), and much like programs, it is ideal if the strategies used to implement programs are described in detail and have a clear rationale for how and why they will be effective to integrate a program into usual care settings (Lewis, Klasnja, et al., 2018; Proctor et al., 2013). Implementation strategies are increasingly evaluated using rigorous designs (Grimshaw et al., 2012; Powell et al., 2019), many of which are described below.

In order to replicate implementation successes and make the necessary changes when implementation failures are identified, it is necessary to carefully document the strategies used to implement a program (Michie et al., 2009; Proctor et al., 2013). Indeed, contemporaneous tracking of implementation strategies is essential given the iterative nature of implementation. Even if implementation strategies are detailed in a study protocol or formal implementation plan, it is often unrealistic to expect that they will not need to be altered as determinants emerge across implementation phases (Aarons et al., 2011; Dunbar et al., 2012; Hoagwood et al., 2011; Powell et al., 2020). For example, during the COVID-19 pandemic, implementation strategies, such as educational workshops, learning collaboratives, and facilitation that were intended to be delivered using an in-person, live format, have needed to be adapted to be delivered online, sometimes using a blend of synchronous and asynchronous delivery.

Another example that is more routine arises when there is a substantial amount of turnover at the leadership or clinical level that necessitates renewed attention to building buy-in and tangible support for an implementation effort, training new staff members, or redefining roles and responsibilities related to the implementation of a program. These challenges and changes to implementation strategies are likely to occur within and between implementing sites in research studies and applied efforts (Boyd et al., 2018; Bunger et al., 2017; Haley et al., 2021; Walsh-Bailey et al., 2021), and without rigorous methods for tracking implementation strategy use, efforts to understand what strategies were used and whether they were effective are stymied. Miller and colleagues (2021) recently extended similar guidance for documenting implementation strategies as has been issued for tracking adaptations to other programs as described above (Wiltsey Stirman et al., 2019). Developing approaches for tracking implementation strategies, and assessing the extent to which they are pragmatic (e.g., acceptable, compatible, easy, and useful) for both research and applied efforts is a high priority (Powell et al., 2019; Walsh-Bailey et al., 2021). Ideally, evaluators would develop and apply methods to track implementation strategies prospectively using structured forms or surveys (e.g., Boyd et al., 2018; Bunger et al., 2017; Haley et al., 2021; Smith et al., 2022; Smith et al., 2023; Walsh-Bailey et al., 2021)—however, in some cases, evaluators may need to rely upon surveys, interviews, or other data sources to assess the use of implementation strategies retrospectively (e.g., Perry et al., 2019; Rogal et al., 2017, 2019; Turner et al., 2021). For example, Rogal et al. (2017, 2019) assessed site-level implementation strategies used by the U.S. Department of Veterans Affairs sites involved in a national collaborative and determined which strategies were associated with treatment initiation.

WHAT KIND OF DESIGNS CAN WE USE TO EVALUATE PROGRAMS AND IMPLEMENTATION STRATEGIES?

This section details some of the research and evaluation designs that can be used to assess the effectiveness of a program, an implementation strategy, or both. We maintain that each of the designs discussed below are relevant to the assessment of *both* program and implementation effectiveness. For example, we might use a cluster randomized controlled trial (RCT) to assess the effectiveness of a school-based prevention program, wherein some schools get the prevention intervention while others receive no intervention or something akin to health education as usual and the primary outcome of interest assessed is adolescents' use of alcohol. We could also use a similar cluster randomized trial involving the aforementioned prevention program to compare two different implementation approaches, such as a trial that compares training to training plus implementation facilitation (Baskerville et al., 2012), wherein the primary outcome of interest is teachers' fidelity to the (presumably evidence based) prevention intervention. Hybrid effectiveness–implementation evaluation designs (Curran et al., 2012, 2022) place an emphasis on both effectiveness and implementation outcomes, and are described in greater detail below. The choice of design depends upon the purpose of the evaluation as well as the degree of control that the evaluators have over the delivery of the program and implementation strategy (Bhattacharyya & Zwarenstein, 2009; Mazzucca et al., 2018; Wensing & Grimshaw, 2020). In general, if the objective of the evaluation is to build generalizable knowledge about whether a program or implementation strategy is effective, then experimental designs are employed. On the other hand, quasi-experimental and observational studies are often appropriate, and more feasible to conduct, when the development of local knowledge (i.e., whether a strategy works here) is the priority (Bhattacharyya & Zwarenstein, 2009; Eccles et al., 2005). It is probably best to "start small," conducting preliminary studies that enhance understanding of the theoretical basis of a program or implementation strategy as well as their feasibility, acceptability, appropriateness, and initial effectiveness. This approach is reflected in the U.S. Department of Veterans Affairs Quality Enhancement Research Initiative (Stetler et al., 2008) and the Medical Research Council's framework for evaluating complex interventions (Craig et al., 2008, 2019). In this section we review some experimental, quasi-experimental, and observational design options. For further discussion of design options, we direct readers to published overviews for discussions of the trade-offs between various implementation designs (Bhattacharyya & Zwarenstein, 2009; Brown et al., 2017; Eccles et al., 2005; Handley et al., 2018; Hwang et al., 2020; Landsverk et al., 2018). These resources describe how these designs can be used in the evaluation of implementation strategies—however, each of these designs is equally relevant to evaluating an intervention or program.

Experimental and Quasi-Experimental Designs

Randomized Controlled Trials

RCTs are commonly considered the "gold standard" for establishing the effectiveness of programs and implementation strategies, largely because they provide the greatest protection against threats to **internal validity**. Indeed, in a review of study protocols published in the journal *Implementation Science*, 164 of 212 (77%) studies evaluating the effectiveness of implementation strategies used RCTs (Mazzucca et al., 2018). Wensing and Grimshaw (2020) argue that randomized designs are especially critical in evaluating implementation, as it is very difficult to adjust for potential confounders in nonrandomized designs given our imperfect knowledge about the potential organizational- and professional-level factors that may impact implementation. While some studies may be able to randomize at the individual level (e.g., patients, students, therapists), many implementation studies are cluster randomized trials, designs that involve clusters of individuals within units (e.g., hospitals, schools, community mental health clinics) that are randomly assigned to an intervention group. For example, 54% (114 of 212) of study protocols published in *Implementation Science* were cluster randomized trials (Mazzucca et al., 2018). This design choice is often made if there are concerns about potential contamination or if the intervention or strategy is targeted at a collective level (e.g., organization, community). Another design choice involves the number of comparison arms and choice of comparators. Two-arm trials either compare two active programs or implementation strategies, or compare an active program or implementation strategy to usual care or a more passive program or implementation strategy. Multiple-arm trials generally involve a true control group (usual care) that is compared to two or more active programs or implementation strategies. Factorial designs compare each program or implementation strategy individually and in combination to a control (e.g., Glisson et al., 2010). Wolfenden and colleagues (2021) provide further guidance using randomized designs to evaluate implementation.

There are several challenges associated with cluster RCTs. First, they are labor-intensive, expensive, and complicated to run well (Davidoff, 2009). Second, as Proctor et al. (2009) acknowledge, implementation research suffers from a "small N" problem, which can be especially problematic for cluster RCTs. In cluster RCTs, statistical power is derived more from the number of clusters than the number of participants in each cluster—thus, difficulty in recruiting at the cluster level may result in an underpowered study. Eccles and colleagues (2005) also caution that when few clusters are available for randomization, there is "danger of imbalance in performance between the study and control groups because of the play of chance" (p. 237). Finally, cluster RCTs introduce the challenge of multilevel data (e.g., student-level data and school-level data, with students nested within schools), which necessitates the use of statistical techniques such as multilevel modeling that account for the fact that observations are not independent (Luke, 2004).

Randomized Rollout Implementation Trials

Brown and colleagues (2017) refer to a broad class of within- and between-site comparisons that involve sites crossing over from one program or implementation condition to another. One version of this design involves all sites starting in a usual practice setting and then crossing over at randomly determined time intervals so that every site eventually receives the program or implementation strategy. Thus, each site serves as its own control (within site) and can be compared with the performance of other sites (between site). These designs are often popular in program or implementation studies in which interest holder groups are unwilling (or unenthusiastic) about being randomized to a true control condition or if it would be unethical to withhold the implementation strategy from study sites (Brown et al., 2017; Landsverk et al., 2018). For example, organizations that are eager to receive a particular program or implementation support for a given program may not be willing to be randomized to a control group in which they receive no program or implementation strategy or a rather passive one such as the dissemination of information or an educational workshop.

Interrupted Time-Series Designs

Interrupted time-series designs involve the repeated collection of data prior to and after a program or implementation strategy is deployed to determine whether it has an effect that is greater than the underlying trend (Bhattacharyya & Zwarenstein, 2009). This design is particularly appropriate when randomization is not possible due to the implausibility of finding a suitable control (Bhattacharyya & Zwarenstein, 2009; Eccles et al., 2005), as is often the case when evaluating health policy changes or systemwide interventions that are implemented at a single point in time. For example, Arrowsmith and colleagues (2014) used an interrupted time-series design to evaluate the impact of a national pay-for-performance policy initiative intended to improve the use of long-acting reversable contraceptives (LARCs). They demonstrated that prescribing rates for LARCs were stable before the introduction of the policy and increased by 4% annually afterward (a change equivalent to an additional 110,000 women being prescribed with a LARC). Two notable limitations of time-series designs are that they don't control for outside influences on outcomes of interest and they are difficult to mount when data are not already routinely collected (Bhattacharyya & Zwarenstein, 2009).

Controlled (and Uncontrolled) before-and-after Designs

Controlled before-and-after studies involve the identification of a suitable control group that is similar to the intervention group, and the collection of data in both groups prior to and after the implementation strategy is instituted. A major challenge with this design is finding a well-matched control group, and these designs are most appropriate when local, not generalizable knowledge is the aim of the study (Bhattacharyya & Zwarenstein, 2009). Uncontrolled before-and-after (or pre–post) designs can be used when evaluating programs or implementation strategies within a single site (e.g., organization, community, or system)—thus, they may be more feasible for evaluations that are more limited in scope or that have limited resources. Pre–post designs compare pre-implementation data to post-implementation data to infer effects of the program or implementation strategy, whereas post designs involve introducing an implementation strategy to integrate an intervention and then evaluating health care processes and utilization (Brown et al., 2017; Landsverk et al., 2018).

Observational Designs

While generally considered weaker designs, observational studies also have a role to play in implementation evaluations (Berwick, 2008; Handley et al., 2018; Landsverk et al., 2011). In particular, observational studies may help bolster our understanding of *how* and *why* programs and implementation strategies are effective in given contexts, as the interaction between context and strategy is not adequately captured in most traditional experimental or quasi-experimental designs. This is problematic given the context-dependent nature of implementation strategies. Davidoff (2009) explains that:

> behavior change interventions are literally created by their interaction with social contexts; that is, in an important and real sense, these interventions do not exist until users instill meaning into them, accept them as valid, and modify them to fit their local situations, a process that has been referred to as "adaptive" work. (p. 2581)

Berwick (2008) echoes that sentiment, "although the OXO model seeks generalizable knowledge, in that the pursuit it relies on—it depends on—removing most of the local details about 'how' something works and about the 'what' of contexts" (p. 1183). He proceeds to laud the contributions of a number of different designs and methods, including ethnography and other qualitative methods, stating emphatically that when used appropriately, they are not compromises but are actually superior to RCTs (Berwick, 2008). In fact, observational designs may be the most responsive for certain evaluations, particularly given that evaluators may often be working with one or a few sites and larger controlled experiments may not be feasible. The following sections provide a few examples of observational designs that have been used to evaluate implementation efforts.

Audit and Monitoring Studies and Developmental Studies

Audit and monitoring studies and developmental studies are essentially types of formative program or implementation evaluation (Bauer et al., 2015). Audit and monitoring studies involve documenting performance before, during, and after a program or implementation strategy is put in place—thus, it is similar to an uncontrolled before-and-after study except that the researcher generally has little control over the study condition (Eccles et al., 2005). They are also characterized by their cyclical nature, as knowledge gained about what is working (and what is not) is often fed back to interest holders (Wensing & Grimshaw, 2020). Developmental studies, such as assessments of barriers and facilitators, can guide the development or refinement of programs and implementation strategies (Wensing & Grimshaw, 2020).

Case Studies

Case studies are generally mixed methods inquiries that incorporate the views of multiple interest holders and incorporate a relatively large number of variables compared to the number of cases (Yin, 2009). Multiple sources of data that are intended to answer the same question (i.e., "triangulation") can enhance validity of the findings (Wensing & Grimshaw, 2020).

Multiple-Case Studies

Multiple case studies (or comparative case studies) can be used to identify change mechanisms by comparing similar cases (Stake, 2005; Yin, 2009). When it is feasible to examine more than one "case," use of this design may be more methodologically robust than a single-case study, and defining hypotheses a priori can protect against associations found by chance (Wensing & Grimshaw, 2020). Sampling is generally purposive (Palinkas et al., 2013) and traditional sampling logic is not used (Yin, 2009). A primary benefit of a multiple-case study is the ability to make comparisons across cases. Individual cases are treated as separate studies that are then compared, allowing for meaningful similarities, differences and site-specific experiences to be identified (e.g., Isett et al., 2007). Admittedly, multiple-case studies may not always be feasible, such as when the "case" is conceptualized at the site level and the evaluation includes only one site.

Effectiveness–Implementation Hybrid Designs

Hybrid effectiveness–implementation designs are intended to shorten the length of time between effectiveness studies that establish that a program works in real-world settings to implementation studies that focus on establishing effective strategies for implementing, sustaining, and scaling those interventions (Curran et al., 2012). They do so by combining elements of both effectiveness and implementation studies. Curran et al. describe three types of hybrid studies. In a hybrid type 1, the primary focus of the study is on testing the program and establishing its effectiveness, whereas a secondary purpose is to observe and gather information about implementation. For example, Beidas and colleagues (2014) assessed whether an evidence-based exercise intervention for breast cancer survivors was safe and effective in a new setting (primary purpose), and also qualitatively assessed barriers to implementation (secondary purpose). In a hybrid type 2, there is a dual (or co-primary) focus on establishing the effectiveness of the program and on evaluating the implementation strategy. One example is the factorial trial of the Availability, Responsiveness, and Continuity organizational implementation intervention and multisystemic therapy (Glisson et al., 2010, p. 26). Finally, in a hybrid type 3 study, the primary purpose is to evaluate the effectiveness of the implementation strategy—however, assessing the outcomes of the program remains a secondary focus (e.g., Kolko et al., 2022; Nguyen et al., 2020; Rogal et al., 2020; Vaughn et al., 2019). These designs can be particularly appropriate if the level of evidence of the program being implemented is not robust or if it is being implemented in new settings. It is worth noting that hybrid designs need to be paired with other formal research designs, such as a cluster RCT (i.e., a hybrid is not a design in and of itself; Curran et al., 2022).

HOW CAN WE ENSURE OUR EVALUATIONS ARE SUFFICIENTLY DETAILED TO INFORM FUTURE EFFORTS?

Publications reporting evaluation efforts often fail to describe the program, context, processes, strategies, and outcomes in adequate detail (Hooley et al., 2020; Michie et al., 2009; Neta et al., 2015; Proctor et al., 2013). Poor reporting limits the power of evaluation by clouding the interpretation of results, precluding replication in research and practice, and limiting our ability to synthesize findings from multiple evaluations (Michie et al., 2009; Proctor et al., 2013). For example, in reporting the results of their systematic review of quality improvement collaboratives, Nadeem and colleagues (2013) note that "reporting on specific components of the collaborative was imprecise across articles, rendering it impossible to identify active quality improvement collaborative ingredients linked to improved care" (p. 355). Generating information that will be useful to relevant interest holders, either locally or more broadly, requires that programs and implementation strategies be reported in greater detail.

A number of **reporting guidelines** could be leveraged to improve descriptions of implementation contexts, processes, strategies, and outcomes. Some of these guidelines focus on general reporting issues. For example, the Standards for Reporting Implementation Studies were developed to increase transparency and accurate reporting of implementation evaluations and include 27 items, from title to discussion, that should be considered when reporting implementation evaluations (Pinnock et al., 2017). Many more guidelines focus specifically on reporting programs or implementation strategies in enough detail so that they can be replicated in research and/or practice (Albrecht et al., 2013; Bragge et al., 2017; Colquhoun et al., 2014; Hoffman et al., 2014; Patient Centered Outcomes Research Institute, 2019; Proctor et al., 2013; Workgroup for Intervention Development and Evaluation Research, 2008). Proctor et al. suggest the importance of naming and defining implementation strategies in ways that are consistent with the published literature, and carefully operationalizing each discrete or component strategy by specifying (1) *actor(s)*; (2) *action(s)*; (3) *action target(s)*; (4) *temporality*; (5) *dose*; (6) *implementation outcomes affected*; and (7) theoretical, empirical, or pragmatic *justification*. Bunger et al. (2016) provide an applied example of reporting a multifaceted implementation strategy, detailing the 11 components of a learning collaborative according to Proctor et al. This guidance is consistent with the Patient-Centered Outcomes Research Institute's recently released Standards for Studies of Complex Interventions (The Methodology Committee of the Patient-Centered Outcomes Research Institute, 2012), which can be applied to programs being evaluated as well as the implementation strategies used to integrate them into routine care. These standards encourage evaluators to (1) fully describe the intervention and comparator and define their core functions (core functions are the intended purpose of the interventions, while forms refer to the intended modes of delivery, providers involved, materials or tools required, dose, and frequency), (2) specify the hypothesized causal pathways and their theoretical basis, (3) specify how adaptations to the form of the intervention and comparator will be allowed and recorded, (4) plan and describe a process evaluation, and (5) select patient outcomes informed by the causal pathway. Evaluators are particularly well positioned to use the aforementioned guidelines to ensure that programs and implementation strategies are tracked and reported in detail, and doing so will ensure that they can be replicated and optimized over time.

CONCLUSION

Implementing effective programs is exceedingly challenging—however, evaluators have an opportunity to play an important role in closing the gap between what we know and what we do. This chapter provides resources to guide the process of specifying programs and associated program theory, monitoring the extent and quality of implementation and other important implementation outcomes, identifying and addressing barriers and facilitators and other process concerns, rigorously evaluating both programs and implementation strategies, and reporting details of programs and implementation strategies in ways that promote replication and the generation of knowledge. The field of implementation research and practice is rapidly developing, and will benefit the most when it draws from the best of theories, methods, and designs from other fields, and when it is inherently innovative. Discussion and critiques along those lines are welcome as readers apply and extend the tools introduced in this chapter.

REFERENCES

Aarons, G. A., Green, A. E., Palinkas, L. A., Self-Brown, S., Whitaker, D. J., Lutzker, J. R., . . . Chaffin, M. J. (2012). Dynamic adaptation process to implement an evidence-based child maltreatment intervention. *Implementation Science, 7*(32), 1–9.

Aarons, G. A., Green, A. E., Trott, E., Willging, C. E., Ehrhart, M. G., & Roesch, S. C. (2016). The role of leadership at multiple levels in sustaining system-wide implementation: A mixed-method study. *Administration and Policy in Mental Health, 43,* 991–1008.

Aarons, G. A., Green, A. E., Willging, C. E., Ehrhart, M. G., Roesch, S. C., Hecht, D. B., & Chaffin, M. J. (2014). Mixed-method study of a conceptual model of evidence-based intervention sustainment across multiple public-sector service settings. *Implementation Science, 9*(183), 1–12.

Aarons, G. A., Hurlburt, M., & Horwitz, S. M. (2011). Advancing a conceptual model of evidence-based practice implementation in public service sectors. *Administration and Policy in Mental Health, 38,* 4–23.

Aarons, G. A., Wells, R. S., Zagursky, K., Fettes, D. L., & Palinkas, L. A. (2009). Implementing evidence-based practice in community mental health agencies: A multiple stakeholder analysis. *American Journal of Public Health, 99*(11), 2087–2095.

Akiba, C. F., Go, V. F., Powell, B. J., Muessig, K., Golin, C., Dussault, J. M., . . . Pence, B. W. (2023). Champion and audit and feedback strategy fidelity and their relationship to depression intervention fidelity: A mixed method study. *SSM–Mental Health, 3,* 100194.

Akiba, C. F., Powell, B. J., Pence, B. W., Muessig, K., Golin, C. E., & Go, V. (2022). "We start where we are": A qualitative study of barriers and pragmatic solutions to the assessment and reporting of implementation strategy fidelity. *Implementation Science Communications, 3*(1), 117.

Akiba, C. F., Powell, B. J., Pence, B. W., Nguyen, M. X. B., Golin, C., & Go, V. (2022). The case for prioritizing implementation strategy fidelity measurement: Benefits and challenges. *Translational Behavioral Medicine, 12*(2), 335–342.

Albrecht, L., Archibald, M., Arseneau, D., & Scott, S. D. (2013). Development of a checklist to assess the quality of reporting of knowledge translation interventions using the Workgroup for Intervention Development and Evaluation Research (WIDER) recommendations. *Implementation Science, 8*(52), 1–5.

Allen, J. D., Shelton, R. C., Emmons, K. M., & Linnan, L. A. (2018). Fidelity and its relationship to implementation effectiveness, adaptation, and dissemination. In R. C. Brownson, E. K. Proctor, & R. C. Brownson (Eds.), *Dissemination and implementation research in health* (2nd ed., pp. 267–284). Oxford University Press.

Arrowsmith, M. E., Majeed, A., Lee, J. T., & Saxena, S. (2014). Impact of pay for performance on prescribing of long-acting reversable contraception in primary care: An interrupted time series study. *PLoS One, 9*(4), 1–6.

Barnett, M., Dopp, A. R., Klein, C., Ettner, S. L., Powell, B. J., & Saldana, L. (2020). Collaborating with health economists to advance implementation science: A qualitative study. *Implementation Science Communications, 1*(82), 1–11.

Baskerville, N. B., Liddy, C., & Hogg, W. (2012). Systematic review and meta-analysis of practice facilitation within primary care settings. *Annals of Family Medicine, 10*(1), 63–74.

Bauer, M. S., Damschroder, L., Hagedorn, H., Smith, J., & Kilbourne, A. M. (2015). An introduction to implementation science for the non-specialist. *BMC Psychology, 3*(32), 1–12.

Baumann, A. A., Powell, B. J., Kohl, P. L., Tabak, R. G., Penalba, V., Proctor, E. K., . . . Cabassa, L. J. (2015). Cultural adaptation and implementation of evidence-based parent-training: A systematic review and critique of guiding evidence. *Children and Youth Services Review, 53,* 113–120.

Becker-Haimes, E. M., Marcus, S. C., Klein, M. R., Schoenwald, S. K., Fugo, P. B., McLeod, B. D., . . . Beidas, R. S. (2022). A randomized trial to identify accurate measurement methods for adherence to cognitive-behavioral therapy. *Behavior Therapy, 53*(6), 1191–1204.

Beidas, R. S., Maclean, J. C., Fishman, J., Dorsey, S., Schoenwald, S. K., Mandell, D. S., . . . Marcus, S. C. (2016). A randomized trial to identify accurate and cost-effective fidelity measurement methods for cognitive-behavioral therapy: Project FACTS study protocol. *BMC Psychiatry, 16*(323), 1–10.

Beidas, R. S., Marcus, S., Aarons, G. A., Hoagwood, K. E., Schoenwald, S., Evans, A. C., . . . Mandell,

D. S. (2015). Predictors of community therapists' use of therapy techniques in a large public mental health system. *JAMA Pediatrics, 169*(4), 374–382.

Beidas, R. S., Paciotti, B., Barg, F., Branas, A. R., Brown, J. C., Glanz, K., . . . Schmitz, K. H. (2014). A hybrid effectiveness–implementation trial of an evidence-based exercise intervention for breast cancer survivors. *Journal of the National Cancer Institute Monographs, 50*, 338–345.

Beidas, R. S., Stewart, R. E., Adams, D. R., Fernandez, T., Lustbader, S., Powell, B. J., . . . Barg, F. K. (2016). A multi-level examination of stakeholder perspectives of implementation of evidence-based practices in a large urban publicly-funded mental health system. *Administration and Policy in Mental Health, 43*, 893–908.

Berwick, D. M. (2008). The science of improvement. *Journal of the American Medical Association, 299*(10), 1182–1184.

Bhattacharyya, O., & Zwarenstein, M. (2009). Methodologies to evaluate effectiveness of knowledge translation interventions. In S. Straus, J. Tetroe, & I. D. Graham (Eds.), *Knowledge translation in health care* (pp. 249–260). Wiley-Blackwell.

Bickman, L. (1987). The functions of program theory. In L. Bickman (Ed.), *Using program theory in evaluation* (pp. 5–18). Jossey-Bass.

Bickman, L. (2008). A measurement feedback system (MFS) is necessary to improve mental health outcomes. *Journal of the American Academy of Child and Adolescent Psychiatry, 47*(10), 1114–1119.

Bickman, L., & Heflinger, C. A. (1995). Seeking success by reducing implementation and evaluation failures. In L. Bickman & D. Rog (Eds.), *Children's mental health services: Research, policy, and intervention* (pp. 171–205). Sage.

Bond, G. R., & Drake, R. E. (2020). Assessing the fidelity of evidence-based practices: History and current status of a standardized measurement methodology. *Administration and Policy in Mental Health, 47*, 874–884.

Boyd, M. R., Powell, B. J., Endicott, D., & Lewis, C. C. (2018). A method for tracking implementation strategies: An exemplar implementing measurement-based care in community behavioral health clinics. *Behavior Therapy, 49*, 525–537.

Bragge, P., Grimshaw, J. M., Lokker, C., Colquhoun, H., & the AIMD Writing/Working Group. (2017). AIMD—a validated, simplified framework of interventions to promote and integrate evidence into health practices, systems, and policies. *BMC Medical Research Methodology, 17*(38), 1–11.

Brown, C. H., Curran, G., Palinkas, L. A., Aarons, G. A., Wells, K. B., Jones, L., . . . Cruden, G. (2017). An overview of research and evaluation designs for dissemination and implementation. *Annual Review of Public Health, 38*, 1–22.

Bunce, A. E., Gold, R., Davis, J. V., McMullen, C. K., Jaworski, V., Mercer, M., & Nelson, C. (2014). Ethnographic process evaluation in primary care: Explaining the complexity of implementation. *BMC Health Services Research, 14*(607), 1–10.

Bunger, A. C., Hanson, R. F., Doogan, N. J., Powell, B. J., Cao, Y., & Dunn, J. (2016). Can learning collaboratives support implementation by rewiring professional networks? *Administration and Policy in Mental Health, 43*(1), 79–92.

Bunger, A. C., Powell, B. J., Robertson, H. A., MacDowell, H., Birken, S. A., & Shea, C. (2017). Tracking implementation strategies: A description of a practical approach and early findings. *Health Research Policy and Systems, 15*(15), 1–12.

Burke, J. G., Lich, K. H., Neal, J. W., Meissner, H. I., Yonas, M., & Mabry, P. L. (2015). Enhancing dissemination and implementation research using systems science methods. *International Journal of Behavioral Medicine, 22*(3), 283–291.

Bussières, A. E., Patey, A. M., Francis, J. J., Sales, A. E., Grimshaw, J. M., & Canada PRIme Plus Team. (2012). Identifying factors likely to influence compliance with diagnostic imaging guideline recommendations for spine disorders among chiropractors in North America: A focus group study using the theoretical domains framework. *Implementation Science, 7*(82), 1–11.

Cabassa, L. J., & Baumann, A. A. (2013). A two-way street: Bridging implementation science and cultural adaptations of mental health treatments. *Implementation Science, 8*(90), 1–14.

Cane, J., O'Connor, D., & Michie, S. (2012). Validation of the theoretical domains framework for use in behaviour change and implementation research. *Implementation Science, 7*(37), 1–17.

Chambers, D. A., Glasgow, R. E., & Stange, K. C. (2013). The dynamic sustainability framework: Addressing the paradox of sustainment amid ongoing change. *Implementation Science, 8*(117), 1–11.

Colquhoun, H., Leeman, J., Michie, S., Lokker, C., Bragge, P., Hempel, S., . . . Grimshaw, J. (2014). Towards a common terminology: A simplified framework of interventions to promote and integrate evidence into health practices, systems, and policies. *Implementation Science, 9*(51), 1–6.

Cook, J. M., Dinnen, S., Thompson, R., Ruzek, J., Coyne, J. C., & Schnurr, P. P. (2015). A quantitative test of an implementation framework in 38 VA residential PTSD programs. *Administration and Policy in Mental Health, 42*(4), 462–473.

Craig, P., Dieppe, P., Macintyre, S., Mitchie, S., Nazareth, I., & Petticrew, M. (2008). Developing and evaluating complex interventions: The new Medical Research Council guidance. *BMJ, 337*, 979–983.

Craig, P., Dieppe, P., Macintyre, S., Michie, S., Nazareth, I., & Petticrew, M. (2019). *Developing and evaluating complex interventions: Following considerable development in the field since 2006, MRC and NIHR have jointly commissioned an update of this guidance to be published in*

2019. Medical Research Council. Available at https://mrc.ukri.org/documents/pdf/complex-interventions-guidance

Crowe, T. (2000). *Crime prevention through environmental design*. Butterworth-Heinman.

Curran, G. M., Bauer, M., Mittman, B., Pyne, J. M., & Stetler, C. (2012). Effectiveness–implementation hybrid designs: Combining elements of clinical effectiveness and implementation research to enhance public health impact. *Medical Care, 50*(3), 217–226.

Curran, G. M., Landes, S. J., McBain, S. A., Pyne, J. M., Smith, J. D., Fernandez, M. E., ... Mittman, B. S. (2022). Reflections on 10 years of effectiveness–implementation hybrid studies. *Frontiers in Health Services, 2*. Available at www.frontiersin.org/articles/10.3389/frhs.2022.1053496

Damschroder, L. J., Aron, D. C., Keith, R. E., Kirsh, S. R., Alexander, J. A., & Lowery, J. C. (2009). Fostering implementation of health services research findings into practice: A consolidated framework for advancing implementation science. *Implementation Science, 4*(50), 1–15.

Dane, A. V., & Schneider, B. H. (1998). Program integrity in primary and early secondary prevention: Are implementation effects out of control? *Clinical Psychology Review, 18*(1), 23–45.

Davidoff, F. (2009). Heterogeneity is not always noise: Lessons from quality improvement. *JAMA, 302*(23), 2580–2586.

Dearing, J. W., & Kee, K. F. (2012). Historical roots of dissemination and implementation science. In R. C. Brownson, G. A. Colditz, & E. K. Proctor (Eds.), *Dissemination and implementation research in health: Translating science to practice* (pp. 55–71). Oxford University Press.

Dopp, A. R., Mundey, P., Beasley, L. O., Silovsky, J. F., & Eisenberg, D. (2019). Mixed-method approaches to strengthen economic evaluations in implementation research. *Implementation Science, 14*(2), 1–9.

Dunbar, J., Hernan, A., Janus, E., Davis-Lameloise, N., Asproloupos, D., O'Reilly, S., ... Carter, R. (2012). Implementation salvage experiences from the Melbourne diabetes prevention study. *BMC Public Health, 12*(806), 1–9.

Durlak, J. A., & DuPre, E. P. (2008). Implementation matters: A review of research on the influence of implementation on program outcomes and the factors affecting implementation. *American Journal of Community Psychology, 41*, 327–350.

Eccles, M. P., Grimshaw, J. M., Campbell, M., & Ramsay, C. (2005). Experimental evaluations of change and improvement strategies. In R. Grol, M. Wensing, & M. Eccles (Eds.), *Improving patient care: The implementation of change in clinical practice* (pp. 235–247). Elsevier.

Eisman, A. B., Kilbourne, A. M., Dopp, A. R., Saldana, L., & Eisenberg, D. (2020). Economic evaluation in implementation science: Making the business case for implementation strategies. *Psychiatry Research, 283*, 1–6.

Escoffery, C., Lebow-Skelley, E., Udelson, H., Böing, E. A., Wood, R., Fernandez, M. E., & Mullen, P. D. (2018). A scoping study of frameworks for adapting public health evidence-based interventions. *Translational Behavioral Medicine, 9*(1), 1–10.

Finley, E. P., Huynh, A. K., Farmer, M. M., Bean-Mayberry, B., Moin, T., Oishi, S. M., ... Hamilton, A. B. (2018). Periodic reflections: A method of guided discussions for documenting implementation phenomena. *BMC Medical Research Methodology, 18*(153), 1–15.

Flottorp, S. A., Oxman, A. D., Krause, J., Musila, N. R., Wensing, M., Godycki-Cwirko, M., ... Eccles, M. P. (2013). A checklist for identifying determinants of practice: A systematic review and synthesis of frameworks and taxonomies of factors that prevent or enable improvements in healthcare professional practice. *Implementation Science, 8*(35), 1–11.

Forsner, T., Hansson, J., Brommels, M., Wistedt, A. A., & Forsell, Y. (2010). Implementing clinical guidelines in psychiatry: A qualitative study of perceived facilitators and barriers. *BMC Psychiatry, 10*(8), 1–10.

Frechtling, J. A. (2007). *Logic modeling methods in program evaluation*. Wiley.

Gertner, A. K., Franklin, J., Roth, I., Cruden, G. H., Haley, A. D., Finley, E. P., ... Powell, B. J. (2021). A scoping review of the use of ethnographic approaches in implementation research and recommendations for reporting. *Implementation Research and Practice, 2*, 1–13.

Glasgow, R. E., & Riley, W. T. (2013). Pragmatic measures: What they are and why we need them. *American Journal of Preventive Medicine, 45*(2), 237–243.

Glisson, C., Schoenwald, S., Hemmelgarn, A., Green, P., Dukes, D., Armstrong, K. S., & Chapman, J. E. (2010). Randomized trial of MST and ARC in a two-level evidence-based treatment implementation strategy. *Journal of Consulting and Clinical Psychology, 78*(4), 537–550.

Gravel, K., Légaré, F., & Graham, I. D. (2006). Barriers and facilitators to implementing shared decision-making in clinical practice: A systematic review of health professionals' perceptions. *Implementation Science, 1*(16).

Green, A. E., & Aarons, G. A. (2011). A comparison of policy and direct practice stakeholder perceptions of factors affecting evidence-based practice implementation using concept mapping. *Implementation Science, 6*(104), 1–12.

Grimshaw, J. M., Eccles, M. P., Lavis, J. N., Hill, S. J., & Squires, J. E. (2012). Knowledge translation of research findings. *Implementation Science, 7*(50), 1–17.

Haley, A. D., Powell, B. J., Walsh-Bailey, C., Krancari, M., Gruß, I., Shea, C. M., ... Gold, R. (2021).

Strengthening methods for tracking adaptations and modifications to implementation strategies. *BMC Medical Research Methodology, 21*(133), 1–12.

Hamm, R. F., Levine, L. D., Szymczak, J. E., Parry, S., Srinivas, S. K., & Beidas, R. S. (2023). An innovative sequential mixed-methods approach to evaluating clinician acceptability during implementation of a standardized labor induction protocol. *BMC Medical Research Methodology, 23*(1), 195.

Handley, M. A., Lyles, C. R., McCulloch, C., & Cattamanchi, A. (2018). Selecting and improving quasi-experimental designs in effectiveness and implementation research. *Annual Review of Public Health, 39*, 5–25.

Hoagwood, K. E., Chaffin, M., Chamberlain, P., Bickman, L., & Mittman, B. (2011, March). *Implementation salvage strategies: Maximizing methodological flexibility in children's mental health research* [Panel presentation]. Fourth Annual NIH Conference on the Science of Dissemination and Implementation, Washington, DC.

Hoffman, T. C., Glasziou, P. P., Boutron, I., Milne, R., Perera, R., Moher, D., . . . Michie, S. (2014). Better reporting of interventions: Template for intervention description and replication (TIDieR) checklist and guide. *BMJ, 348*(g1687), 1–12.

Hooley, C., Amano, T., Markovitz, L., Yaeger, L., & Proctor, E. (2020). Assessing implementation strategy reporting in the mental health literature: A narrative review. *Administration and Policy in Mental Health, 47*(1), 19–35.

Hoomans, T., & Severens, J. L. (2014). Economic evaluation of implementation strategies in health care. *Implementation Science, 9*(168), 1–6.

Hovmand, P. S., & Gillespie, D. F. (2010). Implementation of evidence-based practice and organizational performance. *Journal of Behavioral Health Services and Research, 37*(1), 79–94.

Huijg, J. M., Gebhardt, W. A., Crone, M. R., Dusseldorp, E., & Presseau, J. (2014). Discriminant content validity of a theoretical domains framework questionnaire for use in implementation research. *Implementation Science, 9*(11), 1–16.

Hwang, S., Birken, S. A., Melvin, C. L., Rohweder, C. L., & Smith, J. D. (2020). Designs and methods for implementation research: Advancing the mission of the CTSA program. *Journal of Clinical and Translational Science, 4*(3), 159–167.

Isett, K. R., Burnam, M. A., Coleman-Beattie, B., Hyde, P. S., Morrissey, J. P., Magnabosco, J., . . . Goldman, H. H. (2007). The state policy context of implementation issues for evidence-based practices in mental health. *Psychiatric Services, 58*(7), 914–921.

Jacobs, J. A., Dodson, E. A., Baker, E. A., Deshpande, A. D., & Brownson, R. C. (2010). Barriers to evidence-based decision making in public health: A national survey of chronic disease practitioners. *Public Health Reports, 125*(5), 736–742.

Kane, M., & Trochim, W. M. K. (2007). *Concept mapping for planning and evaluation*. Sage.

Kendall, P. C., Robin, J. A., Hedtke, K. A., Suveg, C., Flannery-Schroeder, E., & Gosch, E. (2005). Considering CBT with anxious youth? Think exposures. *Cognitive and Behavioral Practice, 12*, 136–150.

Khadjesari, Z., Boufkhed, S., Vitoratou, S., Schatte, L., Ziemann, A., Daskalopoulou, C., . . . Hull, L. (2020). Implementation outcome instruments for use in physical healthcare settings: A systematic review. *Implementation Science, 15*(1), 66.

Kirk, M. A., Haines, E. R., Rokoske, F. S., Powell, B. J., Weinberger, M., Hanson, L. C., & Birken, S. A. (2021). A case study of a theory-based method for identifying and reporting core functions and forms of evidence-based interventions. *Translational Behavioral Medicine, 11*, 21–33.

Kolko, D. J., McGuier, E. A., Turchi, R., Thompson, E., Iyengar, S., Smith, S. N., . . . Kilbourne, A. M. (2022). Care team and practice-level implementation strategies to optimize pediatric collaborative care: Study protocol for a cluster-randomized hybrid type III trial. *Implementation Science, 17*(1), 20.

Krause, J., Van Lieshout, J., Klomp, R., Huntink, E., Aakhus, E., Flottorp, S., . . . Baker, R. (2014). Identifying determinants of care for tailoring implementation in chronic diseases: An evaluation of different methods. *Implementation Science, 9*(102).

Landsverk, J., Brown, C. H., Rolls Reutz, J., Palinkas, L. A., & Horwitz, S. M. (2011). Design elements in implementation research: A structured review of child welfare and child mental health studies. *Administration and Policy in Mental Health, 38*, 54–63.

Landsverk, J., Brown, C. H., Smith, J. D., Chamberlain, P., Curran, G. M., Palinkas, L., . . . Horwitz, S. M. (2018). Design and analysis in dissemination and implementation research. In R. C. Brownson, G. A. Colditz, & E. K. Proctor (Eds.), *Dissemination and implementation research in health: Translating science to practice* (2nd ed., pp. 201–227). Oxford University Press.

Lengnick-Hall, R., Gerke, D. R., Proctor, E. K., Bunger, A. C., Phillips, R. J., Martin, J. K., & Swanson, J. C. (2022). Six practical recommendations for improved implementation outcomes reporting. *Implementation Science, 17*(1), 16.

Lengnick-Hall, R., Proctor, E. K., Bunger, A. C., & Gerke, D. R. (2021). Ten years of implementation outcome research: A scoping review protocol. *BMJ Open, 11*(6), e049339.

Lewis, C. C., Fischer, S., Weiner, B. J., Stanick, C., Kim, M., & Martinez, R. G. (2015). Outcomes for implementation science: An enhanced systematic review of instruments using evidence-based rating criteria. *Implementation Science, 10*(155), 1–17.

Lewis, C. C., Klasnja, P., Powell, B. J., Lyon, A. R.,

Tuzzio, L., Jones, S., & Walsh-Bailey, C. (2018). From classification to causality: Advancing understanding of mechanisms of change in implementation science. *Frontiers in Public Health*, 6(136), 1–6.

Lewis, C. C., Mettert, K. D., Stanick, C. F., Halko, H. M., Nolen, E. A., Powell, B. J., & Weiner, B. J. (2021). The Psychometric and Pragmatic Evidence Rating Scale (PAPERS) for measure development and evaluation. *Implementation Research and Practice*, 2, 1–6.

Lewis, C. C., Proctor, E. K., & Brownson, R. C. (2018). Measurement issues in dissemination and implementation research. In R. C. Brownson, R. A. Colditz, & E. K. Proctor (Eds.), *Dissemination and implementation research in health* (2nd ed., pp. 229–244). Oxford University Press.

Lobb, R., Pinto, A. D., & Lofters, A. (2013). Using concept mapping in the knowledge-to-action process to compare stakeholder opinions on barriers to use of cancer screening among South Asians. *Implementation Science*, 8(37), 1–12.

Luke, D. A. (2004). *Multilevel modeling*. Sage.

Luke, D. A., Powell, B. J., & Paniagua-Avila, A. (2024). Bridges and mechanisms: Integrating systems science thinking into implementation research. *Annual Review of Public Health*, 45(1), 7–25.

Lyon, A. R., & Bruns, E. J. (2019). User-centered redesign of evidence-based psychosocial interventions to enhance implementation: Hospitable soil or better seeds? *JAMA Psychiatry*, 76(1), 3–4.

Malone, S., McKay, V. R., Krucylak, C., Powell, B. J., Liu, J., Terrill, C., . . . Newland, J. G. (2021). A cluster randomized stepped-wedge trial to de-implement unnecessary post-operative antibiotics in children: The optimizing perioperative antibiotic in children (OPerAtiC) trial. *Implementation Science*, 16(29), 1–11.

Mazzucca, S., Tabak, R. G., Pilar, M., Ramsey, A. T., Baumann, A. A., Kryzer, E., . . . Brownson, R. C. (2018). Variation in research designs used to test the effectiveness of dissemination and implementation strategies: A review. *Frontiers in Public Health*, 6(32), 1–10.

McLaughlin, J. A., & Jordan, G. B. (1999). Logic models: A tool for telling your program's performance story. *Evaluation and Program Planning*, 22, 65–72.

The Methodology Committee of the Patient-Centered Outcomes Research Institute (PCORI). (2012). Methodological standards and patient-centeredness in comparative effectiveness research: The PCORI perspective. *Journal of the American Medical Association*, 307(15), 1636–1640.

Mettert, K., Lewis, C., Dorsey, C., Halko, H., & Weiner, B. (2020). Measuring implementation outcomes: An updated systematic review of measures' psychometric properties. *Implementation Research and Practice*, 1, 2633489520936644.

Metz, A. (2016). *Practice profiles: A process for capturing evidence and operationalizing innovations*. National Implementation Research Network.

Metz, A., & Easterling, D. (2016). Using implementation science to translate foundation strategy. *Foundation Review*, 8(2), 116–137.

Michie, S., Fixsen, D. L., Grimshaw, J. M., & Eccles, M. P. (2009). Specifying and reporting complex behaviour change interventions: The need for a scientific method. *Implementation Science*, 4(40), 1–6.

Michie, S., Johnston, M., Abraham, C., Lawton, R., Parker, D., & Walker, A. (2005). Making psychological theory useful for implementing evidence based practice: A consensus approach. *Quality and Safety in Health Care*, 14, 26–33.

Miller, C. J., Barnett, M. L., Baumann, A. A., Gutner, C. A., & Wiltsey Stirman, S. (2021). The FRAME-IS: A framework for documenting modifications to implementation strategies in healthcare. *Implementation Science*, 16(36), 1–12.

Nadeem, E., Olin, S., Hoagwood, K. E., & Horwitz, S. M. (2013). Understanding the components of quality improvement collaboratives: A systematic literature review. *Milbank Quarterly*, 91(2), 354–394.

National Cancer Institute. (2018). *Qualitative methods in implementation science*. National Cancer Institute, Division of Cancer Control and Population Sciences.

Neta, G., Glasgow, R. E., Carpenter, C. R., Grimshaw, J. M., Rabin, B. A., Fernandez, M. E., & Brownson, R. C. (2015). A framework for enhancing the value of research for dissemination and implementation. *American Journal of Public Health*, 105(1), 49–57.

Nguyen, M. X. B., Chu, A. V., Powell, B. J., Tran, H. V., Nguyen, L. H., Dao, A. T. M., . . . Go, V. F. (2020). Comparing a standard and tailored approach to scaling up an evidence-based intervention for antiretroviral therapy for people who inject drugs in Vietnam: Study protocol for a cluster randomized hybrid type III trial. *Implementation Science*, 15(64), 1–16.

Overbeck, G., Sofie Davidsen, A., & Brostrøm Kousgaard, M. (2016). Enablers and barriers to implementing collaborative care for anxiety and depression: A systematic qualitative review. *Implementation Science*, 11(165), 1–16.

Palinkas, L. A., Aarons, G. A., Horwitz, S., Chamberlain, P., Hurlburt, M., & Landsverk, J. (2011). Mixed methods designs in implementation research. *Administration and Policy in Mental Health*, 38, 44–53.

Palinkas, L. A., Horwitz, S. M., Green, C. A., Wisdom, J. P., Duan, N., & Hoagwood, K. (2013). Purposeful sampling for qualitative data collection and analysis in mixed method implementation research. *Administration and Policy in Mental Health*, 42(5), 533–544.

Palinkas, L. A., & Zatzick, D. (2019). Rapid assessment procedure informed clinical ethnography (RAPICE) in pragmatic clinical trials of mental health services implementation: Methods and applied case study. *Administration and Policy in Mental Health, 46,* 255–270.

Patient Centered Outcomes Research Institute. (2019). *PCORI standards for studies of complex interventions.* Available at *www.pcori.org/research-results/about-our-research/research-methodology/pcori-methodology-standards#Complex*

Perry, C. K., Damschroder, L. J., Hemler, J. R., Woodson, T. T., Ono, S. S., & Cohen, D. J. (2019). Specifying and comparing implementation strategies across seven large implementation interventions: A practical application of theory. *Implementation Science, 14*(32), 1–13.

Pinnock, H., Barwick, M., Carpenter, C. R., Eldridge, S., Grandes, G., Griffiths, C. J., . . . Taylor, S. J. C. (2017). Standards for reporting implementation studies (StaRI) statement. *BMJ, 356*(i6795).

Powell, B. J., Beidas, R. S., Lewis, C. C., Aarons, G. A., McMillen, J. C., Proctor, E. K., & Mandell, D. S. (2017). Methods to improve the selection and tailoring of implementation strategies. *Journal of Behavioral Health Services and Research, 44*(2), 177–194.

Powell, B. J., Fernandez, M. E., Williams, N. J., Aarons, G. A., Beidas, R. S., Lewis, C. C., . . . Weiner, B. J. (2019). Enhancing the impact of implementation strategies in healthcare: A research agenda. *Frontiers in Public Health, 7*(3), 1–9.

Powell, B. J., Hausmann-Stabile, C., & McMillen, J. C. (2013). Mental health clinicians' experiences of implementing evidence-based treatments. *Journal of Evidence-Based Social Work, 10*(5), 396–409.

Powell, B. J., Mandell, D. S., Hadley, T. R., Rubin, R. M., Evans, A. C., Hurford, M. O., & Beidas, R. S. (2017). Are general and strategic measures of organizational context and leadership associated with knowledge and attitudes toward evidence-based practices in public behavioral health settings? A cross-sectional observational study. *Implementation Science, 12*(64), 1–13.

Powell, B. J., McMillen, J. C., Hawley, K. M., & Proctor, E. K. (2013). Mental health clinicians' motivation to invest in training: Results from a practice-based research network survey. *Psychiatric Services, 64*(8), 816–818.

Powell, B. J., McMillen, J. C., Proctor, E. K., Carpenter, C. R., Griffey, R. T., Bunger, A. C., . . . York, J. L. (2012). A compilation of strategies for implementing clinical innovations in health and mental health. *Medical Care Research and Review, 69*(2), 123–157.

Powell, B. J., Patel, S. V., Haley, A. D., Haines, E. R., Knocke, K. E., Chandler, S. P., . . . Aarons, G. A. (2020). Determinants of implementing evidence-based trauma-focused interventions for children and youth: A systematic review. *Administration and Policy in Mental Health, 47,* 705–719.

Powell, B. J., Stanick, C. F., Halko, H. M., Dorsey, C. N., Weiner, B. J., Barwick, M. A., . . . Lewis, C. C. (2017). Toward criteria for pragmatic measurement in implementation research and practice: A stakeholder-driven approach using concept mapping. *Implementation Science, 12*(1), 118.

Powell, B. J., Waltz, T. J., Chinman, M. J., Damschroder, L. J., Smith, J. L., Matthieu, M. M., . . . Kirchner, J. E. (2015). A refined compilation of implementation strategies: Results from the Expert Recommendations for Implementing Change (ERIC) project. *Implementation Science, 10*(21), 1–14.

Power, T. J., Blom-Hoffman, J., Clarke, A. T., Riley-Tillman, T. C., & Manz, P. H. (2005). Reconceptualizing intervention integrity: A partnership-based framework for linking research with practice. *Psychology in the Schools, 42*(5), 495–507.

Prasad, V., & Ioannidis, J. P. A. (2014). Evidence-based de-implementation for contradicted, unproven, and aspiring healthcare practices. *Implementation Science, 9*(1), 1–5.

Proctor, E. K., Landsverk, J., Aarons, G. A., Chambers, D. A., Glisson, C., & Mittman, B. S. (2009). Implementation research in mental health services: An emerging science with conceptual, methodological, and training challenges. *Administration and Policy in Mental Health, 36,* 24–34.

Proctor, E. K., Powell, B. J., & Feely, M. (2014). Measurement in dissemination and implementation science. In R. S. Beidas & P. C. Kendall (Eds.), *Dissemination and implementation of evidence-based practices in child and adolescent mental health* (pp. 22–43). Oxford University Press.

Proctor, E. K., Powell, B. J., & McMillen, J. C. (2013). Implementation strategies: Recommendations for specifying and reporting. *Implementation Science, 8*(139), 1–11.

Proctor, E. K., Silmere, H., Raghavan, R., Hovmand, P., Aarons, G. A., Bunger, A., . . . Hensley, M. (2011). Outcomes for implementation research: Conceptual distinctions, measurement challenges, and research agenda. *Administration and Policy in Mental Health, 38*(2), 65–76.

Reeves, P., Edmunds, K., Searles, A., & Wiggers, J. (2019). Economic evaluations of public health implementation-interventions: A systematic review and guideline for practice. *Public Health, 169,* 101–113.

Roberts, S. L. E., Healey, A., & Sevdalis, N. (2019). Use of health economic evaluation in the implementation and improvement science fields: A systematic literature review. *Implementation Science, 14*(72), 1–13.

Rogal, S. S., Yakovchenko, V., Morgan, T., Bajaj, J. S., Gonzalez, R., Park, A., . . . Chinman, M. J. (2020). Getting to implementation: A protocol for a hybrid III stepped wedge cluster randomized evaluation of using data-driven implementation strategies to improve cirrhosis care for veterans. *Implementation Science, 15*(92), 1–10.

Rogal, S. S., Yakovchenko, V., Waltz, T. J., Powell, B. J., Gonzalez, R., Park, A., . . . Chinman, M. J. (2019). Longitudinal assessment of the association between implementation strategy use and the uptake of hepatitis C treatment: Year two. *Implementation Science, 14*(36), 1–12.

Rogal, S. S., Yakovchenko, V., Waltz, T. J., Powell, B. J., Kirchner, J. E., Proctor, E. K., . . . Chinman, M. J. (2017). The association between implementation strategy use and the uptake of hepatitis C treatment in a national sample. *Implementation Science, 12*(60), 1–13.

Saldana, L., Chamberlain, P., Bradford, W. D., Campbell, M., & Landsverk, J. (2014). The cost of implementing new strategies (COINS): A method for mapping implementation resources using the stages of implementation completion. *Children and Youth Services Review, 39*, 177–182.

Schoenwald, S. K., Garland, A. F., Chapman, J. E., Frazier, S. L., Sheidow, A. J., & Southam-Gerow, M. A. (2011). Toward the effective and efficient measurement of implementation fidelity. *Administration and Policy in Mental Health, 38*, 32–43.

Shelton, R. C., Cooper, B. R., & Wiltsey Stirman, S. (2018). The sustainability of evidence-based interventions and practices in public health and health care. *Annual Review of Public Health, 39*, 55–76.

Smith, J. D., Merle, J. L., Webster, K. A., Cahue, S., Penedo, F. J., & Garcia, S. F. (2022). Tracking dynamic changes in implementation strategies over time within a hybrid type 2 trial of an electronic patient-reported oncology symptom and needs monitoring program. *Frontiers in Health Services, 2*. Available at *www.frontiersin.org/articles/10.3389/frhs.2022.983217*

Smith, J. D., Norton, W. E., Mitchell, S. A., Cronin, C., Hassett, M. J., Ridgeway, J. L., Garcia, S. F., Osarogiagbon, R. U., Dizon, D. S., Austin, J. D., Battestilli, W., Richardson, J. E., Tesch, N. K., Cella, D., Cheville, A. L., DiMartino, L. D., & IMPACT Consortium (2023). The Longitudinal Implementation Strategy Tracking System (LISTS): feasibility, usability, and pilot testing of a novel method. *Implementation Science Communications, 4*(1), 153.

Stake, R. E. (2005). *Multiple case study analysis.* Guilford Press.

Stanick, C. F., Halko, H. M., Dorsey, C. N., Weiner, B. J., Powell, B. J., Palinkas, L. A., & Lewis, C. C. (2018). Operationalizing the "pragmatic" measures construct using a stakeholder feedback and a multi-method approach. *BMC Health Services Research, 18*(882), 1–12.

Stanick, C. F., Halko, H. M., Nolen, E. A., Powell, B. J., Dorsey, C. N., Mettert, K. D., . . . Lewis, C. C. (2021). Pragmatic measures for implementation research: Development of the Psychometric and Pragmatic Evidence Rating Scale (PAPERS). *Translational Behavioral Medicine, 11*, 11–20.

Stetler, C. B., McQueen, L., Demakis, J., & Mittman, B. S. (2008). An organizational framework and strategic implementation for systems-level change to enhance research-based practice: QUERI series. *Implementation Science, 3*(30), 1–11.

Taylor, M. J., McNicholas, C., Nicolay, C., Darzi, A., Bell, D., & Reed, J. E. (2014). Systematic review of the application of the plan-do-study-act method to improve quality in healthcare. *BMJ Quality and Safety, 23*(4), 290–298.

Turner, K., Weinberger, M., Renfro, C., Powell, B. J., Ferreri, S., Trogdon, J., . . . Shea, C. M. (2021). Stages of change: Moving community pharmacies from a drug dispensing to population health management model. *Medical Care Research and Review, 78*(1), 57–67.

Vale, L., Thomas, R., MacLennan, G., & Grimshaw, J. (2007). Systematic review of economic evaluations and cost analyses of guideline implementation strategies. *European Journal of Health Economics, 8*, 111–121.

Vaughn, A., Studts, C. R., Powell, B. J., Ammerman, A. S., Trogdon, J. G., Curran, G. M., . . . Ward, D. S. (2019). The impact of a basic vs. enhanced GoNAPSACC on child care centers' health eating and physical activity practices: Protocol for a type 3 hybrid effectiveness–implementation cluster-randomized trial. *Implementation Science, 14*(101), 1–15.

W. K. Kellogg Foundation. (2004). *Logic model development guide: Using logic models to bring together planning, evaluation, and action.* Author.

Walsh-Bailey, C., Palazzo, L. G., Jones, S. M. W., Mettert, K. D., Powell, B. J., Wiltsey Stirman, S., . . . Lewis, C. C. (2021). A pilot study comparing tools for tracking implementation strategies and treatment adaptations. *Implementation Research and Practice, 2*, 1–14.

Waltz, T. J., Powell, B. J., Matthieu, M. M., Damschroder, L. J., Chinman, M. J., Smith, J. L., . . . Kirchner, J. E. (2015). Use of concept mapping to characterize relationships among implementation strategies and assess their feasibility and importance: Results from the Expert Recommendations for Implementing Change (ERIC) study. *Implementation Science, 10*(109), 1–8.

Weiner, B. J., Lewis, C. C., Stanick, C. S., Powell, B. J., Dorsey, C. N., Clary, A. S., . . . Halko, H. M. (2017). Psychometric assessment of three newly developed implementation outcome measures. *Implementation Science, 12*(108), 1–12.

Wensing, M., & Grimshaw, J. (2020). Experimental designs for evaluation of implementation strategies. In M. Wensing, R. Grol, & J. Grimshaw (Eds.), *Improving patient care: The implementation of change in health care* (3rd ed., pp. 345–356). Wiley-Blackwell.

Williams, N. J., Ehrhart, M. G., Aarons, G. A., Marcus, S. C., & Beidas, R. S. (2018). Linking molar organizational climate and strategic implementation climate to clinicians' use of evidence-based psychotherapy techniques: Cross-sectional and lagged analyses from a 2-year observational study. *Implementation Science, 13*(85), 1–13.

Wiltsey Stirman, S., Baumann, A. A., & Miller, C. J. (2019). The FRAME: An expanded framework for reporting adaptations and modifications to evidence-based interventions. *Implementation Science, 14*(58), 1–10.

Wiltsey Stirman, S., Gutner, C. A., Crits-Christoph, P., Edmunds, J., Evans, A. C., & Beidas, R. S. (2015). Relationships between clinician-level attributes and fidelity-consistent and fidelity-inconsistent modifications to an evidence-based psychotherapy. *Implementation Science, 10*(115), 1–10.

Wiltsey Stirman, S., Miller, C. J., Toder, K., & Calloway, A. (2013). Development of a framework and coding system for modifications and adaptations of evidence-based interventions. *Implementation Science, 8*(65), 1–12.

Wolfenden, L., Foy, R., Presseau, J., Grimshaw, J. M., Ivers, N. M., Powell, B. J., . . . Yoong, S. L. (2021). Designing and undertaking randomised implementation trials: Guide for researchers. *BMJ, 372*(m3721), 1–14.

Workgroup for Intervention Development and Evaluation Research. (2008). *WIDER recommendations to improve reporting of the content of behaviour change interventions.* Available at *http://interventiondesign. co.uk/wp-content/uploads/2009/02/wider-recommendations.pdf*

Yamey, G. (2012). What are the barriers to scaling up health interventions in low and middle income countries? A qualitative study of academic leaders in implementation science. *Implementation Science, 8*(11), 1–11.

Yin, R. K. (2009). *Case study research: Design and methods* (4th ed.). Sage.

Zimmerman, L., Lounsbury, D., Rosen, C., Kimerling, R., Trafton, J., & Lindley, S. (2016). Participatory system dynamics modeling: Increasing engagement and precision to improve implementation planning in systems. *Administration and Policy in Mental Health, 43,* 834–849.

Chapter 13

Examining Outcomes and Impacts
Designs and Strategies in Theory and Practice

Laura R. Peck
R. Bradley Snyder

CHAPTER OVERVIEW

Two lines of summative evaluation involve assessing outcomes and assessing impacts. This chapter discusses the notion of cause and effect as fundamental to summative evaluation, along with the related concepts of the counterfactual and threats to the internal validity of an evaluation design. After defining key measurement concepts, we review the program logic model, which serves as a foundation for any outcome or impact evaluation. Impact evaluations fall into two main types: experimental and quasi-experimental. Experimental evaluation designs use random assignment to designate access to treatment. This produces a quality representation of the counterfactual and thereby results in a strong estimate of the program's impact. Quasi-experimental evaluation designs use other mechanisms for creating a counterfactual, either a reflexive or comparative group, where some of the threats to internal validity limit interpretation of the estimated impacts as causal. We discuss strengths and weaknesses of the varied design options along with the conditions under which they are optimally used.

This chapter discusses how evaluators use outcomes and impacts as metrics of a program's success. To begin, it is essential to define what we mean by "outcomes" and "impacts." We define **outcome** as the construct that a given program aims to achieve either as the ultimate goal of the program or as a step toward the program's ultimate goal. We define **impact** as the change in an outcome that is attributable to the program. In many circumstances, identifying and measuring outcomes is beneficial to policymakers and program administrators, regardless of whether it is certain that the program is responsible for changes in those outcomes. In other circumstances, it is critical for policy or practice purposes to be able to attribute a change in outcomes directly to the program.

This distinction between outcome and impact is part of a larger discussion within program evaluation that involves classifying types of evaluation. These typologies tend to make a distinction between formative and summative evaluation. **Formative evaluation**—which includes process or implementation evaluation—considers a program's processes, operations, and implementation. As such, it tends to be descriptive in nature, commonly comparing programs as designed to programs as implemented, with critical examination of any differences and explanations for those differences. In comparison, **summative evaluation**—which includes outcome, impact, and economic (cost-related) analyses—considers the documented results of a program's activity, or its "summative" products. This chapter focuses on outcome and impact evaluations as key tools of summative evaluation, and uses the terms as they are commonly used across the field.

Attributing change to a program, the concept of cause and effect, is fundamental to the field of program evaluation. As policymakers and program administrators establish, implement, and evolve public programs in an environment of scarce resources, measuring a program's causal relationship with an outcome—its impact—often is essential to endorsing ongoing funding, to informing how to enact policy changes or program improvements, or to justifying program termination. While **outcome evaluation** is concerned with how to measure a construct that a program aims to achieve, **impact evaluation** is concerned with isolating the change in outcomes that the program caused from the many other possible explanations that exist. Often, estimating how much of the change in an outcome is due to the program involves estimating the "counterfactual." A **counterfactual** is what would have happened in the program's absence. The impact evaluation design challenge is to construct a representation of the counterfactual that permits ruling out plausible, rival explanations for changes in outcomes.

So far, we have introduced the key concepts of outcomes, impacts, and counterfactuals. Next, we present a bullying prevention program and a job training program as two illustrative program examples (see Box 13.1) that we use throughout the chapter to explain and apply concepts. Following that, we address the importance of measuring outcomes to help ascertain whether a program is achieving its goals. From there, we discuss impact evaluation and briefly list experimental and quasi-experimental approaches for measuring a program's impacts. This discussion addresses the conditions for selecting a given evaluation design and the strengths and weaknesses associated with each design in common practice. We conclude by identifying challenges that arise in carrying out outcome and impact evaluations, and we suggest responses and point to other useful research for furthering one's familiarity with outcome and impact evaluation.

BOX 13.1. Example Programs Used in This Chapter

To illustrate the concepts and challenges involved in examining and measuring program outcomes and impacts, this chapter considers two examples: a bullying prevention program and a job training program.

• **Bullying prevention program.** The bullying prevention program we offer as an example is typical among bullying prevention and cessation programs. At its core, it seeks to reduce school-based bullying by educating students on how to recognize bullying and how to respond when they do witness bullying. Among other things, the program directs bystanders, those students who are neither the bully nor the victim, to inform a trusted adult (i.e., a teacher, a coach, a school counselor, other faculty) when they witness bullying occurring. The program assumes that informing a trusted adult will illicit an appropriate response that will eliminate current bullying and prevent it from happening in the future.

• **Job training program.** The job training program we offer as an example also is typical among such programs. It seeks to increase employment by training unemployed or underemployed adults for positions that pay living wages in job sectors that have jobs that pay well. At its core, this job training program is a credentialing program that teaches adults the skills they need to qualify for the jobs in question that lead to greater earnings and self-sufficiency.

MEASURES

We address outcome evaluations and impact evaluation separately but both rely on measurement of outcomes where these outcomes represent the construct of primary program interest. A **measure** is a representation of the construct of a program outcome. Measures are typically judged by two criteria: validity and reliability. We also introduce the concept of parsimony, as relevant to measurement in the context of outcome and impact evaluation in practice.

Validity

The **validity** of a measure is the extent to which the measure actually reflects or represents the underlying construct that it purports to reflect or represent. A digital thermometer, for example, can be used to obtain a valid measure of the surface temperature of an item in Celsius (or

Fahrenheit) because digital thermometers are calibrated to uniformly measure temperature using a universally agreed-upon standard. An evaluator could lay digital thermometers end to end to measure the length of an item, but that would not be a valid measure because there is not an agreed-upon length of digital thermometers. A math test might be an accurate measure of a student's ability to apply certain mathematic concepts. However, the same math test might be a poor measure of that student's knowledge of history or geography.

Reliability

The **reliability** of a measure is the extent to which the measure will produce the same result for the same construct regardless of who is administering the measure and on whom or what it is being administered. Again, a digital thermometer is reliable because it displays the same results regardless of who points the digital thermometer. Reliability is not a characteristic of a measure in isolation but instead it is dependent on context and population, ideally responsive to real changes.

The classic illustration of the relationship between validity and reliability is that of a dartboard. A reliable dart thrower might be able to hit the double eight nine times out of 10 but the goal is to hit the bullseye. That dart thrower is reliable but not valid. A valid dart thrower would hit the bullseye. A valid and reliable dart thrower would hit the bullseye routinely.

Parsimony

A concept that is seldom addressed in discussions of measurement that we believe is increasingly important is parsimony. **Parsimony** is the best possible measure that requires the least amount of measuring. The concept of parsimony is easiest to understand when applied to surveys. As the number of questions a respondent is asked increases, the quality of each additional answer decreases. Generally, this is known as **survey fatigue**, and it is a well-researched phenomenon illustrating the need for parsimony in outcome and impact evaluations (DeVellis, 2012). Good rules of thumb for creating inventories, tests, or surveys that help evaluators achieve parsimony are:

1. If a particular question is not reflected in a program's logic model, then researchers should revise the logic model—which represents the theorized connections between program inputs, activities, outputs, and outcomes, as elaborated later in this chapter and also by Frechtling (see Chapter 20, this volume)—or avoid asking the question.

2. If the response to a particular question will not be used to measure an outcome of interest or important correlate needed for analysis, then researchers should not ask the question.

Another illustration of the need for parsimony—the pursuit of the best possible measure with the least amount of measuring—is testing bias. **Testing bias**—sometimes referred to as **reactivity**—occurs when the act of measuring a construct actually changes the outcome or even the construct being measured. For example, it is well documented that some individuals who agree to be a "Nielson household"—and record data about their television viewing—change their television viewing behaviors after agreeing to be monitored (e.g., Schwindt, 2016; Woodward, 1991). The fact that their viewing was being "tested" changed their viewing outcomes. The possibility of testing bias can increase as the measuring itself increases in intensity, in intrusiveness, in overtness, and so on. Like survey fatigue, testing bias threatens the validity of a measure. Testing bias is just one of the forces that can compromise the credibility of evaluation results that is addressed later in the chapter in the discussion of impact evaluations. At this point, it is enough for evaluators to understand the importance of parsimony in measurement to avoid testing bias.

The final argument for parsimony is a practical one. Measurement takes time and resources to conduct and to analyze. If time and resources were unlimited and if the field, policymakers, program administrators, and the greater good were not affected by the results of an evaluation, then **fishing** (looking for patterns in measures without guidance from a theory, a logic model, or a hypothesis) might be acceptable. However, the best evaluations are relevant, and timeliness is a condition of relevance (see also Harbatkin et al., Chapter 16; Pham et al., Chapter 17, this volume, for more information about measurement issues).

Next, we discuss outcome evaluation. The discussion refers to logic models frequently because we believe that logic models are the best tool for illustrating the relationship between a program's activities and its output, between a program's outputs and its outcomes, and between a program's outcomes and its impacts. For a detailed discussion of how to formulate logic models, refer to Frechtling (see Chapter 20, this volume).

OUTCOME EVALUATION

Identifying the desired outcome for a given program often is relatively easy. It typically is prominent in the program's description, in the parent organization's mission statement, or even in the name of the organization. For example, the U.S. Department of Labor aims to influence "labor" outcomes; and Saint Mary's Food Bank provides food assistance. We have defined *outcome* as the construct that a given program aims to achieve. Interest holders of a given program might think of the outcome as the program's goal, or they may simply think of it as what that program does. More formally, interest holders' conception of all of the activities that constitute "what the program does" can be thought of as the "program theory," defined as "interest holders' implicit and explicit assumptions on what actions are required to solve a problem and why the problem will respond to the actions" (Chen, 2005, p. 15).

With this in mind it is easy to distinguish between an outcome and an "output." An **output** is the direct product of a program. In our bullying prevention program example, the output is the number of students who attended the bullying prevention instruction. Note that *providing instruction* is not the goal of the program, nor is providing instruction likely to be mentioned in the program's mission statement. After all, it is a bullying prevention program, not an instruction provision program. Likewise, the output of our job training program example is the people who completed a training program.

The ultimate goal of the bullying prevention program example is to reduce bullying at the school level—therefore its outcomes address attitudes, actions, and incidents related to bullying. This is reflected in the program's logic model, as illustrated in Figure 13.1. The ultimate goal of the job training program is that its participants will have greater labor market earnings. This is reflected in the program's logic model, as illustrated in Figure 13.2.

In this sense, initially identifying an outcome of interest is among the easiest steps of an outcome evaluation. However, as researchers start to consider how to measure an outcome, they might realize that many outcomes as stated in program descriptions, mission statements, or even in program names are inconveniently expansive or nearly impossible to measure.

As its name implies, our bullying prevention program aims to reduce school-based bullying but neither the program's name nor its description specifies whether the bullying it seeks to reduce is in-person or cyber. It is a school-based program but it does not specify whether it targets elementary schools, middle schools, or high schools. The program description does not even specify a geographic location. A researcher reviewing the bullying literature would quickly discover that bullying at the elementary school level differs from bullying at the high school level. The same researcher would discover that

Inputs	Activities	Outputs	Short (Outcomes)	Medium (Outcomes)	Long (Outcomes)
Students, staff, training materials, training space, etc.	Instructing students on how to recognize and respond to bullying	Students who complete the bullying prevention instruction	Students' knowledge of bullying and how they should respond	Students acting on the knowledge and reporting bullying	Bullying experienced by students

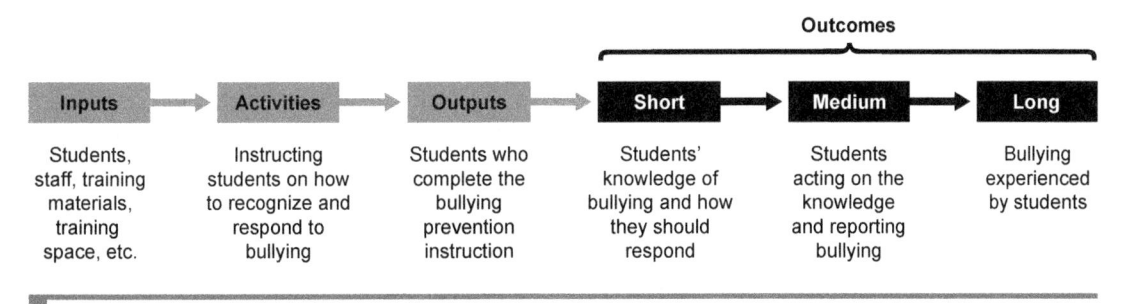

FIGURE 13.1. Bullying prevention logic model.

Job training program logic model

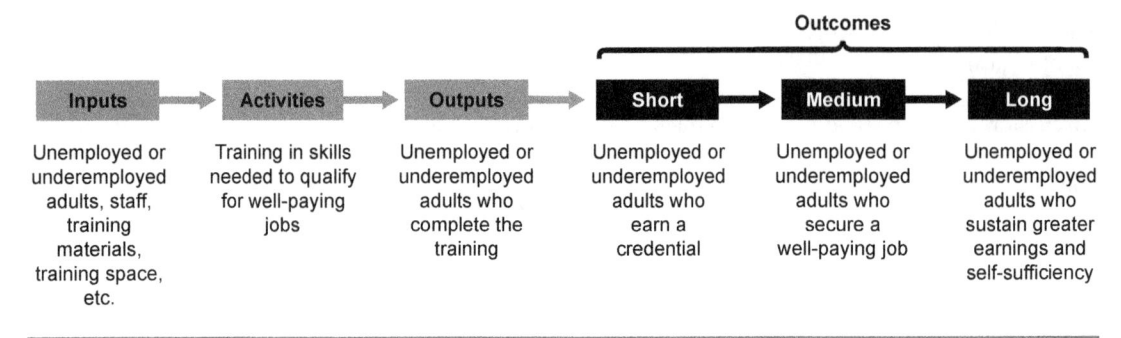

Inputs	Activities	Outputs	Outcomes		
			Short	Medium	Long
Unemployed or underemployed adults, staff, training materials, training space, etc.	Training in skills needed to qualify for well-paying jobs	Unemployed or underemployed adults who complete the training	Unemployed or underemployed adults who earn a credential	Unemployed or underemployed adults who secure a well-paying job	Unemployed or underemployed adults who sustain greater earnings and self-sufficiency

FIGURE 13.2. Job training program logic model.

in-person bullying is different from cyberbullying.

Likewise, if our job training program is located within a community college, then it might have different activities and objectives from those a private company might offer as part of on-the-job training (OJT). A community college-based program might have associates' degree completion as an initial program output, whereas a private company's OJT program might aim to enhance workers' skills so that it has more of a certain type of worker for a given task.

The outcomes often suggested by program descriptions, mission statements, and program names can fail to address the who, what, where, and when that researchers need to construct measures. As described by Frechtling (see Chapter 20, this volume), articulating a program logic model is extremely helpful in answering these questions because a logic model not only defines the inputs (the *who* and *where* of a program) but it also describes the activities (the *what* of the program). Finally, and most importantly to our discussion of outcome evaluation, a logic model can help an evaluator decide not only what outcomes to measure but also *when* to measure them.

For reasons that we hope will become apparent, we recommend dividing outcomes into three categories—short-term outcomes, intermediate outcomes, and long-term outcomes—each of which we discuss next.

Short-Term Outcomes

For programs where the output is a person who has received education or training, it is useful to think of the short-term outcomes as the program participants' knowledge, awareness, or attitudes. For example, the output for our bullying prevention program are the students who attended the bullying prevention instruction on how to recognize bullying and how to respond when they witness it. A short-term outcome for the bullying prevention program, therefore, is that student's knowledge of bullying and how they should respond.

A short-term outcome for our job training program might be a participant who has attained a credential that signals that they are qualified for employment in a specified sector.

Conceived this way, these short-term outcomes are contained within program participants. They are constructs of knowledge, attitude, or achievement. Subjecting program participants to individual assessments, exams, or surveys often is the best way to measure a short-term outcome.

One way to ensure a measure's validity and reliability when subjecting program participants to individual assessment, exams, or surveys is to use existing instruments that have been validated. A validated survey instrument is one that has been subjected to independent research and shown to accurately measure the construct it purports to measure.

It also may be useful to review prior research to ascertain what assessments, exams, or surveys are already employed to measure similar short-term outcomes. Using survey questions that are widely used provides additional data for researchers. This can allow researchers to compare the prevalence or values of a construct among the population being evaluated with other populations that have been previously analyzed. For example, to measure the short-term outcomes of our bullying prevention program (i.e., the extent to which the students who underwent the program recognize bullying and know how to respond when they witness it), it might be useful to use questions from other published evaluations of bullying prevention programs with similar populations.

Intermediate Outcomes

It is useful for evaluators to think of intermediate outcomes as those outcomes that logically follow the short-term outcomes. If the short-term outcomes are changes in a subject's knowledge, awareness, or attitudes, then the subsequent outcome that could logically be expected would be changes in the subject's behaviors. In the bullying prevention program example, where the intervention is educating students on how to recognize bullying and how to respond when they witness it, the short-term outcome is the student's knowledge of bullying and how they should respond, and the intermediate outcome, therefore, might be acting on that knowledge. For this program, evaluators might examine school records and collect data on how often bullying was reported and by whom; and if such data (e.g., school records) are not readily available, then to devise an approach for collecting them (e.g., via observations or some other primary data collection).

In our models, changes in actions follow changes in knowledge, awareness, or attitudes. For some programs the change in behaviors may follow immediately after this change. For other programs, measurable changes in actions may occur long after a change in knowledge. This is especially true in instances where subjects have little control over when they can act on their new knowledge. For example, measurable changes in a subject's knowledge of a new profession, as reflected in a credential, may occur immediately after completing a job training program, but an opportunity to use that knowledge to obtain a new job may not occur until weeks or months after the training is complete.

Here it is important to note that intermediate outcomes are still not the long-term outcomes that we often find in a program's mission statement, in a program description, or, as mentioned, even in the name of the program. The goal of the bullying prevention program, for example, is not to get students to report more bullying. The goal is to prevent and stop bullying. The goal of the job training program is not merely to help people get hired but to help them get jobs where their earnings increase, which occurs when a person retains the job for a period of time after obtaining that job.

Long-Term Outcomes

Simply put, long-term outcomes are those outcomes that programs ultimately want to achieve. For programs that target humans and therefore have participant experiences as the output, it may be useful to think of the long-term outcomes as a state of being. For example, for our bullying prevention program that has students who attended the bullying prevention instruction as the output and knowledge of bullying and how to respond and acting to prevent bullying as the short-term and intermediate outcomes, respectively, the long-term outcome is actual incidents of bullying. Again, this is stipulated in the logic model, which hypothesizes that students who receive the training on how to recognize and report bullying will have that knowledge and then act on that knowledge and, ultimately, experience less bullying in their environment.

For the job training program, the logic model hypothesizes that the short-term outcome of an acquisition of new skills, as indicated by earning some credential, relates to an intermediate outcome of acquiring a job that requires the skills, which, in turn, will affect the long-term outcome of having higher earnings.

As with measuring an intermediate outcome, timing is also important to understanding when to measure a long-term outcome. Evaluators must decide the correct time to measure a long-term outcome in order to ascertain whether the ultimate state of being has been achieved. For example, if obtaining a job is not the ultimate goal of an employment program and if maintaining employment is, then the evaluator needs to decide at what point in time sustained employment is achieved. Once again, the researcher may find it useful to look outside the logic model to other research or to other industry standards for assistance in determining when to measure a long-term outcome—that is, for deciding when to measure for a change in a state of being. For our job training program example, previous research may have determined how long an individual must be employed for that employment to be considered stable. Likewise, financial institutions might employ a metric for determining when an individual's length of employment might make them creditworthy. Outside of the logic model, external insights such as these can inform measurement in practice.

In the bullying prevention program example, the state of being of bullying experienced by students may be measured by using school incident reports that document the number of bullying incidents that occur. Once again, the notion of when to measure is critically important. The bullying prevention program educates students to get them to report bullying so that trusted adults can respond. The logic model illustrates that the reporting would occur temporally before the response and the subsequent reduction. If an evaluator attempts to measure the long-term outcome too soon, then that evaluator might be measuring the reporting (the intermediate outcome) and not the reduction in bullying that is hypothesized to occur after the trusted adults are given time to respond. Again, when to measure a long-term outcome needs to consider program timelines—in this case how much time adults need to respond to reports of bullying—because the further out in time a long-term outcome is, the more difficult it can be to causally connect it to the program. This is another example of the importance of a well-thought-out logic model.

Logic models are useful for determining where to look for evidence on when to measure long-term outcomes in two ways. First, they make long-term goals explicit. Second, they provide a framework that can be generalized. For example, the generalized version of the bullying prevention program is education that leads to knowledge, which leads to action in the form of reporting, which leads to changes in a state of being. This generalized description of a program can help evaluators learn from research on other topics. Many community crime prevention and cessation programs have a similar general description to our bullying prevention programs. They rely on community education to spark reporting so that law enforcement professionals can intervene. Based on the similarities between the logic models, an evaluator may decide to refer to the literature on community crime prevention and cessation programs. Evaluation research in that field lends insights on when long-term outcomes are realized relative to short-term and intermediate outcomes, and it shows that crime rates increase as people act on their new knowledge (intermediate outcome) before crime rates actually decrease (long-term outcomes) (e.g., Kelling et al., 1974). They might reasonably expect something similar to occur with bullying prevention programs and decide to measure for bullying experienced by students (long-term outcome) well after students acting on knowledge and reporting is present (intermediate outcome).

Outcome Monitoring

Documenting *outputs* and measuring *outcomes*—which we have just identified as distinct—is not only useful for understanding the overall success of the program but the process also can help administrators determine the extent to which a program is being implemented as intended. Regularly monitoring outputs and measuring outcomes, especially short-term outcomes, can help program managers make adjustments to ensure that a program is operating as designed and has the greatest opportunity possible to achieve its long-term outcome (the ultimate state of being). Evaluation research takes place because it is unknown with certainty that a program is achieving its goals. Regular monitoring of a program using outcome measures may not *prove* that program's impact, but a manager can use outcome monitoring to discern the opposite: a program that is *not* producing its intended output or meeting its desired short-term, intermediate, and long-term outcomes, will *not* achieve its desired impact. Powell et al. (see Chapter 12, this volume) detail how to conduct implementation monitoring to help ensure the program is properly implemented.

In the private sector world of video game development, the evaluation credo is "test early and test often." Basically, in developing a product for the market, companies do not want to wait until all of the money is invested and the product is available for purchase before finding out whether the product even works. A video game developer wants to know as soon as possible about bugs in the programming, difficulties with the labeling, inefficacies in the gameplay, and other problems that would compromise that video game's appeal so that the problems do not affect the final product. The same should be said of public and nonprofit programs. The "test early and test often" equivalent for public programs is to document outputs and measure short-term outcomes as soon as and as regularly as possible. It is useless to conduct an outcome evaluation on a program that is not producing its outputs. It is similarly useless to evaluate long-term outcomes for a program that is not meeting its short-term outcomes. Finally, as stated above, it is pointless to evaluate the impact of a program that is not fully implemented and where desired outcomes are not present. An evaluability assessment (see Rog, Chapter 11, this volume) is a means for identifying when the time is right to engage in an impact evaluation. Commonly, an implementation evaluation accompanies an outcome or impact evaluation, and we would contend that an implementation evaluation should precede any summative evaluation. Epstein and Klerman (2012, 2016) suggest the use of the "falsifiable logic model" as a means for identifying when a program is ready for a rigorous impact evaluation.

IMPACT EVALUATION DESIGNS

Once it is established that a program is generating outputs and achieving short-term, intermediate, and long-term outcomes as intended, an evaluator can reasonably consider an impact evaluation. The goal of an impact evaluation is to examine whether the program created the desired change in outcomes. Further, an *impact evaluation* isolates the change in outcomes that the program caused from the many other possible explanations for that change. It is important to recognize that outcomes exist in the world independent of evaluation and often change regardless of whether a program does anything to try to affect change. It is the impact evaluation challenge to identify the appropriate design that causally links a change in an outcome to a program's efforts. While there are techniques to qualitatively or theoretically posit a causal link between a program and its outcomes, such as the theory of change or program theory approach to evaluation (Connell et al., 1995; Connell & Kubisch, 1998), we have opted to summarize the quantitative approaches that are common in the field.

Experimental Evaluation Designs

To assess program impacts, experimental evaluation design involves randomly allocating access to a program to create two groups whose average experiences are the same except for access to the program. One group is the "treatment group," which has access to a program or is subject to a policy. The other group is a "control group," excluded from the program or policy for research purposes. In other cases, two or more groups are assigned to alternative treatments, such as "A/B testing" that is common in the private sector (e.g., Manzi, 2012). If we do not know what impact a policy has and resources are scarce, then entering individuals into a lottery to gain access is a fair way both to ration access and to learn about program impacts. Peck (2020) elaborates on issues of ethics and experimental evaluations—the circumstances under which it is ethical to deny access to experimental treatment is an area of debate.

What exactly does randomization involve? The process of randomly assigning units—be they individuals, classes, schools, organizations, cities, and so on—to gain access (or not) to a program involves something akin to a coin toss or a roll of the dice. In practice, randomization is done via a computer program. The evaluation follows and measures both treatment and control groups. Comparing the two groups' outcomes provides an estimate of a program's "impact." Mathematically, the mean outcome for the control group is subtracted from the mean outcome for the treatment group.[1] Because theoretically the only systematic difference between the groups is the presence of an intervention, that impact is unbiased by other sources (those "threats to internal validity" discussed in Box 13.2) and can be interpreted as the intervention's causal impact.

---

[1] Although only this subtraction is needed, often evaluators use multiple regression to estimate impacts. Doing so increases the precision with which impacts are estimated because it accounts for random variation in baseline characteristics between the experimental groups.

BOX 13.2. Threats to Internal Validity

As noted in the text, the "plausible rival explanations" for why a change in outcomes might occur are referred to as "threats" to an evaluation's "internal validity." Internal validity refers to an evaluation design's ability to support causal claims. Several threats to the internal validity of an evaluation exist.

- **History**. Historical forces include political, social, and economic events or trends that influence outcomes of interest. These events or trends can be the underlying reasons for changes in outcomes: People find jobs more quickly in a strong economy than in a weak one. People feel more patriotic around Election Day. Specific violent events—such as school shootings—influence public acceptance of gun safety laws.
- **Selection bias.** Selection bias refers to the likelihood that people who choose to participate in a program differ from those who do not, or that programs may engage in "creaming" to select participants. In brief, the people who are most likely to succeed in and benefit from a program are those who enroll, by their own choice or through selective program processes.
- **Maturation**. Maturation refers to the reality that people and institutions evolve over time. Indeed, this observation matters because people learn and grow in ways that affect their outcomes. For example, many human behaviors that concern policymakers are associated with adolescence, but humans grow out of adolescence regardless of policy initiatives. This maturation process may be mistaken for program impact.
- **Regression artifacts**. Regression artifacts as a threat to internal validity refers to the likelihood that program targets are chosen for being exceptional in some way, either at the top or the bottom of a distribution. People who enroll in programs to help them are there because they are at an extreme low point in their lives and will improve ("regress" to the mean) even without a program's help. On the flip side, test-preparation programs for students, for example, have little additional upward room to move those children who already test at the highest levels and are therefore more likely to report worse outcomes by simple *regression to the mean*.
- **Testing bias**. The sheer process of collecting data on a given outcome might serve to change that outcome. For example, if people are interviewed about whether they eat their "five a day," they might be more likely to start eating more fruits and vegetables because of the interview's focus. In that case, it would be testing that generates some change in the outcomes and not necessarily a nutrition education program.
- **Instrumentation bias**. Consistent measurement matters, and changing measures or data collection procedures over time can result in mistaking instrumentation for impact. For example, in *How Big Is a Foot?*, Myller (1991) illustrates that using the carpenter's foot, relative to the king's foot, to make a bed for the queen, results in the wrong size bed; indeed, a standardized measure of a "foot" is needed. As measures become more sensitive or differently calibrated over time, those changes can mask program impacts.
- **Interactions** among these threats to internal validity exist as well: Selection of the "best" people to participate during an expanding economy brings selection, regression artifacts, and historical threats together to generate a complex interaction of factors, each of which—alone and together—might otherwise take credit for changes in outcomes, in lieu of true program impacts.

Experimental evaluation designs can overcome these above factors because randomization means that the treatment and control groups are alike in all ways, both measurable and unmeasurable. Having a strong counterfactual permits ruling out these factors as plausible rival explanations for a program's influence on outcomes of interest. That said, the one threat to internal validity that experiments cannot overcome is what's referred to as experimental mortality or differential attrition.

- **Differential attrition** occurs when there are different rates of follow-up data collection for treatment and control groups, resulting in nonequivalent groups. This differential attrition can introduce bias into impact estimates because the treatment and control group are no longer alike in all ways measurable.

Quasi-experimental evaluation designs also construct an estimate of the counterfactual but that estimate often does not permit ruling out as many of the threats to internal validity as plausible rival explanations for observed changes in outcomes (see Table 13.1).

Evaluation textbooks, such as Shadish et al.'s (2002) *Experimental and Quasi-Experimental Designs for Generalized Causal Inference*, provide a fuller treatment of this topic.

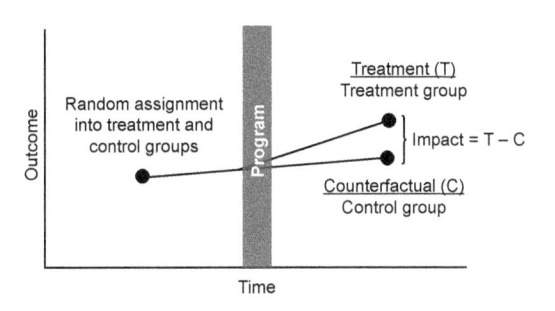

FIGURE 13.3. Graphic depiction of experimental evaluation design.

A basic, two-armed experimental evaluation design involves treatment–control or treatment–treatment contrasts, the latter being commonly used in the private sector where they are referred to as "A/B testing" (e.g., Manzi, 2012; Thomke & Manzi, 2014) or in a health setting as "comparative effectiveness" research (e.g., Sox & Goodman, 2012). The treatment–control contrast involves randomizing to a treatment group and to a control group, where the control group gets no services or can represent "business as usual" or "usual care." In the public policy arena, treatment–treatment (or A/B) testing involves randomizing to two treatment groups, where one can be a standard and the other an enhanced version of a program, or the two treatments can reflect different models of service provision (Peck, 2020).

Figure 13.3 provides a graphical depiction of this evaluation design.[2] For this figure (as well as the ones that follow), the horizontal axis is time: it indicates the introduction of a program, with pre- and postprogram windows where observations might take place. The vertical axis is a measure of the outcome of interest. Each figure shows the treatment outcome along with the counterfactual outcome to which the treatment outcome is compared for impact computation.[3]

---

[2]These visualizations are motivated by and adapted from the graphs that appear in Bingham and Felbinger's (2002) *Evaluation in Practice: A Methodological Approach*.

[3]Although these figures show that computation as simple subtraction, it is more common in the field—especially with quasi-experimental impact analyses—to use multiple regression. Doing so permits controlling for other known factors, including those related to threats to the evaluation design's internal validity.

There are many other experimental evaluation designs involving multiple groups or "arms," staggered introduction and multistage designs, and factorial designs, each of which addresses its own set of research questions (e.g., Bell & Peck, 2016; Shadish et al., 2002; Peck, 2020). The key to each of these is identifying the point of randomization that creates a treatment and a control group whose later differences in outcomes can be interpreted as the impact of access to the treatment.

Quasi-Experimental Evaluation Designs

Quasi-experimental evaluation designs also aim to assess the impact of a program or policy, and they do so by approximating a counterfactual, or what would have happened and does happen in the program's absence. The main ways of constructing a counterfactual without using randomization involve making reflexive comparisons or using untreated comparison groups.

Reflexive Designs

A reflexive comparison involves using a preprogram outcome as the counterfactual, a representation of what the world would be like in the absence of treatment. The simplest of these is a **one-group pretest–posttest design**. This is an appropriate design when the intervention is direct and focused, with relatively short-term outcomes of interest and limited threats to internal validity. When multiple preprogram measures of the outcome are available over time, a **simple interrupted time-series design** can be used. If there are historical, socioeconomic, and/or political trends that might influence the outcome, being able to project into a future time from an underlying baseline trend can improve upon a single preprogram measure and help rule out some plausible rival explanations for observed changes. Figures 13.4 and 13.5 offer a graphic depiction of these two evaluation designs.

Comparison Group Designs

Comparison group designs include the following: posttest-only comparison group design, pretest–posttest comparison group design, comparative interrupted time series, and regression discontinuity designs. Any comparison

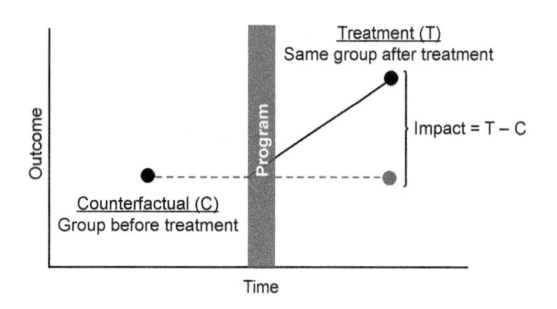

FIGURE 13.4. Graphic depiction of one-group pretest–posttest design.

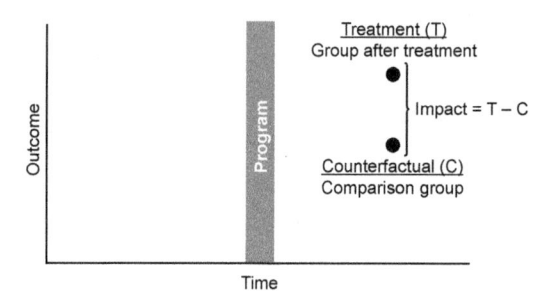

FIGURE 13.6. Graphic depiction of posttest-only comparison group design.

group design requires establishing a plan for constructing the comparison group, usually by some kind of matching strategy. Each of these points is elaborated next.

A **posttest-only comparison group design** (see Figure 13.6) identifies a comparison group, whose postprogram mean outcome is compared to the treatment group's postprogram mean outcome. Without a pretest measure or other preprogram characteristics of the two groups, it is uncertain how comparable the groups are, and any number of plausible rival explanations for differences in the treatment and comparison group means might exist. In cases where a comparison group does not exist, an external, agreed-upon standard or other evidence can be used as a benchmark. This may be all the information available and it is better to have some comparison or benchmark than to have only a free-floating treatment group outcome with no context (e.g., Peck et al., 2004).

Next, a **pretest–posttest comparison group design** (see Figure 13.7), as the name suggests, includes both pretest and posttest measures for the treatment and comparison groups. The associated analysis of impacts subtracts the control group's pretest–posttest difference in outcomes from the treatment group's pretest–posttest difference in outcomes to attempt to net out the effects of a variety of factors represented in the counterfactual. If a comparison group is relatively well matched, then the number and extent of threats to internal validity can be reduced. The next section elaborates quasi-experimental designs (see Table 13.1).

The **comparative interrupted time-series (CITS) design** (see Figure 13.8) includes multiple preprogram measures, permitting the use of a trend to project into a future time a counterfactual that can additionally account for economic, political, and secular trends that influence outcomes.

A **regression discontinuity** design, sometimes called a **"cut-point" design**, involves the use of a nonmanipulable continuous variable to determine selection into or out of a treatment. This

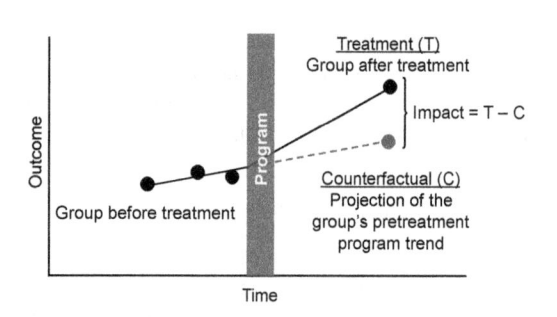

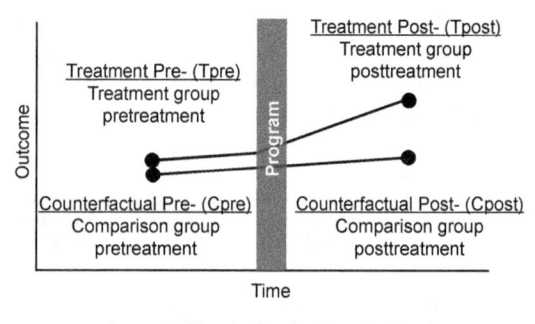

FIGURE 13.5. Graphic depiction of simple interrupted time-series design.

FIGURE 13.7. Graphic depiction of pretest–posttest design with a comparison group.

TABLE 13.1. Summary of Impact Evaluation Designs, including Ideal Conditions, Threats Addressed, and Implementation Challenges

	Reflexive designs		Comparison group designs				Experimental designs
	One group pretest–posttest	Interrupted time-series	Posttest-only comparison group	Pretest–posttest comparison group	Comparative interrupted time-series	Regression discontinuity	Randomized treatment–control group
Conditions ideal for using	Intervention is direct; follow-up is short	Stable, preprogram trend data exist	No other design options exist; outcome benchmark exists	Pretest and posttest data exist on both treatment and matched comparison group	Preprogram trend and posttest exist on both treatment and matched comparison group	A nonmanipulable running variable determines eligibility	Eligible units can be randomized (see chapter for more details)
Threats to internal validity generally addressed							
History		✓		✓	✓	✓	✓
Selection bias				✓	✓	✓	✓
Maturation		✓			✓	✓	✓
Regression artifacts					✓	✓	✓
Testing				✓	✓	✓	✓
Instrumentation				✓	✓	✓	✓
Differential attrition	NA	NA	NA				
Common implementation challenges	Ruling out plausible rival explanations	Baseline data do not create a useful trend	Ruling out plausible rival explanations	Comparison group data and matching strategies	Comparison group data and matching strategies	Few opportunities exist	Ethical and feasibility concerns; site cooperation

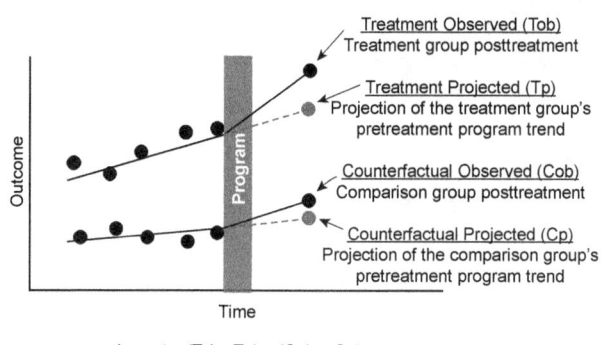

FIGURE 13.8. Graphic depiction of comparative interrupted time-series design.

variable is sometimes referred to as a "**running variable**" or a "**ranking variable**." For example, high school students who achieve a certain score on the Preliminary Scholastic Aptitude Test earn the designation as national merit finalists, making them eligible for a whole host of college scholarships. In this example, the evaluation considers the impact of being named a national merit finalist. The cut point for national merit finalist designation is now known in advance, and students cannot "game" or select into the finalist or "treatment" group: They must earn it by achieving a high score, the specifics of which are determined only after the test is taken. Having a selection criterion such as this means that the regression discontinuity design is strong in overcoming the threat to internal validity of selection bias: The selection procedure is fully known, and so selection does not bias impact estimates, at least close to the cut point. If this year's cutoff for national merit finalists was a score of 204, then the outcomes of those students who achieved a score of 203 would be compared to the outcomes of those students who achieved a score of 205, for example. The just-above and just-below the cutoff groups are the treatment and comparison groups, respectively, and the differences in their characteristics are considered inconsequential. In turn, the differences between their mean outcomes provide a strong estimate of the treatment's impact. In addition to selection bias, the regression discontinuity design also successfully deals with other threats to internal validity, such as maturation, history, testing, or instrumentation bias. This is especially the case when there is a reasonably large sample around the cutoff for analysis. Only when the research aims to generalize results far from the cutoff are there potential concerns about the design's ability to establish causal claims.

Figure 13.9 provides a graphical depiction of the regression discontinuity design. Along the horizontal axis is the running variable, and, where Figures 13.3–13.8 demarked a "program" window, the regression discontinuity design demarks an eligibility cutoff. Those on one side of the cutoff gain access to the treatment, and those on the other do not. Within a band around the cutoff, those who gain access to treatment and those who do not are quite similar, and the differences between their mean outcomes is the estimated impact of the treatment. The further from the cutoff one gets, the more likely plausible rival explanations for differences in outcomes exist.

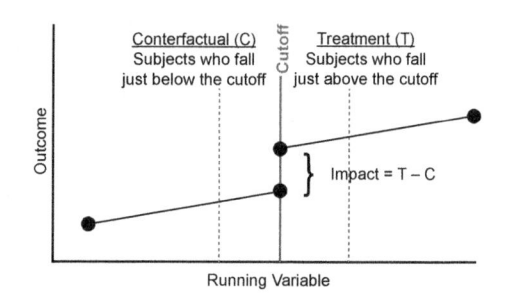

FIGURE 13.9. Graphic depiction of regression discontinuity design.

Identifying the Comparison Group

In implementing a quasi-experimental evaluation that uses a comparison group, the evaluator must choose a specific matching strategy that is feasible and will result in a good match with the treatment group. The exception to this is the regression discontinuity design, which has a built-in process for identifying a comparison group by way of the running variable's cutoff. Other designs' strategies for constructing a comparison group can include single-dimensional matching, multidimensional matching, propensity score matching, or other clustering or latent class techniques. The details of these strategies are beyond the scope of this chapter, but we summarize briefly what each is.

Single-dimensional matching involves using a single trait on which to match treatment and comparison groups. For example, if the treatment group comprises only girls, then the control group would be selected on the basis of sex. It is rare that a single-dimensional matching will be the ideal choice because samples of inference populations of interest—be they people or some aggregation of people such as schools or communities—are multifaceted. **Multidimensional matching** involves matching on additional characteristics in an effort to ensure that the average characteristics of the treatment and comparison groups are comparable. For example, if the treatment targets second-grade girls who excel at math, then these three criteria would be used to identify a matched comparison group. In practice, approaches to multidimensional matching include **coarsened exact matching (CEM)**, **propensity score matching**, and data-driven methods. CEM involves prespecifying the variables to be matched on, and how they should be matched—whether by exact values or within a range of values. Tiebreaker variables for selecting matches can be used as well. Distinct to CEM is that treatment–comparison balance on one variable has no effect on the treatment–comparison balance on another variable (Iacus et al., 2009).[4] Propensity score matching uses regression analysis where many characteristics are used to model treatment group membership, and that prediction model identifies nontreated cases that share the same predicted likelihood of treatment (e.g., Guo & Fraser, 2010). Many decisions must be made in the process of implementing propensity score methods (including both matching and weighting), and other sources can provide guidance on those details (e.g., Guo & Fraser, 2010). Finally, **cluster analysis** or **latent class analysis**—two data-driven analytic methods—can also be used to identify comparison group cases that are similar to treatment group cases (e.g., Peck et al., 2009).

All of these matching strategies aim to achieve the same end: that a matched comparison group is a close proxy for a randomized control group in providing an estimate of the counterfactual, against which the treatment group's outcomes can be compared in estimating a program's impact.

Choosing among Impact Evaluation Designs

Table 13.1 summarizes the reflexive, comparison group, and experimental evaluation designs discussed above and identifies the following about them: ideal conditions for their use, the threats to internal validity that they generally deal well with, and the most common challenge to implementing the design in practice. Moving from left to right across the table, it is evident that the designs increase in their ability to overcome internal validity threats, but any chosen design must be well executed to do so.

Beyond the considerations implied in Table 13.1, certain additional conditions dictate when to use an experimental evaluation design, in particular. A randomized experiment is appropriate under the following conditions (as elaborated in Peck, 2021):

- When getting an unbiased, causal estimate of the policy/program impact matters.[5]
- When randomization is feasible, legal, and ethical.
- When the evaluation is prospective.

---

[4] Gary King's website (*https://gking.harvard.edu*) offers useful resources, including a program for implementing CEM.

[5] Using the term unbiased, we mean that the impact estimate is not biased by any of those internal validity threats. An unbiased impact estimate is one that can plausibly claim that it is the intervention that is responsible for the observed change in outcomes (or impact) as opposed to some other factor.

- When the resulting information will be timely enough to make a difference.
- When the cost of the evaluation is commensurate with the value of the information produced.

In contrast, there are circumstances when it is not appropriate to use an experimental evaluation design. In those cases, a quasi-experimental or other evaluation design should be used. These circumstances include:

- When effects are so large that causality is obvious.
- When a quasi-experimental or other evaluation design could provide a highly reliable answer and at a lower cost.
- When a program may not be ready for an impact evaluation.

The Evaluation Policy Task Force of the American Evaluation Association (n.d.) is further considering the optimal conditions for use of experimental evaluation designs.

CONCLUSION

This chapter examines outcome and impact evaluation as a way to assess the value of a program, policy, or intervention of some sort. Other kinds of evaluation questions—about program processes or operations—demand other kinds of evaluation approaches, discussed elsewhere in this handbook. In considering outcomes and impacts, an important first evaluation step is to identify outcome measure and determine how and when to measure them. Identifying these outcomes is often done as part of a logic modeling exercise (see Frechtling, Chapter 20, this volume), where relationships among program inputs, activities, outputs, and outcomes are articulated. Determining how and when to measure these outcomes—including the sources for data—follows in the evaluation process. Extending the analysis to outcome evaluation and outcome monitoring involves using the logic of the logic model to make conditional statements about the attribution of changes in outcomes to the program itself. In the face of the several threats to internal validity discussed in this chapter, attribution of changes in outcomes to programs can be strengthened by using impact evaluation design strategies that aim to overcome those threats.

Although experimental evaluation designs can overcome most threats to internal validity when implemented properly, no experimental or quasi-experimental design is in and of itself a panacea for establishing causal claims. Regardless of the specific design, a quality evaluation requires thoughtful practice. Very often the reality of circumstance demands that a certain evaluation design be used, and an evaluator might have to sacrifice the rigor of a design to accommodate those circumstances. For example, although local comparison groups—those drawn from geographically proximal pools—tend to be better matched to treatment groups than nonlocal comparison groups, there might not be an option for collecting data from an appropriate local source. Further, sometimes program administrators or funders may choose to evaluate a program well after it has been implemented. This implies a retrospective design, which precludes the possibility of random assignment as part of the evaluation.

Bamberger (see Chapter 24, this volume) discusses the cost trade-offs associated with evaluation design quality. Although we recognize that costs are a major factor in executing an evaluation, we flag concerns over undertaking a less-than-ideal evaluation for cost reasons alone. Very often program administrators and funders want to know about the outcomes and impacts that their programs are achieving. There is value in having that information. Perhaps most importantly, if a program cannot establish its value (either because it is ineffective or because the chosen evaluation design cannot generate the quality evidence needed), then those program resources would be better spent on program redesign, reallocation, or even on a different program.

Our closing point is this: Perhaps the most important step in a program evaluation is to align the evaluation questions to their appropriate design—that is, the question should always drive the design and interest holders should always prefer the design for a given circumstance that can best answer the question(s) of interest. We hope that this chapter has provided guidance on how to think about outcome and impact evaluation, offering an array of design options and strategies for carrying out evaluations of this sort in the field.

REFERENCES

American Evaluation Association, Evaluation Policy Task Force. (n.d.). *Evaluation policy initiative.* Available at *www.eval.org/p/cm/ld/fid=129*

Bell, S. H., & Peck, L. R. (2016). On the "how" of social experiments: Experimental designs for getting inside the black box. *New Directions for Evaluation, 152,* 97–107.

Bingham, R. D., & Felbinger, C. L. (2002). *Evaluation in practice: A methodological approach* (2nd ed.). Seven Bridges Press.

Chen, H.-T. (2005). *Practical program evaluation: Assessing and improving planning, implementation, and effectiveness.* Sage.

Connell, J. P., & Kubisch, A. C. (1998). Applying a theory of change approach to the evaluation of comprehensive community initiatives: Progress, prospects, and problems. In K. Fulbright-Anderson, A. C. Kubisch, & J. P. Connell (Eds.), *New approaches to evaluating community initiatives, volume 2: Theory, measurement, and analysis* (pp. 14–44). Aspen Institute.

Connell, J. P., Kubisch, A. C., Schorr, L. B., & Weiss, C. H. (1995). *New approaches to evaluating community initiatives: Concepts, methods, and contexts.* Aspen Institute.

DeVellis, R. F. (2012). *Scale development: Theory and applications* (Vol. 26). SAGE.

Epstein, D., & Klerman, J. A. (2012). When is a program ready for rigorous impact evaluation? *Evaluation Review, 36*(5), 373–399.

Epstein, D., & Klerman, J. A. (2016). On the "when" of social experiments: The tension between program refinement and abandonment. *New Directions for Evaluation, 152,* 33–45.

Guo, S., & Fraser, M. W. (2010). *Propensity score analysis: Statistical methods and applications.* SAGE.

Iacus, S. M., King, G., & Porro, G. (2009). CEM: Software for coarsened exact matching. *Journal of Statistical Software, 30*(9), 1–27.

Kelling, G. L., Pate, T., Dieckman, D., & Brown, C. E. (1974). *The Kansas City preventive patrol experiment: A summary report.* Police Foundation.

Manzi, J. (2012). *Uncontrolled: The surprising payoff of trial-and-error for business, politics, and society.* Basic Books.

Myller, R. (1991). *How big is a foot?* Yearling.

Peck, L. R. (2020). *Evaluation design for program improvement.* SAGE.

Peck, L. R. (2021, August 13). When is randomization right for evaluation? [Blog post]. Abt. Associates Perspectives. Available at *http://tinyurl.com/When2Experiment*

Peck, L. R., Camillo, F., & D'Attoma, I. (2009). A promising new approach to eliminating selection bias. *Canadian Journal of Program Evaluation, 24*(4), 31–56.

Peck, L. R., Hall, A., & Heller, J. (2004). *Evaluation report on the operations and outcomes of Arizona's marriage and communication skills program.* Arizona Department of Economic Security, Arizona Marriage and Communication Skills Commission.

Schwindt, O. (2016). Confessions of a millennial Nielson viewer: Here's what it feels like to decide what stays on TV. *International Business Times.* Available at *www.ibtimes.com/confessions-millennial-nielsen-viewer-heres-what-it-feels-decide-what-stays-tv-2385002*

Shadish, W. R., Cook, T. D., & and Campbell, D. T. (2002). *Experimental and quasi-experimental designs for generalized causal inference.* Wadsworth.

Sox, H. C., & Goodman, S. N. (2012). The methods of comparative effectiveness research. *Annual Review of Public Health, 33*(1), 425–445.

Thomke, S., & Manzi, J. (2014). The discipline of business experimentation. *Harvard Business Review, 92*(12), 17.

Woodward, R. B. (1991). Television: True confessions of a Nielson "family." *New York Times.* Available at *www.nytimes.com/1991/07/14/arts/television-true-confessions-of-a-nielsen-family.html*

Chapter 14

Combining Costs and Results
Designs, Strategies, and Analysis

Robert Shand
A. Brooks Bowden
Henry M. Levin

CHAPTER OVERVIEW

Social interventions show widely different costs. By choosing interventions without considering both their costs and impacts, agencies often face a much higher cost than would be imposed by selecting those that are most effective relative to cost. Adding an economic component to evaluation, employing a method such as cost analysis, cost–feasibility analysis, cost-effectiveness analysis, cost–utility analysis, or benefit–cost analysis, can provide aid in decision making based on evaluation results. In this chapter, we discuss ways these methods can enhance evaluation and provide an overview of how to utilize one such method—cost-effectiveness analysis—illustrated with several examples from the field of education.

In order to serve social policy, the field of evaluation attempts to provide information on the effectiveness of a reform or specific intervention to improve one or more social outcomes. Most evaluations seek to provide useful information on evidence of effectiveness in addressing a social issue. But, even when evaluations are competently undertaken, they typically lack crucial information for the user: information on costs. To achieve the same desired result of almost any intervention there are usually alternatives but some are likely to produce a given outcome at lower cost than others. By choosing a lower-cost alternative that can obtain similar or higher effectiveness, it is possible to spare resources that can then be allocated to other needs or can be used to reduce overall cost burdens of the intervention.

The purpose of this chapter is to introduce different methods for applying cost analysis to evaluation, with particular emphasis on **cost-effectiveness analysis**, their importance, and guidance on their application. The method of cost-effectiveness analysis can be applied to virtually any endeavor for which effectiveness results are claimed, including education, health, criminal justice, nutrition, security, and a wide range of other applications. Further, cost-effectiveness analyses can be helpful in understanding and contextualizing the implementation and effectiveness of an intervention, along with comparability of those results with alternative interventions, and typically require relatively modest additional resources when included as a part of a larger evaluation. However, cost analysis is rarely done, perhaps because persons trained and experienced in evaluation lack training in the estimation of costs and their analysis in a decision framework and because decision makers rarely request it (Levin, 2001). Similar methodological principles apply in cost analysis across applied domains. Hence, reviewing competent cost-effectiveness evaluations in one field can provide useful guidance and insight that can be applied more generally. Since we have done most of our cost-effectiveness analyses for education, we focus primarily on that setting in providing illustrations and examples, but the principles outlined in this chapter can apply to virtually any type of intervention for which an evaluation can be undertaken.

The goal of cost-effectiveness analysis is to ascertain the costs of reaching particular goals (effectiveness) in the most parsimonious way. This does not mean the least cost per se but only relative to the effectiveness of the alternative interventions that are under consideration. A key prerequisite is that reliable measures of effectiveness can be obtained or estimated using sound methods that provide information on the statistical confidence and magnitudes of results; methods for obtaining such estimates are beyond the scope of this chapter but are discussed in other chapters in this handbook and other references (e.g., Murnane & Willett, 2010). These can be combined with costs, but unfortunately useful cost information is often not readily available and is distorted or incomplete with the use of conventional accounting data, such as programmatic or departmental budgets or expenditure reports. In this chapter we address a straightforward and standard method from economics to estimate costs, a method that we have adapted for cost-effectiveness analysis and have used for several decades and that other organizations have adopted, such as the World Bank (Levin, 1975; Levin & McEwan, 2001; Levin et al., 2018).

There are many cost tools that can be applied to evaluation. These tools, collectively known as methods of **economic evaluation**, include cost–feasibility, cost-effectiveness, benefit–cost, and cost–utility analyses. Table 14.1 summarizes the types of economic evaluations, including the advantages, disadvantages, and intended applications for each. The cost analysis that provides the economic foundation for each of these analyses follows the same methodology: the ingredients method (Levin et al., 2018, Chapters 4–6). While each method has advantages and disadvantages, each should be considered in terms of its particular purposes. The basic details of how to perform these analyses, with emphasis on the foundational cost analysis and cost-effectiveness analysis, are discussed in the next section.

Cost–feasibility analysis compares estimated costs to available sources of support and political constraints to determine whether an intervention is feasible. Cost-effectiveness, as noted earlier, refers to the cost comparison of alternative interventions aimed at meeting the same objectives. **Benefit–cost analysis** represents a comparison of the costs of an endeavor with the monetary value of the benefits that interested parties and broader society will receive. **Cost–utility analysis** compares the subjective values of a given set of outcomes with their costs. All of these are reviewed in Levin et al. (2018; see specifically Chapter 1). For this handbook, we focus on how to apply cost-effectiveness, using applications from the education area. We focus on how the method can be applied to enhance evaluation and decision making, with a brief overview of the method and several examples, which can help the reader determine when economic methods can enhance an evaluation, which method to choose, and what resources to consult to learn more, although readers will likely need additional resources and further guidance beyond this chapter to independently conduct a cost-effectiveness analysis. These resources include freely available resources sponsored by federal agencies, such as the Institute of Education Sciences of the U.S. Department of Education (2003)[1] and the U.S. Department of Health and Human Services;[2] resources from organizations with an international focus, such

---

[1] *https://ies.ed.gov/seer/cost_analysis.asp*

[2] *www.acf.hhs.gov/sites/default/files/documents/cb/cost_analysis_guide.pdf*

TABLE 14.1. Overview of Types of Economic Evaluation

Type of analysis	Question(s) to be answered	Outcome measure	Advantages	Disadvantages
Cost analysis	What is the full resource cost of each intervention?	None	Describes all resources used for each intervention, regardless of who pays for them	Cannot establish if each intervention is worth that resource use or which option is most efficient
Cost–feasibility	Can a single intervention be carried out within the existing budget?	None	Permits alternatives that are not feasible to be immediately ruled out, before evaluating outcomes	Cannot judge overall worth of intervention, because it does not incorporate outcome measures
Cost-effectiveness	Which option yields a given level of effectiveness for the lowest cost (or highest level of effectiveness for a given cost)?	Units of effectiveness	• Easy to incorporate standard evaluations of effectiveness • Useful for comparing among multiple interventions with a single or small number of objectives	• Difficult to interpret results when there are multiple measures of effectiveness • Cannot judge overall worth of a single intervention; only useful for comparing two or more alternatives
Cost–utility	Which intervention yields a given level of utility at the lowest cost (or the highest level of utility at a given cost)?	Units of utility	• Incorporates individual preferences of constituencies with units of effectiveness • Can incorporate multiple measures of effectiveness into single measure of utility • Promotes constituency participation in decision making	• Sometimes difficult to arrive at consistent and accurate measures of individual preferences • Cannot judge overall worth of a single intervention; only useful for comparing two or more alternatives
Benefit–cost (BC)	• Which intervention yields a given level of benefits for the lowest cost (or the highest level of benefits for a given cost)? • Are the benefits of a single alternative larger than its costs?	Monetary value of outcomes	• Can be used to judge absolute worth of a project • Can compare BC results across projects in education or other areas (e.g., health, infrastructure)	Often difficult to place monetary values on all relevant benefits

Note. Based on Levin et al. (2018).

as the World Bank[3] and the Abdul Latif Jameel Poverty Action Lab (J-PAL) at the Massachusetts Institute of Technology;[4] examples and training materials offered through the Center for Benefit–Cost Studies of Education at the University of Pennsylvania;[5] several textbooks (e.g., Boardman et al., 2018; Levin et al., 2018); and many others.

---

[3] *https://openknowledge.worldbank.org/handle/10986/2561*

[4] *www.povertyactionlab.org/resource/conducting-cost-effectiveness-analysis-cea*

[5] *cbcse.org*

HISTORY OF ECONOMIC EVALUATION

All of these tools have a relatively recent history. With growth in the role and scope of government in the United States in the wake of the Great Depression, World War II, and the Great Society programs of the 1960s, there was growing demand for attention to outcomes and efficiency in social programs, giving rise to the evaluation field (Hogan, 2007; Rossi et al., 2003, pp. 8–15; Russell & Taylor, 1998). It is only more recently, however, that economic evaluation, encompassing cost, cost-effectiveness, benefit–cost, and cost-utility analysis, has become ingrained as a formal part of the evaluation process (Levin, 1975; Phillips, 1996). The application of economic methods to evaluation of public policies, programs, and investments began with the evaluation of public water investments via benefit–cost analysis by weighing the value they created against their costs during the Great Depression (Porter, 1995), codified in the Federal Navigation Act of 1936. Cost-effectiveness analysis began in earnest during the Cold War with congressional investigation of the efficiency of weapons systems (Quade, 1971). The notion that social decisions ought to be made on the basis of economic or **opportunity costs**—what is sacrificed or given up in order to achieve an objective—and how those compare to the value of the outcome was embraced by the federal government. Executive Order No. 12291, 3 C.F.R. p. 127 (1981) mandated that regulatory changes likely to have significant economic impact of $100 million or more undergo cost–benefit analysis.

Landmark evaluations in health, crime, youth development, employment assistance, and other fields have incorporated cost-effectiveness or benefit–cost analyses that have influenced policy. Some of the earliest and most influential social benefit–cost analyses came in conjunction with the adoption of **randomized controlled trials (RCTs)** in social service provision. Evaluations of interventions in the 1970s and 1980s designed to help individuals on welfare transition to the workforce laid the foundation for more rigorous use of evidence to guide social policy, with an emphasis on RCTs but also including benefit–cost analysis as a critical component (Couch, 1992; Gueron, 1988; Gueron & Pauly, 1991; Gueron & Rolston, 2013; Hamilton, 2002). Highly influential evaluations in areas such as early childhood education (Barnett, 1985), teenage pregnancy (Maynard, 1996), and job training programs (Bell & Orr, 1994; Bloom et al., 1997) solidified the growing importance of rigorous causal evidence in evaluations of social programs and its natural fit with economic evaluation to enhance decision making (see, e.g., Cave et al., 1993, on JOBSTART; Levin, 1970; Levin et al., 1987, the latter two with early examples in education on teacher selection and computer-assisted instruction, respectively, among many others). In recent years, economic evaluation has been increasingly applied to programs in juvenile justice,[6] public health,[7] and development.[8] In a leading example of how economic evaluation has directly influenced policy, the Washington State Institute of Public Policy has valued costs and benefits of public investments to the Washington State Legislature and applied those methods to numerous programs, particularly in the areas of youth development and juvenile justice.[9]

Historically, the primary aim of economic evaluation has been to support decision making in the service of efficient allocation of resources—achieving the outcome at the lowest possible cost and directing resources to where they will provide the most good for society. In the field of education, which according to the World Bank (2016) encompasses public and private investments totaling nearly 5% of global economic activity, that is not a trivial consideration. Given inequities in access to resources and opportunities and disparities in outcomes among groups of students and between countries, channeling resources to their most productive uses is a necessary step to improving educational quality and equity. Nonetheless, in recent years more attention has been paid to how adding an economic component to evaluation enhances evaluation itself by highlighting not just issues of efficiency, **sustainability**, and scale but also helping to shift the focus from whether an intervention "works" to *how, under what conditions*, and *for whom* it works by emphasizing how theories of action translate into resources, how resource use varies, and the distributional consequences of who pays the costs and who receives the benefits of an intervention. Focusing on costs from a resource (and not just financial) perspective, as we do in this chapter, helps to highlight issues of implementation, treatment contrast, site-level variability, and replicability, among other factors—in other words, the question is not just whether an intervention is effec-

---

[6] *https://documents.ncsl.org/wwwncsl/Center%20 for%20Results%20Driven%20Governing/Using-Data-Evidence-Budget-Decisions_v02.pdf*

[7] *www.cdc.gov/cardiovascular-resources/php/training/ economic-evaluation.html*

[8] *www.betterevaluation.org/resources/guides/develop_ cost_benefit_tool*

[9] *www.wsipp.wa.gov/ReportFile/1050/Wsipp_ Washington-State-Institute-for-Public-Policy-Origins-and-Governance_Full-Report.pdf*

tive or even whether it is cost-effective but what the intervention *is* and what it takes to make it effective (Belfield & Bowden, 2019). Emphasizing distributional considerations in benefit–cost analysis also provides a pathway to center equity in evaluating the impacts of policies and programs, though much more work remains to be done to consistently implement this stance in practice (Liscow, 2021).

PURPOSE OF ECONOMIC EVALUATION

The most fundamental purpose of economic evaluation is to support decision making through adding an economic component to an evaluation. Adding an economic component focused on either the costs to achieve a particular outcome, or the costs of one or more outcomes relative to how much society values those outcomes, can support decision making in at least three ways (Hollands & Levin, 2017, p. 2):

- Identifying "what it takes," either prospectively, to successfully implement a new program, or retrospectively, to identify what needs to be in place to replicate a successful program.
- Making difficult decisions about existing programs—replicating or scaling up what's working, and making adjustments to or discontinuing what's not.
- Identifying particularly effective and efficient sites, subgroups, particular practices, or particular resources or "ingredients" that appear to be tied to success.

A second purpose for economic evaluation is to consider the trade-offs among program options. As the J-PAL notes (Carter, 2017), when there are multiple ways to achieve the same objective, cost-effectiveness analysis provides a clear and objective framework for considering trade-offs and weighing different objectives against their resource requirements. As part of a larger framework that considers other programmatic and contextual factors, cost-effectiveness analysis can help identify strategies and programs that offer the greatest value for money and direct resources to where they can do the most good.

Performing rigorous cost, cost-effectiveness, or benefit–cost analyses as part of an evaluation confers additional benefits as well. Economic costs are not defined in a vacuum and are always measured relative to achieving a particular outcome, in a specific context and under a specific implementation. Outcomes are not produced by an intervention "in general" or by any particular application of an intervention but rather by a specific intervention, implemented in a specific way, with specific ingredients, to a specific population. By highlighting the costs of replicating a particular effect, cost analysis emphasizes issues of implementation, differences in resource usage, target population, dosage, and other factors that affect both costs and effects. These issues pertain to effectiveness evaluations as well. Ultimately, by more clearly articulating what is being estimated and under what conditions, a well-executed cost analysis can clarify issues of construct validity and external validity—exactly what is being measured, and what population and contexts it generalizes to. Because cost-effectiveness analysis in particular is inherently comparative, it has the challenge and advantage of highlighting issues of comparability when deciding among two or more programmatic choices. When comparing two programs using cost-effectiveness analysis it is critical that they target the same outcome, measured in identical or materially similar ways, for a similar target population, and assessed using a rigorous experimental or quasi-experimental causal framework (Levin & Belfield, 2015). These considerations of implementation, appropriate measure of effectiveness, and comparability of outcomes and interventions in a decision-making framework are not exclusive to cost-effectiveness analysis—however, adding an economic dimension to an evaluation brings these considerations to the forefront of the analysis. They highlight the selection of a single outcome measure, the alternatives and comparison conditions under consideration, what ultimately led to the measured outcomes, and how that varies (e.g., across sites, over time, or by subgroups).

A third purpose of economic evaluation is to highlight issues of the distribution of who bears the costs and who receives the benefits of an intervention, which can have implications for equity as well as for political feasibility of scaling or replicating interventions. A well-designed cost study separately analyzes the full economic costs of the resources required to replicate a measured outcome, regardless of who provides or pays for them, with an analysis of who bears those costs or how they are financed. For that reason, traditional accounting methods, such as budgets, are inadequate and inappropriate to capture the full social and economic cost of an intervention. Capturing the full cost of an intervention from all interested parties, including the hidden costs (e.g., costs that are provided in-kind, are reallocated from a different purpose, or are provided by a different constituency than the primary intervention sponsor), is an important question that is separate from who pays for or bears the burden of an intervention. Separate analysis of costs and financing enables analysis according to multiple interested party perspectives—for instance, a program staffed primarily by volunteers may have a very low financial cost to program sponsors but high-quality and well-trained volunteers must be available to staff the program as a prerequisite to its success. In analyses that tie costs to multiple outcomes—benefit–cost and cost–utility analysis—those outcomes, and costs per unit of outcome, can be partitioned among multiple constituency groups as well. Box 14.1 provides an example of different types of costs and why it is important to consider costs beyond budgetary expenditures using a coding program.

> **BOX 14.1. Coding Program Costs**
>
> A school district is implementing a new after-school coding class. The class is taught by area volunteers. The district purchased a set of computers while a foundation contributed a set of tablets and the curriculum.
>
> **Hidden costs.** The school is reallocating classrooms for the club. These rooms cannot be used by teachers for prep work or by other after-school programs during this time.
>
> **Budget.** The school has budgeted only for the purchase of computers. The volunteer time, the reallocated classrooms, and the donated tablets do not appear on the budget. The full purchase price of the computers appears in one budget year, even though they will be used in multiple years.
>
> **Distribution of costs.** Costs are borne by the school district, the volunteers, and the tech company.

ECONOMIC EVALUATION: A HOW-TO GUIDE

The first task in a cost analysis, which serves as a foundation for other forms of economic evaluation, is to determine the resources or ingredients that were used to operationalize a **theory of action** and implement an intervention that is being evaluated via the **ingredients method** (Levin, 1975; Levin et al., 2018). It is helpful to first consider ingredients in resource terms—what did it take under a particular implementation of an intervention to achieve a measured effect—and only then apply **market** and **shadow prices** based on qualitative descriptions of the ingredients to estimate the costs in monetary terms. For each ingredient, this entails documenting the amount used—for personnel, this might be in person hours or full-time equivalents; for facilities this might be a space with specific features for a percentage of time, and so on—and the characteristics that were observed to produce the effect, such as qualifications, training, and experience for personnel, or special characteristics for facilities. This process is repeated for all ingredients, regardless of who provides or pays for them, as the analysis of financing the costs is separate from the determination of costs. The analysis should also be based upon the specific implementation that led to a particular effect, as subtle differences in resource use and qualities may have implications for both costs and effects. It is not just broad categories of resources that drive measured effects but rather the specific ingredients tied to a program's theory of change, with their descriptive characteristics and qualities that should be documented (see Box 14.2). A template outlining major categories of ingredients—personnel, facilities, materials and durable equipment, and other categories as relevant to the type of intervention—based on program functions, descriptions, and theory of action can be a useful organizational device for ascertaining the ingredients. One example of the types of ingredients that might be considered, and their categories is included in Table 14.2.

It may seem at first glance that such a detailed tabulation of resources is itself a burdensome endeavor, as costs are presumably incorporated in budgets and other types of expenditure reports. While budgets may be an acceptable starting point for establishing the scope and

> **BOX 14.2. Coding Program Ingredients**
>
> The theory of change indicates that by spending time with volunteer instructors from the tech industry, students will both gain coding skills and will better envision themselves in tech careers. The volunteers receive mentorship training. The program curriculum requires a space with desks and chairs as well as some flexible open space. Computers and tablets must meet curriculum specifications.
>
> **Personnel:** Tech professionals with 3–7 years of experience
>
> **Training:** 6 hours mentorship training
>
> **Facilities:** Classrooms with desks, chairs, projector, screen, and flexibility for open space for activities
>
> **Materials:** 2019 iPads, 2019 MacBook Pros

TABLE 14.2. Example Ingredients List for Wilson Reading System

Ingredients	Cost per student	% of total costs
Personnel total	$6,060	90%
Wilson Reading System teacher	$5,340	
Substitute teacher	$360	
Local district coordinator	$30	
Wilson Reading System trainers/coaches	$300	
Testers to screen students	$30	
Facilities total	$470	7%
Classroom and training facilities	$470	
Materials and equipment total	$70	1%
Wilson Reading System lesson materials	$50	
Classroom materials	$10	
Screening tests	$ <10	
Training materials	$ <10	
Other inputs total	$100	2%
Travel costs for training	$100	
Grand total	$6,700	100%

Note. Based on Hollands et al. (2013).

overall parameters for some interventions, they are in fact incomplete and unreliable sources of information about costs for a variety of reasons. Unfortunately, most references to costs in education neither define what is meant by cost nor use a cost accounting system that measures costs consistently among alternatives. Revenue and expenditure accounting in education was established mainly for public control and accountability, not for ascertaining costs of specific programs or interventions (Allison, 2015). Their intended purpose to support auditing and public oversight creates serious obstacles for using the "official" accounting documents of school entities as elaborated in Levin et al. (2018, pp. 54–55).

For these reasons, ingredients data specific to resource utilization are needed for a cost analysis. There are three main sources of such data: descriptions found in program reports and evaluations, interviews with personnel who participated in the interventions, and direct observation of the intervention. Program documentation, such as detailed descriptions, grant proposals, stated theories of change or logic models, and the like can provide a useful starting point but it is often necessary to supplement this information with focused questioning of informed staff with direct knowledge of program implementation. Depending on the nature of the intervention and the amount of information available from other sources, semistructured interviews or surveys can be used, and the roles and number of informants might vary. It is often useful to begin with program developers or leaders who might provide general background and recommend individuals closer to the intervention to provide detailed information. The process is akin to triangulation, by which additional information is obtained to corroborate or add detail to other sources of information until necessary details have been aligned. Ideally, such data collection can be performed in conjunction with an implementation study to limit additional burden on evaluators and participants, and potentially enhance both the implementation and cost analyses through complementarities.

The preferred method of obtaining ingredients information is to collect such data in the evaluation effort at the same time that the evaluation of effectiveness is convened. Since evaluators wish to document the details of the intervention process, it is easiest to capture data on the ingredients that were used, both quantity and quality, simultaneously with the evaluation of effectiveness impact—that is, collection of the effectiveness and cost information and analysis can be integrated. For this purpose, observation protocols, and time and activity logs can be used by program implementers. This approach also provides details on program implementation that offers interpretive information on effectiveness results.

Questions specifically about quantities and qualities of resources required, such as number of hours of personnel time and associated qualifications and fringe benefits, can be appended to existing data collection instruments. Table 14.3 provides an example of the wide range of potential data sources that were used to create a preliminary ingredients list in an evaluation of a university–school–community partnership (Shand et al., 2018). With such a detailed starting point, follow-up questions via survey or interviews can be quite parsimonious and targeted at resolving apparent disparities and filling specific gaps in the data. More details on measuring the ingredients used to determine costs can be found in Levin et al. (2018, Chapter 4). Sufficient background information on the program can help guard against excessively burdensome data collection on costs likely to be irrelevant to the analysis, including costs that would be incurred anyway regardless of the intervention or evaluation; costs that could be double-counted if they are both itemized and included as part of a general overhead rate; and costs that are trivially small, unlikely to make a difference in the analysis or any decisions that stem from it, and are thus not worth expending significant efforts on the part of evaluators or participants to collect, analyze, or report. As a general rule of thumb, the efforts focused on gathering cost data should be roughly proportional to the magnitude of the cost relative to the total cost.

After the ingredients and their associated quantities and qualities have been established, the next step is to apply an appropriate economic value, represented by a market or shadow price, for each ingredient. We recommend using average market prices whenever available, as the market value approximates the opportunity cost value of the resource. The qualitative

TABLE 14.3. Sources of Ingredients Data for University Partnership Program

Data source	Information contained
Documents	
Implementation evaluation report	• Detailed description of program implementation • Types and qualifications of human resources • Types of training and professional development activities that program offers to partnering schools
Professional development (PD) session attendance record	• Dates, number of hours for PD sessions • Attendance of invited teachers for each session • Cumulative attendance hours by school
List of contractors	• Name and description of contractors • Schools for which the contractors work • Contract values for each contractor • Sources of funding and distribution (percentage) for each contract
List of graduate student workers	• Name and description of all graduate student worker positions • Schools for which each student worker works • Hours worked and hourly or yearly rate
School work plans	• Targets for the type and quantity of services to be delivered • Personnel that are involved in implementing these services
Interviews/email communication	
Program staff	• Rough estimates of how each staff member distributes their time across different domains • Activities at each school site and the frequencies of each activity
Sponsoring university staff	• Estimates of administrative support • Description of roles and responsibilities performed by senior program managers
School personnel	Description of the type and quantity of personnel, materials and equipment, facilities, training, and other resources involved in implementation of program at each school site

Note. Based on Shand et al. (2018).

information on each ingredient, such as qualifications, training, and experience for personnel, can be used to identify an appropriate market price. National or regional surveys, such as the National Compensation Survey by the U.S. Bureau of Labor Statistics (*www.bls.gov/ncs*), can provide good estimates of market prices based on representative samples, and the Center for Benefit–Cost Studies of Education at the University of Pennsylvania, has assembled a large, database of educational resource prices, available to users in its software platform (Hollands et al., 2014). For personnel ingredients, it is critical to include fringe benefits in addition to salary to fully capture the opportunity cost value of personnel time. Detail on the cost of ingredients is found in Levin et al. (2018, Chapter 5).

In some cases, ingredients do not come from competitive markets and will require a cost estimate based upon other methods that provide what is called a "shadow price." For instance, a program that employs volunteer services will not pay a market wage to the volunteers but the value of their time can be ascertained based on what it would cost to hire a person with comparable skills on the labor market to perform the same service. Developing a shadow price for volunteer services both accounts for the value of volunteer time and the fact that a replacement would need to be hired if volunteers were unavailable. Even if the program could be staffed by volunteers in perpetuity, it is important to still note volunteer time as an input into the production process and an opportunity cost to the volunteers themselves. School-owned facilities also present a special case that may require careful consideration of the shadow price. If there is a strong rental market for the type of facilities used for an intervention, then the rental rate for the square footage and time used of a particular type of space is a good proxy for the opportunity cost, as the opportunity cost of using a facility for one purpose is indeed the foregone rent that could have been earned if the facility were leased out for a different purpose. However, for many of the types of facilities used in social service interventions, such as schools, the facility space is too unique for there to be a robust rental market to estimate the opportunity cost of using the space. In this case there are methods of determining the annual cost of use of a facility with specific features in Levin et al. (2018, pp. 86–90). Other durable goods, such as equipment, technology, furniture, and the like, along with human capital investments in training, can likewise be **annualized** to divide the costs over the useful life of the resource.

As prices may require adjustment in order to be comparable to one another, we generally recommend using national average prices to make general comparisons rather than local prices so that differences in costs can be attributed to real differences in resource usage, not differences in regional price levels. Prices for ingredients that are derived in different years need to be adjusted to a single year for comparison to correct for changes in price levels over time. If costs are only needed for a locality such as a school district, they can rely on price information for that locality or region, which are generally available from government sources. Most importantly, and notably distinct from inflation, costs that occur in future years for multiyear programs, or benefits that are incurred in the future in a benefit–cost analysis, need to be **discounted** to present value, or adjusted for the fact that benefits received, or costs incurred in the future have less social value than when they are registered at the present. Discounting accounts for time preference—the tendency to prefer the present over the future—and the opportunity cost of capital—that is, economic benefits received sooner, or costs deferred later are preferred over later benefits or earlier costs because interest could be earned in the interim. Because researchers have found that society at large has a lower discount rate than individuals, following guidance from U.S. government agencies, and for the sake of consistency across interventions (Moore et al., 2004), we generally recommend a relatively low discount rate (around 2–5%) for social investments, which can then be tested in **sensitivity analysis** (see Box 14.3). Spreadsheet software, such as Microsoft Excel, can be easily adapted to categorize and document ingredients and their prices, along with necessary adjustments, and to tabulate the final cost by multiplying each ingredient quantity by its price and summing across ingredients. A number of tools have been developed to facilitate the process of tabulating ingredients, attaching appropriate market prices, and making necessary adjustments for comparability across programs and over time.

> **BOX 14.3. Finite Discounting Example**
>
> $PV = FV/(1 + r)^t$
> (PV: present value, FV: future value, R: discount rate, t = time period)
>
> The coding program has an average benefit in terms of increased wages of $10,000, 5 years after graduation
>
> The present value of the $10K in 5 years using a 3.5% discounting rate is calculated below:
>
> $\$8,714 = \$10K/(1 + 3.5\%)^4$
>
> If we want to test for sensitivity to our selection of rate, we can use a discount rate of 3% and 4% as well:
>
> $\$8,884 = \$10K/(1 + 3.0\%)^4$
> $\$8,548 = \$10K/(1 + 4.0\%)^4$
>
> We can see from the sensitivity test that the estimate is not highly sensitive to a change in the discount rate.

Costs are often borne by more than one government unit (e.g., state, school district, health departments) or private sources, such as philanthropies, community organizations, and volunteers. After the ingredients and their costs have been established, we proceed to an analysis of who provides or finances the ingredients. This can be done on an ingredient-by-ingredient basis, documenting who contributes or pays for each resource. A separate analysis can also be performed to capture payments that shift the overall burden, rather than providing particular ingredients—for example, if one level of government subsidizes another, or if users are charged fees to participate in a program, that would affect who pays the cost across all ingredients but not impact the cost itself. It is important to emphasize that payments such as user fees and intergovernmental subsidies represent transfers, and not costs, as they affect the distribution of who pays but not the overall social cost. The analysis of who pays for a program (and, in a benefit–cost analysis, who receives the benefits) can have important implications for the politics and feasibility of a program, in addition to implications for equity (see Levin et al., 2018: Chapter 6). For instance, in both the Reading Partners (Jacob et al., 2016) and Raising Educational Achievement Coalition of Harlem (Shand et al., 2018) programs, a resource-rich program is provided to schools that pay only about 20% of the costs, with the remainder provided by partner agencies or borne by volunteers who expend the work effort with no financial cost to schools. Of course, if the schools were unable to obtain the volunteers, the costs of equivalent personnel would have to be absorbed by school costs. Table 14.4 provides an example from the evaluation of Reading Partners to demonstrate how ingredients are analyzed along with the distribution of how they are financed.

The total costs of a program can be summarized in several different ways. The most straightforward approach is to multiply each ingredient's quantity by its market or shadow price and sum across all ingredients for the **total cost** of the intervention. This total cost can be divided among the number of participants for an **average cost per participant**. In the presence of attrition or other differences between planned and actual service delivery, we recommend dividing the costs among the number of participants who actually complete the intervention, akin to a "treatment on the treated" estimate in a causal impact evaluation framework. This is to err on the side of a conservative estimate of the cost—in essence, we assume that attrition is a natural phenomenon that occurs as part of any program, and therefore, to deliver the program to, say, 35 participants you may need to plan for and fund 45 slots. However, these costs should only then be divided among the 35 who actually completed the intervention—in other words, the costs of attrition are "baked in" to the per student costs for the completers. Costs can also be divided by what is **fixed** over some number of participants and what is **variable** based on the number of participants to determine the **marginal cost** of serving one additional unit. Continuing with the example above, for the program with 35 participants but capacity for 45, the physical space and time for a facilitator, such as a teacher, may be fixed regardless of whether the program is fully subscribed, but additional participants may only require minimal variable costs, such as materials, meaning that the average cost would be high but the marginal cost of serving one additional participant may

TABLE 14.4. Example of Estimation of Ingredients and How They Were Financed

Cost of Reading Partners per Program Group Student

Cost	Cost per Student	Cost to School	Cost to Volunteers	Cost to Reading Partners	Cost to AmeriCorps
Ingredients					
Reading Partners staff	690			690	
AmeriCorps members	930			930	
School staff	90	90			
Volunteer time and transportation	1,520		1,520		
Facilities	300	300			
Materials and equipment	80			80	
Total ingredients	**3,610**	**390**	**1,520**	**1,700**	**0**
Fee for service ($)		320		−320	
AmeriCorps grant ($)				−270	270
Net cost per student (Total ingredients + fee for service + AmeriCorps grant) ($)		710	1,520	1,110	270
Portion of net cost per student (%)	20	42	31	7	

Note. Data from Jacob et al. (2016).

be low. Such insights can be useful for distinguishing between replicating or scaling up an existing program.

COMBINING COSTS AND EFFECTS

Costs per participant can also be divided by an effectiveness measure for a **cost-effectiveness ratio**. This ratio provides the cost per unit of outcome, which can then be used to compare interventions that have the same intended outcome. An analyst can also compute the **yield**, the units of effect per dollar (which can be scaled to, e.g., $1,000). Note that this is not the sole criterion on which interventions should be judged, so the cost-effectiveness ranking should not be interpreted as a hard-and-fast decision rule—rather, the relative efficiency of interventions for major outcomes provide an important data point to guide decision makers.

Cost-effectiveness analysis provides a convenient and easy-to-interpret, single metric for each program but it also has some limitations in its applicability. For one, it is purposively a comparative method of ranking alternatives. Such cost-effectiveness comparisons must be made with much caution. Even programs that appear to target the same outcome may employ very different outcome measures that reflect different subskills, measures that are tailored to a particular intervention, or different levels of underlying population variance. For example, assessments for three different math interventions may target rote facts versus complex problem solving, or an assessment may be highly tailored to a particular intervention without measuring whether the skills gained transfer to other settings—these three assessments may appear comparable at first glance but a cost-effectiveness comparison based on them would be misleading. Furthermore, while cost-effectiveness analysis requires selection of a single outcome measure of effectiveness, that does not imply that it should be limited to just standardized test scores. In education, cost-effectiveness analysis has been applied to high school graduation or dropout (Hollands et al., 2014), postsecondary outcomes, social and emotional outcomes, and many others. Therefore, the most important considerations for the suitability of cost-effectiveness analysis to an evaluation relate to whether the effects are measured in a rigorous way that lends itself to a valid comparison. Many interventions and evaluations have more than one intended or measured outcome. This can be accommodated in cost-effectiveness analysis by calculating a separate cost-effectiveness ratio for each outcome but that can inflate the cost per unit of outcome because the full cost of the intervention must generally be ascribed to each individual outcome unless there is a logical and defensible way to separate the intervention into components. In such cases, methods that allow for multiple outcomes—benefit–cost analysis or cost–utility analysis—may be preferable to cost-effectiveness analysis.

As an example, the 2015 reauthorization of the Elementary and Secondary Education Act of 1965, known as the Every Student Succeeds Act, requires educators to use "evidence-based" interventions, applying different standards of evidence to decisions at different stakes—for example, a decision to launch a small pilot program may require "promising evidence," whereas a decision to adopt a curriculum across a large school district would require "moderate" or "strong" evidence (*https://ed.gov/policy/elsec/leg/essa/guidanceuseseinvestment.pdf*).

One source of evidence for policymakers and practitioners is the What Works Clearinghouse (WWC), a compendium of vetted research findings in 12 areas, ranging from early childhood to higher education and including research and evaluation on programs and practices in several subject areas and targeting several specific populations. As of this writing, of 228 literacy programs, 28 targeted alphabetics outcomes, comprising phonemic and phonological awareness, letter identification, and phonics, or the basic reading skills required to translate printed text into spoken words. These programs vary widely in format, duration, and target audience, making comparisons among them particularly challenging. The WWC helps to facilitate these comparisons on effectiveness, conditional on targeting the same outcome for the same population. The WWC evaluates the quality of evidence supporting results but lacks cost information for judging efficiency among the alternatives. Given the broad range of approaches, evidence on costs and cost-effectiveness can significantly aid the decision-making process.

Table 14.5 shows the target population, cost per student, effect sizes in alphabetics and

TABLE 14.5. Cost-Effectiveness Ratios for Early Literacy Programs

Programs by grade level	Reading ability of target students	Total cost per student	Literacy outcome	Effect size gain	Cost per unit of effect size
Kindergarten average readers					
Kindergarten Peer-Assisted Learning Strategies	All	$27	Alphabetics	0.61	$38
Kindergarten struggling readers					
Stepping Stones	Struggling; behavioral disorders	$479	Alphabetics	0.84	$570
Sound Partners	20–30th percentile	$791	Alphabetics	0.34	$2,093
			Fluency	0.48	$165
First-grade struggling readers					
Fast ForWord Reading 1	Slightly below average	$282	Alphabetics	0.24	$601
Reading Recovery	Bottom 20th percentile	$4,143	Alphabetics	0.70	$1,480
			Fluency	1.71	$606
Third-grade struggling readers					
Corrective Reading	Bottom 25th percentile	$10,108	Alphabetics	0.22	$38,135
			Fluency	0.27	$6,364
Wilson Reading	Bottom 25th percentile	$6,696	Alphabetics	0.33	$13,392

Note. Based on Hollands et al. (2013).

other early literacy outcomes, and the cost-effectiveness ratio for each of seven early literacy programs with rigorous evidence of effectiveness in the WWC. Since effects are measured as effect sizes, the cost-effectiveness ratio can be interpreted as the cost per standard deviation increase in measured skills on a particular early literacy outcome. It is initially quite striking how widely variable the cost-effectiveness ratios are, ranging from approximately $40 per standard deviation increase to nearly $40,000. However, caution must be exercised in interpreting these results, as the programs target different ages, different populations of readers (average readers or struggling readers), different comparison groups using different research designs, and different outcomes even within the same domain. Nonetheless, even limiting comparisons to within the same population and outcome, adding costs and considering effects relative to those costs provides useful additional information to decision makers. For instance, a school district official seeking to improve outcomes for struggling first-grade readers may choose Fast ForWord over Reading Recovery, as even though it is less effective, it is also far less costly, providing greater impact per dollar of cost. The cost-effectiveness ratio alone should not be the sole information for the decision but it should carry some weight and be visible to the decision maker—Reading Recovery targets more outcomes and more struggling readers, partially explaining its higher cost, and Fast ForWord may simply not be effective enough, even at a much lower cost.

While the method of determining costs is the same for all of the economic evaluation methods, benefit–cost analysis also requires measures of effectiveness to be converted into monetary values. If the outcome of an intervention is something that is traded on a market, such as labor market earnings for educational interventions, or access to health care services with a market price for health interventions, then its value can be readily ascertained. However, for nonmarket goods, as is most often the case for social interventions, the social value needs to be estimated using **shadow pricing**, a range of methods for estimating nonmarket values as noted earlier. When possible, observing people's behavior and choices yields more valid and reliable shadow price estimates than directly asking for stated preferences, though the latter is sometimes unavoidable (Diamond & Hausman, 1994). Describing methods for developing shadow pricing methods are beyond the scope of this chapter but readers may consult one of several standard texts on the subject, including Levin et al. (2018, pp. 207–217) and Boardman et al. (2018).

Readers may note that economic evaluation methods require a high degree of professional judgment, similar for any research and evaluation method, where details of sampling, data collection instruments, coding, and analytic models are subject to assumptions and decisions by the evaluator. However, economic evaluation methods are distinguished by the sheer number of decisions that must be made: how many sites or informants are "enough" before additional participants stop adding useful new details to the analysis, what discount rate to use to bring future costs and benefits to the present value, whether to use local or national prices, over what time period to amortize or annualize a facility or piece of capital equipment, whether effects of the program fade in the long term, and ad infinitum. The method requires informed judgment by an evaluator but the key virtues of the ingredients method for economic evaluation are its straightforwardness and transparency. Because the resources and steps used to calculate their costs are so clearly documented, it can become a routine matter to test the sensitivity of results to assumptions about costs and benefits using sensitivity analysis (see Box 14.4). If there are only a few assumptions with a great deal of uncertainty around them, this can be a simple matter of testing a range of plausible values for each one to determine whether those changes substantively alter results. When there is more uncertainty about a large number of assumptions, the problem of dimensionality (varying not just each individual parameter but a wide range of combinations of them) can become unwieldy. In these cases, **break-even analysis** (at what point would the costs of one intervention equal the benefits, or what combination of assumptions would change the rank order of programs in a cost-effectiveness comparison?), or **best-case and worst-case scenario testing** (what are the most and least favorable combinations of assumptions, and which are more plausible?) can serve to simplify the analysis to a clear decision

> **BOX 14.4. Coding Program Costs Sensitivity Analysis**
>
> You wonder about the sensitivity of your results on three assumptions:
>
> 1. You estimated the wage for the tech volunteers to be too high.
> 2. You assumed the computers would be used for 5 years but now wonder if it is really closer to 3 years.
> 3. You valued the classroom using a national rate, but think they may be more specialized than a typical classroom, impacting the quality of instruction.
>
> You can test for the sensitivity of your result on these assumptions by changing the values and re-running your analysis three times, with one of the following changes each time:
>
> 1. Re-estimate the costs with a lower wage rate for the volunteers.
> 2. Annualize the computer cost over 3 years instead of 5 years.
> 3. Increase the cost of the classroom space by a percentage that reflects the increase in quality.
>
> After reestimating the costs using each of the above changes you see that only the change in volunteer wages meaningfully changes your average cost estimate. You can gather more information to see which rate is the most accurate for the analysis.

problem. In particularly complex cases where a wide range of assumptions vary not just in their means but in their distributions, these assumptions can be analyzed using simulation methods of sensitivity analysis. These simulation methods can include **bootstrapping** methods for hypothesis testing and **Monte Carlo analysis**, by which several variables in the analysis are varied simultaneously by randomly drawing them from distributions as specified by the evaluator. Since there is not a clear analogue to classical statistical inference testing for cost, cost-effectiveness, and benefit–cost analysis, simulation-based methods like this can be used to quantify uncertainty around point estimates.

While the additional effort to conduct an economic evaluation may seem extensive, much of the additional burden of time to incorporate this perspective into an efficacy evaluation is in the collection of detailed data on ingredients and their associated market or shadow prices. For this reason, the additional costs and disruption can be minimized when, as suggested above, data collection on ingredients is integrated into other data collection efforts, such as interviews, surveys, and observations documenting implementation. Primarily because of the additional data collection requirements, a standalone economic evaluation—for instance, a prospective cost analysis for a proposed program, or a retrospective cost-effectiveness analysis for a program that has already undergone impact evaluation—requires substantially more effort to design and conduct the study. Parsimony in data collection is a strong argument for the simultaneous approach in combining the ingredients method into designs for effectiveness (Levin & Belfield 2015).

HOW ECONOMIC EVALUATION ENHANCES EVALUATION

The most obvious way that adding an economic dimension can enhance evaluation is by providing additional evidence on resource efficiency in producing an educationally effective result. Often evaluation has the purpose of seeking an implicit selection among alternatives. A benefit of economic evaluation is that it makes that selection more explicit, whether it is in choosing between different ways of achieving the same objective in a cost-effectiveness analysis, or determining whether to continue, expand, or discontinue a single program in a benefit–cost analysis. Economic evaluation also features ways to explicitly include constituent perspectives. For instance, because cost-effectiveness analysis focuses on comparing alternatives for a single outcome, a cost-effectiveness evaluation can stimulate a conversation among constituents at the outset of the evaluation on the intended outcome of an intervention and how it should be measured. Along similar lines, when a cost analysis is supplemented by a distributional analysis of financing—who pays for the costs, and who receives the benefits—the perspectives of multiple interested parties can be explicitly included. Thus, the evaluation can focus on how multiple groups fare in the intervention, perhaps with an eye toward equity or redistribution of resources. Finally, an economic evaluation increases focus on not just whether something works in an impact evaluation but by drawing attention to the resources required it raises the important questions of *how, under what conditions,* and *for whom* something works.

As part of a comprehensive evaluation framework, an economic evaluation provides a critical link between a theory of change, program implementation, and measured impacts, as the resources used are in effect the channel through which impacts are achieved and as a basis for valuing an intervention and its impacts. Resource utilization can provide additional clues on implementation, how a theory of change is operationalized, and how implementation in practice may differ from program design. For instance, Table 14.6 shows the distribution of costs of a university–school–community partnership across five schools and the five domains, or programmatic areas, of the partnership. The Expanded Learning Opportunities domain, which comprises tutoring and enrichment programs, represents about half of the total cost of the program, suggesting it is a major part of the program's theory of change (Shand et al., 2018).

A related benefit of economic evaluation derives from the practice of measuring costs incrementally—the costs of the treatment above and beyond business as usual. Effects in impact evaluation are implicitly defined as incremental, as outcomes are measured relative to some control or comparison condition but there is seldom much attention paid to what the control or comparison condition looks like. Economic evaluation can help address this concern by highlighting the treatment contrast, as the costs to produce an impact are what the treatment group receives minus what the control group receives. For example, the City Connects program entails the assessment of the strengths and needs of every student in a school, provisions of tailored interventions delivered by the school, and a wide range of community partner organizations to help address student needs. However, simply estimating the costs of the program, including induced services, will likely overstate the true costs as nearly all schools have some degree of diagnostics of student needs and community partnerships. Therefore, analyzing how comparison group schools comprehensively address student needs and the types of partnerships they pursue not only helps arrive at a more accurate estimate of the true social costs of a program like City Connects but it also more clearly delineates how the program differs from traditional practice, thus providing greater insight into causal mechanisms (Bowden et al., 2020).

Further, by raising the salience of comparisons between programs and the need to have comparable effectiveness estimates for a cost-effectiveness analysis, or effectiveness measures that can be monetized for a benefit–cost analysis, economic evaluation also highlights the importance of selecting valid and comparable outcome measures. In many ways, programs, research designs, outcomes, and measures that are good candidates for cost-effectiveness analyses are also simply indicators of strong impact evaluations in their own right (see Levin & Belfield, 2015, for more discussion of valid cost-effectiveness comparisons and lessons cost-

TABLE 14.6. Costs of University–School Partnership by Domain

	Leadership	Teaching and learning	Health	Expanded learning opportunities	Family	Total
School A	$59,480	$85,380	$45,150	$263,630	$55,120	$508,760
School B	$47,840	$83,290	$122,680	$447,220	$46,270	$747,290
School C	$61,710	$97,160	$130,960	$173,430	$59,570	$522,830
School D	$63,440	$88,760	$215,260	$220,030	$55,470	$642,970
School E	$5,120	$5,120	$90,120	$203,650	$7,120	$311,110
Total	$237,590	$359,710	$604,160	$1,310,960	$223,560	$2,732,970

Note. Based on Shand et al. (2018).

effectiveness can provide on making impact evaluations more useful for decision makers broadly). The selection and potential monetization of outcomes also ties to the important issue of valuation in evaluation, discussed by Gates and Schwandt (see Chapter 5, this volume). Cost-effectiveness analysis implicitly addresses issues of valuation by forcing interested parties to select a single, valid, and comparable outcome in advance, whereas cost–utility and benefit–cost analysis explicitly place values on potentially diverse outcomes using economic methods. One limitation to conducting a benefit–cost analysis is that not all outcomes can be monetized but the approaches can provide transparent and testable methods for assessing how much society values different outcomes, encouraging the allocation of resources to the interventions where they will do the most social good. They certainly do not provide the final word on valuation of outcomes—individuals may disagree, some outcomes may be omitted because they are not measured or not monetized, other outcomes may be double counted or miscounted—but they provide an evidence-based starting point for a more objective discussion about valuation.

The Center for Benefit–Cost Studies of Education has estimated the social value of a number of outcomes in education and related fields, such as the prevention of high school dropouts (Belfield et al., 2012) and a variety of social-emotional outcomes (Belfield et al., 2015). Much work has been done estimating the wide variety of benefits of early childhood education, including Perry Preschool project (Belfield et al., 2006) and the Chicago Parent–Child Centers (Reynolds et al., 2001).

For multisite interventions, an economic analysis can also provide insight into site-level variation in resource usage, tied to differences in implementation and outcomes. For example, an analysis of a federal program demonstrated that site-level costs and the resulting resources available to students varied widely (Bowden & Belfield, 2015). The program, Talent Search, is one of the federal TRIO educational opportunity programs that aims to improve educational outcomes among students who will be the first in their families to attend college and who are often from low-income households. The program raises their knowledge and uptake of Pell Grant funding and other available financial aid for college. Table 14.7 demonstrates the wide variation found among sites implementing Talent Search. This variation in resources provides valuable information for future policy and efforts to share information across sites to improve the production of outcomes for the program as a whole. With enough sites and site-level variation in costs, implementation, and impacts, statistical analysis could be used to analyze connections between resource use and effectiveness, and potentially to engage in scenario analysis to predict potential future outcomes with design changes. Of course, any such analysis would need to be undertaken with significant caution and reported with appropriate caveats, as variation in resource use and outcomes are likely endogenous to other factors, may not generalize to other settings, and predictions may entail out-of-sample extrapolation that could present real-world complications in implementation.

Finally, economic evaluation can provide insight into the design of evaluations themselves (Belfield & Bowden, 2019). The most notable example relates to the issue of statistical power—when determining the necessary sample size to detect a particular minimum effect size, evaluators often struggle to determine what the minimum detectable effect size

TABLE 14.7. Talent Search Site-Level Variation in Costs

Sites	Annual cost per student	Cost per student (6-year total, PV)
Texas		
Site 1	$660	$5,190
Site 2	$570	$3,120
Site 3	$430	$2,890
Site 4	$770	$5,150
Site 5	$650	$2,800
Site 6	$730	$4,000
Florida		
Site 1	$690	$2,960
Site 2	$700	$3,830
Site 3	$630	$2,730
Pooled	$640	$3,580

Note. Based on Bowden and Belfield (2015). 2010 dollars. PV, present value. Copyright © 2015 Cambridge University Press. Adapted with permission.

or hypothesized effect should be. Ideally, this would be guided by theory and prior research, as well as the minimum effect that would be of policy relevance or substantive significance. Cost-effectiveness analysis can provide evidence on the latter point, as the minimum effect that is policy relevant might be the minimum effect at which a policy is cost-effective relative to alternatives, or the minimum effect at which the benefits exceed the costs. That implies, perhaps surprisingly, that cheaper interventions actually require larger evaluations because even a very small effect could be justified for a very low-cost intervention. This also implies that the cost of the evaluation should not generally be tied to the cost of the intervention—a very low-cost intervention with outsized effects relative to its costs may well justify extensive evaluation, as evidence in support of such an intervention could do much good in efficiently allocating resources.

CONCLUSIONS

Decision makers are constantly urged to use evidence in making choices among approaches to address specific social challenges. To this point the emphasis of most evaluation studies has been to ascertain the effectiveness of alternatives for different populations and at different dosage levels and different approaches to implementation. In addition, we need to recognize explicitly that all decision makers are constrained by available resources. Accordingly, placing the evidence in a framework that explicitly and appropriately accounts for the cost of producing results is a key part of the decision–evidence for choosing among alternatives. Although the applications of the analysis and presentation of Levin et al. (2018) are mainly applied to educational evaluations, the methods are readily applicable to other fields, such as criminal justice, health, environment, transportation, and many other social challenges. If evidence on effects is not coupled with accurate cost information on resource requirements, it will not serve fully the needs of decision makers. Accordingly, we believe that cost analysis when combined with excellent effectiveness studies will increase the usefulness of the evidence for social decisions.

REFERENCES

Allison, G. S. (2015) *Financial accounting for local and state school systems: 2014 Edition* [NCES 2015347]. National Center for Education Statistics, U.S. Department of Education. Available at *https://nces.ed.gov/pubsearch/pubsifo.asp?pubid=2015347*

Barnett, W. S. (1985). Benefit–cost analysis of the Perry Preschool program and its policy implications. *Educational Evaluation and Policy Analysis, 7,* 333–342.

Belfield, C., Bowden, A. B., Klapp, A., Levin, H., Shand, R., & Zander, S. (2015). The economic value of social and emotional learning. *Journal of Benefit–Cost Analysis, 6*(3), 508–544.

Belfield, C. R., & Bowden, A. B. (2019). Using resource and cost considerations to support educational evaluation: Six domains. *Educational Researcher, 48*(2), 120–127.

Belfield, C. R., Levin, H. M., & Rosen, R. (2012). *The economic value of opportunity youth.* Center for Benefit Cost Studies of Education. Available at *cbcse.org*

Belfield, C. R., Nores, M., Barnett, S., & Schweinhart, L. (2006). The High/Scope Perry Preschool program: Cost–benefit analysis using data from the age 40 followup. *Journal of Human Resources, 41*(1), 162–190.

Bell, S. H., & Orr, L. L. (1994). Is subsidized employment cost effective for welfare recipients? Experimental evidence from seven state demonstrations. *Journal of Human Resources, 29*(1), 42–61.

Bloom, H. S., Orr, L. L., Bell, S. H., Cave, G., Doolittle, F., Lin, W., & Bos, J. M. (1997). The benefits and costs of JTPA Title II-A programs: Key findings from the National Job Training Partnership Act study. *Journal of Human Resources, 32*(3), 549–576.

Boardman, A. E., Greenberg, D. H., Vining, A. R., & Weimer, D. L. (2018). *Cost–benefit analysis: Concepts and practice* (5th ed.). Cambridge University Press.

Bowden, A. B., & Belfield, C. (2015). Evaluating the Talent Search TRIO program: A benefit–cost analysis and cost-effectiveness analysis. *Journal of Benefit–Cost Analysis, 6*(3), 572–602.

Bowden, A. B., Shand, R., Levin, H. M., Muroga, A., & Wang, A. (2020). An economic evaluation of the costs and benefits of providing comprehensive supports to students in elementary school. *Prevention Science, 21,* 1126–1135.

Carter, S. (2017, October 23). *Cost-effectiveness for informed decision-making* [Blog]. Available at *www.povertyactionlab.org/blog/10-23-17/cost-effectiveness-informed-decision-making*

Cave, G., Bos, H., Doolittle, F., & Toussaint, C. (1993). *JOBSTART. Final report on a program for school dropouts.* MDRC. Available at *https://files.eric.ed.gov/fulltext/ED363774.pdf*

Couch, K. A. (1992). New evidence on the long-term effects of employment training programs. *Journal of Labor Economics, 10*(4), 380–388.

Diamond, P. A., & Hausman, J. A. (1994). Contingent valuation: Is some number better than no number? *Journal of Economic Perspectives, 8*(4), 45–64.

Gueron, J. M. (1988). Work–welfare programs. *New Directions for Program Evaluation, 1988*(37), 7–27.

Gueron, J. M., & Pauly, E. (1991). *From welfare to work*. Russell Sage Foundation.

Gueron, J. M., & Rolston, H. (2013). *Fighting for reliable evidence*. Russell Sage Foundation.

Hamilton, G. (2002). *Moving people from welfare to work: Lessons from the national evaluation of welfare-to-work strategies*. MDRC. Available at https://files.eric.ed.gov/fulltext/ED469794.pdf

Hogan, R. L. (2007). The historical development of program evaluation: Exploring past and present. *Online Journal for Workforce Education and Development, 2*(4), 5.

Hollands, F., Bowden, A. B., Belfield, C., Levin, H. M., Cheng, H., Shand, R., . . . Hanisch-Cerda, B. (2014). Cost-effectiveness analysis in practice: Interventions to improve high school completion. *Educational Evaluation and Policy Analysis, 36*(3), 307–326.

Hollands, F. M., & Levin, H. M. (2017). *The critical importance of costs for education decisions*. REL 2017-274. National Center for Education Evaluation and Regional Assistance.

Hollands, F. M., Pan, Y., Shand, R., Cheng, H., Levin, H. M., Belfield, C. R., . . . Hanisch-Cerda, B. (2013). *Improving early literacy: Cost-effectiveness analysis of effective reading programs*. Center for Benefit-Cost Studies of Education, University of Pennsylvania.

Jacob, R., Armstrong, A., Bowden, A. B., & Pan, Y. (2016). Leveraging volunteers: An experimental valuation of a tutoring program for struggling readers. *Journal of Research on Educational Effectiveness, 9*(S1), 67–92.

Levin, H. M. (1970). A cost-effectiveness analysis of teacher selection. *Journal of Human Resources*, 24–33.

Levin, H. M. (1975). Cost-effectiveness analysis in evaluation research. *Handbook of Evaluation Research, 2*, 89–122.

Levin, H. (2001). Waiting for Godot: Cost-effectiveness analysis in education. *New Directions for Evaluation, 2001*(90), 55–68.

Levin, H. M., & Belfield, C. (2015). Guiding the development and use of cost-effectiveness analysis in education. *Journal of Research on Educational Effectiveness, 8*(3), 400–418.

Levin, H. M., Glass, G. V., & Meister, G. R. (1987). Cost-effectiveness of computer-assisted instruction. *Evaluation Review, 11*(1), 50–72.

Levin, H. M., & McEwan, P. J. (2001). *Cost-effectiveness analysis: Methods and applications*. Sage.

Levin, H. M., McEwan, P. J., Belfield, C., Bowden, A. B., & Shand, R. (2018). *Economic evaluation in education, cost-effectiveness and benefit–cost analysis* (3rd ed.). SAGE.

Liscow, Z. (2021). *Equity in regulatory cost–benefit analysis*. Symposia on Cost–Benefit Analysis, Law and Political Economy Project. Available at https://lpeproject.org/blog/equity-in-regulatory-cost-benefit-analysis

Maynard, R. A. (1996). *Kids having kids: A Robin Hood Foundation special report on the costs of adolescent childbearing*. U.S. Department of Education.

Moore, M. A., Boardman, A. E., Vining, A. R., Weimer, D. L., & Greenberg, D. H. (2004). "Just give me a number!" Practical values for the social discount rate. *Journal of Policy Analysis and Management, 23*(4), 789–812.

Murnane, R. J., & Willett, J. B. (2010). *Methods matter: Improving causal inference in educational and social science research*. Oxford University Press.

Phillips, J. (1996). *Accountability in human resource management*. Butterworth-Heinemann.

Porter, T. M. (1995). *Trust in numbers: The pursuit of objectivity in science and public life*. Princeton University Press.

Quade, E. S. (1971). *A history of cost-effectiveness* (No. P-4557). RAND Corp.

Reynolds, A. J., Temple, J. A., Robertson, D. L., & Mann, E. A. (2001). Long-term effects of an early childhood intervention on educational achievement and juvenile arrest: A 15-year follow-up of low-income children in public schools. *JAMA, 285*(18), 2339–2346.

Rossi, P. H., Lipsey, M. W., & Freeman, H. E. (2003). *Evaluation: A systematic approach* (7th ed.). SAGE.

Russell, R. S., & Taylor, B. W., III. (1998). *Operations management: Focusing on quality and competitiveness* (2nd ed.). Prentice Hall.

Shand, R., Muroga, A., Rodriguez, V., & Levin, H. M. (2018). *REACH cost analysis report*. Center for Benefit Cost Studies of Education. Available at cbcse.org

U.S. Department of Education. (2003). *Identifying and implementing educational practices supported by rigorous evidence: A user-friendly guide*. U.S. Department of Education, Institute of Education Sciences, National Center for Education Evaluation and Regional Assistance. Available at www2.ed.gov/rschstat/research/pubs/rigorousevid/rigorousevid.pdf

World Bank. (2016). *Government expenditure on education, total (% of GDP)*. World Development Indicators. Available at https://data.worldbank.org/indicator/SE.XPD.TOTL.GD.ZS

Chapter 15

Evaluation as Storytelling
Using a Qualitative Design

Sharon F. Rallis
Janet Usinger

CHAPTER OVERVIEW

Every program has a story to tell. Evaluators discover and tell that story to inform and guide program decisions and actions. Qualitative methods used in evaluation can tell the story from various angles: developmentally, formatively, summatively. Stories can take many forms: descriptive, critical, appreciative, naturalistic, responsive. The process begins with framing the story: examining the perspective from which the theory of change is expected to play out in practice. The second step is discovering the story by meticulously generating data through a variety of qualitative techniques including interviews, observations, focus groups, documents, and artifacts. Analysis and interpretation make sense of the data and build the story. Finally, the story must be brought to life by clearly and transparently constructing the narrative that portrays the program story. This chapter shares many of the lessons we have learned from telling program stories after conducting countless evaluations, often in highly complex situations.

Every program has a story to tell. Developing a credible story about the program involves a systematic, rigorous, criteria-guided evaluation. Our role as evaluators is to discover and tell that story as grounding for value judgments about the program. Many references exist that focus on how to conduct a wide variety of evaluations; our intent in this chapter is to share our own, usually unwritten *lessons learned*, having conducted countless evaluations, often in highly complex—and sometimes contentious—situations.

In this chapter we argue that our goal in evaluation work is almost always to generate "explicit or tacit sequence of events or interpretation of events" (House, 2017, p. 184) (*the story*), to share that understanding with other people (*storytelling*) in order to guide their valuing of the program and related actions (*use*). To do so, House suggests that evaluators "stand closer to the program, as reflected in the evaluator's voice, and describe events in greater detail, sometimes quoting the words of program participants and observers" (p. 184). Such close descriptions of programs rely on qualitative methods that place evaluators in the field with the programs so they may see, hear, and read (and often taste, smell, and feel) what is happening. The story they capture contains detail and context necessary to produce evaluation results capable of allowing interest holders to see the program in a new light, even altering the reader's beliefs or attitudes, and opening potential for action.

A long line of researchers has argued that qualitative inquiry is a form of storytelling (e.g., Christensen, 2012; Clandinin & Connolly, 2000). For example, in narrative analysis, the stories are the source of data; ethnographers often present findings in the form of stories; and grounded theories are themselves stories, either implicit or explicit. Similarly, evaluators use story when they articulate program theory and how it is operationalized in specific programming.

Qualitative methods used in evaluation can tell the story from various angles: developmentally, formatively, or summatively. Stories can take many forms: descriptive, critical, appreciative, naturalistic, or responsive. Qualitative techniques can be used to describe the context within which evaluation work takes place, can document actions as they occur, and can record the voices and varying perspectives of the actors involved. In short, we argue that evaluators who seek to conduct evaluations that produce credible and actionable knowledge can use qualitative thinking and methods to produce evidence as a basis for learning and also to communicate findings to facilitate meaningful change. A well-told story can inspire people toward improving "policy and programming for the well-being of all" (Weiss, 1998, p. ix).

How do you, the evaluator, design a study to capture the story? Generating a credible and actionable story requires a design grounded in principles of systematic inquiry. According to Carol Weiss's (1998) classic definition: "Evaluation is the *systematic assessment* of the *operation* and/or *outcomes* of a program or policy, compared to a set of *explicit* or *implicit standards*, as a means of contributing to the *improvement* of the program or policy" (p. 4, emphasis in original). Thus, in our chapter we explore various qualitative approaches to systematic scientific inquiry: framing the story; discovering the story; making sense of the story; and bringing the story to life. Within each of these sections, we include practical recommendations for conducting rigorous and credible evaluations that include qualitative methods.

FRAMING THE STORY

By definition, a story is a narrative that relates a sequence of events constructed around a setting (the time, place, and environment within which a story takes place) and characters (the people, objects, and places that have agency within the story). As an evaluator, you need to choose where to focus among the events related to the program. Often the best place to start is with the program itself: what is the program intending to accomplish, and what will the program *do* to accomplish its purpose? This expected cause–effect relationship can be referred to as the *program theory, theory of change,* or *theory of action* (see Frechtling, Chapter 20, and Peck and Snyder, Chapter 13, this volume). Program decision makers choose interventions that they expect will make a positive difference in the context. "Social programs are based on explicit or implicit theories about how and why the program will work" (Weiss, 1998, pp. 66–67). A theory of change is phrased as a causal statement: If we implement X intervention, then Y outcomes will result—and in itself tells a story. Figure 15.1 illustrates the links between intention, action, and result in a theory of change.

A program would be easy to evaluate if it consisted of an explicit purpose or goal, a few objectives, and a set of actions that could be

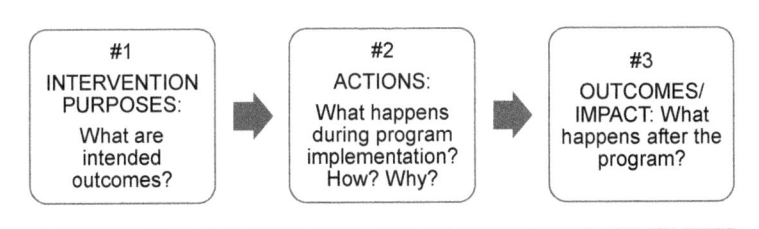

#1 INTERVENTION PURPOSES: What are intended outcomes? → #2 ACTIONS: What happens during program implementation? How? Why? → #3 OUTCOMES/IMPACT: What happens after the program?

FIGURE 15.1. Theory-of-change model.

implemented faithfully; we would simply assess whether the outcomes/impact were consistent with the theory of change (connecting Box 1 with Box 3). Easy! Unfortunately, anyone with any program experience knows that it is seldom simple. The challenges lie in Box 2 because plans are just that—plans; even when they are carefully constructed, the best-laid plans are never implemented flawlessly. The underlying reason for this lack of simplicity is that programs are designed by humans, often in response to complex human conditions or actions; they are implemented by humans, usually in messy environments or circumstances; and they involve human participants who may have their own ideas about how to meet their needs. As well, programs are supported by humans with varied understandings of the purposes, contexts, and participants. Finally, programs and all of their components are permeated with different meanings for each individual associated with the program. Indeed, programs we now evaluate are usually very complex and implemented in dynamic environments.

In other words, the story lies in asking about and exploring the complex interactions that take place as the program plays out in practice with real participants. What activities and events occur? What do they mean to people involved? These questions open up Box 2 and are informed through the descriptive data that qualitative methods provide. Given interest holders' interests, participant needs, and available resources, your design may identify several evaluation questions. Furthermore, you may start with your own evaluation questions but working with interest holders (e.g., policymakers, program leaders, practitioners, users) may generate questions that direct the evaluation toward their particular focus or interest. Often the program purposes, goals, objectives, and planned activities develop and change during

---

BOX 15.1. Uncovering Perspectives through Formative Evaluation

A small but growing foundation devoted to improving the quality and availability of clean water made the strategic decision to expand their program efforts into East Africa, specifically for people living in extreme poverty. To identify firsthand the most important water quality issues that the foundation resources could address, staff were sent into the field. However, once in the field, staff disagreed on the issues—thus program development was delayed. As well, critical contacts in several sites suggested that local people were not engaging with these foundation field teams and questioned whether the proposed programs would actually address local water needs. Before investing further, the foundation asked their evaluators to explore what was happening.

The evaluation team held focus groups of field staff who had returned from program sites. The data told a story that exposed unexpected and troubling perspectives among the staff that created obstacles to effective implementation of the foundation's growth strategy. For example, unintended bias was heard when one team member explained:

"My degree is in environmental science and ecology. So, you can imagine how upset I was when I saw everybody throwing away their trash on the ground. I didn't know what to do. It just really turned me off. And you know how committed I am to the environment—see this eco-friendly bush vest I bought for my granddaughter in the airport on the way out? I wanted to support local industry. But the trash!! And the diesel fumes—my God!"

An equal problem of romanticizing the local situation was also uncovered:

"Oh, the people in the village were so marvelous! Those people are just so welcoming and gracious. Everyone went out of their way to make me feel like a true African! I really learned a lot about them and their wonderful culture. Like, their food was so good—and so exotic. I'd never eaten matoke and, you know, once you get used to it, it's just yummy!! And their native clothes—those dresses with batwings. Fabulous!! I brought some home! And see my kikoy? It's so authentic—and all the village women wear them!"

Using these and other perspectives shared in the focus groups, the evaluators told the story of naïve staff that lacked cultural knowledge. The foundation leaders realized that staff were unable to interact productively with locals and thus could not hear authentic needs and concerns about water. Based on these findings, the foundation leadership realized the critical need to complement environmental science with cultural sensitivity before embarking on their plan to expand their reach into East Africa.

implementation. As evaluator, you will be capturing the story as it develops.

As overall questions are generated, it is important to consider *whose* questions will be explored. Will funders or policymakers, those with decision-making power, choose the questions and frame the evaluation design? Such evaluations usually seek to learn whether the intervention was implemented with fidelity: Are the actions and events consistent with the program goals? Formative evaluations focus on the program itself: How can we improve program activities? Alternatively, will the evaluation be framed through a participant lens? These evaluations are designed to discover what the program means to participants and how it serves their needs. Unintended bias must be considered as well. House (2017) warns of the need to consider whether the design has a *white racial frame*—that is, "an overarching white worldview that encompasses a broad and persistent set of racial stereotypes, prejudices, images, interpretations and narratives, emotions, and reactions" (Feagin, 2013, p. 3).

> Such racial framing can bias programs, policies, and evaluations. Strong evidence indicates that some programs and policies have racist effects that evaluators overlook. Evaluation may even inadvertently contribute to the racist effects. By being aware of racial framing, evaluators could be better prepared to anticipate, discover, and deal with the biases, much as we deal with other threats to validity. (House, 2017, p. 167)

Because every story reflects a particular point-of-view, evaluators make decisions about the positionality of themselves and others within a story. These decisions are important because everyone involved in the program (e.g., funders or policymakers, program leaders, practitioners, you as evaluator) brings an individual perspective, interacting with the others. According to the philosophy of *perspectivism*, "knowledge claims are grounded in the experience of the 'knower'" (Tebes, 2005, p. 220)—and a program has many "knowers." As Weiss (1998) reminds us, effective program evaluation depends on the ability to delve below the surface of human behavior and social relationships and into an understanding of communities and the people who live in those communities. Storytelling facilitates the narrator's **perspective taking**, which is what can make the evaluator as storyteller so effective in conveying a program's value from multiple points of view. Because alternative perspectives are often in play, you need to articulate the criteria or standards you will use to make sense of the data, to judge the value of what happens in the program.

In short, you must ask, "Whose story is it? What contributes to the story? and How will you tell the story?" Your evaluation design reveals decisions you have made about point of view, narrative voice (how to represent multiple perspectives in the text), and narrative construction (setting, characters, events, and sequence). You explore:

- What actions take place in the setting? How do people perform these actions? Why?
- What do these actions mean to the participants—both during and afterward?
- What are the perceived effects of these actions?
- In what ways do the actions relate to one another and to external forces?
- Are these actions and meanings organized into patterns that indicate norms for this setting?

By recognizing the multiple knowers, perspective taking also aligns with the ethical principles of respect, beneficence, and justice. These three principles are generally accepted in Western traditional culture as a guide to the ethics of research involving human subjects (see National Commission for the Protection of Human Subjects of Biomedical and Behavioral Research, 1978; see also Seiber, 2009; Hemmings, 2006; Brothers et al., 2019; Pritchard, 2021). Because your design uses qualitative methods, your data will come from natural settings usually through face-to-face encounters with participants. How you treat these people affects the data and the story that builds.

Ultimately, you want the evaluation to make a difference in policy or practice. To produce evidence that results in a story that affects how readers/audiences view the program and participants, your design makes transparent the many decisions you have reasoned through about purposes, questions, data sources, analysis and interpretation, and reporting. Throughout the entire design process, you attend to **rigor** (adherence to established standards for conducting inquiry), **probity** (wholeness, integrity, and moral soundness), and **transparency** (open and detailed documentation or display of all decisions and actions). In other words, do you understand how I arrived at the story and does the story I'm telling you ring true?

DISCOVERING THE STORY: GENERATING DATA

We discover the program story by intentionally seeking information that can shed light on what people are really doing in a program. This information does not fall from the sky, it is not invented, nor is it created in the evaluator's mind. Information is built from data that are carefully generated through meticulous processes that can be identified (e.g., observations, interviews, and documents, which are described later in the chapter). The term *generate* is intentionally used here, as opposed to *collect* data. As Mason (2002) notes, qualitative inquiry seldom involves data that already exist in their complete and final forms for an evaluation. Rather, **data**, the basic units or building blocks of information, are found in many forms: images, sounds, written words, spoken words, documents, numbers, smells, and actions. Grouped into **patterns**, data become information to be interpreted (analyzed and synthesized). When the process is clear and applied to the evaluation purposes or questions, we can say we have learned something about the program and that the evaluation has produced knowledge. "The process is analogous to building a house. Like data, cinder blocks are not particularly useful by themselves, but they can be placed together to make a wall. Like information, the wall can be used to build a house" (Rossman & Rallis, 2017, p. 3).

Evaluators must determine the types of data appropriate to the evaluation questions. Then they design the manner in which the data will be gathered, knowing that some of the data exist, but that much must be generated through observing program events and talking to people involved with the program. The data are captured in a tangible form using various techniques that allow the data to be recorded: interviews are transcribed and dated, observations become field notes, and artifacts and photos are labeled with participant permission and appropriate attention to confidentiality.

> Data gathering, then, is a deliberate, conscious, systematic process that details both the products (the data) and the processes of the research activities so that others may understand how the study was performed and can judge its adequacy, strength, and ethics. Recording what is learned takes persistence and effort, but as a researcher, you undertake this discipline so that you may analyze the data and others may decide if they are convinced that the processes, evidence, and conclusions are sound. The data are not unexamined impressions that speak for themselves but are strong, complete, detailed documentation that includes the interpretive material of the researcher's perspectives and values [evaluator's criteria]. (Rossman & Rallis, 2017, p. 153)

Finally, evaluators analyze and interpret the data in relation to the focus of the evaluation: What do these words, actions, or images mean for the program? Because the evaluator is so integral to the process, the concept of trustworthiness is essential to the discussion. Rossman and Rallis (2017) ask two inextricably linked questions in relation to whether a study is trustworthy: Is the study conducted in a competent manner and Is the study conducted ethically? Both are required to discover and tell a credible story.

When conducting a qualitative evaluation, data collection and generation, analysis, and interpretation are distinct activities but are woven together in an iterative fashion. As data are accumulated, it is essential to reflect upon what the data represent before moving to the next step. For instance, do the data represent a policymaker's "ideal" or the client's plan—or do they explain what is actually happening in the field? Whose reality do they illuminate? Do they represent an authentic need? Do the "numbers" make sense? Put simply, what story are the data telling? Finally, what additional information is needed to answer the evaluation question(s) and what are the most appropriate ways to obtain those data?

Although iterative, an explicit data management plan is essential as an evaluator thinks about the implementation of a sound evaluation. Consistent with how the evaluation is framed, information must be gathered from specific sources in an intentional manner to credibly discover the story. The chart found in Table 15.1 is drawn from a study that explores the effects of teacher training on special education referrals and illustrates how a plan aligns questions with information on data gathering activities, materials needed, and expected costs (see Bickman, Chapter 21, this volume, for more details on estimating costs and budgets). Although plans generally include numbers, they are collected for the purpose of describing and are not intended for statistical analysis. Estimating costs ensures that your design is feasible given your funding.

The most common techniques for generating qualitative data are interviews, focus groups, observations, surveys, and documents or artifacts. Each is used in an evaluation for a specific purpose—however, data management plans commonly incorporate more than one of these techniques as they may complement each other and/or provide different perspectives of what is happening in a program. While we introduce these common methods, covering each technique fully in a chapter on design is impossible. To learn the details of each method, we recommend referring to specific publications that focus on individual techniques. The American Evaluation Association is an excellent source for the most complete and up-to-date evaluation approaches. Our intent is to offer you what you are unlikely to find in these references—summaries and tips drawn from our own evaluation experiences that can help you plan ahead. Knowing what these strategies involve can help you choose and can prepare you to include sufficient time to generate appropriate data and to schedule appropriate locations to find relevant documents or artifacts.

Interviews

One-on-one interviews are conducted with individuals specifically selected for their perspectives or knowledge of some aspect of the program. That knowledge can be positive or negative. For instance, if the evaluation seeks to understand the program from the participants' lens, interviews with people who have had negative experiences are as valuable as interviews with people who rave about the endeavor; we also include nonparticipants who either support or oppose the program for one reason or another. Indeed, we almost always seek contrary views of a program so we can get a balance of viewpoints. Likewise, if the evaluation is formative for program improvement, the various perspectives of staff members can reveal sides of the program not visible to participants. For example, when generating data in schools, we always find time to talk with secretaries or others at the school who often have the backstory of a situation. Use your evaluation focus and questions to guide your selection of individuals to interview.

Conducting effective interviews is not always what is taught. Students and new evaluators often spend an inordinate amount of time crafting the perfect questions—making sure their grammar is perfect and their word choice is exact and consistent with the theory of change associated with the program under evaluation. They approach the task much like human resource personnel recommend when conducting job interviews: Ask everyone the exact same *perfect* questions to avoid showing favoritism to one person or another. In other words, evaluators want to do the tasks associated with *their* job perfectly. Unfortunately, this approach is focused in the wrong direction.

What is essential is establishing the right atmosphere for a conversation. People are willing to tell their stories or describe their experiences when they feel that the other person is open to understanding their perspective, whatever it may be. Settings that allow for this sharing tend to be friendly, informal, and nonthreatening. You are engaging people in a conversation, not subjecting them to a barrage of questions. Remember the first and second principles of conducting any ethical study: respect for persons and beneficence. Do your best to create a safe space for people to voluntarily open up and share their thoughts without fear of being judged or misinterpreted. Consider choosing a location for interviews where power dynamics won't be in play (such as a coffee shop). Consider concerns such as: Do you appear to bring a set agenda or are you open to alternatives? How might participants fear harm from your report?

Becoming an effective interviewer means doing your homework on the program and the evaluation context. In addition to reading formal documents, it is critical to consider political and environmental factors that may influence

TABLE 15.1. Sample Management Plan

Evaluation questions	Data collection tasks in five schools (evidence sources)	Responsible personnel	Dates	Materials needed	Associated costs
Intervention: Have teachers been trained? Scope of the training—who and how many Timeframe of the training Nature of the training (state of art)	Review of training curriculum Review of implementation records	RA	5 half-days in January	Checklists Computer	2.5 days at RA cost = $ Computer already owned
Application: How have teachers used the assessment and intervention strategies they learned in training?	Observations of classroom practices and materials	PI and RA	10 days each in February and March	Protocols based on training curriculum	10 days at PI cost = $ 10 days at RA cost = $ Travel (X miles × cost/mile) = $
Outcome: How is student learning performance improving?	Review of teacher-assigned student work; teacher tests; performance measures of student work	PI and RA	10 days each in February and March (same as above)	Protocols based on training curriculum	(See row above)
Effect: What changes have occurred in special education referrals? Number and percentages of referrals Reasons for referrals	Review of school records Interviews with principal and counselor(s)	RA PI and RA	5 half days in April 5 days each in April	Checklists Computer Interview guides Digital tape recorder	2.5 days at PI cost = $ 7.5 days at RA cost = $ Digital tape recorder = $
Capacity building: Has regional capacity for improvement been built? Evidence of new collaborative programs and materials Evidence of new opportunities for joint planning	Review of records Interviews with key interest holders (e.g., principals, superintendent, regional professional development staff)	PI and RA	5 days in April (same as above)	Checklists Computer interview guides Digital tape recorder	(See row above)

the program. Who are the "players" and where does the power lie—and how is power exerted? Whose interests are represented in the program design? Why was this particular community selected?

Being an effective interviewer also takes intention and is developed through experience. Of utmost importance is working with a curious and open mind-set. You are talking with the interviewees because they possess specific information based on their experiences about the program. You want to learn what they know. Put simply, you enter the interview with the assumption that the person has an important and distinctive way of experiencing and interpreting events, activities, interactions, and relationships. Your job is to discover those unique perspectives.

Certainly, the evaluator must have a deep sense of where the interview needs to go to make sure that all the appropriate questions/topics are explored. In many respects, that's the easy part because if you know what you want to cover, you can engage in an authentic conversation. To get their unique perspectives, however, building relationships with the participants is crucial, focusing on their words so you know when to ask follow-up questions, to clarify responses or words chosen, or to probe an undeveloped idea. You are aware of body language to assess how the conversation is unfolding. Does a question evoke a natural willing response? Or does the participant seem to withdraw? Or become confused or defensive? Attending to the participant's reactions, as you would in any interesting conversation, allows you to engage the participant in a conversation they *want* to be part of. In essence, an effective interview is an intense activity conducted under the guise of casualness. The only way to accomplish this is to be laser focused on the participant, not on yourself.

Consider using a variety of prompts during an interview. Photographs can trigger thoughts and memories. Journaling or asking people to write their thoughts is a particularly respectful way to engage individuals who are introverted or quiet. Using art and creative activities can allow the person you are interviewing to express and expand on ideas they may not be able to access verbally. Even people who do not consider themselves artists can voice their thoughts cogently as they are drawing something.

No matter how well prepared you may be, you can expect to face several challenges that are inherent in the interviewing process: participants can go off on what you, the evaluator, consider to be a tangent; they can misrepresent what was supposed to happen in a program; they can be disrespectful of staff or of the program purposes; and some can be just plain obnoxious. These situations are not times to become defensive or discount what the participant portrays. Keep in mind that their words and behaviors are still data that contribute to the story. Knowing the program theory helps you to respond respectfully, probing and asking for clarification to explore factors underlying these responses.

Similarly, because interviews generate data, you are already analyzing what you hear. At times, responses can make you question whether the participant is being truthful. Sometimes participants misrepresent events or actions intentionally for a reason, and you are challenged to unpack those reasons. Other times, what seems untrue is really how individuals make sense of their experiences. It is best to start with the assumption that whatever your participants are telling you is *their* truth. You may not agree with—or even understand—how they arrived at their thoughts or decisions. Again, you engage with individuals to discover how an idea makes sense to them and what it might mean for the program. Some questions that might help you explore in a nonthreatening manner are "Help me understand what you mean by . . ."; "There are lots of definitions of . . . but what do you mean when you say . . . ?"; and "I know how I think about . . . but I would like to hear your understanding of it." These questions acknowledge that among the different ways to interpret something, what you want to know is how that person interprets it.

Location can also influence responses. To illustrate, we relate our experience evaluating a medical training program. We suspected that nurses and doctors might have different views about their experiences with training events, so we scheduled the interviews on different days in the hospital. We assumed that talking with nurses near where they worked on the floors would be most natural—and thus, most comfortable. During initial interviews we sensed tension as the nurses gave what seemed to us hyperbolic praise for the program: They emphasized that they needed the knowledge and skills and that they used what they learned regularly. When asked for specifics, their responses came directly from what we had read in the training manuals. At one point a nurse commented that we could just wait to ask the doctors when they came to the floors. We realized that the nurses might not feel they could talk freely there, so we moved the location to the visitor coffee shop where doctors seldom came. The conversations with the nurses about the training changed substantively.

Although we emphasize accepting that people have unique perspectives about any situation, a word of caution is in order. People often make trite statements or use platitudes because to do otherwise might be considered inappropriate or, to use a cliché, *politically incorrect*. Examples can be found in every field but an example in education is the overused statement that "all students can learn" regardless of their circumstances. When the evaluator has a sense that the person is simply restating what is expected, probing to explore the issue from a different angle is essential. Another way to break through banal statements is through other sources of data, particularly observations, which is described after a discussion of focus groups.

Focus Groups

Unlike interviews that provide a window into the thinking of an individual, focus groups allow evaluators to capture how thoughts are socially—that is, collectively—developed. Many of the same principles associated with interviews (e.g., establishing a safe space and not judging) apply. What differs is that in focus groups participants share and develop ideas through their interactions; they refine their thinking by bouncing ideas off of one another. An effective evaluator facilitates interaction among the members around the topic discussion rather than ticking off a series of questions that everyone answers separately. Through rich dialogue, responses evolve as individuals build on the ideas of others in the group. In addition to building and developing ideas collectively, focus groups can also uncover nuanced variations in how individuals think about or experience something. This process can be particularly valuable when conducting a formative evaluation for program improvement because focus groups often gen-erate new ideas. For example, a program in its formative stages is often vaguely or even poorly designed. Focus groups provide an opportunity for those involved to clarify together details in their theories of action.

The challenge to focus group success comes when power dynamics are at play. Thus, as you construct the focus group experience, be aware of potential power differences. Bauer and Abma (2014) describe creating *homogeneous* (focus) groups with people who share similar experiences as a means of allowing the group to develop their ideas collectively in a safe environment. Then, following idea generation among similar individuals, facilitated discussions among the homogeneous groups as a *heterogeneous* group (consisting of members from each of the individual homogeneous groups) can take place. In this way, individuals with less *voice* or power can speak their truths and share their ideas with others who hold greater perceived power. For example, focus groups conducted in schools can initially involve separate homogeneous groups of teachers, parents, students, or administrators, depending upon the issue at hand. Once each group has formulated their ideas, members from the different groups can meet together as a heterogeneous group. Students or parents can present their ideas first, as typically they have the least amount of "power" in the school. They can be followed by teachers and finally administrators, who typically hold the most power.

Of course, focus groups are not for every situation. Some individuals, particularly those who are introverted, quiet, or have anxieties about speaking in a group, can be reluctant to share their thoughts in a group. A related problem can occur if one or two individuals dominate the focus group discussion. To avoid these problems, focus groups must be carefully constructed and facilitated by people who have knowledge about the individuals invited to the focus group.

Observations

Intentionally incorporating observations in evaluations is often overlooked for fear that observations are too subjective for a rigorous evaluation. To avoid this subjectivity, some evaluators use **rubrics** for observations, particularly in K–12 educational settings. Rubrics that consist of checking off a predetermined list of items or actions that should be seen in a program can limit the value of the data and are considered more quantitative than qualitative. In contrast, observations that document what people do (often called field notes) can provide critical clues about the unfolding story of the program. The most obvious way observations are used in an evaluation is to describe the physical setting of a program, and what staff and participants see while they are part of the program. The external environment can also offer vital information for programs designed to address community issues. For example, a needle-exchange program implemented at a research hospital is quite different from the exact same needle-exchange program implemented in a struggling clinic in a resource-deprived urban area. Neither of these should be confused with the same program being implemented in a tight-knit rural community. In discovering and portraying the story of this program, context matters.

Observations can provide insight into the various relationships operating in the program. Interactions among staff members shed light on how the program functions and indicate strengths and weaknesses in organizational decision making and problem solving. Seeing how people interact provides insight into power dimensions and why participants describe their experiences in a particular way. Reactions when outsiders enter the setting can be very revealing. As the evaluator, your presence can affect behaviors. The more familiar you become in the setting, the less people react to you as external—thus, be sure to plan for enough time in the field to avoid being the focus of attention.

Observations can triangulate other data, both by complementing information gathered during an interview or focus group or by challenging it. The following are examples of each. In a districtwide alternative professional development program, teachers received salary credit for courses that were directly related to the subjects they taught. The metalworks/welding teacher in the vocational high school took a course in blacksmithing that he claimed informed his teaching. Based on his description of his urban students, we had doubts that the course was directly related; we could not imagine that he had a forge installed in the room. Had he simply taken a course for his own interests? Then we visited the high school and saw the students at work. While no actual forge was visible, he showed us a firepot set and smithing tools. When students showed us objects they had made—items they could actually use such as lamps and bike parts, our reaction was "Now I see—I get it!" Seeing made us believers.

In another case that involved psychological services for women inmates, our observations supported changes to improve cultural competence. While interviewing therapists about handling client disclosures of discrimination, we heard them say, "We can't help these women." We wondered what was actually going on. Then, observing sessions revealed the cultural context and that the therapists were not trained to serve this inmate population. The descriptions we took to program leaders fostered insights into specific areas where training was needed.

An example of how observations can challenge other data occurred during an evaluation of safety strategies implemented at a public middle school with a documented history of bullying. During an interview, the principal was proud to explain how the learning of all of the students had improved because of the safety measures that had been implemented. The impression was that the strategies had allowed the school to realize its stated mission of being a safe place where all students could learn and thrive. After the interview, we walked the hallways to see cameras that had been strategically placed throughout the building. While walking, the principal kept pointing out various students who came from "bad families and were destined to go nowhere in life" or were "troublemakers." Particularly notable during our walk through the hallways filled with students was that the principal made no references to students developing their potential to thrive as described in the interview. This observation of an apparent disconnect between the principal's response to questions and his behavior in the hallway caused us to probe more deeply in subsequent interviews. For instance, we asked questions about how the improved learning could be the result of the safety measures that had been implemented. We also asked about what messages teachers and administrators used to reinforce that all students could be successful at the school. This example illustrates how the evaluator makes sense of the data while collecting and adjusts accordingly.

Surveys

We often think of surveys as quantitative data, but there are ways to obtain rich qualitative data by surveying a large number of respondents. Asking people to rate their answers on a scale or ask them the degree to which they agree or disagree can provide more nuance than questions with yes or no or other binary response choices. Surveys are much more directed than **open-ended questions** that allow participants to choose their own words in their responses. Open-ended questions can be embedded in a survey to allow participants to share in a sentence or short paragraph their personal thoughts beyond specific survey questions. This can be tricky, however, because it is fairly common for respondents to write in one- or two-word answers that provide little more information than the survey response. When responses are long and many, analysis can be time-consuming.

Another issue particularly important to consider when administering surveys is timing. Unlike an interview or focus group that is interactive, allowing you to gauge responses and ask follow-up questions, surveys are administered with little or no personal interaction. The findings capture the participants' feelings at the time of the survey, opinions that may or may not be relevant for the evaluation in the long run. A dramatic example for us was a case where our program was being evaluated—we were the focus of the evaluation. The ministry of education in an embattled country contracted us to transform the faculty mind-set and instruction from teacher centered to learner centered. Our program theory of change was *If we model learner-centered instruction whereby teachers learn and use action research in the workshops, they will understand and become learner-centered instructors in their classes.* The evaluators administered a **Level 1 questionnaire** (often called *smiley face*) to capture faculty reaction immediately following the first workshop (see Kirkpatrick, 1996). Participants' reactions were uniformly negative: "You did not tell us how to do it [learner-centered instruction]"; and "We needed you to give us directive steps to follow." We were concerned until we returned for the follow-up workshop during which the teachers would present and discuss their action research. Remarkably, we were greeted with hugs and smiles—and many thanks. Once they had a chance to put their learning into practice in their classrooms, they understood and appreciated what they had learned and how we had taught it. Clearly, telling the story of this program called for more than the initial survey.

Documents and Artifacts

Your evaluation design should include existing material that contributes to the story the program tells. Written material can be in many forms: formal, semiformal, or informal. Formal documents (e.g., proposals, handbooks, technical manuals) are most often used to describe how a program has been designed: the goals, objectives, implementation plan, evaluation, budget, and so on. These formal documents serve as baseline information for understanding the initial intent of any program. Similarly, meeting agendas and minutes, as well as formal correspondence, provide insight into the formal implementation of a program. Semiformal written documentation (e.g., email, Twitter [now known as X], Facebook, and other social media) can shed additional light on program implementation and internal communication and reveal alternative views of what is happening. Care must be taken, however, because although social media is technically public information, many individuals consider it private communication, particularly if the content is sensitive.

MAKING SENSE OF THE STORY: ANALYSIS AND INTERPRETATION

As we stated in the previous section, "Discovering the Story," data gathering and analysis, while separate activities, are interwoven. You move back and forth between the two because making sense of qualitative data requires both **deductive and inductive thinking**. The program goals and logic guide your deductive thinking—that is, to begin the evaluation, an agreed-upon program/intervention is understood to have a stated goal and specific objectives; that understanding serves as the purpose of the evaluation. Thus, you do not enter the field with a blank mind. Your inductive reasoning begins when you are actually in the field, looking at and listening to the data. In other words, initially, you have a theory of what is happening; as soon as you interact with the data, you begin to draw a picture and construct a story that shapes and elaborates the ideas you brought in with you. Saldaña (2015) develops the interaction in more detail, adding further reasoning:

- Deduction—you have an idea of what you are looking for (*program theory*).
- Abduction—examining the possibilities and selecting those you want to pay attention to (*purpose and focus*).
- Induction—discovering what is going on in what you see and hear (*data collection and generation and analysis*).
- Retroduction—reconstructing what happened (*telling the story*). (pp. 22–23, emphasis added)

The process is both sequential and iterative: You follow steps and recursively revisit your decisions as you learn more. The theory and data inform each other.

This analytic, interpretive process is not magic. Themes or findings do not emerge as if you can wave a wand—rather, a more apt metaphor is a puzzle. You question and name (code) and group (categorize) the individual pieces (data), trying out ways to fit them together into patterns (themes) that ultimately form a coherent whole (the story). To be credible, your story also shows how your data became the patterns that informed your findings; your readers have to know how you discovered the story. Credibility can be established by (1) documenting each decision and (2) providing **thick descriptions** (Geertz, 1973) that allow your readers to see what you see.

As you analyze your data, you will make decisions both large and small. Essential to making sense of the data are the *criteria* you use to place meaning or value on particular data. Each criterion represents a principle or standard by which something may be judged or decided. These must be made transparent so that your readers can make their own judgments. Your entire reasoning process reflects the program logic that you have articulated with the relevant program personnel.

Building transparency is grounded in your design, which details what you are doing, why, and with whom. This program logic directs the sequencing of questions and discovery. Figure 15.2 offers an example of a program logic that was developed for an evaluation of a state-level intervention to improve primary-grade teachers' skills in assessing and addressing student reading needs through knowledge of instructional strategies and tools. The intervention, a *best-practices* training, was chosen in response to an identified problem: referrals to special education of students in grades K–2 exceeded percentages set in federal guidelines. The rationale of the state education leadership was that because these early-grade teachers had not been adequately trained to teach reading skills to their students, they referred students who were slow to read to special education. The design recognized that several action steps must be completed (and evaluated) before the final outcome could be considered.

The matrix reveals how data gathering and preliminary analyses (i.e., beginning to put the pieces of the puzzle together) are interwoven, deductively and inductively. What the design does not reveal are the many steps/actions you take to manage your data to support your analyses and findings. Keeping data organized and accessible facilitates your process—and, importantly, serves as an audit trail to support the credibility of your findings. Each piece of data is labeled and stored. If your data sources are large and/or numerous, you probably want to use data management software[1] (which, by the way, do not analyze the data for you!). Creating a log of each date and the amount of time spent in the field—or among documents—is critical to record specific activities, noting the date, what you did, names, times, and places. As soon as possible, clean up your observations that have been reported as field notes and transcribe interviews. "Consider creating tables or matrices to record and store data according to research questions, initial codes or categories, theoretical perspectives, dates, or any other organizing tactic" (Rossman & Rallis, 2017, p. 230).

Organizing your data in a timely manner helps you find connections among the individual sources. This facilitates **coding** and subsequently sorting data into categories. Each code

---
[1] Examples of qualitative data management software: Atlas.ti, NVivo, MAXQDA, Dedoose, and others.

Theory of change: If teachers are trained in reading strategies and then use the strategies to address student needs, their instruction will improve student reading performance, thus reducing the need for inappropriate referrals to special education.			
Objective-based activity	Evaluation question	Data source for evidence	Criteria for analysis
Delivery of training	1. Were teachers trained according to plan (see criteria for analysis)?	Training records and observations	X number of relevant teachers are trained The curriculum is consistent with *best practices* Fidelity to the curriculum Readiness/engagement of participants
Teachers' use of assessment tools and instruction strategies learned in training	2. How do teachers use tools and strategies learned during the training in their instruction?	Observations and review of class practices and materials	Instructional practices/materials used in classes align with training
Student performance and learning in reading	3. Is there evidence of improved student performance and learning?	Review of student work, tests, and relevant performance measures	Student work aligns with strategies taught in training Improvement in reading skills and performance
Teachers' decisions regarding special education referrals	4. What changes occurred in special education referrals? 5. To what do teachers attribute these changes?	School records of referral number, percentages, and documented reasons Teacher interviews or surveys	Referrals decrease Teachers report confidence in addressing student reading needs due to training

FIGURE 15.2. Example of program logic matrix.

must convey meaning. "A code . . . is . . . a word or short phrase that symbolically assigns a summative, salient, essence-capturing, and/or evocative attribute for a portion [of your] . . . data" (Saldaña, 2015, p. 3). Codes do not occur naturally; they do not emerge or sprout. You deliberately decide upon codes based on your deductive–inductive reasoning. It is essential to refer regularly to the program logic, which can inform and shape preliminary codes and categories. Keep the evaluation questions in mind. Remember what the intervention is supposed to do. Above all, be open to insights and alternatives.

The coded data are grouped into particular categories that, again, are often generated from the program theory and logic. Note that the same piece of data may fall into more than one category. For instance, in an evaluation of a college-readiness program, students described the college visits as simultaneous hopes and fears of leaving home, being on their own, and pursuing their dreams. Initially these statements were coded under "possibilities," "apprehensions," and "transition" because we were not sure how the rest of the data would play out. As more data were analyzed, the codes became clearer.

As you immerse yourself in the data, you will begin to see patterns—sets of characteristics, traits, or activities distinctly arranged or organized according to some rule that identifies them as a discreet meaningful phenomenon—what quantitative researchers call a variable. Patterns are observed—as you see them in the data, you interpret and begin to construct themes.

> Since a theme implies some claim or assertion as a result of the process, themes take the form of a declarative statement describing a process, a connection, or an insight. Think of a theme as an abstraction that explains the pattern you see in or across categories. In a theme, you often state an argument regarding your interpretation. (Rossman & Rallis, 2017, p. 240)

The **theme** conveys a learning, a finding. What learning does the theme convey? What surprises? What makes the theme worth presenting? In the college-readiness example above, the theme became "roller coaster of emotions" associated with college visits.

Because themes do not emerge magically nor are they produced through a preconfigured procedure, as in quantitative analysis, you want to show the systematic process you engaged to find the theme—so, when you present a theme or preliminary finding, you will consider and state the following:

- What evidence supports this finding? What data contributed to its formation?
- How are you representing the theme/finding? Will others (participants, funders) see it as you do?
- How does this finding relate to the questions and the program theory?
- What alternative interpretation might exist?

We want to make note of the mental energy and time each recursive step in this process takes. Indeed, time is often cited as a reason to avoid choosing an evaluation approach that relies on direct interaction with participants. Perhaps the more relevant question to ask is "What is the purpose of the evaluation?" If it is simply to comply with a demand from a funder, collecting and analyzing qualitative data are a lot of work. If the evaluation aims to produce credible and actionable knowledge as a basis for learning, any methodology will take considerable time and mental energy.

Throughout the analysis process, you will become deeply immersed in interview transcripts, field notes, and other materials you have collected. The notes you write and the quotes you capture all contribute to what is referred to as **thick description** (Geertz, 1973), which fully details the physical surroundings, the nature of the actions or events taking place, the time, effects of actions, the people present and involved, words spoken, and interactions. "This deep description generates insights that lead to identifying patterns and can suggest or hint at intentions and meaning. Thick description makes analysis and interpretation possible, and it allows your readers to see what you see" (Rossman & Rallis, 2017, p. 233).

As you get deep into analysis and develop thick descriptions of what is happening in the program, we encourage you to engage in ethical reasoning. Ethics are moral principles that guide your practice. Remember, you are the one who gathered the data, you organized it, you assigned codes and identified patterns, and you wrote the thick descriptions included in your findings. You are the intermediary between the people directly associated with the program and those who want to know about the program. This actually is a perilous position, in large part because of the initial evaluation design and the question posed at that point: *Whose story is it?* It is not your story; it is the program story. In telling the story, ask yourself, In what ways am I demonstrating respect for the people related to the program?; How might the evaluation benefit them?; How might it harm them?; Has the evaluation been designed and conducted in fairness and justice to all involved?; What evidence do I have that I am capturing the appropriate voices?; and Have I reflected the various, multiple perspectives that contribute to the story of the program?

The following example of an ethical lapse resulted in serious damage to almost all parties involved, including the institution. The focus of a dissertation was an evaluation of a reading program conducted in a chronically underperforming elementary school located in an economically disadvantaged community. Throughout the findings, the teacher was described as engaged in *learned helplessness*. Upon reading the final (and approved) dissertation, this teacher was horrified; she believed her words and actions had been misrepresented and misinterpreted. The teacher filed a complaint with the institutional review board (IRB) that the teacher's professional reputation had been compromised with the publication of the dissertation. The IRB concurred—with a great deal of fallout.

The problem was that the researcher/evaluator did not thickly describe the actions and interactions that were occurring in the classroom and at the school; instead, the researcher inserted interpretations in the findings that constituted an opinion about the teacher and not what was actually happening in the classroom.

In essence, it became the story of the researcher, not the story of the classroom.

Disrespect and harm could have been prevented if the ultimate analysis and interpretation had been undertaken with caring reflexivity. Rallis and Rossman (2010) define caring reflexivity as "enacted through relationships that recognize and honor the participants within their specific context" (p. 496). It involves establishing relationships with participants and requires thinking deeply about the ethical considerations at every phase of an evaluation, not just how to gather data but also how those data are analyzed and reported. In our example, rather than the investigator drawing the conclusion that learned helplessness was in evidence and attributing that characteristic to the teacher, thick descriptions could have illustrated what the teacher was doing, with a focus on the repeated obstacles encountered and the attempts to overcome the obstacles. The interpretations could have been explored with the teacher. The conclusion could have indicated that this is how learned helplessness may happen, rather than assigning a pejorative label to someone as their professional practice is described.

Rallis (2010) describes the effort involved in building these relationships with participants:

> I always share my drafts with my participants (qualitative researchers generally do not call the people in their studies subjects) as a validity check. The process is referred to as member checks—not so that members can change the results but so that the researcher can ensure that her interpretations are ones others share.
>
> Yes, this takes time. Often unbelievable amounts of time. In fact, I recently finished a chapter for *The Sage International Handbook of Educational Evaluation*—the chapter is based on the work of the Superintendents Network, and I must have run 5 or 6 different drafts by them, making many changes—both minor and major—never changing the findings but the way in which I represented them. The final result is one that they and I are deeply pleased with. And we did have a deadline, but the publishers felt it was critical that the chapter offer a trustworthy representation of what actually happened in the network. (p. 445)

In summary, making sense of the story, which includes both analysis and interpretation, is a complex and time-consuming endeavor. Taking shortcuts at this stage can undermine a high-quality and rigorously conducted evaluation.

BRINGING THE STORY TO LIFE

Now that you have gathered and analyzed your data, it is time to think about clearly and transparently constructing the narrative that will portray the program story. This step should not be taken lightly—and also needs **foreshadowing** in a design that has articulated the *what*, *how*, and *why* of the evaluation. You begin the storytelling when you design the evaluation. Qualitative researchers and evaluators are often criticized for drawing conclusions from a series of quotations or descriptions without explaining or supporting their conclusions. The story is only credible if it is grounded in the reality of the program that is recognizable to the program participants. As you approach telling the story the question to ask is: Can the reader not only see and hear what you, as the evaluator, saw and heard, but can the reader follow your logic in reaching your conclusions? This question is important because your findings matter; they can affect people's lives and can influence public policy.

Before tackling creative reporting approaches, we focus on the content of the narrative. Erickson (1986) offers a practical outline to guide meaningful evaluation reporting that incorporates qualitative data—or mixed methods using both qualitative and quantitative data. His outline is posed in four questions:

1. What is happening?
2. What does this mean to the participants?
3. What patterns are in evidence?
4. How does it connect to larger issues?

For many evaluations, the first question, What is happening? might more aptly be stated as What is supposed to happen (the plan)?; What really happens (the reality)?; and What factors contribute to the discrepancy (the why)? Formal documents are used to describe what *should* be happening in the program. Funding proposals outline the project, with goals, objectives, an implementation plan, staffing plans, evaluation plans, and a detailed budget that describes how funds are allocated to various parts of the program. If available, handbooks or technical manuals provide details about the implementation activities.

While these documents provide a description of what should happen, actual implementation rarely follows the formal plan without deviation. In many cases, the program is better for its departure from what was proposed; understanding why things changed and whether data guiding the changes are important for making sense of the program. In fact, your data may question whether the proposed efforts actually serve those they were meant to. Here is where we draw on the thick descriptions of what you hear in interviews and/or focus groups as well as what you see in the field. They provide the evidence that tells the story.

If the program is implemented more or less as planned, the nuances between what is planned can be interspersed with the nuances of what happens. It is important, however, to clearly distinguish between the two and provide thick descriptions (with reference to the appropriate data sources) about the differences. On the other hand, if what occurs differs greatly from what is planned, you may have two narratives, with detailed analyses of where the differences happen and why.

You may encounter incidences where funders demand fidelity to the initial design without consideration of changes during implementation. This puts an evaluator in a difficult position. Your challenge as evaluator is to determine whether the funder is genuinely committed to a meaningful evaluation—that is, an evaluation that tells the story of what actually happened during implementation.

Next, Erickson's (1986) questions address perspective: What does this mean to the participants? This is where using caring reflexivity (Rallis & Rossman, 2010) is important. Indeed, Erickson's question might be rephrased, How would they (e.g., participants, staff, others) describe what is happening to them? This too comes from the thick descriptions of the analysis of interviews and focus groups. The benefit of the third question (What patterns are in evidence?) is obvious because it encourages you to move beyond the details and look for the patterns.

Finally, the question of how the actions and patterns connect to larger issues brings you back to why you are spending all of this time with these data—the evaluation and the story the program has to tell. After all, evaluations are not conducted as basic or applied science primarily to contribute to the general body of knowledge. Evaluations are conducted because people are sufficiently concerned about an issue or situation so they take the time and energy to design and implement a specific program or intervention. Evaluations are conducted because people participate in the intervention, usually to improve their lives. Evaluations are conducted because others may want to appropriately (considering context) learn and replicate programs and interventions that demonstrate positive results. Therefore, the final question to be addressed is how the program story can be used (see Alkin & Vo, Chapter 8, this volume).

Use of evaluation findings seldom just happens. As Michael Patton (2008), who wrote an entire book on *utilization-focused evaluation* argues, use is both a mandate and a challenge. Whatever the reason that motivated your evaluation, whatever approach you chose, you will produce findings. You want interest holders to use what the evaluation discovers, to take some action based on the evidence produced. Yet, how often are findings conveyed in inaccessible formats—or not seen as meaningful? How many evaluation reports sit on shelves, unread? We encourage you to plan for use from the start, as you design, as you build relationships in the field, as you make sense of the data, and as you communicate what you learned. Three questions can help you facilitate use throughout the process: *What is the message? Who needs to hear?* and *How can the story be told to inspire action?*

While you cannot know in advance what you will learn, you do know the purposes of the evaluation. We refer to purpose in the plural because different people or groups involved with the program bring varying interests. The purposes and program theory not only guide your data gathering and analyses, they also indicate who cares and why and what types of findings they might expect. So, you continually revisit the message and the audience. For example, Do people hope to learn program strengths and weaknesses so they might make changes for improvement? Are they more concerned with whether the program was implemented with fidelity? Do they need evidence to inform decisions about program continuance (a high-stakes situation)? Do some want the findings to influence how key people—policymakers, foundations, agencies, funders—think about the program or issues related to the program? Or, is the evaluation conducted merely because it is required? Considering both expressed purposes along with other possible purposes can shape your relationships and guide your inquiry along the way.

As you make sense of the data, the message becomes clear; you discover the story. You also discover people who need to hear the story. The *who* is anyone who cares about or needs to act upon the issues related to the program or policy. The *who* could be funders, policymakers, concerned community members, staff, and participants, just to name a few. These people are both players in the story and audiences for the story.

One evaluation where we were present from the proposal writing illustrates how programs develop over time, often with changing purposes and changing players (see Lawrence et al., 2018). The proposed program was a complex and ambitious plan that aspired to build the capacity of teachers in a state's public charter schools to serve English language learners (ELLs) and students with disabilities (SWDs). A nongovernmental agency wrote the proposal and was in charge of its implementation. How exactly the program would do this was ambiguous because the proposal was written to please several groups: the funder, the agency leadership, state education department, and the schools. The agency hired personnel to coordinate and deliver services. Meanwhile, the original authors of the proposal left the agency and new people were hired. As evaluators, we watched program leadership and practitioners struggle with what activities and services best met the schools' and teachers' needs—and witnessed the evaluation purposes change from summative to formative to developmental. We continued to conduct interviews and observations as planned; what we did with the data changed. We used the data as a source of ongoing feedback to the directors to discuss what the data meant and what changes needed to be made. The program evolved. The story that unfolded was an affirmation of the knowledge, skills, and willingness to learn by both the program providers and the professionals in the charter schools. The program leaders learned how to provide what the teachers needed, and the teachers did build capacity to serve ELLs and SWDs. The agency leadership determined to capture the story in a "white paper" to be written collaboratively by the directors and evaluators and disseminated widely. We believe this story contributed to changes in attitudes toward charter school teaching in the state.

This example also illustrates how the evaluation process itself can inspire action and how findings can be communicated to facilitate use. The most common way to tell the story is through a written evaluation report. Particularly for programs that are funded either though public (governmental) or private (foundation or corporate) sources, a written report is required. These written reports generally follow fairly specific guidelines and expectations—but do not have to be dry or boring! The power of the story depends on how deeply the reader can be absorbed into the story: The more engaged the reader, the greater the influence the story has on the reader's real-world beliefs (Green & Brock, 2000). In essence, the story transports the reader into the narrative world, thus altering the reader's perspective. Thick descriptions can be a very powerful means of bringing the story to life.

Sometimes a traditional written report is not the best way to represent the story. Face-to-face meetings where the evaluator can display and discuss findings is often effective. Photographs can be used much like observations conducted during data generation—as a substitute for words to describe the physical setting of the program, how program participants interact with staff members, or the expressions of program participants as they engage in program activities. (Do not forget to obtain permission if you use photographs of people.) Graphics can be used to support the story; they can be used to display timelines associated with qualitative data: what happened when, where deviations occurred (and why), and how adjustments were made.

In some situations, the story can be told verbally. This might be particularly helpful for a formative evaluation that is designed for program improvement. The story can be told (from a basic script or PowerPoint) with time allowed for discussion and brainstorming. Likewise, a preliminary report can be told verbally to program participants as a means of member checking to make sure you have captured the details of the experiences from their lens. Sometimes a story is best told through performance. An evaluation of a poetry writing workshop conducted in a women's prison was "reported" by the women reading their poems and describing how writing affected their individual sense of self. Final decisions about how to communicate findings do not need to be made until you have the findings. Still, thinking ahead about and with potential audiences can open possibilities for effective ways to tell the program story.

SUMMARY AND CONCLUSION

We began the journey of this chapter with the argument that an evaluator's responsibility is to generate and tell the program story. The story is neither random nor haphazard. Developing a credible program story is a systematic, criteria-guided process that demands ethical considerations throughout. To learn the details of specific techniques for conducting an evaluation, we direct you to appropriate resources; our intent in this chapter has been to share our own, usually unwritten *lessons learned*, having conducted countless evaluations, often in highly complex—and sometimes contentious—situations.

You begin the process by focusing the purpose of your evaluation. While the purpose may change as the evaluation progresses, purpose suggests approach and thus it is your starting point. Will it be developmental, formative, or summative? If it is a long-term project, will the evaluation have multiple purposes? For example, it could start out formative but ultimately want to learn outcomes. Whose voice(s) will be represented? Taking time with relevant interest holders to appropriately frame the evaluation at the outset will save time and frustration, as well as help you avoid ethical missteps in the long run.

The program theory of change is articulated at the outset and guides the design, implementation, and evaluation of the program; the program story unfolds and captures the actions, the actors, and the relationships between the people and the events. Capturing the humanness of a program relies on qualitative methods that involve face-to-face interaction with people and events in the field where decisions are enacted. Only by hearing and seeing what is happening in the actual program context can you, the evaluator, discover the story.

Making sense of the program story is like putting together a jigsaw puzzle without looking at the top of the box. The process requires that you, as evaluator, gather and analyze the pieces of the puzzle (i.e., the data) in an iterative fashion to construct the story that is both true to the people directly involved in the program and can be used by others to affect appropriate change. Deductive and inductive reasoning are involved as you look for patterns in the distinct pieces of data. As with any meaningful process, this takes time and concentrated focus.

> **BOX 15.2. When a Theory of Change Goes Awry**
>
> A state Department of Education discovered that a number of charter schools each had small but significant populations of students with special needs. Reviews of faculty preparation and licensure revealed that few charter schools had teachers who were adequately trained to address the various needs of these students. The state developed a *theory of change*: If they created regional networks and documented the various resources that each school had, expertise could be shared throughout the network, thus reducing the need to replicate resources in each school.
>
> The first step in the *action plan* was to administer a survey at each school to determine existing expertise and resources that could later be shared within the network. The *outcome* of this initial step was that several schools refused to contribute information to the regional database. The evaluators, who regularly employ qualitative methods, observed at regional network meetings that the staff from different schools were not engaging with one another. To generate the data to solve the perplexing puzzle, the evaluators conducted individual interviews with leadership of the various schools in the network. When analyzing the interview data, a clear pattern was identified: Each charter school had been established to reflect a specific ideological stance. The deep differences among the schools made it difficult for staff to share resources among schools that were not aligned philosophically.
>
> After bringing the story to life, the evaluators worked with the state Department of Education personnel to *redesign their action plan* to be more sensitive to the realities of the critical interest holders in this important effort.

Because the data come from people in real-life settings, ethical reasoning is ongoing; decisions about respect, benefits to participants, and justice need to be continually revisited and renewed throughout every phase of the evaluation (see Hemmings, 2006). For example, a place that felt safe and nonjudgmental at one time for an early interview may not remain so at a later time—or feel safe to another person. Also, remember that the story is not yours; it belongs to the people and the program. The question of *whose voice is represented* often gets lost as we make sense both of multiple events and of multiple participants' experiences. Being transparent about decisions and sharing your thick descriptions reveals how you arrived at the story you tell about the program—and thus allows audiences to appraise its credibility and value.

Finally, the primary importance of telling the program's story is to affect change. The story could inspire nearly countless intended and unintended results: specific program improvements; a replicable model to alleviate some form of human suffering; giving voice to groups that are not often heard in public debate; or legitimizing a new method. How the story is told and to whom can make all the difference in how people respond to and use learnings from the evaluation.

In conclusion, a program is designed and implemented for specific purposes. Those purposes are important to the program participants, to the community, and often to the broader public. You, as evaluator, play a critical role in whether all of the time, energy, and effort is heard and acted upon by others. Through qualitative methods, you can help bring the program story to life.

ACKNOWLEDGMENTS

We acknowledge and thank our colleague Ezekiel Kimball for initial conversations during which we framed evaluation as storytelling. We also appreciate the feedback and suggestions Bethany Rallis provided on early drafts.

REFERENCES

Baur, V. E., & Abma, T. A. (2014). Dealing with asymmetric relations between stakeholders: Facilitating dialogue and mutual learning through qualitative inquiry. In L. Goodyear, J. Jewiss, J. Usinger, & E. Barela (Eds.), *Qualitative inquiry in evaluation: From theory to practice* (pp. 167–188). Jossey-Bass.

Brothers, K. B., Rivera, S. M., Cadigan, R. J., Sharp, R. R., & Goldenberg, A. J. (2019). A Belmont reboot: Building a normative foundation for human research in the 21st century. *Journal of Law, Medicine and Ethics, 47*(1), 165–172.

Christensen, J. (2012). Telling stories: Exploring research storytelling as a meaningful approach to knowledge mobilization with Indigenous research collaborators and diverse audiences in community-based participatory research. *Canadian Geographer, 56*(2), 231–242.

Clandinin, D. J., & Connolly, F. M. (2000). *Narrative inquiry: Experience and story in qualitative research*. Jossey-Bass.

Erickson, F. (1986). Qualitative methods in research on teaching. In M. C. Whittrock (Ed.), *Handbook of research on teaching* (3rd ed., pp. 119–161). Macmillan.

Feagin, J. R. (2013). *The White racial frame* (2nd ed.). Routledge.

Geertz, C. (1973). *The interpretation of cultures: Selected essays*. Basic Books.

Green, M. C., & Brock, T. C. (2000). The role of transportation in the persuasiveness of public narratives. *Journal of Personality and Social Psychology, 79*(5), 701.

Hemmings, A. (2006). Great ethical divides: Bridging the gap between institutional review boards and researchers. *Educational Researcher, 35*(4), 12–18.

House, E. R. (2017). Evaluation and the framing of race. *American Journal of Evaluation, 38*(2), 167–189.

Kirkpatrick, D. L. (1996). *Evaluating training programs: The four levels*. Berrett-Koehler.

Lawrence, R. B., Rallis, S. F., Davis, L. C., & Harrington, K. (2018). Developmental evaluation: Bridging the gaps between proposal, program, and practice. *Evaluation, 24*(1), 69–83.

Mason, J. (2002). *Qualitative researching* (2nd ed.). SAGE.

National Commission for the Protection of Human Subjects of Biomedical and Behavioral Research. (1978). *The Belmont report?: Ethical principles and guidelines for the protection of human subjects of research?: Appendix*. Department of Health, Education, and Welfare.

Patton, M. Q. (2008). *Utilization-focused evaluation* (4th ed.). Sage Publications.

Pritchard, I. A. (2021). Framework for the ethical conduct of research: The ethical principles of the Belmont report. In S. Panicker & B. Stanley (Eds.), *Handbook of research ethics in psychological science* (pp. 3–21). American Psychological Association.

Rallis, S. F. (2010). "That is NOT what's happening

at Horizon!": Ethics and misrepresenting knowledge in text. *International Journal of Qualitative Studies in Education, 23*(4), 435–448.

Rallis, S. F., & Rossman, G. B. (2010). Caring reflexivity. In G. B. Rossman & S. F. Rallis (Eds.), *Qualitative Studies in Education: Research Ethics in the Everyday, 23*(4).

Rossman, G. B., & Rallis, S. F. (2017). *An introduction to qualitative research: Learning in the field.* SAGE.

Saldaña, J. (2015). *Thinking qualitatively: Methods of mind.* SAGE.

Seiber, J. E. (2009). Planning ethically responsible research. In L. Bickman & D. J. Rog (Eds.), *The Sage handbook of applied social science research* (pp. 106–140). SAGE.

Tebes, J. K. (2005). Community science, philosophy of science, and the practice of research. *American Journal of Community Psychology, 35*(3–4), 213–230.

Weiss, C. H. (1998). *Evaluation: Methods for studying programs and policies.* Prentice Hall.

Chapter 16

Planning, Data Collection, and Data Preparation for Quantitative Analysis

Erica Harbatkin
Gary T. Henry
Lam D. Pham

CHAPTER OVERVIEW

This chapter addresses planning, data collection, and data preparation for a quantitative program evaluation. The goal of quantitative data collection is to obtain data that are valid, reliable, and credible—such data are essential to conducting a quantitative program evaluation. This chapter covers all aspects of the planning process, beginning with engaging interest holders to obtain and understand quantitative data, determine relevant outcomes, and establish ownership and expectations around data and sample decisions as well as release of findings. This chapter includes a particular focus on analyst considerations for sampling, data, and measures; understanding quantitative data structure; and data screening and cleaning. It provides specific guidelines for data screening in order to help analysts identify missingness and inaccuracies early in the evaluation process to avoid inaccurate or biased results. A common phrase in data analysis is "garbage in, garbage out"—meaning that collecting inaccurate or insufficient data will yield ineffectual results regardless of how rigorous the analytic strategy may be. This is especially salient in the context of program evaluation, where evaluators often have one opportunity to plan for and collect the necessary data. This chapter provides the necessary framework to help evaluators avoid the "garbage-in" part in order to set them up for a rigorous, impactful program evaluation.

This chapter addresses planning, data collection, and data preparation for an evaluation whose primary data are quantitative. Quantitative data and analysis can be marshalled for many different evaluation purposes: to understand the needs and assets of members of a particular group or population, examine a program's implementation, estimate the effects of a program, or identify the mechanisms behind a program's success or failure. The goal of quantitative data collection is to obtain data that are valid, reliable, and credible—terms that we describe in detail later. Generally, obtaining valid and reliable quantitative data requires that the evaluator (1) obtain measures for which there is evidence of validity and reliability prior to the collection of the data for the evaluation, and (2) implement consistent data collection procedures (Rossi et al., 2019). Where qualitative data collection can take on more flexible and adaptive approaches in order to collect data that best represent the experiences of program participants (see Rallis & Usinger, Chapter 15, this volume), a hallmark of quantitative data collection is the consistency of the data collection process, although some qualitative data collection can be consistently collected as well. These differing approaches to data collection underscore differences in the goals of quantitative and qualitative evaluations. Whereas qualitative analysis allows evaluators an opportunity to dive deeply into the experiences of program participants or interest holders but usually limits the number of individuals from whom data are collected and may intentionally vary the data that are collected, quantitative data collection allows evaluators to examine a key set of variables for a population or sample of participants or other interest holders.

Evaluators may conduct quantitative analysis on its own or in combination with qualitative analysis (see Azzam & Jones, Chapter 18, this volume, for a description of designs that combine both approaches). One way to think about the two analytic approaches is that quantitative analysis provides a high-level view of a program often focusing on averages (whether across a population, sample, or subgroups) or trends over time, whereas qualitative analysis can detail the variety of experiences and reactions from a closer and more personal perspective. Quantitative evaluation is most likely to be an appropriate approach if an evaluator is interested in examining the needs of a population or computing the average effect of a program and has access to existing data or the means for consistently collecting original data. In addition, quantitative analysis may be the only viable approach to retrospectively describing a program or estimating its effects using secondary or administrative data collected during the time the program was being implemented.

Before making decisions regarding the most suitable quantitative analytic approach, evaluators must clearly ascertain the purpose of the evaluation. Estimating an overall program effect can be one major purpose of quantitative analysis. An evaluation designed to isolate the effect of a program, policy, or intervention on an outcome of interest to the interest holders is referred to as an **impact evaluation**. Impact evaluations, which answer questions about the extent to which a program is effective on some measure, can be conducted in order to influence decisions about expanding, continuing, or terminating the program or for better understanding of the outcomes of particular subgroups of program participants. Usually, we focus on the impact evaluations' influence on decisions about the program; however, when programs are designed to investigate new approaches to solving a social problem or to better understand the nature of such a problem, impact evaluations can also provide evidence that expands the existing knowledge base and influences decisions about adopting the program in other locations. It is helpful to clearly distinguish between impacts and outcomes. An **outcome** is one of the measures of social conditions that a program is intended to change, or in other cases, a possible unintended consequence. An **impact** is the change in those conditions that can be attributed to the program. In other words, the impact is the program's effect on the outcome of interest. It is possible to conduct an outcome evaluation before the intervention is carried out on, for example, the baseline outcomes. But it is only possible to conduct an impact evaluation after the intervention has taken effect.

In addition to estimating program impacts, quantitative evaluations can have other purposes, including program improvement, outcome monitoring, or assessing program needs (Rossi et al., 2019). **Process evaluations** are designed to assess program operations and implementation in order to help the program improve. **Outcome monitoring** evaluations are designed to inform judgments about program performance in order to help program leaders make management decisions, including whether to modify or even discontinue the program (see also Peck & Snyder, Chapter 13, this volume, on examining outcomes). Finally, quantitative analysis can be conducted as part of a needs assessment to determine the magnitude of the social problem that a program is intended to confront, or the size and other characteristics of the **target population** (i.e., those intended to be served by a program). No matter the type of evaluation or its intended purpose, the quantitative analysis should be designed to meet the highest feasible methodological standards.

Quantitative evaluation data can be used for three types of analyses that relate to the purposes above: exploratory, descriptive, and correlational/causal. The decision about which type of quantitative analysis to conduct is based on the purpose for the evaluation. **Exploratory data analysis** investigates a social problem or situation, often using existing data, including displaying trends over time and applying graphical methods to help visualize data. **Descriptive** analytic methods are used to investigate characteristics of programs, participants, and other relevant program features. Correlational and causal analysis are used to investigate program effects. **Correlational analysis** focuses on estimating the association between two or more variables, including the association between participating in a program and outcomes. **Causal analysis** seeks to establish how a change in one variable (often participation in a program) causes another variable (usually the outcome of interest) to change. The three categories are not **mutually exclusive**, and many quantitative evaluations use multiple analytic techniques at different stages of the evaluation process. For example, an evaluation may describe both a program and its participants (descriptive analysis) as well as estimate its effect (causal analysis). Deciding which analytic strategy or combination of analytic strategies to implement requires evaluators to closely attend to the evaluation purpose and the availability or collectability of data. Pham et al. (Chapter 17, this volume) provide a detailed treatment of each of these evaluation analyses. The goal of this chapter is to prepare the evaluator to plan a quantitative analysis for an evaluation, collect or obtain the data, and prepare the data to carry out the analyses.

In this chapter, we focus on planning and data collection for quantitative analysis and refer readers to Part IV of this volume for more information on planning other aspects of the evaluation. We begin by discussing interest holder engagement, a necessary first consideration before engaging in the evaluation planning process. We proceed by describing evaluation planning for quantitative evaluation, including research design, sampling, and data collection. We then discuss important concepts for understanding the quantitative data for the evaluation—including **data structure**, levels of measurement, and variable distributions—and processes and decisions related to data screening and cleaning. We conclude with a summary of key points.

ENGAGING INTEREST HOLDERS

Ascertaining the purpose of an evaluation often requires evaluators to work in close collaboration with key interest holders while remaining sensitive to the intended purpose and audience for the findings. The evaluation team should collaborate with interest holders to specify key evaluation questions, outline the research design, organize the data acquisition strategy, plan the approach to data analysis, and agree on a plan for communication. Interest holders may include program participants, program staff, policymakers, or others affected by the program. To fully detail these issues and topics, evaluators are encouraged to write evaluation plans at the beginning of the evaluation and to revisit the plan throughout the evaluation process. Evaluators may choose to engage interest holders throughout the process. For example, a change in available data may require a change to the evaluation plan. After schools switched to remote learning at the end of the 2019–2020 school year due to the COVID-19 pandemic, they were no longer required to administer the end-of-grade and end-of-course assessments on which evaluators often rely for student achievement measures. Evaluators of education programs that intended to use these assessments as outcome measures have needed to find alternative approaches to measuring learning during this period or in some cases reconsider the feasibility of including learning outcomes.

Across all evaluation types and purposes, evaluators must remain sensitive to the interests and needs of multiple relevant interest holders. With formative evaluations, interested audiences often comprise program participants, program leaders, managers, and funders who tend to work closely with evaluators throughout the research process in order to produce findings that can be immediately actionable. With summative evaluations, interested audiences may include evaluation sponsors, program management, and the wider communities of scholars and policymakers. Knowledge-generating summative evaluations often involve transparent collaboration between these various interest holders. Indeed, interest holders may play an important role in helping to identify relevant outcomes to measure in the planning stage, helping evaluators to unpack results, describing potential data challenges, and even encouraging participation in data collection activities (see Box 16.1 for an example of such a collaboration in a Michigan school and district turnaround evaluation). Program management may provide input in summative evaluations but quantitative evaluators should remain relatively independent in planning, executing, and reporting the evaluation findings to produce formal findings that are credible when shared with the public and policymakers. An **independent evaluation** is one in which the evaluator is primarily responsible for developing the evaluation questions, conducting the evaluation, and disseminating the results—but it can still involve input from and cooperation with interest holders throughout the process (Rossi et al., 2019). Evaluator independence helps to reduce the risk that evaluation decisions introduce bias into the process and to retain its credibility with diverse audiences interested in the findings. However, maintaining evaluator independence does not require that evaluators

---

BOX 16.1. Michigan's Partnership Model of School and District Turnaround

In 2016–2017 and 2017–2018, the Michigan Department of Education (MDE) identified two cohorts of low-performing schools that it would target for school turnaround. A team of researchers planned an evaluation of this intervention in partnership with program managers at MDE.

Because this project involved a partnership between researchers and state program staff and policymakers, it involved several layers of **interest holder engagement**. Researchers engaged with MDE staff to ensure the research would answer questions that were relevant to them and build trust. Researchers engaged with district leaders, whose support was needed to conduct research with teachers and leaders in their schools. Interest holder conversations occurred at the outset of the project and were also ongoing. When researchers released public-facing reports, they also posted a response from MDE in which program leaders were able to provide their perspective on the findings and describe how they were engaging with the findings (see, e.g., https://epicedpolicy.org/partnership-turnaround-year-four-report for an annual report and MDE response). The early interest holder conversations supported initial planning, including development of a theory of change that would ultimately help to inform the **outcome measures** the research team would collect and create. The ongoing conversations allowed researchers to (1) ask questions about findings (e.g., What was going on in a particular context that the research might be able to look into to explain this effect?), and (2) provide formative feedback to program managers and policymakers about the intervention. For example, program staff drew on research findings in developing program priorities in later years of the intervention.

In the initial planning stage, the research team settled on collecting two types of quantitative data. One would be **secondary data** in the form of statewide administrative data on students and educators in intervention schools and districts as well as other similarly low-performing schools that could serve as a comparison group. This **longitudinal data** allowed researchers to track outcomes over time, from the pre-intervention period through the intervention. The other was **primary data** in the form of surveys to teachers and principals in intervention districts. Researchers elected to administer surveys to the full sample of teachers and principals in intervention districts rather than sampling in order to maximize the sample size. Researchers developed survey items in alignment with the theory of change in order to create both **process measures** and outcome measures that were not available in the administrative data.

Evaluators were able to draw on survey data to answer questions about implementation and outcomes. For example, survey data allowed for **descriptive analysis** of implementation before outcome measures from statewide administrative data were available. Administrative data allowed for both descriptive analysis and **impact evaluation**. Additionally, researchers were able to link administrative and survey data by including a unique identifier in the survey database that was also in the administrative data. Planning for this linkage allowed researchers to combine primary and secondary measures in their analyses—for example, by examining the extent to which school climate (measured using survey data) appeared to be associated with outcomes (measured using administrative data).

Using a difference-in-differences (event study) design (see Pham et al., Chapter 17, this volume, for more on this design), researchers found positive effects of the intervention using the administrative data. Importantly, the survey data allowed them to unpack these results and understand the mechanisms that might have contributed to the positive effects (Burns et al., 2023; Harbatkin et al., 2025).

operate in isolation without engaging interest holders. In fact, interest holders can be valuable partners in gaining access to data and program participants, understanding program context, and interpreting or unpacking the findings from an evaluation (e.g., through informal conversations, presentations, and engagement of expert practitioners). Planning in particular can engage partners to ensure the findings are relevant and to incorporate a clear understanding of the program, theory of change, and context.

Evaluators should develop a communication plan at the outset of an evaluation that lays out plans for internal briefings and public release of findings. This agreement between the evaluator and interest holders is critical for all parties to assure shared understanding of their respective rights in access to and public release of study findings. To that end, two components of these plans are essential. First, the plan should identify who controls publication and dissemination of the report and the findings, including the public release of evaluation findings. To avoid disagreements about publication, which can occur when interest holders are sensitive about the findings, these matters should be included in a plan agreed to by the key interest holders and evaluators before the evaluation commences. Second, timing of the access to the report and its findings should be agreed to in advance. It is common practice for the plan to include language that allows for program management and sponsors to review the report and its findings prior to public release. The plan generally lays out a specific amount of time interest holders will have to review the materials, during which they can provide comments and note any inaccuracies in the materials. It is paramount that evaluators and interest holders reach agreement on these factors before the evaluation begins because negotiating ownership of evaluation findings can be difficult after the findings are known. For example, if the evaluator finds that a program did not have its intended effect, program management or sponsors may be wary about releasing the findings at all. A clear and thorough communication plan can help to avoid conflicts between the evaluators and key interest holders. If the evaluation includes a contract (e.g., if it is funded by a grant), some of these parameters, including opportunities to review findings before public release, ownership of findings, and ownership of data, may be included in the contract.

In an independent evaluation, data planning responsibilities including sample selection, data cleaning decisions, and the analysis itself should remain under the evaluator's purview though interest holders may inform such decisions by sharing information on data collection procedures. Interest holders such as program managers and staff, while knowledgeable about program operations, may not have the background or training to understand how data quality issues may affect the findings or the credibility of findings and may feel the need to respond to other pressures in the workplace. In general, it is important to cultivate a climate of transparency and of "no surprises." Though outside the scope of this chapter, we also note that some evaluations are initiated because of ulterior political motives, which can compromise the credibility of the research findings. We urge evaluators to avoid evaluations based on these hidden agendas and refer the reader to Chapters 5–8 of this volume for further reading on these issues and how these concerns may be constructively navigated with the interest holders.

PLANNING FOR QUANTITATIVE ANALYSIS

Preparing an evaluation plan is a necessity for all evaluations. An evaluation plan, which is often the culmination of extensive discussions about the goals, objectives, and methods for the evaluation, guides the evaluators in conducting the evaluation by defining the main purposes for the evaluation, the research question(s), the types of data and measures that will be obtained, the analyses that will be conducted, the resources to be allocated, how the project will be managed, and plans for communicating about the project and its findings (Rossi et al., 2019). Russ-Eft (see Chapter 19, this volume) provides a detailed discussion of evaluation planning for program evaluation. An additional resource for evaluation planning is Chapter 11 of *Evaluation: A Systematic Approach* (Rossi et al., 2019). In the current chapter, we highlight essential planning components for quantitative analysis in particular, including research design, sampling, collecting or otherwise obtaining data, measures, units of measurement and analysis, and data storage.

Research Design

For quantitative analysis, the plan includes a section on research design that identifies the evaluation purpose and the methods the evaluator will use to achieve the stated goal(s). The intent of quantitative analysis may be exploratory, descriptive, or correlational/causal, as described above. An evaluation may have a single purpose or multiple purposes. In practice, causal designs usually include a descriptive component as well, such as examining implementation.

Sampling

After identifying the research design, the plan for quantitative analysis will describe the sample to be studied. The primary goal of sample selection is to identify a study sample that adequately represents the target population for the evaluation and will thus provide sufficiently **generalizable** and precise information on key study measures. A **sample** is the subset of the target population about which the evaluation will collect and analyze data. In some cases, evaluators may have access to population data, which is data from all participants in a program. When researchers are evaluating a very large or geographically dispersed program, or are collecting their own data, it can be necessary to select a subset of the full population participating in the program. For example, in an evaluation of School Improvement Grants (SIGs) awarded under President Barack Obama for states throughout the country to turn around their lowest-performing schools, Dragoset et al. (2017) selected a sample of about 60 districts across 22 states out of the 420 districts and 51 states (including Washington, DC) that received SIG funding. While there are many approaches to sampling, two broad categories are **probability sampling**, which draws on probability theory to construct a sample that models the population of interest, and **nonprobability sampling**, which prioritizes convenience, availability of subjects, or purposeful selection of subjects. A sufficiently large probability sample will allow evaluators to make inferences about the relevant population from which the sample was drawn, whereas a nonprobability sample will limit the findings to a description of the sample itself. The sampling process will depend on a combination of available resources (Do you have sufficient resources to collect data from a large probability sample?) and the evaluation goals (Are you interested in generalizing to a larger population to answer broad questions?). While sampling theory is beyond the scope of this chapter, an introduction to sampling logic and methods can be found in Chapter 7 of *The Basics of Social Research* (Babbie, 2016). Ultimately, an evaluator's approach to sampling may depend on the purpose of an evaluation. If the purpose is to obtain a causal effect of a program through an impact evaluation, the sample should reflect program participants and nonparticipants similar to the individuals who were eligible for program participation. If the purpose is a needs assessment, it is critical to identify a sample that contains members of the population of interest that have characteristics similar to the entire population of interest.

In concert with the sampling process, **power analysis** is often an important step to ensure the sample size is sufficiently large for the analysis to detect an effect if one occurs. **Statistical power** is the probability of rejecting a false null hypothesis in a study (Cohen, 1992). The **null hypothesis** states that there is no difference between two populations on a measure of interest. In the case of program evaluation that seeks to estimate program impacts, a null finding could be that the treatment and comparison groups performed similarly on some outcome measure. Rejecting the null would therefore be finding that the treatment and comparison groups did not perform equally on the outcome measure. If the null is false, then the difference in the program and comparison outcomes is large enough to rule out random chance as an explanation; if the null is not rejected, then random chance alone could explain the amount of the difference. Without population data, it is not possible to know for certain whether a null is true or false; the best an evaluator can do is reject or fail to reject the null hypothesis in the study sample. As such, an evaluator cannot *prove* that a program worked, even if they find a positive effect using a rigorous study design. Instead, the evaluator can say with some predetermined degree of confidence that program participants fared better than nonparticipants.

Broadly, there are two types of power analysis. Using the study design combined with effect sizes found in prior studies, one type of power analysis allows evaluators to calculate the sample size needed to be reasonably confident in finding a difference if a difference does occur. This type of power analysis occurs in the planning stage because it helps determine the sample size for an evaluation, or whether the sample size is sufficient to move forward with an impact evaluation. A second type of power analysis involves computing the minimum detectable effect size based on sample size and method. This second type of power analysis may be carried out either during the planning phase or even in the analysis phase to better understand the reasons that the null hypothesis was not rejected. It may also be useful in pilot studies where there are not yet good estimates of the potential effect size—though evaluators planning data collection often draw potential effect sizes from closely related literature as a guidepost for determining necessary sample size. An imperfect estimate of effect size in power analysis can be preferable to no estimate because it provides a starting point for data collection planning. While the details of power analysis are beyond the scope of this text, *PowerUp!* is a popular power analysis tool that provides a step-by-step method for determining sample size (Dong & Maynard, 2013).

Primary and Secondary Data

Part of the planning process involves determining whether data will be collected from primary sources or made available from secondary sources. **Primary data** are data that evaluators collect themselves for the purposes of an evaluation. Data collection activities for primary data usually consist of observations, interviews, focus groups, surveys, or direct assessments—and often combine multiple strategies. While many of these activities produce qualitative data, there are conditions under which each can be quantified—for example, by coding structured observations or interviews—and then analyzed quantitatively. **Secondary data** are data that evaluators acquire from another source that was originally collected for purposes other than the evaluation at hand. Examples of secondary data sources include program administrative data; databases of student test scores from states, districts, and schools; unemployment data from the U.S. Bureau of Labor Statistics or individual states; and public health survey data collected by health agencies from the residents of developing nations. Administrative databases such as tax records, unemployment records, censuses, medical records, and state educational data systems are valuable secondary data sources in many evaluations. Evaluations may draw exclusively from available secondary data, exclusively from primary data, or they may combine data sources. Decisions about the data to collect depend on evaluation goals, program context, data availability, cost, time, and quality. Even in cases where secondary data are available, these data may not be useful if they are incomplete, or were collected inconsistently or in an unreliable way. As part of the planning process, evaluators should consider what secondary data are available and of sufficient quality (e.g., not too much missing data, data meet purposes of evaluation), and then focus any primary data collection activities on important measures they cannot obtain from extant datasets. For impact evaluations, it is important to collect data on factors that might be correlated with both participation in that program or adoption of the policy and the outcome(s), as we discuss in Pham et al. (see Chapter 17, this volume). This is because the goal of an impact evaluation is to isolate the effect of an intervention from other factors that may contribute to the outcome of interest and be correlated with program participation.

Measures

Study **measures** are variables representing program outcomes, processes, or other characteristics of participants and the services they receive that may be relevant to the evaluation. This section outlines several key concepts for understanding and collecting data for quantitative study measures. **Outcome measures** are variables that the program is intended to influence or may influence unintentionally. For example, outcome measures for a school tutoring program may include student test scores or whether a student graduates from high school in four years. Outcome measures for a job training program may include earnings six months after program completion or a measure of whether each participant has a full-time job.

Process or implementation measures are measures that characterize the services delivered or received, the extent to which a program was implemented as intended (also known as implementation fidelity), exposure to a program, or other measures capturing how or to what extent a program was carried out. For example, in an evaluation of a professional development program supporting teachers tasked with implementing college- and career-ready writing standards, Gallagher and colleagues (2017) collected process data on the number of hours teachers participated in professional development activities. They used these data to construct measures of dosage—that is, the amount of program exposure participants received. Both outcome and process measures generally have either a positive or negative valence—for example, higher test scores, graduation, and participation in a program for the prescribed number of hours have a positive valence, whereas higher recidivism rates for corrections programs and high school dropout rates have a negative valence. Because a core function of program evaluation is to make judgments about programs, descriptive measures without explicit valence should be identified and justified based on the importance of the contextual information they will provide in the evaluation plan. Therefore, in addition to delineating outcome and process measures, the evaluation plan should describe any measures such as those that will be used as covariates to adjust for differences between the treatment and comparison groups.

In quantitative evaluation, most study measures—whether outcome, process, or other—must be quantified. Some variables are quantitative in their original form, such as test scores, recidivism rates, or hours of professional development. Others need to be quantified—for example, survey responses from Likert scale items that ask study participants to indicate whether they strongly disagree, disagree, neither disagree nor agree, agree, or strongly agree can be coded on a scale of 1 (*strongly disagree*) to 5 (*strongly agree*) or dichotomized as 1 for agree or strongly agree and 0 for any other response. Given a set of variables measuring a similar construct, evaluators may also combine multiple responses into composites—for example, through means, summations, or factor analyses. How these measures are quantified may depend in part on the unit of observation. For example, researchers evaluating a recidivism reduction program may have prison-level data on recidivism rates or they may have inmate-level data denoting whether each inmate reoffended during a specific period of time after release from a correctional facility. The former example is already quantitative because it is a continuous measure representing the proportion of inmates who reoffend within some predefined time period. But the latter is a yes/no measure that the evaluators need to measure, most likely as a dichotomous measure, such as coding a recidivism variable as 1 if an offender commits another crime and as 0 if the individual does not commit another crime during the period. When dichotomous variables such as this are collected, the mean represents the proportion of observations for whom the answer is yes.

Units of Observation and Analysis

The **unit of observation** in an evaluation is the level at which evaluators will collect data. Units of observation can be thought of as rows in a dataset or spreadsheet: person-level data has one row per person, with the spreadsheet having as many rows as there are people in the study sample; organization-level data has one row per organization, with the spreadsheet having as many rows as there are organizations in the evaluation. Generally, data need to be collected at least at the level of the program being implemented (e.g., firm level for a program implemented in firms), though evaluators may collect data at any level at or below the level of program implementation. When feasible, collecting data at a level lower than the unit of analysis (e.g., employee level for a program implemented in firms) can improve power and allow for more precise estimates. For example, in an evaluation of a school reform program carried out in low-performing schools throughout North Carolina, Henry and Harbatkin (2020) drew from school-, principal-, teacher-, and student-level data (see Box 17.1 in the next chapter). Unit of observation should not be confused with **unit of analysis**, which is the level at which the data are analyzed, often the level at which the intervention was implemented. For example, the unit of analysis in an evaluation of the effect of the school turnaround intervention on student test scores would be schools, because the intervention was carried out in entire schools, but the unit of observation could be student level if the evaluators collected individual student test scores or school if they collected school-level averages. It is important to consider unit of observation in planning an evaluation because it informs how study measures are collected and defined as well as how much statistical power the evaluators have to detect an effect of an intervention.

Data Security

Regardless of the type of data being collected, data security is paramount both during the data transfer process and in data storage. Data security addresses unintentional breaches of sensitive data, such as inadvertently identifying a respondent who was promised confidentiality, and intentional breaches, such as hacking into the files containing identifiable information. Mitigating the risk of unintentional disclosure of personally identifiable information requires careful consideration of how data will be aggregated and reported, including minimum number of units within cells, suppressing data below preset thresholds, and rounding. A set of recommendations for protecting personally identifiable data can be found in Abouelmehdi et al. (2018), though evaluation teams will need to make their own decisions based on the nature of their data and the risks involved. A discussion of data security and privacy strategies to mitigate intentional breaches can be found in Bertino (2015). In the case of primary data collection, evaluators should make plans to de-identify sensitive data—for example, by assigning unique IDs to all participants and sites that are attached to all data collection activities, and remain consistent through the study period to ensure participants can be tracked over time. Daries and colleagues (2014) provided a suggested approach to de-identifying data collected as part of social science research through a running example involving student records from massive open online courses.

UNDERSTANDING YOUR DATA

Once the data are collected but before any data analysis begins it is critical for the analyst to ensure they have a clear and thorough understanding of the data, including the nature of the observations, variables, and dataset itself. In this section, we provide an overview of data structure and variable types and distributions. We then discuss the importance of, and strategies for, data screening and cleaning. Before we begin, it is important to understand some basic vocabulary around quantitative data. An **observation** is a row in a dataset representing a person, institution, state, country, or any other observational unit (e.g., person by year, institution by month) on which the evaluators acquire data. The number of rows in a dataset is the number of observations. A **variable** is a column in a dataset representing a measure and each column contains a value for each observation. Examples of variables that might be included in an evaluation of a job training program include age, gender, education level, and annual earnings. A quantitative **dataset** is a collection of values for observations and variables. It is organized in a tabular, rectangular format, similar to the format of a spreadsheet, and generally contains a unique identifier for each observation and a label for each variable. A unique identifier is a numeric, alphabetical, or alphanumeric value that is different for each observational unit in the study sample. The variable names must be unique across the entire dataset and may be limited by the format of the program that is used for storing the data. Often, the variable name is limited to relatively few characters with no spaces—but most programs used for analysis may allow for a longer, more descriptive label for reference or for use in presenting tabular information.

Data Structure

Program evaluation data, such as the rectangular data files described above, are often referred to as **cross-sectional data**. Cross-sectional data contain variables collected during a specific period of time from different units, such as individuals, sites, or organizations. For example, the National Center for Education Statistics administers the National Assessment of Educational Progress (NAEP) in math and reading to a nationally representative sample of students each year. The NAEP data can be aggregated to the district and state levels, allowing researchers to track districts, states, and national trends. However, due to the selection of a unique sample for each administration of the NAEP, analysts cannot track student-level trends over time. On the other hand, many evaluations collect or obtain longitudinal data on units such as program participants or organizations. Longitudinal data follow the units over time and a longitudinal dataset therefore contains multiple observations on each unit. For example, an evaluator examining the effects of a tutoring program may be interested in measuring student knowledge before the program (the baseline or pretest) and then after the program (the posttest) in order to evaluate how much participants learned.

There are two types of formats for longitudinal datasets: long and wide. A **long dataset** contains a separate row for each unit of observation and time period. In the above example of a program evaluation with a pretest and posttest, each participant would have two rows: one with a pretest score and one with a posttest score. Importantly, both of those rows would contain the participant's unique ID and a variable that denotes whether the test score in that row applies to the pre- or posttest. In the NAEP example, a state-level dataset in long format would contain one row for every state-by-year combination. A **wide data structure** contains one row for each unit of observation, regardless of how many time periods are observed. The number of rows in a wide dataset for the pretest- and posttest example would be equal to the number of units in the evaluation and would contain separate pretest and posttest variables. A state-level NAEP dataset in wide format would contain one row per state, with separate variables for each year the NAEP was administered.

It is important for evaluators to understand the format of their dataset before beginning any analysis task. In some cases, it will be necessary to reorganize data from its original form. For example, regression methods for longitudinal analysis require data to be in long format, whereas graphical analyses may in some cases be easier with wide data. This reorganization of data from one format to another is known as **reshaping**. Analysts should reshape data using a statistical package such as Stata, SAS, or R, rather than by hand, which is more cumbersome and prone to human error. Figure 16.1 provides an example of both long and wide data formats for a dataset that contains a pretest (Time Period 1) and posttest (Time Period 2) for k students. The unique student ID appears once per student in the wide dataset and twice per student in the long dataset (because there are two time periods, each of which has its own row). The long dataset contains a single test score (*test score*) variable and a separate time period variable (*time period*) to denote the time period for which the observed test score applies. The wide dataset contains a separate test score variable (*test_score1* and *test_score2*) for each of the two time periods.

Levels of Measurement

The four levels of measurement for a variable are nominal, ordinal, interval, and ratio. As shown in Figure 16.2, these levels are nested in one another: all ordinal variables are nominal, all interval variables are ordinal, and all ratio

Long dataset		
student_id	test_score	time_period
101	84	1
101	91	2
102	72	1
102	76	2
...		
k	88	1
k	89	2

Wide dataset		
student_id	test_score1	test_score2
101	84	91
102	72	76
...		
k	88	89

FIGURE 16.1. Data format.

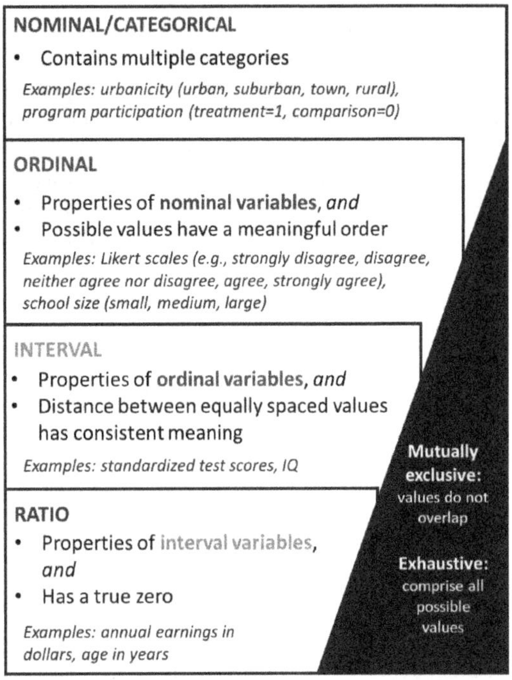

NOMINAL/CATEGORICAL
- Contains multiple categories

Examples: urbanicity (urban, suburban, town, rural), program participation (treatment=1, comparison=0)

ORDINAL
- Properties of **nominal variables**, *and*
- Possible values have a meaningful order

Examples: Likert scales (e.g., strongly disagree, disagree, neither agree nor disagree, agree, strongly agree), school size (small, medium, large)

INTERVAL
- Properties of **ordinal variables**, *and*
- Distance between equally spaced values has consistent meaning

Examples: standardized test scores, IQ

RATIO
- Properties of **interval variables**, *and*
- Has a true zero

Examples: annual earnings in dollars, age in years

Mutually exclusive: values do not overlap

Exhaustive: comprise all possible values

FIGURE 16.2. Levels of measurement and their properties.

---

variables are interval. A **nominal measure** is a variable representing a particular characteristic. Examples include gender (where possible values may be, e.g., male, female, other, or prefer not to say), race/ethnicity (where possible values may be, e.g., White, Black, Hispanic or Latin/a/e/x, Asian or Pacific Islander, multiple races, other, or prefer not to say), and college major (where possible values will be all possible majors in the sample). However, it is important to note that in recent years, the broader social science field has become more aware of nuance in measures related to gender, race, and ethnicity. A variable that combines race and ethnicity into a single variable with only six or seven possible values is a coarse measure that may not accurately capture the racial and ethnic identities in a dataset of diverse individuals, and a dichotomous gender variable cannot be accurate for those who do not identify as male or female. A researcher using administrative data is constrained by the categories collected and reported by the data collection and reporting agencies—although it may be possible to use more inclusive terminology than the reporting agency. A discussion of how researchers can measure race and ethnicity to better reflect individual identities can be found in Viano and Baker (2020).

In program evaluations that include a comparison group, analysts construct a nominal measure that takes a value of 1 for the treatment group and 0 for the comparison group. Nominal variables have no meaningful order—in other words, a value of 1 is no better or worse than a value of 0 or 2. Two important properties of each of these examples are that their possible values are (1) mutually exclusive and (2) exhaustive. **Mutually exclusive** values are those that do not overlap—for example, an observation cannot be coded as part of both the treatment and comparison groups. In cases in which variables may take on multiple values, such as race/ethnicity or college major, the analyst must make reasonable and consistent decisions about how to code those values. In some cases, these decisions can be made prior to data collection (e.g., requiring respondents to select only one from a predetermined list of race/ethnicity options), while in others it can be useful to collect more nuanced, open-ended responses and then collapse values to a smaller number of categories (e.g., allowing respondents to choose multiple race/ethnicity options and then coding into categories for analysis by the evaluators). Evaluators should make these decisions based on their evaluation goals and analysis plan while considering sensitivity to respondent preferences. To qualify as **exhaustive**, the values of a variable must comprise all possible values of a given measure for the study sample. For example, a college major variable that includes only science, technology, engineering, and mathematics (STEM) and humanities would not qualify as exhaustive unless the study sample had only participants who identified as STEM or humanities majors.

Two important types of nominal variables are race and gender. Race, ethnicity, and gender are nuanced measures but quantitative analysis requires the evaluator to make decisions in order to turn them into nominal variables. There has been added attention to this topic in recent years given a growing understanding that racial and ethnic groups are not monoliths, and intersectional identities are important to individual experiences. To that end, data collection and coding procedures around race, ethnicity, and gender that were previously considered a standard may no longer be appropriate. However, it is also important to consider data quality and sample size in planning for data collection. Asking respondents for their race, ethnicity, and gender without any parameters may lead to data that are not sufficiently consistent across individuals for quantitative analysis. Strategies to engage in more inclusive data collection may include multiple collections to allow for changing identity over time, providing a more comprehensive list of race and ethnicity options (and collapsing in the analysis stage if, e.g., there are no or few members of a particular group), and potentially asking a follow-up question to those selecting multiple identities about which identity best represents their lived experience (Viano & Baker, 2020). After data collection occurs, a small sample size overall or within a particular subgroup may ultimately necessitate collapsing smaller, more precise subgroups into larger, coarser groups. It would not be appropriate, for example, to report results about a subgroup with a very small number of respondents.

An **ordinal measure** is a variable that contains categories that can be assigned a rank order. For example, Likert scale items that range from 1 (*strongly disagree*) to 5 (*strongly agree*) are often considered ordinal. Ordinal variables can also be simplified continuous measures—for example, a school-size variable might be broken into three categories representing buckets of school sizes (e.g., small, medium, and large). Like nominal measures, ordinal measures must also be mutually exclusive and exhaustive. For example, a measure for number of books in a household defined as 0–5 books, 5–10 books, and 10 or more books would not qualify as mutually exclusive because households with 5 or 10 books would each fit into two different categories, while the same measure defined as 1–5 books, 6–10 books, and 11–15 books would not qualify as exhaustive because it excludes households with less than 1 and more than 15 books. Both ordinal and nominal measures are also sometimes referred to as **categorical**, which simply means that they represent categories of a variable and can be reorganized as a set of dichotomous or indicator variables, which are each coded 1 or 0 for membership within the category or not, respectively.

Interval and **ratio measures** are both continuous variables in which the distance between two equally spaced values has the same meaning regardless of where those values are located on the scale of the variable. Standardized test scores, IQ, and annual earnings are examples of these measures. The distinction between interval and ratio measures is that ratio measures contain a true zero that represents the complete absence of the characteristic being measured. For example, annual earnings is a ratio variable because a zero value represents the absence of earnings. In contrast, IQ does not qualify as a ratio measure because an IQ of zero would not represent the complete absence of intelligence. A more detailed treatment of levels of measurement can be found in Chapter 5 of Babbie (2016).

Level of measurement in both the dependent and independent variables will inform decisions about how to analyze and interpret data. For example, the interpretation of a binary predictor in regression is different from the interpretation of a continuous predictor. The coefficient on a binary predictor or independent variable is the difference in the mean of the dependent variable for the group coded 1 on the variable and the mean of the dependent variable for the group coded 0, conditional on any other covariates in the model. The coefficient on a continuous predictor variable represents the change in the dependent variable for each unit change in the predictor variable. Nominal measures with multiple categories need to be recoded into a set of binary variables, with 1 designating an observation within the category and 0 designating an observation that is not within the category (e.g., 1 for Black and 0 for all other races), before using them as covariates in regression analysis. Analysts need to make decisions about whether to treat ordinal variables as continuous or as a series of dichotomous or indicator variables. These decisions will depend on evaluation priorities and field-specific norms.

Variable Distributions

In addition to identifying the level of measurement of all variables in a dataset, it is important to understand how those variables are distributed. The **frequency distribution** of a variable is the range and frequency of values it takes. The classic example is a normal distribution, shaped like a bell curve in which the mean and median are equal to each other, about two-thirds of observations are within one standard deviation, plus or minus, of the mean, 95.0% are within two, and 99.7% are within three. But variable distributions can take many shapes. An introduction to normal curves and frequency distributions can be found in Cohen (2013). The distributions of nominal and ordinal variables look different from the distributions of interval and ratio variables. For example, a gender variable coded as male or female can only take two values, while a gender variable coded as male, female, or other can take three. It is important to understand the distribution of your variables because those distributions can inform analytic decisions. If, for example, you have a survey item on which all respondents answered the same way, then that item is not useful for analysis, or if responses were mostly clustered in a few response categories, then you might consider combining response options (e.g., collapsing strongly agree and agree into one "agree" variable) for analysis.

One challenge for analysis of categorical variables involves whether the original categories should be maintained in a single variable or divided into several dichotomous variables. It is necessary for regression analysis to transform nominal variables, such as race, gender, urbanicity, and others, into separate dichotomous (indicator) variables that take a value of 1 for observations that have a particular characteristic and 0 for otherwise. For example, an urbanicity variable with categories for urban, suburban, town, and rural would be transformed into four separate variables, with one taking a value of 1 for study participants in an urban setting and 0 for study participants in any of the other three settings, another taking a value of 1 for study participants in suburban settings and 0 for all others, and so on. But it is not possible to include all four of those urbanicity variables in a regression analysis. One variable will drop out because it is **perfectly collinear** with the other three—that is, its value can be determined with 100% certainty from the combination of other indicator variables due to the exhaustive and mutually exclusive requirements. Regression coefficient estimates for these dichotomous variables are always in reference to the single reference category that is omitted in order to avoid perfect collinearity. In the case of a categorical variable, the reference category will be one of the categories of that variable, which forces the data analyst to make a choice, which is sometimes made in favor of the category with the most observations or the relevance of comparing all other groups to one of the groups.

DATA SCREENING AND CLEANING

Data screening and cleaning are two of the most important steps in any quantitative analysis because the validity and reliability of all subsequent analyses depend on the quality of the data and the decisions made in the cleaning process. Analysts need to undertake the data screening and cleaning processes before beginning any analysis. This section highlights only the fundamental tasks and foci involved in the data screening and cleaning processes for program evaluation. A thorough treatment of data screening and cleaning—including the planning process, strategies for dealing with missing data, and strategies for analyzing responses to questions that are only offered to a subset of survey respondents—is available in Osborne (2013). In dealing with secondary data, as much of the data screening process as possible should occur on available data prior to beginning any data collection activities for several reasons. First, important measures that are missing may need to be collected as part of the primary data collection process. Second, there may be issues with how secondary data are collected or reported that necessitate additional data collection by the evaluator.

Data screening involves carefully investigating the data to check for missing values, missing observations, out-of-range values, and other unanticipated anomalies that may be present in a dataset. **Missing values** are cells that are blank for a given observation—in other words, you may have a dataset that includes 100,000 students but test scores may be missing for 5,000 of those students. **Missing observations** occur when the dataset excludes entire observations that should be included in the dataset—for example, the student dataset contains 95,000 observations but the study population included 100,000 students. It is the responsibility of the analyst to attempt to determine why those test scores or observations are missing. If the missingness is systematic (e.g., the school district didn't provide test scores for 11th graders, or specific schools or classrooms are missing test scores), then it is necessary to request the missing data from the data providers or to determine the reason for missingness if the data are not available. Sometimes data are missing by design—for example, the district may not have provided 11th-grade test scores because 11th graders do not take any tests. Any systematically missing data must be explained, and even if explained, statistics calculated from those data are subject to bias due to omitting some units from the calculations.

At some point in the data cleaning process, there will likely be missing data remaining that the data providers cannot explain. The **ignorability** of the missing data, which refers to the extent to which the missing data can be ignored and the cases without missing data analyzed without concern for the bias that missing cases cause, depends on the reason they are missing. Missingness will not introduce bias if data are **missing completely at random (MCAR)**. Data are MCAR if they are missing in a pattern that is independent of all other variables. In other words, missingness and patterns of missingness are not correlated with variables that are observed or unobserved in the dataset. While it is impossible to know for certain that data are MCAR, a formal test is provided in Little (1988). Data are unlikely to be MCAR. A lower bar to clear is **missing at random (MAR)**, in which missingness may be explained by the observed and unobserved values of other variables but cannot depend on unobserved variables after conditioning on observed variables. When a variable is MAR, it is possible to use values of other variables in the data to calculate the probability of missingness. Importantly, missing values for a particular variable may not be explained by the variable itself. If a variable's missingness is a function of the variable itself—for example, if an evaluator is less likely to have data on program participants under a certain income level or over a certain test score—then the data are **missing not at random (MNAR)** and the missingness is non-ignorable, which means any statistics calculated from the data may be biased.

It is easy to know if a value is missing because the cell that should contain that value will be blank, unless missing values have been coded with a "." or using some other convention. It is less easy to know that an entire observation is missing. How can you know that an entire observation or observations are missing from your dataset? The short answer is you usually cannot know exactly which observations are missing from your dataset unless you have a list of the full sample that ought to be in your dataset. For example, if you know you have a complete list of all program participants and you administer a survey to all of them, you can easily observe which participants did not respond. On the other hand, if you do receive a list of program participants but have not confirmed exactly who should be on that list, identifying missing observations is to some degree uncertain. While you may not be able to confirm with 100% certainty that an observation is missing, there are some useful questions to ask during the data screening process that will help you identify missingness:

1. How many observations did I expect? If you are evaluating a program with 1,000 participants and only have data from 500, you know you are missing data from about half of the participants. Similarly, if the number of students in an educational dataset or patients in a health dataset is much lower in the current year than in prior years and you have no reason to expect a decrease, you may be missing data.

2. Are there variables in the dataset that I expect to have similar means from one period to the next or to have particular frequency distributions? If you are evaluating a tutoring program with sixth-, seventh-, and eighth-grade participants, you can tabulate a grade-level variable to ensure you have data on all three grade levels and that the breakdown approximately matches your expectation.

3. Are there multiple sites represented in my study? In a multisite study, you can confirm you have data from all sites and that you have approximately the expected number of participants from each site.

4. Do certain groups appear to be missing from the database? If you know from publicly available aggregated data or other reports that your population is about 10% special education students, or 20% non-English speakers, for example, you can use available data on special education and language, respectively, to examine whether the data include the expected share of each group.

The data screening process should also include a check for **out-of-range values**. Out-of-range values are values of a variable that are either impossible or highly unlikely. For example, an evaluation of a healthy eating program might include a survey about participant demographics and daily caloric intake. A value of 100 for the age variable or a value of 25,000 for the daily caloric intake variable are examples of out-of-range values because it is unlikely that the participant is truly 100 years old (unless the intervention is targeting a geriatric population) or that they consume 25,000 calories per day. Similarly, values of 2 for the age variable and 100 for the calorie variable would also raise red flags. One approach to identifying out-of-range values is to determine an expected possible range of values and flag observations that fall outside that range. There is no bright-line rule for where to set the expected range that can apply to all studies; you would set a different expected age range for a study of preschoolers, for example, than for a study of senior citizens. But what do you do with the 100-year-old program participant who consumes 25,000 calories per day? Again, there is no hard-and-fast answer. Your approach depends in part on whether you have primary or secondary data: In the case of primary data you should first check for an error in data entry. In the absence of data entry errors, the evaluator may be able to request clarifying information from participants. It also depends on your level of comfort with making assumptions based on the data you do have. For example, you may or may not be comfortable assuming the calories variable has an extra zero and ought to be set at 2,500. Once you make a decision rule, it is critical to (1) apply it consistently, and (2) document it clearly. Without clear and thorough documentation, a decision rule that seems obvious today can become a mystery 6 months after the recoding is completed. Clear and thorough documentation also allows for more seamless transition across data analysts (without documentation, an individual analyst's decision rules leave the building with them) and provides the necessary information to transparently report findings.

It may be useful to note that there is no singular best software to use for data screening and cleaning. Analysts should select software that (1) they are familiar with, (2) allows for a clear record of cleaning decisions made, and (3) allows for replicability. Replicability in this case means another analyst would be able to use the original analyst's code to generate an identical analytic dataset from the raw data. For example, statistical packages such as Stata and R allow the analyst to write code that carries out their selected cleaning rules. Regardless of software used, any data cleaning process should involve creating a new analytic dataset while retaining a copy of the original dataset.

Different types of data tend to present different challenges for the analyst. Secondary data, for example, are likely to have more unexplained missing values and observations than primary data. Evaluators can be more confident in the quality of secondary data that are used for administrative purposes. For instance, a "years-of-experience" variable that is used to compute salary amounts for teachers' pay may be more likely to be accurate than a "years-of-experience" variable that is self-reported by teachers. However, even secondary data are subject to inaccuracies because humans entering the data make mistakes or make inaccurate assumptions. Primary data may have missing values that can be explained—for example, data from a survey designed with skip logic will contain missing values by design. Human error in data entry leads to out-of-range values in both primary and secondary data. The data collection process is a good time to prevent problems from arising later—for example, by assigning unique IDs, planning data entry formats and processes that involve careful quality control, and designing surveys to minimize out-of-range and missing values. Online survey platforms include options for skip logic, data validation rules, requiring selected responses, and piping (dropping, or "piping" values from one part of the survey into subsequent survey questions or response options). But these strategies come at a cost: tightly defined data validation rules or requiring responses for questions not relevant to all respondents may frustrate respondents and lead them to give up on the survey or to select responses without regard to accuracy. For example, a survey respondent who encounters an error after choosing to skip a question and clicking "next" on an online survey may assume the error was a technical glitch rather than the result of the survey requiring a response to the item and may simply close out of the window rather than scrolling up to find the language indicating a response to the item is required before moving to the next questions. It is therefore important to carefully plan and test these rules, and then to pilot the survey with respondents who are similar to the target respondents. Even with careful planning, primary data collection may yield values that appear unlikely. In these cases, it is necessary to make decision rules based on available information and apply those rules consistently. In some cases, the evaluator may choose to run sensitivity analyses in which they check the robustness of results when they include and exclude certain observations.

SUMMARY AND CONCLUSION

Throughout this chapter, we have outlined processes related to planning a quantitative program evaluation; defined key concepts related to quantitative program data; and laid out processes for collecting, screening, and cleaning data. The first step in planning a quantitative program evaluation is, like other program evaluations, to develop an evaluation plan. This process often involves engaging interest holders, though the level of interest holder involvement may vary depending on the goals of the evaluation. Of particular importance to an evaluation plan that involves interest holders is a communication agreement that clearly delineates who controls the release of evaluation findings. The evaluation plan also includes a section on research design that identifies the evaluation purpose and the methods that will be used to achieve that purpose. The purpose may be exploratory, descriptive, or correlational/causal. Pham et al. (see Chapter 17, this volume) provide a breakdown of evaluation purposes and common analytic techniques for each purpose. Another key research design decision is selecting the sample to be studied. In some cases, the study sample may include the entire population of interest (e.g., all program participants) but in many cases—and in particular when the program contains a large number of participants and primary data collection—includes only a subset of the population.

Quantitative data for an evaluation may come from **primary data sources**, **secondary data sources**, or a combination of both. Secondary data sources, such as administrative databases, provide evaluators with access to data for a large group of observations—in some cases the entire population of interest—but are limited in detail and evaluation relevance by the scope of the agency or organization that collected the data. Primary data can be tailored to the evaluator's specific purposes but require a large investment to develop a data collection instrument, collect the data, and follow up to obtain sufficient response rates. Regardless of whether the evaluation uses primary data, secondary data, or both, assuring data security before any data are collected or obtained is critical to the integrity of the evaluation. Data security considerations include both having the infrastructure and other capacity to keep data secure and making plans to de-identify sensitive data.

A precondition for any quantitative analysis is that the evaluator has as complete an understanding of the dataset as possible, including data structure and variables. Even the most well-designed and executed quantitative analysis could yield inaccurate findings if the evaluator misunderstood the data structure or the way a measure was defined in the data. Both are particularly salient with secondary data because the evaluators may not be as familiar with data structure and variables in a dataset they did not collect, though primary data collection can also be subject to errors related to misunderstanding data (e.g., an analyst might miss a duplicate survey response from the same respondent or survey software may code a variable in reverse of what the analyst expects). To minimize errors that can arise from an incomplete understanding of the data, evaluators must engage in a thorough data screening and cleaning process that involves visualizing data structure, summarizing all variables, cross-checking variables against any available codebooks, investigating missingness, checking for out-of-range variables, and making and documenting all decision rules. Maintaining an archive of decision rules is critical in all cases, and especially in the case of longitudinal or multisite studies in order to ensure consistent application of rules over time and across sites. The analysis of quantitative data should not take place until after the evaluator has carefully completed all of these steps. By taking the appropriate steps in the planning, data collection, and data screening and cleaning processes, an evaluator can compile a robust dataset that allows them to undertake an accurate and rigorous quantitative program evaluation.

REFERENCES

Abouelmehdi, K., Beni-Hessane, A., & Khaloufi, H. (2018). Big healthcare data: Preserving security and privacy. *Journal of Big Data, 5*(1), 1.

Babbie, E. R. (2016). *The basics of social research.* Cengage Learning.

Bertino, E. (2015). Big data—security and privacy. 2015 IEEE International Congress on Big Data, 757–761.

Burns, J., Harbatkin, E., Strunk, K. O., Torres, C., Mcilwain, A., & Frost Waldron, S. (2023). The efficacy and implementation of Michigan's Partnership Model of school and district turnaround: Mixed-methods evidence from the first 2 years of reform implementation. *Educational Evaluation and Policy Analysis, 45*(4), 622–654.

Cohen, B. H. (2013). *Explaining psychological statistics* (4th ed.). Wiley.

Cohen, J. (1992). A power primer. *Psychological Bulletin, 112*(1), 155.

Daries, J. P., Reich, J., Waldo, J., Young, E. M., Whittinghill, J., Dean Ho, A., . . . Chuang, I. (2014). Privacy, anonymity, and big data in the social sciences. *Communications of the ACM, 57*(9), 56–63.

Dong, N., & Maynard, R. (2013). PowerUp!: A tool for calculating minimum detectable effect sizes and minimum required sample sizes for experimental and quasi-experimental design studies. *Journal of Research on Educational Effectiveness, 6*(1), 24–67.

Dragoset, L., Thomas, J., Herrmann, M., Deke, J., James-Burdumy, S., Graczewski, C., . . . Giffin, J. (2017). *School improvement grants: Implementation and effectiveness.* NCEE 2017-4013. National Center for Education Evaluation and Regional Assistance. Available at *https://eric.ed.gov/?id=ED572215*

Gallagher, H. A., Arshan, N., & Woodworth, K. (2017). Impact of the National Writing Project's College-Ready Writers Program in high-need rural districts. *Journal of Research on Educational Effectiveness, 10*(3), 570–595.

Harbatkin, E., Burns, J., & Cullum, S. (2025). The role of school climate in school turnaround. *Teachers College Record.*

Henry, G. T., & Harbatkin, E. (2020). The next generation of state reforms to improve their lowest performing schools: An evaluation of North Carolina's school transformation intervention. *Journal of Research on Educational Effectiveness, 13*(4), 702–730.

Little, R. J. A. (1988). A test of missing completely at random for multivariate data with missing values. *Journal of the American Statistical Association, 83*(404), 1198–1202.

Osborne, J. W. (2013). *Best practices in data cleaning: A complete guide to everything you need to do before and after collecting your data.* SAGE.

Rossi, P. H., Lipsey, M. W., & Henry, G. T. (2019). *Evaluation: A systematic approach* (8th ed.). SAGE.

Viano, S., & Baker, D. J. (2020). How administrative data collection and analysis can better reflect racial and ethnic identities. *Review of Research in Education, 44*(1), 301–331.

Chapter 17

Conducting a Quantitative Analysis

Lam D. Pham
Gary T. Henry
Erica Harbatkin

CHAPTER OVERVIEW

This chapter describes methods and approaches for conducting a quantitative analysis. We separate these methods into three categories: exploratory, descriptive, and correlational or causal analysis. While these three approaches are not mutually exclusive, we describe all three so that the quantitative evaluator can decide which approach (or combination of approaches) is most appropriate depending on the purpose of the evaluation, the availability of data, and the needs of relevant interest holders. Exploratory analyses involve discovering and documenting trends and patterns in data. Descriptive analyses aim to describe and summarize data. Correlational and causal analyses allow the evaluator to test a hypothesis (e.g., whether a program had a statistically significant effect). Regardless of the approach or methods used, we emphasize throughout the chapter how the evaluator's quantitative analyses should be carefully designed to meet the highest feasible methodological standards of rigor.

In this chapter, we describe three broad categories of quantitative data analysis. The first, **exploratory analysis**, involves the process of discovering trends or patterns in data. The second, **descriptive analysis**, aims to describe and summarize data. While exploratory and descriptive analysis approaches employ similar methods (e.g., visualizing and summarizing data), they differ in their analytic goal. Babbie (2020) described three goals of exploratory analysis: (1) build a better understanding of a topic or issue, (2) examine the feasibility of a study employing more rigorous methods, and (3) inform the development of methods to use in a later study. Exploratory analyses provide quicker, more preliminary information, which may be a function of limited time and resources. Descriptive analysis, by contrast, aims to accurately and with acceptable precision describe a program, its context, its participants, or the **target population**. The third set of methods we describe, **correlational** and **causal analysis**, involve testing a hypothesis—often whether a given program had its intended effect. Correlation designs have weaker causal warrants and should be more cautiously interpreted to imply a program effect, whereas causal analyses are designed to attribute any differences in outcomes to the program.

As discussed in Harbatkin et al. (see Chapter 16, this volume), these three approaches are not **mutually exclusive,** and many quantitative evaluations use a combination of these methods at different points in the evaluation process. The decision between which approach or combination of approaches to use depends on the purpose(s) of the evaluation, the availability of data, and the interests and needs of relevant interest holders. In order to prepare the available data for the analytic methods described here, the quantitative evaluator should carefully attend to cleaning, preparing, and understanding the data as described in Chapter 16. Regardless of the chosen approach or its intended purpose, the quantitative analytic approach should be designed so that it meets the highest feasible methodological standards.

EXPLORATORY ANALYSIS

Exploratory analysis can be part of a larger evaluation or can constitute an entire evaluation. For example, a **needs assessment** can be an exploratory analysis that assesses the nature, magnitude, and distribution of a social problem to determine whether an intervention is needed as well as what type of intervention may best fit the actual problem. Because the goal of the needs assessment is to determine the gap between the current social condition and the condition judged to be acceptable to society or a particular community, it provides a useful framework for considering exploratory analysis even though exploratory analysis can take many forms other than needs assessment. The specific details of the needs assessment process are beyond the scope of this chapter but Chapter 2 of Rossi et al. (2019) provides a detailed description of the needs assessment process.

Suppose a researcher is conducting a needs assessment of low-performing schools to help inform a school improvement program. The goal of this needs assessment is to describe the issues surrounding low performance to support program designers in structuring a program to address the specific issues identified in the needs assessment. Drawing from secondary data on all schools in the state or district, the analyst might begin by computing summary statistics that compare low-performing with non-low-performing schools on a range of available **measures,** such as teacher and principal turnover, student transfer patterns, absenteeism, course taking, school composition, per pupil expenditures, and others. After examining these summary statistics, the analyst will likely conduct graphical analyses in order to better visualize trends and patterns suggested by the summary statistics. Graphical analysis can be helpful in visualizing data and identifying trends by plotting timelines and correlations in the data using scatter plots—it is often easier to discover patterns by examining several graphs than through summary statistics alone.

Graphical Analysis

The type of graphs to examine depend on **variable** type, variable distribution, and whether the evaluator is interested in understanding the distribution of a single variable or visualizing a relationship between variables. Figure 17.1 provides a breakdown of the most common and useful types of graphical displays, including when they are most useful, and an example of each. Graphs that provide useful information on the distribution and central tendency of a single variable include box plots, sometimes called box-and-whisker plots, histograms, and kernel density plots. A box plot provides a visual representation of the central tendency of a variable, the range in which most values fall, and outliers. Box plots are particularly helpful for identifying outliers in the data, which may artificially skew averages in the direction of the outliers. Histograms group **observations** in "bins" based on their values on a particular continuous variable and then represent the proportion of observations—or "density"—within each of those bins by bar height. It is sometimes useful to overlay a kernel density plot (a representation of the distribution that smooths out noise), on a histogram to examine the distribution of a variable more critically.

Two common graphs that provide information about the relationship between two variables are scatter plots and bar graphs. In particular, scatter plots are useful when the evaluator is interested in visualizing the relationship be-

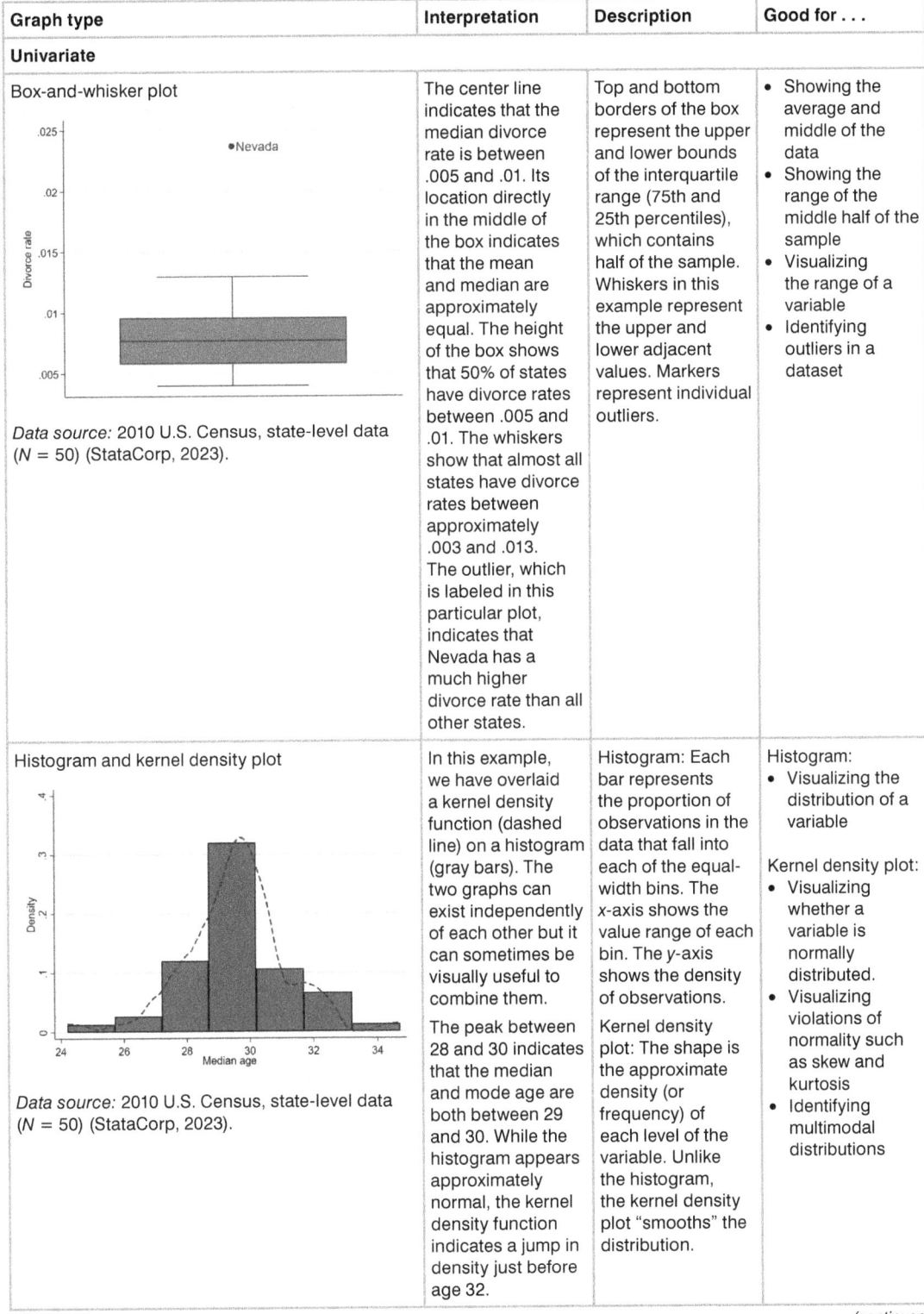

Conducting a Quantitative Analysis 327

Graph type	Interpretation	Description	Good for . . .
Univariate			
Box-and-whisker plot *[Box plot showing Divorce rate from .005 to .025, with Nevada labeled as outlier near .023]* *Data source:* 2010 U.S. Census, state-level data (*N* = 50) (StataCorp, 2023).	The center line indicates that the median divorce rate is between .005 and .01. Its location directly in the middle of the box indicates that the mean and median are approximately equal. The height of the box shows that 50% of states have divorce rates between .005 and .01. The whiskers show that almost all states have divorce rates between approximately .003 and .013. The outlier, which is labeled in this particular plot, indicates that Nevada has a much higher divorce rate than all other states.	Top and bottom borders of the box represent the upper and lower bounds of the interquartile range (75th and 25th percentiles), which contains half of the sample. Whiskers in this example represent the upper and lower adjacent values. Markers represent individual outliers.	• Showing the average and middle of the data • Showing the range of the middle half of the sample • Visualizing the range of a variable • Identifying outliers in a dataset
Histogram and kernel density plot *[Histogram with overlaid kernel density plot, Density on y-axis (0 to .4), Median age on x-axis (24 to 34)]* *Data source:* 2010 U.S. Census, state-level data (*N* = 50) (StataCorp, 2023).	In this example, we have overlaid a kernel density function (dashed line) on a histogram (gray bars). The two graphs can exist independently of each other but it can sometimes be visually useful to combine them. The peak between 28 and 30 indicates that the median and mode age are both between 29 and 30. While the histogram appears approximately normal, the kernel density function indicates a jump in density just before age 32.	Histogram: Each bar represents the proportion of observations in the data that fall into each of the equal-width bins. The *x*-axis shows the value range of each bin. The *y*-axis shows the density of observations. Kernel density plot: The shape is the approximate density (or frequency) of each level of the variable. Unlike the histogram, the kernel density plot "smooths" the distribution.	Histogram: • Visualizing the distribution of a variable Kernel density plot: • Visualizing whether a variable is normally distributed. • Visualizing violations of normality such as skew and kurtosis • Identifying multimodal distributions

(continued)

FIGURE 17.1. Graphical displays of data.

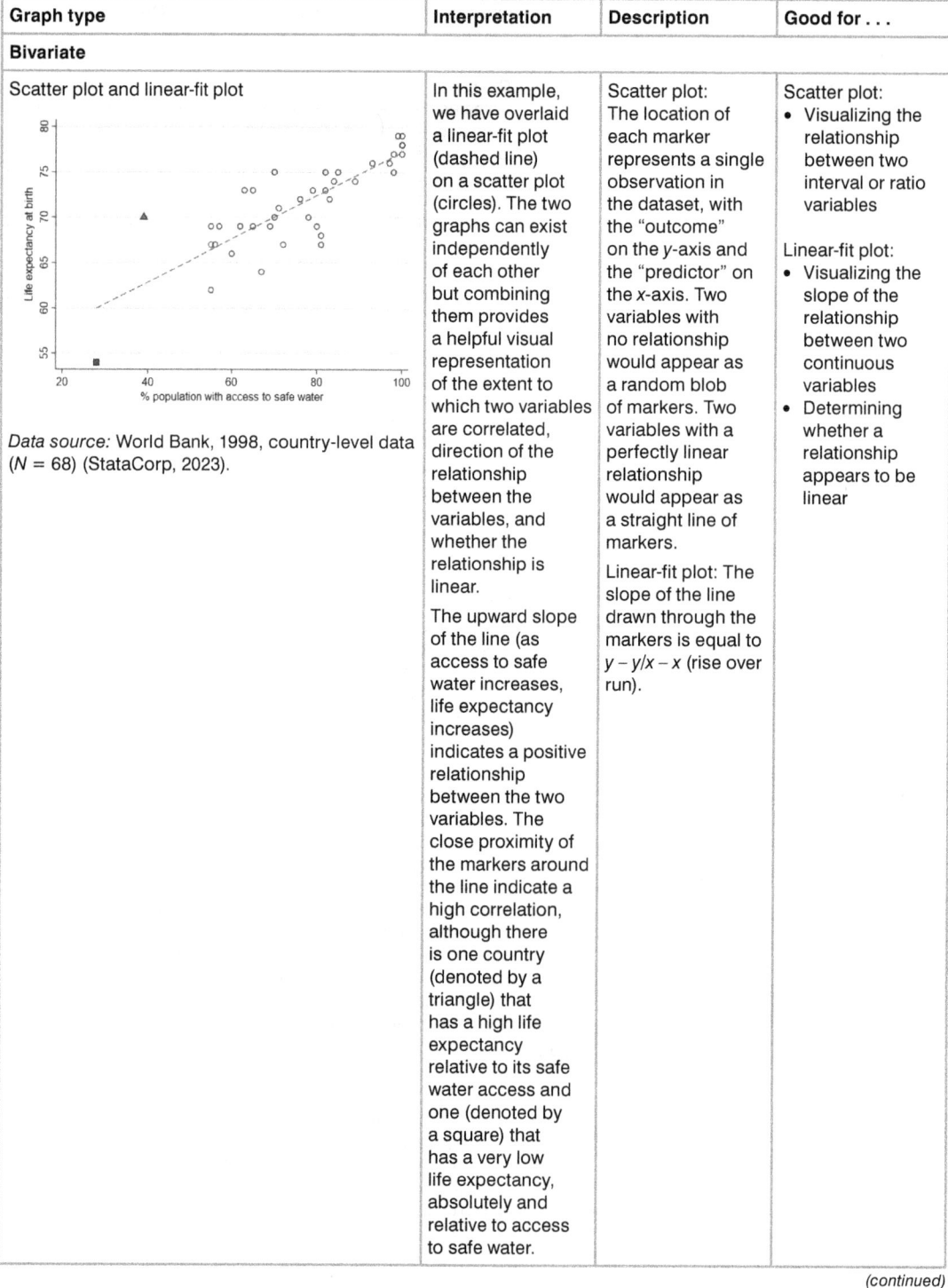

Graph type	Interpretation	Description	Good for . . .
Bivariate			
Scatter plot and linear-fit plot *Data source:* World Bank, 1998, country-level data (*N* = 68) (StataCorp, 2023).	In this example, we have overlaid a linear-fit plot (dashed line) on a scatter plot (circles). The two graphs can exist independently of each other but combining them provides a helpful visual representation of the extent to which two variables are correlated, direction of the relationship between the variables, and whether the relationship is linear. The upward slope of the line (as access to safe water increases, life expectancy increases) indicates a positive relationship between the two variables. The close proximity of the markers around the line indicate a high correlation, although there is one country (denoted by a triangle) that has a high life expectancy relative to its safe water access and one (denoted by a square) that has a very low life expectancy, absolutely and relative to access to safe water.	Scatter plot: The location of each marker represents a single observation in the dataset, with the "outcome" on the *y*-axis and the "predictor" on the *x*-axis. Two variables with no relationship would appear as a random blob of markers. Two variables with a perfectly linear relationship would appear as a straight line of markers. Linear-fit plot: The slope of the line drawn through the markers is equal to $y - y/x - x$ (rise over run).	Scatter plot: • Visualizing the relationship between two interval or ratio variables Linear-fit plot: • Visualizing the slope of the relationship between two continuous variables • Determining whether a relationship appears to be linear

(continued)

FIGURE 17.1. *(continued)*

Conducting a Quantitative Analysis 329

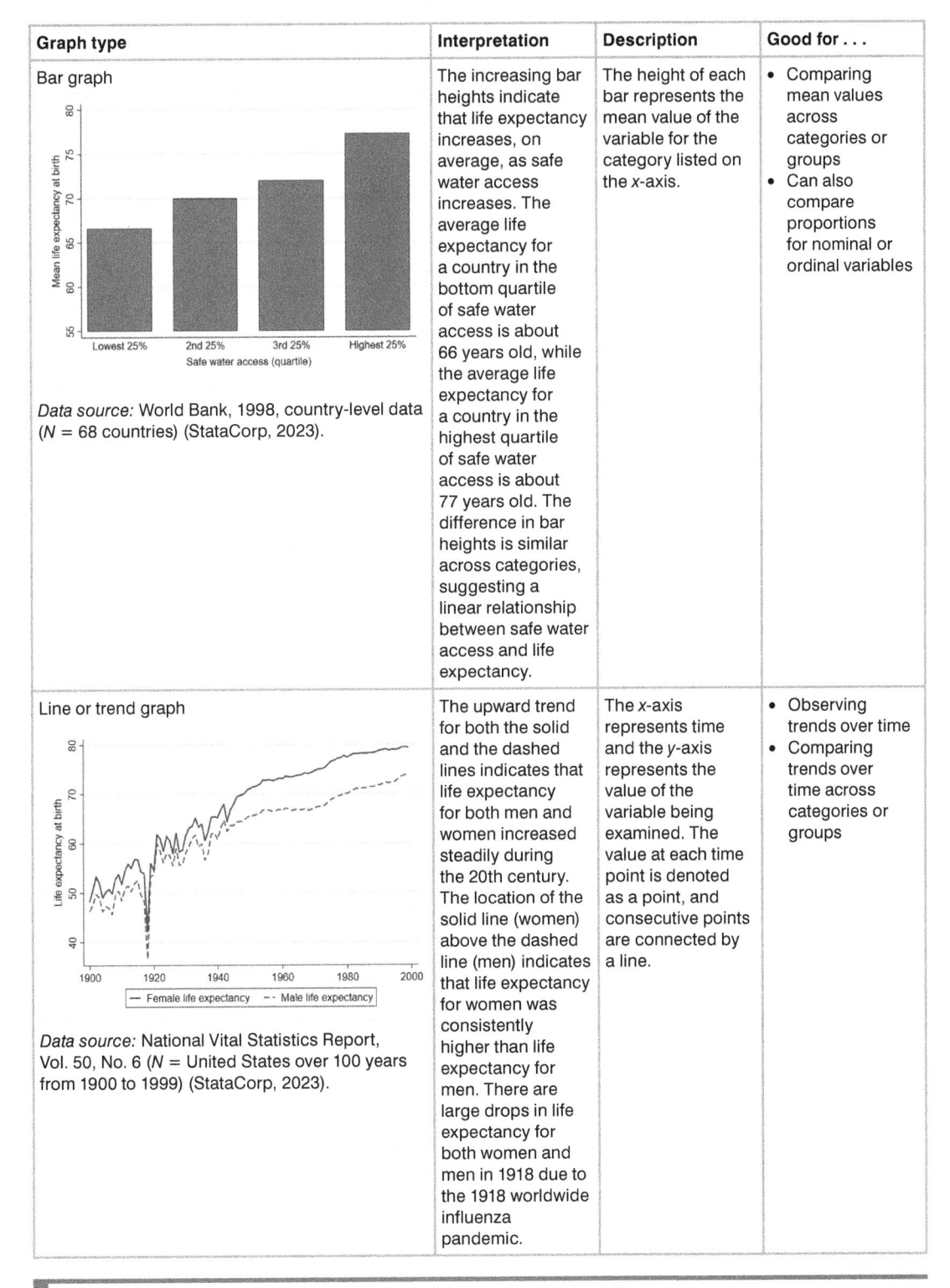

Graph type	Interpretation	Description	Good for . . .
Bar graph *Data source:* World Bank, 1998, country-level data (*N* = 68 countries) (StataCorp, 2023).	The increasing bar heights indicate that life expectancy increases, on average, as safe water access increases. The average life expectancy for a country in the bottom quartile of safe water access is about 66 years old, while the average life expectancy for a country in the highest quartile of safe water access is about 77 years old. The difference in bar heights is similar across categories, suggesting a linear relationship between safe water access and life expectancy.	The height of each bar represents the mean value of the variable for the category listed on the *x*-axis.	• Comparing mean values across categories or groups • Can also compare proportions for nominal or ordinal variables
Line or trend graph *Data source:* National Vital Statistics Report, Vol. 50, No. 6 (*N* = United States over 100 years from 1900 to 1999) (StataCorp, 2023).	The upward trend for both the solid and the dashed lines indicates that life expectancy for both men and women increased steadily during the 20th century. The location of the solid line (women) above the dashed line (men) indicates that life expectancy for women was consistently higher than life expectancy for men. There are large drops in life expectancy for both women and men in 1918 due to the 1918 worldwide influenza pandemic.	The *x*-axis represents time and the *y*-axis represents the value of the variable being examined. The value at each time point is denoted as a point, and consecutive points are connected by a line.	• Observing trends over time • Comparing trends over time across categories or groups

FIGURE 17.1. *(continued)*

tween two continuous variables because they graph each observation in the **dataset** based on the values of both variables. Bar graphs are more appropriate with one continuous and one categorical (nominal or ordinal) variable because a scatter plot with categorical variables would simply overlay all observations with a particular value on top of one another. Finally, if you are interested in a bivariate relationship between a variable and time—visualizing trends over time—the most common display is a line graph with time on the x-axis (horizontal axis) and the variable of interest on the y-axis (vertical axis). The line graph can reveal trends over time as well as anomalies. For example, the linear graph in Figure 17.1 shows a precipitous drop in life expectancy in 1918. Further investigation would reveal that this drop occurred during the worldwide influenza epidemic of 1918 that caused half a million deaths in the United States. In exploratory analysis, an anomalous drop or upswing in a variable should lead the analyst to explore the potential explanation behind or correlates of the sudden change.

BOX 17.1. The North Carolina Transformation Initiative

In 2015, the North Carolina Department of Public Instruction began an intervention to turn around its lowest performing schools. The North Carolina Transformation Initiative (NCT) targeted 75 low-performing schools for coaching support. The intervention, carried out by staff from the state District and School Transformation office, provided tailored instructional and leadership coaching for teachers and principals, respectively, that was intended to be tailored to the specific needs of the school. The state set a maximum number of elementary, middle, and high schools it would support through NCT. Before selecting schools for treatment, the state narrowed the **target population** based on specific parameters; to be eligible, a school needed to be a traditional public schools that scored a D or F on the school report card, could not be in the largest 10 school districts in the state or an 11th district that was already receiving services, and did not exceed growth as defined by the school value-added measure. The state then selected schools for support based on their prior year proficiency rates, which is the rate of end-of-grade and end-of-course exams administered in the school that students passed at grade-level proficiency or above. Schools with proficiency rates below a specified cutoff would receive services, while schools with proficiency rates above the cutoff would not. This proficiency measure provided researchers with a **quantitative assignment variable**, which is required for a **regression discontinuity** (RD) design. The NCT evaluation began as a research-practice partnership in which evaluators provided formative feedback to program staff on implementation as the intervention began and later on outcomes. Prior to conducting any correlational and causal analyses, evaluators conducted exploratory analyses on the schools selected for treatment, followed by process evaluation and outcome monitoring in addition to causal analysis using RD.

The **exploratory analysis** involved grouping treatment schools using data on the barriers they faced in the year they became low performing. This grouping, which is known as cluster analysis, allowed evaluators to place schools into groups based on barriers such as teacher turnover, proportions of novice teacher in the schools, student mobility, and other factors correlated with low performance. Evaluators shared these groups with program managers, who used the information to brainstorm strategies for supporting schools with different types of challenges.

The **descriptive analysis** involved both **process evaluation** and **outcome monitoring**. As part of process evaluation, evaluators examined fidelity of implementation, dosage, and implementation quality. The fidelity of implementation analysis required the evaluation team to iterate with program managers to develop a theory of change reflecting the intervention process. Drawing on the theory of change, evaluators developed an implementation index that quantified each dimension of implementation and placed schools on a four-point scale from no implementation to high implementation. Evaluators aligned data collection to the implementation index by designing principal and teacher surveys that would generate data to situate all schools on the implementation scale. While dosage was not a component of fidelity of implementation, evaluators also collected and coded data on dosage through coaching reports from program implementers. In order for evaluators to produce accurate measures of program dosage, implementers needed to diligently record coaching visits in a shareable format, including dates, coaching foci, and coaching content. Evaluators then coded these reports to quantify implementation dosage.

As part of the **outcome monitoring** process, evaluators examined intervention outcomes while the inter-

> vention was still in progress. The intervention began in the 2015-16 school year and continued through the 2016-17 school year. As such, it was possible to examine outcomes after one year of supports and share those findings with program implementers. In particular, evaluators examined student test scores, as well as more immediate outcomes such as teacher and principal turnover, chronic absenteeism, and use of exclusionary discipline. These analyses involved means and standard deviations of outcomes, line graphs showing trends over time on relevant outcomes, and comparisons between treatment and comparison schools.
>
> Finally, the **causal analysis** involved **RD** to examine the outcomes in treatment and comparison schools. Using the baseline proficiency rate—that is the proficiency rate at the time of assignment to treatment—as the forcing variable, evaluators conducted RD analyses to establish the causal effect of NCT. Because there was noncompliance on both sides of the cutoff—in other words, the state served some schools above the cutoff and did not serve some schools below the cutoff—evaluators used a fuzzy RD design. Based on this fuzzy RD design, the evaluators found a negative effect of NCT on student test scores (Henry & Harbatkin, 2020).
>
> Evaluators were able to draw from implementation findings to contextualize these results. Because the intervention was implemented with high fidelity, researchers could conclude that the failure of the intervention was not simply a failure of implementation; the state had implemented NCT as intended. Instead, evaluators suggested the findings may point to a theory of change failure. By contrast, if the program had failed to produce the intended effect but also had low implementation, evaluators would not have been able to distinguish between these two possibilities.

DESCRIPTIVE ANALYSIS

Similar to exploratory analysis, descriptive techniques can include basic statistical as well as graphical analysis. While descriptive analysis cannot be used to estimate program impact, it is a necessary complement to any causal analysis and can provide useful context on its own about a program being evaluated. It includes many of the same techniques as exploratory data analysis but may be focused on a more definitive description of programs, their context, participants, or the target population for a particular intervention.

Descriptive analysis is often conducted for a **process evaluation**. Process evaluation examines what a program is, the activities undertaken, who receives services or other benefits, and the consistency with which it is implemented in terms of both its design and across sites. Process evaluation may provide a neutral description but the measures may also have a valence for program interest holders—for example, in the case of fidelity of implementation, which is the degree to which an intervention was implemented as intended. Fidelity of implementation has a positive valence because high implementation indicates a high level of adherence to the program design. While Powell et al. (see Chapter 12, this volume) provide a detailed framework for examining program implementation, we highlight the role of quantitative analysis in this process.

Rossi and colleagues (2019) wrote that process evaluation answers at least one of two key questions: (1) Is the program reaching its target population? and (2) Is service delivery consistent with program design? Answers to both of these questions are quantifiable. As part of the first question, an evaluator could address whether and to what extent the target population received services. Measures for this construct are important and often understudied. These measures could include the proportion of the target population that received services and whether the characteristics of the program participants match target population characteristics. Gaps between program participants and those eligible to participate may indicate disparities or inequities in delivery of the services. As part of the second question, an evaluator could address the extent to which the target population received an adequate dosage as well as the quality of the services they received. Measures for these dosage and quality constructs could draw from service logs from program implementers or survey responses from program participants about the amount and quality of the services received. As part of the second question, the analyst can develop a set of measures aligned with the **theory of change** guiding the program and assess the extent to which the program's service delivery conformed with each of the measures. Multiple measures such as these can be combined into a single construct using factor analysis methods or forming an index by simply taking the mean of a set of identically scaled measures. Combining multiple measures into a single construct or a smaller set of constructs is a useful strategy for reducing the number of measures to be reported, especially if measures are highly correlated with one another.

Although process evaluation does not attempt to isolate the effects of the program on its recipients, it does provide formative findings that can be shared with program implementers for program improvement and can be a crucial element in interpreting effect estimates from impact evaluations. Process findings would provide context if, for example, an impact evaluation found no effect of a program on its intended recipients, by helping to explain whether the lack of impact stemmed from a theory of change failure or a failure to fully implement the program as intended. Moreover, process evaluation that also includes the control condition can help determine whether there is spillover in the program effects or whether there is a lack of contrast between the program condition and the control condition. For more details on process evaluation, see Peck and Snyder (Chapter 13, this volume) as well as Powell et al. (Chapter 12, this volume) on implementation.

A second type of descriptive analysis is **outcome monitoring**, which focuses on the proximal, intermediate, or longer-term outcomes, whether intended or unintended, rather than the intervention process. Analyses of outcomes may focus on either outcome level or outcome change. The outcome level is simply the value of the outcome at a given point in time. The outcome change is the difference between the outcome level from one time period to the next. Evaluators should identify appropriate outcomes (in consultation with relevant interest holders and as outlined in the program's theory of change) and determine the process for measuring those outcomes as part of the evaluation plan, as described in Chapter 16. Once the evaluator establishes relevant outcomes and collects data, they can begin the outcome monitoring process by summarizing and reporting those outcomes for program managers and other interest holders. Such reporting is descriptive in nature because it does not account for numerous factors, some of which have nothing to do with the program, that may contribute to the amount or change in an outcome, and findings must therefore be reported and interpreted without attributing the amount or change in the outcome measures to the program.

When conducting descriptive analysis, whether for process monitoring, outcome monitoring, or some other purpose, evaluators usually want to provide information about the averages or central tendency for a group, to contrast averages across groups. An evaluation for a multisite program may provide average process or outcome measures by site. For example, an evaluation of No Child Left Behind, a federal education policy focused on closing achievement gaps between subgroups of students, could calculate average test scores for students in these various subgroups to allow for comparison across subgroups or for computing differences between subgroups across multiple sites (schools in the case of the example).

The average test score for participants in a tutoring program is an example of **univariate analysis** because it involves the analysis of one variable without regard to its relationship with other variables. Univariate analysis involves simply reporting summary statistics for a single variable and may involve graphical as well as statistical analysis. Statistics you may compute as part of univariate analysis include central tendency (mean, median, mode), dispersion (standard deviation, variance, interquartile range, percentiles), and distribution (frequency, skewness, kurtosis). The summary statistics you choose to report depends on variable type, variable distribution, and audience. For example, frequency distributions are more interpretable for categorical variables than for continuous variables, which can have as many unique values as there are observations in the dataset. Consider an evaluation of a job training program in which you are interested in reporting the central tendency and dispersion of baseline earnings for participants. Given a single continuous income variable, either the mean or median would provide a reasonable measure of central tendency and the standard deviation or interquartile range would provide a reasonable measure of dispersion. A frequency tabulation, by contrast, would tell you very little because it would produce as many rows of frequencies as there are unique values of income. Suppose, however, that instead of a single continuous income variable, you have a categorical variable that takes eight possible values representing different amounts of income. In this situation, a mean or median would not tell you much at all because it would represent the mean of eight values that do not necessarily have intrinsic meaning, while the standard deviation and variance would only describe the spread of incomes across those eight categories. But frequency tabulation would provide useful information about central tendency (e.g., the mode is the value that appears with the highest frequency) and dispersion of the categorical variable.

In calculating the central tendency of a continuous variable, it is important to remember that the mean of a variable with one or two very high outliers may be skewed, making the median a more appropriate measure. For example, the mean annual income of a **sample** with Bill Gates and 99 people who make $40,000 per year is about $80,000—twice the income level of 99% of the sample. By contrast, the median is $40,000, a more accurate measure of the sample. Table 17.1 provides an overview of summary statistics on central tendency and variation, and contexts in which they may and may not be appropriate measures.

TABLE 17.1. Measures of Central Tendency and Dispersion

Measure	Brief description	Good for . . .	Not good for . . .
Central tendency			
Mean	The average value, calculated as the sum of all observation values divided by the number of observations.	• Continuous variables without extreme values or large enough sample sizes • Dichotomous variables for which you want to know the proportion of observations with a given characteristic	• Variables with extreme values that skew the mean • Ordinal variables in which the distance between equally spaced values does not have consistent meaning
Median	If the data were sorted smallest to largest, the value of the observation in the middle.	• Continuous variables with extreme values	• Categorical variables (nominal or ordinal)
Mode	The value that occurs most often for a variable in a dataset.	• Categorical variables (nominal or ordinal)	• Continuous variables that can take an infinite number of values
Dispersion			
Variance and standard deviation	The variance is the sum of squared deviations from the mean. In other words, subtract the value of each observation on a given variable from the mean of that variable, square it, and add all those squared deviations together. The standard deviation is simply the square root of the variance.	• Continuous and dichotomous variables • Any time you are reporting a mean	• Variables with extreme values that skew the mean may also skew the variance and standard deviation • Categorical variables (nominal or ordinal)
Interquartile range	The value at the 25th percentile of a given variable and the value of the 75th percentile. In other words, the range in which the middle 50% of observations fall on a given variable.	• Continuous variables with extreme values	• Categorical variables (nominal or ordinal)

Bivariate analysis includes many of the same approaches as univariate analysis but involves two variables instead of one. Instead of calculating a single arithmetic mean for an entire sample, you may calculate conditional means, which are simply arithmetic means under the condition that some other characteristic is true. For example, an evaluation of a job training program might include calculating the mean earnings for all participants, but then also calculating the mean earnings separately for female and male participants, or separately for different individuals with different levels of education (e.g., less than high school completion, high school completion, some college). These latter analyses are a form of bivariate analysis, which is an analysis of two variables at a time. The same measures of dispersion apply in this type of analysis but they are relative to the subgroups rather than the full sample. Another type of bivariate analysis is a simple correlation, which we describe in more detail below.

Descriptive analysis, both univariate and bivariate, may include the same types of graphs as exploratory analysis. Once you have computed measures of central tendency and dispersion, it is often useful to visualize some of those measures using graphical analysis. For example, seeing box-and-whisker plots for different subgroups next to one another allows the analyst to show how central tendency and dispersion vary from group to group. Line graphs with time on the x-axis and a continuous variable on the y-axis can show clearly how multiple groups change over time on average and in relation to one another. Bivariate analysis in a program evaluation may include bar graphs or box-and-whisker plots showing how process and outcome measures differ for the program participants and a comparison group. It could also compare means and standard deviations on these measures of interest for the treatment and comparison groups. However, these comparisons between the treatment and comparison groups should not be confused with program impacts. Outcome measures may vary for reasons other than program participation, and descriptive analysis does not isolate the program impact from those other reasons. Estimating program impacts is the domain of causal analysis, which we discuss in the next section.

CORRELATIONAL AND CAUSAL ANALYSIS

One of the most common goals for program evaluation is to isolate the effect of the program on various outcomes of interest. This particular type of program evaluation is often referred to as an **impact evaluation**. A high priority among multiple key interest holders from policymakers to program managers to funders is whether the program brings about better outcomes for participants relative to what those outcomes would have been in the absence of the program, which is called the **counterfactual**. Therefore, a primary goal of impact evaluation involves determining whether the program has caused a difference in the outcome for the target population that would not have occurred otherwise, and estimating the amount of this difference, what evaluators often call a **program effect** (Rossi et al., 2019). An overarching framework for understanding the issues involved in obtaining a credible estimate of the program effect, known as the potential outcomes framework, is discussed in the next section.

A GENERAL APPROACH TO IMPACT EVALUATION: THE POTENTIAL OUTCOMES FRAMEWORK

According to the **potential outcomes framework**, each individual has two potential outcomes, one if they are exposed to the program and one if they are not exposed to it (Rubin, 1974, 2008; VanderWeele, 2018). These outcomes can be the same or different. The average of the differences in the outcomes for each member of the target population is the average treatment effect. A central issue with determining the average treatment or program effect (what is known as the **fundamental problem of causal inference**) is that outcomes for a single individual cannot be simultaneously observed with and without exposure to the program (Holland, 1986).

For each individual, the fundamental problem of causal inference means that the outcome for an individual can only be observed as either participating or not participating in the program. Since an individual cannot be observed under both conditions simultaneously, the unobserved counterfactual is missing data. Although we cannot simultaneously observe the outcome for both conditions for each individual, it is possible to observe the average outcomes for individuals who are exposed to the program and the average outcomes for individuals who are not exposed to the program—that is, we can observe outcomes for two groups: the exposed (treatment) group and the unexposed (comparison or control) group. If it is reasonable to assume that in the absence of exposure to the program, the outcomes of the two groups would have been the same, then it is possible to estimate the average treatment/program effect. The credibility of an estimate of a program effect hinges on the reasonableness of this assumption.

However, the reasonableness of this assumption cannot be empirically verified since it would require simultaneously observing both outcomes for the same individual, which is impossible due to the fundamental problem of causal inference. Therefore, evaluators must use the average outcomes from individuals who were not exposed to the program to represent the potential outcomes for program participants had they not been program participants. If the selection into one of the two groups—those exposed and those unexposed to the program—is unrelated to the program outcomes, then the counterfactual is valid and the differences in outcomes can be reasonably attributed to program exposure. However, the selection process used to decide which members of the target population have access to the program could lead to different outcomes among participants and nonparticipants even in the absence of the program, an issue known as **selection bias**. For example, some studies find that students who attend charter schools tend to have better outcomes than students attending traditional public schools (Buddin & Zimmer, 2005; Epple et al., 2016). However, a fundamental concern with these studies is that parents must exert additional effort in order to withdraw their children from a traditional public school and find and apply for admission into a charter school. Under these conditions, it is highly probable that these parents would have put forth more effort to ensure that their children have higher-quality educational opportunities regardless of the charter school. Therefore, it is difficult to ascertain whether the difference in student outcomes is due to the charter school or due to the efforts of more motivated parents. Selection bias can represent both initial differences between participants and nonparticipants and differences in how the participants and nonparticipants would have responded to the program (Morgan & Winship, 2015). Both sources of selection bias are salient issues that must be resolved in order to establish credible estimates of program effects.

All attempts to estimate the effects of programs, policies, or interventions rest on four conditions for establishing causality—that is, in order to establish a causal relationship between a hypothesized cause and a hypothesized outcome, evaluators must establish that (1) the cause precedes the effect (temporal precedence), (2) the cause has a statistically significant relationship with the effect (observed covariation), (3) likely alternative explanations are ruled out (nonspuriousness), and (4) a plausible process exists to explain the observed relationship (a probable mechanism). Hence, evaluators hoping to make credible causal claims must use a combination of design and analyses to satisfy all four criteria.

We also note that the conditions and assumptions laid out below tend to focus on issues of bias, or the **internal validity**, of the estimated program effect. A separate issue of whether the program effects would widely apply beyond the study sample from which it is estimated is **external validity**. As we discuss below, some designs tend to offer higher internal validity but raise concerns for external validity, while others may offer greater external validity but more concerns for internal validity. In the next two sections, we describe two strategies for estimating program effects, which impose strict controls on program access and additional strategies that do not impose controls on program access.

Designs That Impose Strict Controls on Program Access

Under the potential outcomes framework, selection bias is a particular concern because nonparticipants (who represent the unobserved counterfactual condition) may be systematically different from program participants either initially or in how they respond to the program. In this section, we describe research designs that eliminate selection bias by strictly controlling which members of the target population have access to the program. There are two designs that can eliminate selection bias: **randomized designs**, including **randomized control trials (RCTs)**, and **regression discontinuity (RD)** designs.

RCTs utilize **random assignment** or **randomization** to designate whether an individual participates in the program. Random assignment requires that each individual be assigned to either the experimental (program participant) or control (nonparticipant) condition based purely on a random process, such as a coin toss. Additionally, in order for experimental estimates to be credible average effects of the program, the integrity of the random assignment process must be strictly observed, so that no individuals switch from their randomly assigned condition. If the integrity of the random assignment is upheld, any differences between individuals in the experimental and control groups are also randomly distributed between the two groups making them, on average, balanced across all factors that may affect their postintervention outcome. With assurance that the experimental and control groups are equivalent on average, mean differences in the outcome between the two groups can reasonably be attributed to the program.

Often considered the gold standard for establishing causal estimates, RCTs provide strong protection against any spurious factors that may bias estimates of the program effect but only if the initial random assignment is not compromised. The random assignment can be compromised by noncompliance or differential attrition. **Noncompliance** occurs when individuals do not comply with their randomly assigned condition (e.g., individuals assigned to participate in the program choose not to participate and vice versa). Relatedly, **differential attrition** occurs when individuals leave either condition for a reason related to their treatment assignment. For example, differential attrition occurs when individuals leave a free community exercise program because they are physically active and already have access to a preferred exercise facility. In this situation, individuals remaining in the experimentally treated conditions may be less active and have poorer health on average than individuals in the control condition. Hence, the differential attrition among healthier individuals will diminish the estimate of any potentially positive health effects coming from the community exercise program. Another important limitation of the RCT is its feasibility. Some social programs cannot be ethically or practically randomized. For example, students cannot be randomly assigned to high-crime versus low-crime schools in order to quantify the impact of unsafe learning environments on academic performance. Other situations, when exposure to a "treatment" that is known to be harmful, cannot be ethically assigned by the evaluators, which means that RCTs cannot be applied in some evaluation settings.

The second strategy that imposes strict controls on exposure to the program is called the regression discontinuity (RD) design. In this respect, the RD design is similar to the RCT. However, unlike in an RCT, individuals in an RD design are assigned to program participation based on a quantitative **assignment variable** (also called a **forcing variable**). In an RD design, all individuals in the evaluation have a value for the assignment variable and then are placed into either the program participant or nonparticipant condition based on whether their value of the assignment variable is above or below some prespecified cut point. In the absence of the intervention, the units just above the cutoff and those just below the cutoff are likely to be very similar. When restricting access to the intervention to individuals close to the cutoff, the difference in the two groups' outcomes can be reasonably attributed to access to the intervention after controlling for the quantitative assignment variable. Controlling for the assignment variable ensures that individuals on either side of the cut point have been effectively randomized and the differences in outcomes are attributable to the intervention.

The RD design has strong internal validity but is subject to some potential sources of bias that the evaluator should examine. Like in RCTs, noncompliance could occur if some individuals assigned to the intervention end up not participating, or vice versa. Noncompliance is easily observed when the assignment variable and participation status are visible to the evaluator. In cases where noncompliance is observed, the evaluator can use a "fuzzy" regression discontinuity design to rescale the program effect estimate in a way that reflects the number of noncomplying individuals (Bertanha & Imbens, 2020; Imbens & Lemieux, 2008). A more difficult problem occurs when the values of the assignment variable are systematically manipulated to ensure that certain individuals who have systematically better (or worse) outcomes have access to the program and/or others who have systematically worse (or better) outcomes do not. Evaluators can assess this possibility by investigating whether a disproportionate number of individuals have scores on either side of the cutoff (McCrary, 2008), which may indicate manipulation of the values of the assignment variable. Other relevant validity checks include examining whether individuals on either side of the cutoff have similar baseline characteristics using **balance tests**, testing whether discontinuities in outcomes occur at values of the assignment variable other than the cutoff, checking for differential attrition, ensuring that the relationship between the assignment variable and the outcome has been properly specified, and checking the sensitivity of the effect estimate to include individuals who are further away from the cutoff (What Works Clearinghouse, 2017).

While both RCTs and RDs have high inherent capacity to produce unbiased (internally valid) estimates of program effects, they may be difficult to implement for ethical or practical reasons. For example, RD designs cannot be implemented in situations where the assignment to the intervention is not done according to values on a quantitative assignment variable. The program effect estimates from these designs may also have questionable external validity since they apply to very specific samples (e.g., RD designs apply only to individuals near the cutoff, and RCTs rely on participants who were recruited or volunteered for a study). When these two **design-based** methods cannot be feasibly applied to the evaluation circumstances, evaluators can turn to more feasible designs that may be more vulnerable to bias but may also offer greater external validity.

Designs That Do Not Impose Strict Controls on Access to the Intervention

The designs that do not impose controls on program access attempt to remove the effects of confounding factors, or factors other than the intervention, which may cause the outcomes of the group that has access to the intervention and those that do not to differ. Often collectively called **quasi-experimental** or **comparison group evaluation designs**, these methods include a variety of strategies to remove, or at least reduce, the effects of potential **confounders** (factors that influence both selection into the program and the relevant outcome). Examples of such methods include covariate-adjusted **regression**, matched sampling, and interrupted time-series designs. We note that these designs continue to be under active development. The decision about which of these designs to apply in any particular evaluation will depend largely on data availability and the evaluation purposes. Because these strategies also tend to be more widely applicable to larger study populations, they often have greater external validity than designs with strict controls but this increased external validity comes with increased concerns for the credibility of the program effect estimates.

Unlike RCTs and RD designs, comparison group designs do not directly manipulate individual exposure to the program and instead rely on a variety of methods to obtain credibly causal estimates under some prespecified assumptions. Without the ability to control individual access to the program, these analytical methods are subject to a number of potential biases in addition to selection bias, including time trends, unobserved treatments, maturation, and mean reversion (Rossi et al., 2019). **Time trends** are a source of bias where external forces lead individuals to change in systematic ways across time. For example, studies of birth rates in some countries can be biased by declining birth rates over time that are unrelated to any one particular program. **Unobserved treatments** occur when an external event affects the evaluation outcomes, independent of the program effects. For example, a sudden heat wave could cause ice cream sales to spike while a new marketing campaign for ice cream is being evaluated. Without attention to the heat wave, increased sales would be inappropriately attributed to the marketing campaign instead of the heat wave. **Maturation** occurs in longitudinal evaluations when the target population changes even in the absence of the program. An example of maturation occurs in evaluations of preschool programs where student test scores at the beginning of the school year are compared with scores at the end of the year. In these comparisons, it is likely that these children would develop cognitively throughout the year even without attending preschool. Maturation threats are relevant in comparison group designs only when there is evidence that program participants and comparison group individuals will differentially mature—if the treatment and comparison groups mature at the same rate, then maturation is not a threat to validity. Finally, **mean reversion** (also known as regression to the mean) occurs when extreme values of a certain outcome at one time period revert to their natural long-term averages in later time periods. An example of mean reversion occurs when a public health campaign is enacted after a particularly strong flu season. The strength of the flu will likely return to less extreme levels in the following year, which would bias the estimated effects of the public health campaign if not properly taken into account when interpreting the differences between the two years as the program effect.

In order to adjust for observed differences between program participants and nonparticipants, evaluators often use **multivariate regression** techniques that control for **covariates**. Multivariate regression models are designed to account for preexisting differences between program participants and nonparticipants that may affect postintervention outcomes, which we refer to as confounders. For instance, the effects of a job training program may be biased by preexisting differences in education levels of participants and nonparticipants. Including education levels as a covariate in the multivariate regression analysis allows the evaluator to essentially condition the outcome comparisons by comparing those in the treatment and comparison groups with similar education levels to each other. An important strength of this strategy is that it allows evaluators to also control for factors that are correlated with observed covariates. For example, education level is likely related to innate academic ability. After controlling for education level, academic ability will also be controlled to the extent that it is related to education level. However, a major limitation of this covariate adjustment approach is that relevant confounders are often unavailable for the analysis of the program effects, either because the measures were not collected or cannot be obtained. The limited availability of measures for relevant confounders means that evaluation results based purely on covariate-adjusted regressions are unlikely to be free of bias. Instead, these estimates are usually considered correlational in that they can help the evaluator to establish that difference exists between the program participants and comparison group on a relevant outcome but are insufficient to conclude that the program caused the observed difference.

Another approach for reducing bias is matched sampling. **Matching** methods typically involve finding comparison subjects who are similar to program participants on variables that have been collected for both groups. Characteristics that are important to use in matching include any factors related to both selection into the program and the relevant outcomes. Consider an evaluation of a volunteer job training program on participants' likelihood of obtaining a job. An important matching characteristic in this evaluation would be prior job experience if individuals with less experience are both more likely to join the program and less likely to obtain a job. The choice of matching variables will depend on theoretical considerations and relevant factors as identified in previous research. To the extent possible, evaluators should strive to measure and include relevant factors correlated with both selection and the outcome—however, just as with covariate adjustment, some matching variables may be highly correlated with each other, relaxing the need to include all correlated factors in the matching process.

Multiple matching methods exist, including propensity score matching, exact matching, nearest neighbor matching, and coarsened exact matching (Abadie & Imbens, 2016; Austin, 2011; Rosenbaum & Rubin, 1983). The most straightforward matching method, **exact matching**, requires evaluators to find comparison individuals who share exactly the same characteristics as each program participant on the chosen set of matching variables. While exact matches serve as a good comparison case, this method is difficult to implement, especially when multiple matching variables are used, because there may not be any comparison individuals in the study who exactly match all program participants. Given the difficulty with finding exact matches, evaluators often choose to use exact matching on only one or two variables as an initial step to matching.

In order to address the difficulty that arises from finding exact matches with multiple covariates, evaluators commonly use a matching method called **propensity score matching** (Abadie & Imbens, 2016; Caliendo & Kopeinig, 2008; Stuart, 2008). In propensity score matching, all relevant matching variables are used to predict the likelihood that an individual will participate in the program. The predicted likelihood of participation is called a **propensity score**, a single value that can be used to match program participants with comparison group members. Once propensity scores are predicted for all study participants, the evaluator would typically compare the distribution of propensity scores for both the program participant group and the comparison sample in order to remove individuals from either group with propensity scores that are either too high or too low to be matched to the other group. This **trimming** process ensures that the two groups have sufficient **overlap** or similarities on the propensity to be program participants. Then, to ensure the matching process worked as expected, the two matched groups should be compared on the most critical covariates that are correlated with the outcome to ensure that they are equivalent. This condition is called **covariate balance**.

The trimming and covariate balancing processes produce a participant group and comparison group that should be similar on observed characteristics that are most likely to be correlated with both selection and the outcome. The matched groups can be compared in a number of ways, including stratification, weighting, or regression adjustment (Rossi et al., 2019). In **stratification**, participants and matched individuals are placed into separate bins, or strata, based on the propensity score (e.g., deciles). Individuals within the same bins have similar propensity scores, so the outcome differences between program participants and comparison individuals can be calculated within each bin and then averaged together. In **weighting**, participants are weighted so that comparison individuals with a higher propensity for joining the program have a larger influence in estimating the program effect. In regression adjustment, the propensity score is directly included as a covariate along with other covariates, thereby controlling for selection into the program to the extent that the variables included in the regression comprise or correlate with all variables that influence both selection and the outcome. Interested readers should consult specific methodological texts on matching for further details (Abadie & Imbens, 2016; Caliendo & Kopeinig, 2008; Rosenbaum & Rubin, 1983; Rossi et al., 2019; Stuart, 2008).

Matching methods have become widely popular comparison group designs because of their broad applicability across multiple evaluation circumstances and available data. The diverse range of matching techniques also provides evaluators with the opportunity to test whether estimates of program effects are robust across multiple matching methods. However, we caution that these methods all rest on the assumption that the differences are causal and that all factors related to both selection into the program and the outcome are highly correlated with a matching variable or a covariate in the regression adjustments. The potential for bias remains when important covariates are omitted or missing and evaluators using matching methods should be careful to acknowledge when potentially critical covariates are missing.

A different type of comparison group design leverages change over time to estimate program effects and includes methods such as interrupted time-series, difference-in-differences, and fixed-effect models. The simplest of these methods, the **interrupted time-series (ITS)** model, compares outcomes for program participants before and after joining the program. The strategy does not require comparisons between program participants and comparison individuals but instead compares participants to themselves before joining the program. Because the ITS model relies on comparison over time, it is most vulnerable to bias from any other changes that occur at approximately the same time as exposure to the program, including time trends, unobserved treatments, maturation, and mean reversion. In order to implement this approach, evaluators need outcome data from participants in at least one time period before they join the program and one time period after they join the program. This approach could be augmented with multiple periods before and after participation in the program and the inclusion of covariates to help control for variables that could affect the outcome, which are potential sources of bias in the estimates of program effects. A common way to extend the ITS model is to compare cohorts of individuals who participate in the program with earlier cohorts that did not participate, often called a **cohort design**. In these cases, the earlier cohorts act as a counterfactual for how the later cohorts would have fared on relevant outcome measures had they not been exposed to the program. For example, a reading intervention for third-grade students can be assessed by comparing student achievement outcomes for third graders in previous years who did not receive the reading intervention with later cohorts of third graders who do participate in the intervention. The validity of this strategy is vulnerable to changes over time that could be affecting successive cohorts in ways unrelated to the program. For example, a reading intervention program may overlap with more concerted efforts to help teachers improve by providing them with more training on literacy instruction. If the implementation of the reading intervention program coincides with steadily increasing teacher effectiveness due to extra training, estimates of the reading intervention could be biased by the improvements in teacher performance.

One way to strengthen the ITS model is to add a comparison group, so that the pre–post differences for program participants can be compared with the same pre–post difference for a group of comparison individuals who did not participate in the program. This strategy is called a **difference-in-differences** (DID) model because it directly calculates a difference between two differences (Athey & Imbens, 2006; Card & Krueger, 1993; Goodman-Bacon, 2018). The advantage of the DID model is the addition of a comparison group that has been exposed to the same time trends and other changes in the environment as the program participants. In the third-grade intervention example, adding a comparison group of similar third graders in the same schools who did not participate in the reading intervention program would help to remove any bias coming from the teacher training effects occurring at the same time, because the comparison third graders would have also benefited from the training the teachers received.

The central identifying assumption for the DID model is that, conditional on covariates, the pre–post changes in the outcomes for the comparison group would have been the same as those for the program participants had they not joined the program. Although there is no direct test of this assumption, evidence that it is likely to hold can be provided by comparing the trends of the participant and comparison groups prior to the interruption of the treatment to see if they are **parallel trends**. Note that the two groups do not necessarily need to have had the same levels of outcomes in the preprogram time periods. Rather, the two groups should behave in similar ways to show that any external events affecting the outcome occurred in both groups, leaving the impact of the program as the only difference. Showing that the program participants and comparison groups are similar on observed characteristics prior to program initiation also provides evidence that the comparison group is likely a valid counterfactual. Other relevant concerns for the DID model include unobserved treatments and mean reversion. Unobserved treatments refer to the possibility of other interventions occurring for the intervention group besides the program of interest (e.g., when an increase in minimum wage coincides with a large company offering new job opportunities in the same area). Mean reversion occurs when program participants exhibit one instance of particularly low or high performance just before joining the program, such that they are likely to revert back to their long-term average performance after joining the program. Evaluators can help address this concern by averaging multiple years of preprogram outcome data so that the measure of preprogram performance is less sensitive to one period of particularly low or high performance.

Along the same lines, the DID model can be strengthened by using multiple time periods of outcome data to model the preintervention trends for participants and nonparticipants prior to the beginning of the program. This approach, called a comparative interrupted time-series (CITS) model, allows the program effect to be estimated as a deviation from the preprogram trends, rather than as an aggregated pre–post difference (Somers et al., 2013). The CITS model requires a longer time series than the DID, but similar to the DID model, the CITS model is vulnerable to bias from a comparison group that may not represent a valid counterfactual trend for how participants would have behaved in the absence of the program. Another consideration for the CITS model is that it assumes the preprogram outcome trends are correctly modeled and that they are a good approximation of post-program trends. This assumption becomes more tenuous when examining long-term outcomes (Bloom, 2003; Hallberg et al., 2018).

The version of the time-series model with the greatest causal warrant uses only the variation of outcomes across time for each individual in the study, rather than both within and between individual variation. This model first calculates the deviation for each person in each time period from that person's average performance across all time periods. These deviations involve both the periods before and after program exposure. Then, the individual deviations for each time period are compared between the periods when the individual participated in the program with comparison periods when the individuals did not participate. The program effect is then the individual-level postparticipation deviations minus preparticipation deviations for those exposed to program minus the individual-level postparticipation deviations minus preparticipation deviations for those *not* exposed to the program, then averaged across all individuals in the sample. This strategy, called a **fixed-effect model,** has an inherent advantage in that it compares individuals with themselves across time. Therefore, any observed or unobserved individual characteristics that do not vary across time (e.g., innate ability) are controlled in the model.

Note that we have been discussing the fixed-effects model using individuals, but fixed effects can be applied to different types of units, including neighborhoods, schools, or states. In these cases, the fixed effects control for any characteristics that do not vary for individuals within the unit. For example, a state fixed effect would control for the confounding effects of statewide characteristics, like minimum wage increases, that affect all individuals living in the state. The fixed-effects model requires that multiple observations be nested within each unit (e.g., multiple individuals within a state). For individual-level fixed effects, the model requires that each individual be observed multiple times in the data. The fixed-effects model also requires that program participants and the comparison group be observed in both the period before and after joining the program. Although the fixed-effects model helps to control for any confounding characteristics shared between observations within a unit, there remains the potential for within-unit differences and time-varying characteristics to bias estimates of program effects. For example, a model that uses state fixed effects does not control for bias from factors that differ between individuals within the same state (e.g., race, education level, income) or factors that vary across time, such as the election of a new governor. As with all other comparison group designs discussed in this chapter, the fixed-effects approach can address some sources of bias under particular assumptions, and it is up to the evaluator to decide whether the quantitative approach used has sufficiently addressed all key sources of bias.

SUMMARY AND CONCLUSION

Throughout this chapter, we have outlined multiple quantitative analyses that serve different evaluation purposes ranging from exploratory to descriptive to correlational and causal analysis. Exploratory analysis uses graphical techniques and foundational measures of central tendency and dispersion to visualize and discover patterns. Using similar methods, descriptive analysis aims to describe and summarize data. Correlation analysis uses techniques such as covariate adjusted regression to establish a relationship between two variables (e.g., participation in an exercise program and physical fitness). In order to isolate an unbiased program effect using causal analysis, the evaluator must be sensitive to key sources of bias and the availability of data. In cases when designs with strict controls on program access (RCT and RD designs) are feasible, they offer the greatest protection against bias when estimating program effects. When these approaches cannot be applied, comparison group designs offer more flexible approaches that can be adapted to many evaluation situations where the estimation of program effects is a goal. In these cases, the evaluator must decide which approach or combination of approaches are most likely to address the most critical sources of biases. In addition, due to the limitations that will likely remain, evaluators should make the audiences for the evaluation aware of these limitations after making concerted efforts to address them. Though imperfect, this careful approach to evaluation provides useful and rigorously obtained knowledge in contribution toward a goal of improving individual and collective well-being.

REFERENCES

Abadie, A., & Imbens, G. W. (2016). Matching on the estimated propensity score. *Econometrica*, 84(2), 781–807.

Athey, S., & Imbens, G. W. (2006). Identification and inference in nonlinear difference-in-differences models. *Econometrica*, 74(2), 431–497.

Austin, P. C. (2011). A tutorial and case study in propensity score analysis: An application to estimating the effect of in-hospital smoking cessation counseling on mortality. *Multivariate Behavioral Research*, 46(1), 119–151.

Babbie, E. R. (2020). *The practice of social research*. Cengage Learning.

Bertanha, M., & Imbens, G. W. (2020). External validity in fuzzy regression discontinuity designs. *Journal of Business and Economic Statistics*, 38(3), 593–612.

Bloom, H. S. (2003). Using "short" interrupted time-series analysis to measure the impacts of whole-school reforms. *Evaluation Review*, 27(1), 3–49.

Buddin, R., & Zimmer, R. (2005). Student achievement in charter schools: A complex picture. *Journal of Policy Analysis and Management*, 24(2), 351–371.

Caliendo, M., & Kopeinig, S. (2008). Some practical guidance for the implementation of propensity score matching. *Journal of Economic Surveys*, 22(1), 31–72.

Card, D., & Krueger, A. B. (1993). *Minimum wages and employment: A case study of the fast food industry in New Jersey and Pennsylvania*. National Bureau of Economic Research.

Epple, D., Romano, R., & Zimmer, R. (2016). Charter schools: A survey of research on their characteristics and effectiveness. In E. A. Hanushek, S. Machin, & L. Woessmann (Eds.), *Handbook of the economics of education* (Vol. 5, pp. 139–208). Elsevier.

Goodman-Bacon, A. (2018). Difference-in-differences with variation in treatment timing. *NBER Working Paper*.

Hallberg, K., Williams, R., Swanlund, A., & Eno, J. (2018). Short comparative interrupted time series using aggregate school-level data in education research. *Educational Researcher*, 47(5), 295–306.

Henry, G. T., & Harbatkin, E. (2020). The next generation of state reforms to improve their lowest performing schools: An evaluation of North Carolina's school transformation intervention. *Journal of Research on Educational Effectiveness*, 13(4), 702–730.

Holland, P. W. (1986). Statistics and causal inference. *Journal of the American Statistical Association*, 81(396), 945–960.

Imbens, G. W., & Lemieux, T. (2008). Regression discontinuity designs: A guide to practice. *Journal of Econometrics*, 142(2), 615–635.

McCrary, J. (2008). Manipulation of the running variable in the regression discontinuity design: A density test. *Journal of Econometrics*, 142(2), 698–714.

Morgan, S. L., & Winship, C. (2015). *Counterfactuals and causal inference*. Cambridge University Press.

Rosenbaum, P. R., & Rubin, D. B. (1983). The central role of the propensity score in observational studies for causal effects. *Biometrika*, 70(1), 41–55.

Rossi, P. H., Lipsey, M. W., & Henry, G. T. (2019). *Evaluation: A systematic approach* (8th ed.). SAGE.

Rubin, D. B. (1974). Estimating causal effects of treatments in randomized and nonrandomized studies. *Journal of Educational Psychology*, 66(5), 688–701.

Rubin, D. B. (2008). For objective causal inference, design trumps analysis. *Annals of Applied Statistics*, 2(3), 808–840.

Somers, M.-A., Zhu, P., Jacob, R., & Bloom, H. (2013). The validity and precision of the comparative interrupted time series design and the difference-in-difference design in educational evaluation. *MDRC*.

StataCorp. (2023). *Stata 18 data management reference manual: Census11 dataset*. Stata Press.

Stuart, E. A. (2008). Developing practical recommendations for the use of propensity scores: Discussion of "A critical appraisal of propensity score matching in the medical literature between 1996 and 2003" by Peter Austin. *Statistics in Medicine, 27*(12), 2062–2065.

VanderWeele, T. J. (2018). On well-defined hypothetical interventions in the potential outcomes framework. *Epidemiology, 29*(4), e24–e25.

What Works Clearinghouse. (2017). *Standards handbook: Version 4.0*. U.S. Department of Education, Institute of Education Sciences, National Center for Education Evaluation and Regional Assistance, What Works Clearinghouse. Available at *https://ies.ed.gov/ncee/wwc/Docs/referenceresources/wwc_standards_handbook_v4.pdf*

Chapter 18

Mixed Methods Design

Tarek Azzam
Natalie D. Jones

CHAPTER OVERVIEW

As a developing methodological approach, mixed methods have the potential to be a useful tool for evaluators and researchers alike. With its ability to help answer various questions through the integration of qualitative and quantitative data, mixed methods have become a preferred design among evaluators. Providing an overview of mixed methods, this chapter discusses the unique decision points that need to be considered as part of the design process, including (1) the priority placed on each data source, (2) the timing of when qual and quant will be collected, and (3) where the actual mixing or integration of the qual and quant will occur. Subsequent sections introduce the common mixed methods designs: convergent/parallel design, explanatory/exploratory sequential designs, and multiphase/complex designs, and describe how they can each be used to answer various evaluation questions. Last, the chapter discusses issues related to the use of mixed methods, worldviews (e.g., constructivist, transformative, pragmatist, and postpositivist), potential tools, and future directions.

Mixed methods has become a widely used evaluation design, with over 70% of evaluators indicating that this is their preferred design (Azzam, 2011). This popularity can be partially explained by the potential usefulness of mixed methods at answering various evaluation questions, such as the following:

1. Why did we get these quantitative survey findings or patterns, and what do they mean?
2. Are the outcomes that were described by participants during qualitative interviews common across the broader population of participants?
3. What additional evidence can we bring to bear to support our quantitative or qualitative evaluation findings?

These questions can be answered through the purposeful integration of **quantitative** (quant) data (e.g., ratings from surveys, scores on a test, attendance numbers; see Harbatkin et al., Chapter 16, this volume) and **qualitative** (qual) data (e.g., interviews, observations, focus groups; see Rallis & Usinger, Chapter 15, this volume) in a design that aims to build on the strength of each data source (Tashakkori & Teddlie, 2010). The key to mixing these two data sources is figuring out what evaluation questions you want answered, what **priority** (or level of importance of each data source) is placed on the different types of data, and the **timing** of the mixing (e.g., will the qual and quant be collected at the same time, or will it happen sequentially where the results of one data source will inform the design and analysis of the other data source?). These are the topics that we discuss in this chapter and delve deeper into how mixed methods can be used to answer various evaluation questions.

OVERVIEW OF MIXED METHODS

The development and acknowledgment of mixed methods as an approach to research and evaluation design is a relatively recent phenomena that essentially emerged during the paradigm debates that started in the 1970s and continued through the mid-1990s (Creswell & Plano Clark, 2017). These debates helped the development of the idea that qual and quant, if mixed in a purposeful manner, can be leveraged to improve our ability to answer research (Bryman, 1988) and evaluation questions (Reichardt & Rallis, 1994). There was also evidence to suggest that we have actually been doing this type of mixing for some time, and even though there has been evidence of mixed methods being implemented, many of these previous efforts at mixing qual and quant were frequently unintentional (Maxwell, 2016). This is important to note because if the different types of data are not integrated in some way, then it's not a mixed methods design. The integration tends to be a core component of mixed methods, and is often incorporated into the multiple definitions of mixed methods that include the following "**[mixed methods research** is] research in which the investigator collects and analyses data, integrates the findings, and draws inferences using both qualitative and quantitative approaches or methods in a single study or a program of inquiry" (Tashakkori & Creswell, 2007, p. 4). There are also different strategies for how to do the integration (Guetterman et al., 2020), and we attempt to cover some of the main ways of doing so in this chapter.

Mixed methods has unique decision points that need to be considered as part of the design process, including (1) the priority placed on each data source, (2) the timing of when qual and quant will be collected, and (3) where the actual mixing or integration of the qual and quant will occur.

The first decision that should be made when designing a mixed method study is the priority placed on each of the data sources. Priority in mixed methods refers to the degree of emphasis or weight placed on a qual or quant data source over the other (Creswell & Plano Clark, 2017). In some cases, it may be ideal for both the qual and quant to have the same degree of emphasis or priority when the data are collected simultaneously. For instance, if the emphasis is on triangulation of qual and quant, an evaluation assessing the effectiveness of a math program on increasing math confidence may place equal priority on the qual and quant data within a mixed methods design. For this design the evaluation team would interview students about their math confidence and ask them to complete a math confidence quant survey. This design would allow for potential alignment between the qual and quant data sources. However, due to several factors related to the training of the researcher/evaluator—the type of questions that are asked, the expense of collecting different types of data, and the quality of the data collected—one can place a higher priority on one data source over the other. If we know that there are methodological issues with how a quant survey was collected (e.g., very low response rate), then we can prioritize the findings from a qual study over the quant findings. This could be a decision made after the fact but ideally it would be better to consider the priority question before the study is implemented. For example, if you know that the resources available for the evaluation would not allow you to conduct a high-quality qualitative study, then you should be explicit about the priority placed on that data source when communicating the design and how discrepant findings would be dealt with.

Next, the timing of when the qual and quant data will be collected is critically important, and in essence defines the type of questions that can be answered and the designs that can be used. Therefore, the timing of the data collection should be carefully considered and planned before carrying out the design. There are two broad timing decisions that should be made: will the qual and quant data be collected at approximately the same time (simultaneous) or will one data source be collected and analyzed, then used to inform the design and collection of the second data source (sequential)? The simultaneous timing of data collection can be used to gather qual and quant data that focus on the same phenomena, such as a program's outcomes, and attain different forms of evidence to better understand the phenomena discussed further in the convergent design section. With simultaneous data collection the integration between the qual and quant usually occurs after each data source has been analyzed independently, then each source is compared to the other. This process should yield a more nuanced or complete understanding of a specific outcome since multiple perspectives are brought to bear on it (Fielding, 2012: Kern, 2018; Turner et al., 2017). For instance, in a study examining depression a convergent design was used to compare physicians' depression ratings of patients (by quant) to actual patient interviews. These two data sources on patient depression helped to identify factors that led to accurate identification of depression (e.g., specific behaviors), and factors that reduced the accuracy of identifying depression (e.g., age of patients; Wittink et al., 2006).

The sequential timing decision can also be relevant to evaluators interested in (1) explaining quant findings through the use of qual data (discussed further in the explanatory design section), or (2) need to understand the program context/process/outcomes through exploratory qual data before the development and use of quant measures (discussed further in the exploratory design section). With sequential timing the integration happens after one type of data source is collected and analyzed. The findings from this initial data source are then used to inform the design and collection of another data source. For example, you may collect grade point average (GPA) quant data from participating students, and after conducting the analysis you notice that male GPAs are significantly lower than female GPAs, even after accounting for hypothesized covariates. This finding may inform the design of a qualitative study that uses interviews or focus groups to help you explain why this difference exists, discussed further in the explanatory design section.

The third critical decision to be made in a mixed methods study is where in the process of the study (i.e., the design, collection, analysis, and/or interpretation of findings) the mixing or **integration** of the qual and quant pieces will occur. There are different integration approaches that are highlighted in this chapter, and often the design dictates when this integration occurs. However, there should be a purposeful effort to consider when the mixing of the qual and quant will occur. For example, the mixing could occur at the last stage of the evaluation after the qual and quant data have been independently collected and analyzed. In this case the findings from each data source could be compared to determine whether there is agreement or disagreement between them. Another option is to mix the data sources during the data analysis stage. Degree of agreement can be estimated by merging the qual and quant into the same database and transforming one data source to match the format of the other. For example, qual interviews discussing participants' satisfaction with the program can be **quantitized** (converted to quant data) by counting the frequency that participants said something good or bad about the program. Similarly, qual data can also be transformed into quant data through the process known as **qualitizing** (e.g., factor analysis). This information can then be linked to the participants' survey responses in the same database to see whether their quant ratings matched their quantitized descriptions of the program. This approach has some advantages but it can also reduce the rich qual data and may violate the essence of qualitative approaches—we discuss this in greater detail in this chapter's section on issues in the use of mixed methods.

A third possible option for mixing qual and quant can occur during the data collection phase of a mixed methods study. The mixing can occur when one form of data informs the design and collection of another form of data. This is also linked to the timing issue and requires the conduct of a sequential approach. For example, an evaluator may use qual data to better understand the experiences of participants, and through the conduct of interviews identifies themes that represent the program's impact on participants. The mixing between the qual and quant occurs when the findings from the qual phase of the evaluation are used to inform the development of quant measures. These quant measures represent an attempt to test the generalizability of the qual findings to a broader sample.

We hope that these examples illustrate the critical decisions that should be made when designing a mixed methods study. The subsequent details presented in the rest of this chapter can increase your awareness and allow you to anticipate critical factors that can contribute to the success of your mixed methods evaluation. However, it should be noted that there are other factors that also inform these key decisions, including access to participants, funding levels, and the amount of time given to the evaluation. It's worth noting that budgeting for a mixed methods study can be more difficult to accurately anticipate, since some designs require that data collection and analysis occur after (and be informed by) an initial round of data collection and analysis. This means that as an evaluator, you might not know exactly what additional qual or quant data you would need in subsequent phases of the design. There are different ways of approaching this issue: The first is to estimate the cost of conducting the full mixed methods study using the best information you have at the time and keep the subsequent qual or quant phases limited within the budget as they are being developed. This is typically the most pragmatic approach in many contexts. The other approach is to budget each phase separately and use the most up-to-date information to ensure that you are able to design each phase to the best of your ability. This option tends to be less common, as budgets are frequently determined months if not years in advance. Therefore, the feasibility and benefit of a particular study design should be considered in light of the potential benefits (see Bickman, Chapter 21, and Bamberger, Chapter 24, this volume). Additionally, evaluators using a multiphase/complex design need to consider the many factors, including the emergent nature of many of the designs and the potential for additional associated costs. Therefore, proposals (e.g., institutional review board and evaluation plans using mixed methods, especially multiphase/complex designs) should include a section discussing the flexible and often emergent nature of such design.

The remaining sections of this chapter introduce you to common mixed methods designs and how they can be used to answer various evaluation questions and provide you with an overview of current tools and issues related to mixed methods.

COMMON MIXED METHODS DESIGNS

The analogy of building blocks might be a good way to think about the different possible design options in mixed methods. Each block is comprised of different qual and quant data sources that can be used simultaneously or sequentially and combined together to answer different research and evaluation questions. There are different taxonomies for mixed methods (Guest, 2013) but none fully capture the possible range of designs. Given this situation, Creswell and Plano Clark (2017) suggest that we focus on three building blocks, which they describe as core designs, and can be combined together in myriad ways (if needed) to form a fourth broad category of more complex mixed method designs. These three core blocks include:

1. **Convergent/parallel designs** (core)
2. **Explanatory sequential designs** (core)
3. **Exploratory sequential designs** (core)
4. They can be combined to form **multiphase/complex designs.**[1]

Throughout this section we take each of these core designs and provide an overview that describes:

- The types of questions that the design is well suited to answer.
- Common implementation procedures.
- Strengths and challenges with the design and its implementation.
- Integration techniques for different types of data within the design.

Then we examine more complex designs that are multiphased to provide a sense of how mixed methods can be adapted to suit different evaluation situations and questions.

---
[1] Multiphase/complex design also encompass multilevel and fully integrated designs.

Convergent/Parallel Designs

The convergent design, also referred to as a simultaneous design, attempts to use qual and quant data sources that focus on answering the same question (see Figure 18.1). For instance, an evaluator could use this design to answer "What additional evidence can we bring to bear to support our quantitative or qualitative evaluation findings?" This design can also be applied to different or related aspects of the question.

One example of this is if an evaluator wants to know more about program participants' intrinsic motivation, then they could use a convergent mixed method design to collect quant and qual data on that outcome. A validated quant intrinsic motivation (e.g., Children's Academic Intrinsic Motivation Inventory [CAIMI]) survey can be distributed to participants and used to provide an overview of the participants' intrinsic motivation level. At the same time the evaluator may also conduct interviews or focus groups with another participant sample during which they ask participants to describe their level of intrinsic motivation and if and how the program may have affected it. The quant and qual data could then be analyzed separately, then compared (or integrated) to see if there is agreement or disagreement between the two different data sources. The comparison can offer some very relevant insights about the program and its potential effects. If there is agreement between the qual and quant that intrinsic motivation is high after participating in the program, then this provides the evaluator with consistent evidence about the program's potential effects given that two different sources of data converged on the same finding.

Even a disagreement between the qual and quant data sources can offer opportunities for learning about the program and its participants. For example, if the qual data suggest that participants had low intrinsic motivation, while the quant data suggest that it's high, then this can lead to additional insights about the appropriateness of the measures used in the evaluation. The quant survey may be measuring something wholly different from what the participants are actually experiencing, and this would suggest a need to use a different quant measure. The same may be true for the collected qual data and can lead to refinements in the types of questions asked. There are also issues of method quality that can come into play, which are discussed later in this section.

To conduct a quality convergent design, you should be familiar (or have someone on your team) with the appropriate methods for each data source. This is a real challenge to the implementation of a convergent design because the evaluator has to design and implement two different studies (quant and qual) with a high

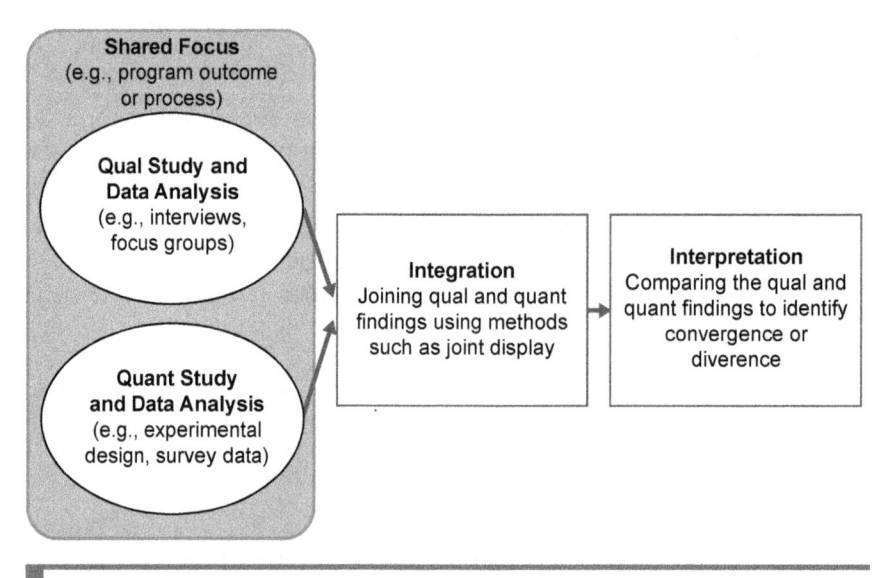

FIGURE 18.1. Convergent mixed method design layout.

degree of rigor and fidelity. It's frequently challenging to carry out one study, and when doing both the challenge is doubled. This is why in a convergent design authors (Feldon & Kafai, 2008) will sometimes talk about the priority placed on the data sources and use it to signal to the reader that the study's emphasis and resources were more focused on one data source versus another. In essence this can imply that one source of data is stronger than another, and this can occur due to how the evaluator allocates data collection resources, or to data quality issues that can emerge as part of the evaluation process. The priority designation adds a level of transparency.

From an evaluation perspective the convergent design is helpful in answering questions about outcomes that can be operationalized in multiple ways. For example, if the program aims to increase motivation, self-esteem, develop interest in science, technology, engineering, and mathematics (STEM) careers, or even lead to improvements in health behaviors, then a convergent design could be applicable. For each of these outcomes there could be a quantitative source of data, such as a validated survey that attempts to measure things such as motivation or self-esteem, and a qualitative way of capturing the same outcomes through interviews or focus groups with a sample of the participants who can provide a more in-depth understanding of how a program affected these same outcomes. The challenge at the end of the data collection phase is how to combine both of these data sources to reach a better understanding of the program's outcomes.

One of the most common ways of combining the qual and quant in a convergent design is to use a **joint display** approach for the analysis of both data sources. The joint display "is a figure or table in which the researcher arrays both qualitative and quantitative data so that the two sources of data can be directly compared. In effect the display merges or connects the two forms of data" (Creswell & Plano Clark, 2017, p. 449). The joint display is often created using the priority placed on the data source or is guided by the main focus of the evaluation. For example, if we use the self-esteem outcome, we can create a joint display that shows the qual interview responses of those who scored high, medium, or low on a quant self-esteem survey. This would allow the evaluator to understand a few important things about the program's impact on self-esteem. First, it would let the evaluator better see how participants with high (or medium, or low) self-esteem scores on the quant measure experienced and expressed this self-esteem level and identify the potential unique program characteristics that contributed to its presence or change (Fetters et al., 2013).

Another way of creating this joint display is to code the qual interviews and identify the self-esteem-related themes that emerge. Then the evaluator can create the joint display around those themes. For example, some of the themes could include (1) increased feelings of self-worth, (2) increased feelings of educational competence, and (3) reduced feelings of social skills. The joint display can be framed around these three themes and include the quant self-esteem scores along with excerpts from the qual interviews that support each of the themes. This joint display framing allows the evaluator to better understand how the self-esteem outcomes were expressed by the participants, how they relate to the quant measures, and may even offer insights about how the program affected these various thematic self-esteem outcomes.

The insights gained from this integration technique is unique to a convergent mixed method design because it systematically combines the quant and qual to provide an improved perspective on how the quant numbers are represented in qual data and how the qual information is expressed in the quant numbers (Guetterman et al., 2015). This design can also be used to tackle other evaluation questions related to the program's processes, such as quality of implementation and responsiveness of staff, and can offer guidance on how specific program components contributed (or hindered) the intended outcomes. However, there is a key potential challenge with using this approach that should be anticipated and planned. The challenge can occur when qual and quant findings contradict each other, and you are left with having to make sense of the divergence (i.e., nonconvergence).

There are options for dealing with the apparent discrepant situation that include an assessment of the quality of the quant and qual data, the collection of additional data, the use of the priority for each data source, or conducting a deeper investigation to understand the factors leading to the discrepancies. The quality assessment of the data is a good initial step to take when contradictory findings emerge. You can examine the sampling techniques used for the qual and quant studies, and this may tell you that your qual sample did not match your larger quant sample, or that the survey data collected during the quant study had a lot of missing data or low reliability that may have biased the analysis. There are also many other factors that can affect the quality of the information collected, and if you are able to systematically assess which source of data was better, in terms of rigor and quality, then this may help inform the data source you will rely on for the evaluation. Unfortunately, this can also mean that you are not doing a mixed methods study anymore since you would be, in essence, dismissing one source of data, and depending solely on another. So optimally, it would be advisable to collect additional data in the domain (qual or quant) where there were serious quality issues. This would enable you to continue the implementation and analysis of a mixed methods study and would most likely lead to a convergence of findings between the qual and quant sources.

There are also decisions about the priority placed on each data source that can help to inform how you deal with contradictory qual and quant findings. If the priority is placed on the quant beforehand, and that phase is conducted with a high degree of quality, then it could be acceptable to rely primarily on that source, while acknowledging that the qual data was not a priority in this study. This is not an optimal solution but it does show a degree of transparency about how each data source was used and the role that it would play in the evaluation. There are also situations where the quality of the data (qual and quant) are equally good, and the priorities are equivalent, but the results from the qual and quant still contradict each other. This can be viewed as an opportunity to better understand what each of the data sources are capturing, since they may be reflecting real variations in how an outcome is experienced or operationalized. For example, a program that aims to increase academic self-esteem could be working according to a quant measure of academic self-esteem—however, the qual interviews may indicate that even though the participants feel better about their academic abilities and capabilities (i.e., self-esteem), their actual academic performance is still suffering, and thus they are not sure how long the feelings of positive academic self-esteem will last. In this case the divergent qual and quant responses can lead to insights about how the program is defining its outcomes (by having them focus on actual academic performance as well as academic self-esteem), and help the evaluation better understand the program's impacts. This situation still remains a potential challenge but the typical advantages of using a convergent design are frequently worthwhile.

Explanatory Sequential Designs

Explanatory sequential mixed method designs have an overarching aim of helping you better understand your quant findings through qual data. This is even reflected in the title of the design, where the main idea is to "explain" the quant findings through the use of qual sources. Unlike the convergent design, where the qual and quant would be collected and analyzed at approximately the same time, the explanatory sequential design requires the collection and analysis of quant data, which is then used to design and collect qual data—hence the use of the term *sequential* in the design title (see Figure 18.2). For instance, an evaluator might use this design to answer the question "Why did we get these quantitative survey findings or patterns, and what do they mean?" With this type of design, evaluators must plan for, or consider, the eventuality of the study's continuation through subsequent collection of qual data.

The key to a well-implemented explanatory sequential design is the identification of relevant quant data patterns or findings, and the purposeful design and implementation of a qual study that can help explain these patterns. The first step in this process has to be done carefully to optimize the utility of the qual phase of this design. There are many studies showing how this design can be used effectively (Ivankova & Stick, 2007). In our own practice, we conducted an evaluation of a college program that aimed to reduce the dropout rates of participating students by developing their academic skills and knowledge. In this evaluation we also had access to a randomly assigned control group that did not receive the dropout prevention program.

```
┌─────────────┐   ┌──────────────┐   ┌──────────────┐   ┌──────────────┐
│ Quant Study │   │Quant Pattern │   │  Qual Study  │   │Interpretation│
│and Data     │──▶│Identification│──▶│and Data      │──▶│The use of    │
│Analysis     │   │Finding a     │   │Analysis      │   │qual data to  │
│(e.g.,       │   │relevant      │   │Conducting a  │   │help explain  │
│experimental,│   │pattern in the│   │qual study to │   │the identified│
│survey data) │   │quant data    │   │help explain  │   │quant pattern │
│             │   │that requires │   │the quant     │   │              │
│             │   │additional    │   │pattern       │   │              │
│             │   │explanation   │   │identified in │   │              │
│             │   │              │   │the previous  │   │              │
│             │   │              │   │step          │   │              │
└─────────────┘   └──────────────┘   └──────────────┘   └──────────────┘
```

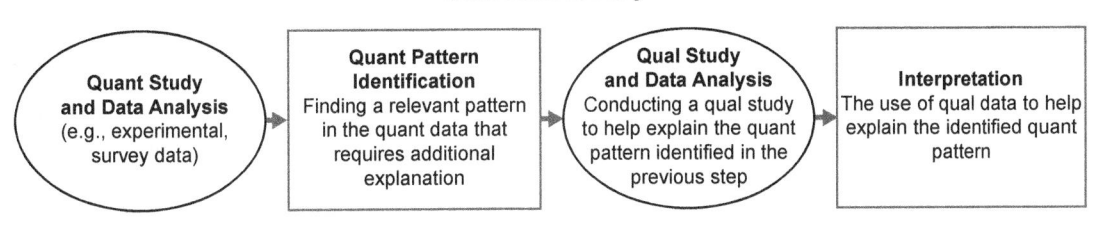

FIGURE 18.2. Explanatory mixed method design layout.

After a year of implementation, we compared the dropout rates of those who participated in the program (treatment group) to those who did not participate in the program (control group), and found that both of their dropout rates were exactly the same, and that the program did not appear to increase the retention rates for participants. After completing this quant analysis, a question emerged about why the treatment group did not have improved retention rates.

The quant analysis did not tell us the reasons why students were dropping out and we needed to know the factors that were contributing to their decisions to drop out of college. This was important for us to understand, and it was even more important for the program to know so that the program operators could modify their activities and focus to respond to the real and relevant factors that led students to drop out. This is where the qual piece of the design was used to help provide information on why students were actually dropping out of college. It's worth noting that we spent a lot of time discussing the quant data and the patterns that emerged, and also conducted various subgroup analysis and looked at other outcomes before deciding to use the qual phase of our study to understand the factors contributing to the dropout decision.

Once this was decided we selected a sample of treatment and control students who had dropped out and conducted semistructured interviews. Students were randomly selected and invited to take part in the interviews. Interviews were conducted until the data had reached saturation (i.e., the point at which collecting more data would not lead to further information related to the research questions). We asked them about the factors and circumstances that led to their decision to drop out. We soon discovered that a minority of the students were dropping out due to academic reasons, and the majority were leaving college because of other factors that included personal health, family tragedies, and financial pressures. The interviews also revealed that it was rarely one of these factors alone, and it was more common to find that two or more situations emerged that compounded the difficulty and led students to leave college. This qual phase of the evaluation was very helpful in *explaining* the quant patterns that emerged, and also helped to reshape how the dropout prevention program supported students, and led them to offer additional supports, including mental health and financial aid counseling. From these findings, we discovered that the control and treatment students were experiencing dropout for similar reasons, leading us to conclude that the program was not well thought out and that changes to the underlying assumptions of the program were required.

This example highlights one implementation process for the explanatory sequential design. There are other variations that can be used in the evaluation that are derived by the types of questions that you want the qual phase to answer. In the previous example the qual phase attempted to explain the quant findings and identify the factors that contributed to college dropout with the hope of understanding why the program did not positively affect this outcome. However, an evaluator can also focus on other quant patterns that emerge, like extreme cases (or outliers), subgroups that have different quant patterns than the larger group, or more commonly examining the average quant findings qualitatively. The point of interpretation in this design occurs after the qual phase is completed because that is when the qual can help explain the quant to offer a fuller perspective on the underlying meaning behind the quant findings.

There are also decisions that have to be made about how to select the qual sample. In the example we discussed, our sample came from students in the treatment and control groups who dropped out of college. If the quant analysis revealed group differences, individual outliers, or different outcomes for certain subgroups, then these are potentially relevant candidates for a deeper qual study.

The main challenge for this design is to determine what to actually pursue in the qual phase, since it is often unknown until the quant phase is completed. When you reach this decision point in the evaluation, we recommend working closely with the interest holders to determine what types of information would be most useful for them to know. For example, if the quant phase results are *as expected* and there is general agreement behind the theory underlying why the intervention worked, then it might be more useful to focus the qual phase on unexpected outliers, or differences in subgroups (if present). This may offer more useful information by helping to explain how the program and its components may have affected people differently. The knowledge gained can both inform theory, practice, and further program development and improvement. This qual phase may also help the program explore and identify unmet needs and interventions. This design is appealing for many evaluations because it is conceptually easy to understand but also relevant in many cases where the quant data alone does not offer enough information about how a program is being implemented and the impacts it is having on participants.

Exploratory Sequential Mixed Methods Designs

Exploratory sequential designs are well suited to helping evaluators better understand the program, its context, and potential outcomes before committing to the development of quant measures. In essence, this design helps the evaluator "explore" relevant program processes or outcomes through the use of qual methods. The findings from the initial qual phase can be synthesized, and then used to help select or develop a quant measure that is distributed to a larger sample of the population to assess whether the themes, issues, and outcomes identified in the qual phase have a broader presence in the program (see Figure 18.3; see Mills, 2006).

This design is particularly helpful when evaluating programs that are new or where there are disagreements among the interest holders about what the program does and what it hopes to accomplish. This design is also useful if and when a program has not been examined in a long time, or when new staff and leadership begin replacing the original staff and leaders. The exploratory sequential design allows you as the evaluator to spend the needed time understanding the program and its activities and outcomes before having to select a quant measure of implementation and/or outcomes. For instance, an evaluator might use this design to answer the question "What are the potential outcomes of a newly developed and implemented program, and how common are they across the broader population of participants?"

This design requires a few important decisions to be made about what the qual phase of the study will focus on. This can be determined through a combination of evaluator judgment and interest holder discussions. For example, the evaluator may note that the stated goals and outcomes are vague and that interest holders are inconsistent in their descriptions of how program participants will change or improve after completing the intervention. Interest holders may also be interested in knowing more about unexpected outcomes or identifying the presence and spread of a developing need among participants. These discussions can inform the qual phase of this design, and it is important to spend the time and effort to achieve some form

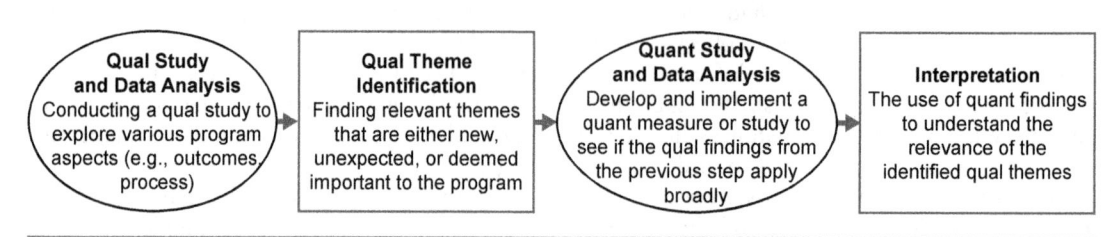

| Qual Study and Data Analysis: Conducting a qual study to explore various program aspects (e.g., outcomes, process) | Qual Theme Identification: Finding relevant themes that are either new, unexpected, or deemed important to the program | Quant Study and Data Analysis: Develop and implement a quant measure or study to see if the qual findings from the previous step apply broadly | Interpretation: The use of quant findings to understand the relevance of the identified qual themes |

FIGURE 18.3. Exploratory mixed method design layout.

of agreement among the interest holders about what the exploration may focus on.

Once these decisions are made then the qual phase can commence and may include various data collection methods ranging from interviews, observations, focus groups, and/or document analysis. In an evaluation we completed, a sample of 52 individuals who were either alumni or current participants in the program were interviewed and asked to describe their experiences with the program (noting specific program activities that were relevant to them), and also describe any outcomes (positive or negative) that can be directly attributed to their participation in this program.

This specific program was attempting to increase career interest in STEM by offering real-world STEM-related experiences (e.g., working in a genetics lab and doing original biological research). The analysis of the qual data highlighted some interesting patterns in how students experienced this program and there were also some unexpected outcomes that emerged. These outcomes included improved team-building skills, the development of technical lab skills, and alumni noting that they were well prepared for a STEM position after entering the job market.

These specific outcomes were not originally part of the program outcomes but clearly emerged from the student interviews. The next phase of this design was the attempt to represent these outcomes through a quant survey measure. We did this through a multiphase process that required the identification of existing validated quant measures, and the revision and development of new quant measures that were customized to the program. By comparing existing measures to the qual themes, we were able to adapt a quant measure of team-building skills and develop a technical lab skill measure that reflected the training received in the program. These quant measures were initially piloted and then distributed to over 300 program participants and a comparison group. Data collected from the quant phase supported the presence of these outcomes across the larger samples, and also provided the program with important information about the intervention elements that they should maintain in the future, which were directly related to these unexpected outcomes.

The strength of this design may also be its biggest implementation challenge. This design requires *time* to decide on the focus of the qual phase and to actually conduct and analyze the qual data. This time is necessary—however, it may be difficult for some programs and evaluations to spend the first 6–12 months on this qual phase, and it would be very difficult to implement this design in a program that has a short implementation cycle. This is more suited for longer-term interventions that are either new and/or complex and that require time to understand before committing to a quant measure of its outcomes. However, if this design can be implemented well, it can contribute to the development of a possibly more impactful evaluation that more readily reflects the program processes and outcomes.

Multiphase/Complex Mixed Methods Designs

The core designs discussed in the previous sections form the building blocks of more complex designs that attempt to answer different evaluation questions. While this chapter discusses a few of these complex designs, it is important to note that there are a multitude of designs that could be labeled a complex design (e.g., multilevel, and fully integrated designs). In this section we focus on two commonly asked questions and attempt to illustrate how mixed methods can be used to answer both. These questions are:

- Program implementation: Is the program doing what it is supposed to do?
- Program outcomes: What are the program's outcomes?

It's worth noting that these are suggested designs and that they would need to be adapted to your own unique context and program. Each question is used as a section heading for ease of reference.

Program Implementation: Is the Program Doing What It Is Supposed to Do?

This evaluation question is often answered by tracking and comparing what the program promised to do (e.g., serve 1,000) with it actually did (e.g., provided services to 998 people). This is a critical question to answer since it can directly relate to the program's outcomes (Alkin & Vo, 2017). An evaluator can approach this question with a multiphase mixed method design that attempts to understand the adherence to the implementation plan, and also identify how the program as implemented is being received by interest holders (see Figure 18.4).

• *Phase 1 of a multiphase mixed methods design: Identifying adherence or fidelity of implementation.* In this initial phase the evaluation assesses whether the program is being implemented as planned, and also gains insights on what issues are present and why they have emerged (and potentially how to fix them). This type of inquiry is well suited for an explanatory sequential mixed methods design, where the evaluator can collect quant information on how the program is being implemented, identify relevant patterns in implementation, and then conduct a qual study to understand why these patterns emerged (see Figure 18.4).

For example, if evaluating a multisite education program that is attempting to offer after-school services to 800 students with a planned target of 40 students per site, you would want to collect attendance data along with the demographics of (1) the students attending, and (2) the schools where the program is implemented. These data may reveal that some sites have higher attendance then others, that there are more males than females in the program across the different sites, and that the majority of students attending the program come from high- to middle-socioeconomic status (SES) families. All these quant patterns can form the basis for a qual study that attempts to explain variations in attendance, and the factors that contribute to males attending more than females, and barriers to access for low-SES students.

Through the conduct of a qual study you may be able to identify critical factors that affect implementation, including lack of staff training in creating a welcoming environment, inaccessibility issues that are due to lack of transportation or narrow program operating hours, and even social/cultural barriers that the program unintentionally propagates (e.g., lack of dual-language speakers in programs located in diverse communities). This phase of the evaluation can help identify and address some of the logistical issues surrounding the program and its ability to implement as planned. However, this phase does not provide as much information on how the program content is being understood or interpreted by participants.

• *Phase 2 of a multiphase mixed methods design: Participants' understanding of the intervention/program.* Attaining a clearer understanding of how an intervention or program is being received by participants is also a critical piece of information that can help clarify the links between what the program does and how that changes or impacts participants. This information allows you to get a sense of what the participants are experiencing and compare it to the intended program experiences, while also noting any unexpected/unanticipated points of confusion, disagreement, or discontent. This type of inquiry is well suited for the exploratory sequential mixed methods design, where the main focus is on the use of qual data (e.g., interviews, observations, focus groups) to capture participant reactions, interpretations, and understanding of what the program is doing. Then use that knowledge to inform the development of a quant measure that can be distributed widely to assess the presence or absence of these findings to a larger population.

For example, when evaluating the same multisite educational program, it would be helpful to select a sample of students and conduct focus groups. These focus groups could explore the accessibility of the curriculum, its applicability to their own academic progress or regular school classes, or particularly effective or ineffective instructional strategies. The findings from this qual inquiry process can then be used to inform the development of a quant measure of curriculum accessibility, applicability, and quality of delivery to see whether the qual findings generalize across sites.

Even though Phases 1 and 2 are described separately, they can be combined for more efficiency (see Figure 18.4). The qual data collection process described in Phase 1 (explanatory sequential design), can also be used as an opportunity to explore the issues raised in Phase 2 (exploratory sequential design). Instead of having to conduct two different qual data collection efforts, an evaluator can develop an interview/focus group protocol that (1) helps to

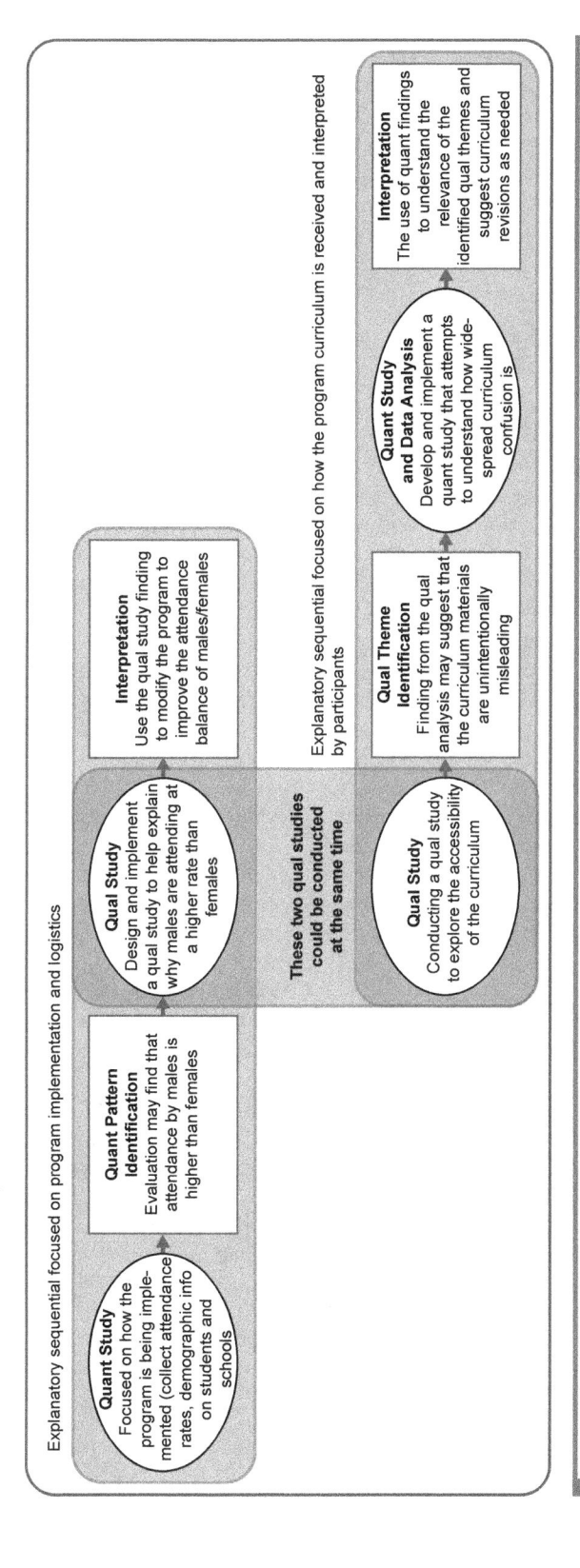

FIGURE 18.4. Multiphase mixed method study examining program implementation.

explain quant data patterns and findings, and (2) explores the program context and the participants' reactions and understanding of what is being delivered. Through this design it may be possible to reduce the time and cost of conducting a process evaluation and yield valuable information about the program and how it's being implemented.

Program Outcomes:
What Are the Program's Outcomes?

There are many design options that can be used to help answer this question, and it is commonly the most requested question from interest holders and funders. Since there are several ways of approaching this question from a mixed methods standpoint, we attempt to categorize it by using two different program contexts (a well-established program and a new program) and exploring how a multiphase mixed methods design can be used to answer the outcome question. These are just two examples of how to use a multiphase mixed method design, and in reality, there would be other factors, such as the priorities of the funders and interest holders, to consider. However, the mixed method design suggestions made for a "well-established program" and a "new program" do reflect a potentially viable and applicable choice for answering questions about program goals and objectives.

Program Context 1: A Well-Established Program

In this context we can assume that the program is well established, with clearly defined activities. The program also has the capacity to collect quant and qual data from program participants, and the evaluation has access to a comparison/control group. In this program context the design can take the form of an experimental (exp) or quasi-experimental (quasi-exp) design that is embedded (i.e., nested) within the multiphase mixed method study, with the qual data supporting the implementation of the exp or quasi-exp design and/or helping to interpret the quant findings. For simplicity, let's assume that you are able to conduct a quasi-exp study to examine the outcomes of the program on participants. In this case the program could be an obesity prevention program, where the core outcome is reduction in body mass index (BMI), along with improved health behaviors (e.g., increase exercise, reduce sugar intake; see Figure 18.5).

The qual phase of this evaluation could come before the quasi-exp design is implemented and used to help with the quant data collection from treatment and comparison group participants. The qual could identify barriers to data collection (e.g., timing, cultural, and/or physical) and discover appropriate incentives or solutions to the barriers. The role of the qual would be supportive in nature during this phase but also relevant to help ensure that the quant phase is optimally designed and implemented. The quant phase would come next and would be the *priority* in this mixed method design as a measure of the program's outcomes. In this phase the evaluation could potentially collect quant data on BMI, minutes spent exercising, and amount of sugar consumed from the treatment and comparison group. Then statistically compare both groups to see whether those in the obesity prevention program performed better than those who did not have access to such a program. Again, the initial qual phase would have helped to ensure that the quant phase was well implemented.

Following the quant data collection and analysis, the evaluator may find that the program had no effect on the treatment outcomes (meaning the comparison and treatment conditions were equivalent) or they conducted a subgroup analysis that revealed differences based on age (e.g., younger people in the program were less likely

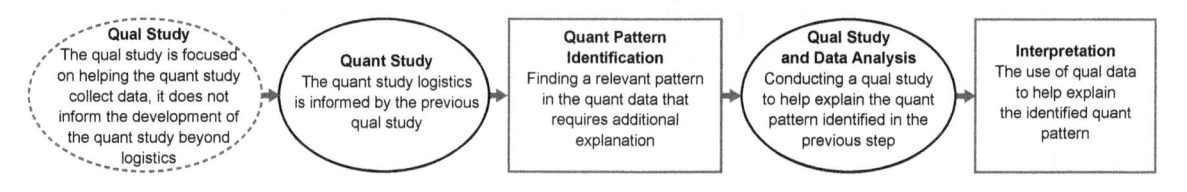

FIGURE 18.5. Multiphase mixed method study examining program outcomes (well-established program).

to perform well on the outcomes). This may lead the evaluator to conduct a follow-up qual study to help explain these patterns of findings, which would also contribute to a better understanding of the program's ability to achieve the stated goals and objectives (see Figure 18.5).

This multiphase mixed method design is a potential example of how mixed methods can be used to evaluate a well-established program. This design may also be useful in other program contexts but may require some modifications to account for the level of development of the program. For example, if it is a new program or recently revised, then an understanding of how the outcomes are operationalized may be necessary.

Program Context 2: A New or Recently Revised Program

If we modify the assumptions of the obesity program and describe it as a newly developed intervention, then it would also be helpful to revise the mixed method design to optimize the evaluation effort. In this case, there would be general agreement around some of the outcomes and their measures (e.g., BMI, exercise, sugar intake)—however, the program could be using new theories or intervention techniques to address obesity that may also yield some short-term outcomes that can help predict longer-term effects. In such a case an evaluator can design and implement a multiphase mixed method design that begins with an exploratory sequential phase, followed by a convergent mixed methods phase (see Figure 18.6).

The purpose of this initial exploratory sequential phase is to identify short-term program outcomes or side effects through qualitative interviews. These initial exploratory interviews or focus groups from the qual study could yield new outcomes or constructs related to improved self-efficacy, improved body image, and/or increased feelings of dietary control. These emerging outcomes could be used to inform the development or adaptation of existing quant measures that can be tested with a broader sample of program participants. These new quant measures can be embedded (i.e., nested) within a new convergent quasi-exp study that attempts to capture the treatment and control condition's outcomes via various quant measures (e.g., BMI, exercise, body image survey, self-efficacy survey) and additional qual interviews and focus groups. The qual piece in this case may appear redundant—however, it is critical to keep tracking these outcomes qualitatively as the program evolves and changes (as many new programs often do) to ensure that the outcomes captured in the exploratory phase of the evaluation are still consistent across time. This design allows the evaluator to reflect changes more accurately in the program and its outcomes at the start of its development, and also provides the opportunity to document and track the evolution of these outcomes as the program matures.

These are suggestions for how to possibly use mixed methods to answer the two most common

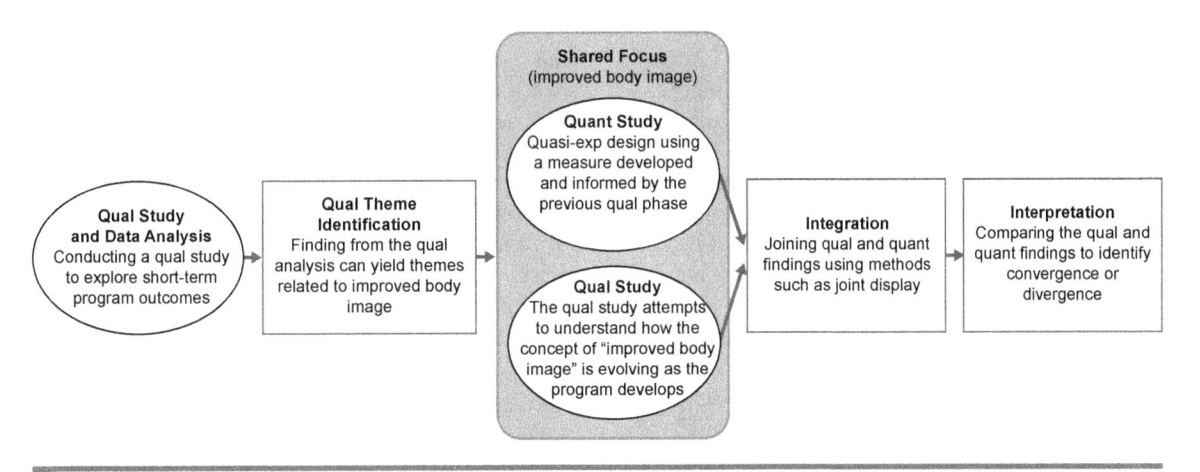

FIGURE 18.6. Multiphase mixed method study examining program outcomes (new program).

evaluation questions. As with any evaluation design, the logistical factors (time and money) can ultimately determine what the evaluation can and cannot do. However, it's important to note that even if the costs are higher upfront for some of these designs, there is also the potential benefit of more accurately understanding and capturing the program's outcomes and providing more useful knowledge.

ISSUES IN THE USE OF MIXED METHODS

The development and evolution of mixed methods as a methodology has generated various controversies about the appropriateness of combining two existing methodological approaches that stem from fundamentally different views on the nature of reality and how we represent it (Creswell & Plano Clark, 2017). This divide is frequently described using the constructivist and postpositivist epistemological positions (Guba & Lincoln, 1994; Morgan, 2007). Within the **constructivist** perspective a researcher or evaluator takes the stance that there are multiple meanings or realities that there should be purposeful attempts to represent them through the qualitative analysis and description process. This worldview highlights the subjective differences between experiences and explicitly acknowledges that bias is inherent in the interpretation of qual data. In contrast, a **postpositivist** worldview assumes that the truth underlying experiences can be measured with a certain degree of accuracy since there is a single and shared reality. This worldview highlights the researcher's ability to be objective and prioritizes the aggregation of information (often in the form of numerical data) as a close approximation of reality. Given how diametrically opposite these two perspectives are, some have argued that they should not be combined (Mastenbroek & Doorenspleet, 2007) since each requires an orientation and perspective that would be challenging for many researchers to switch between (Furlong & Marsh, 2002).

A common example of the potential difficulty of balancing the qual and quant worldviews is the tendency of many mixed method studies (especially convergent designs) to quantitize the qual data (Sandelowski et al., 2009). The quantitizing process entails converting qual data to numerical values, often to represent the frequency of themes or ideas that emerge from the rich experiences captured in qual information. This process allows for easier comparison and mixing with quant data sources using statistical techniques and approaches but it often comes at the cost of reducing or eliminating many of the details, contextual variations, and meanings generated from talking to different interest holders. At its core, the quantitizing process can be helpful, but it prioritizes the postpositivist approach to knowing to the detriment of the constructivist worldview. Often researchers engage in this process without the full awareness of what they are doing and the potential loss of rich perspectives that may better reflect what is happening on the ground. If pursuing this approach, then it would be appropriate to acknowledge this loss of rich qual data in your evaluation, and to clearly state the *priorities* (qual or quant) used in the evaluation to help guide the reader.[2]

There are also approaches used to convert quant data to qual information and it is becoming more present in the mixed method literature (Onwuegbuzie & Dickinson, 2008; Onwuegbuzie & Teddlie, 2003; Tashakkori & Teddlie,1998). Using this approach, the evaluator would attempt to create descriptive profiles that represent the numerical values captured in a quant measure(s). These profiles can be used to describe the average or normative responses or even quant outliers in the data. For example, quant findings from different measures of self-efficacy, self-esteem, and locus of control can be used to create a descriptive profile representing the average performance and relationship (correlation) between these measures. These profiles can describe the "typical" responses to these measures and provide insights into how the "typical" responders might think or behave in different situations. This qualitizing process can be used to support and aid the interpretation of qual data by providing potential themes, behavioral patterns, and attitudes/beliefs that can be used to understand collected qual data and in-

---

[2] Note that it still is possible to use the qual richness in some aspect of the evaluation but to quantitize the qual data for the purposes of merging or integrating the data.

formation. It should be noted that this approach can produce profiles that are overgeneralized with few if any contextual information to help explain the factors that contributed to the development of the described attitudes, behaviors, and beliefs.

The qualitizing and quantizing procedures are attempts aimed at bridging the divide between the constructivist and postpositivist worldviews. Even though each has inherent limitations that prevents them from neatly fitting into one category or another (e.g., quantitizing reduces rich experiences to numerical values, qualitized profiles may oversimplify the numerical responses), they do represent a **pragmatic** worldview and approach to research and evaluation. This pragmatic worldview has been described as oriented toward problem solving, with an emphasis on identifying practical solutions and methods that can best answer the research or evaluation questions (Creswell & Plano Clark, 2017). At its core a pragmatic orientation tends to work well for a mixed method design because it allows for multiple worldviews and attempts to take advantage of the benefits of each one. This stance also prioritizes the question or questions, rather than the method, and requires the evaluator to consider how qual and quant data and procedures can be leveraged to answer the questions. Even though pragmatism may be a preferred worldview for mixed methods, many of the biases (e.g., prioritization of quant data) can still remain (Maxwell & Mittapalli, 2010), and thus need to be directly discussed as a part of any mixed method report or article. This push for transparency by declaring a specific perspective has also evolved to encompass approaches to mixed methods that highlight issues of social inequity, promote social justice, and aim to transform society.

The **transformative worldview** is an approach to mixed methods that explicitly acknowledges a cultural or social position that aims to identify power dynamics that privilege or oppress different groups and work toward social justice through collaborative and participatory practices (Sweetman et al., 2010). In mixed methods this worldview can be part of any of the core and complex designs discussed but with the added focus on a group that has historically been oppressed or ignored. For example, this transformative/social justice approach to mixed methods can take on a feminist or critical race theory when designing and conducting a mixed methods evaluation. This orientation can be operationalized in who the evaluator chooses to talk to in a program context (e.g., an evaluator using feminist theory may work to ensure that women are selected and heard in interviews and/or surveys), the types of questions asked about experiences (e.g., a feminist theory evaluator may probe deeper into how women are perceived and treated in a specific program context), and how the data are analyzed and used (e.g., a feminist theory evaluator may make sure that the quant analysis compares results for women and men, that the interpretation of the data is conducted collaboratively, and that women have a voice in how the findings are used). At its core this orientation and approach to mixed methods prioritizes advocacy and the use of the knowledge gained from evaluation and research to bring about change for the purposes of social betterment.

These worldviews are critically important to acknowledge when using mixed methods in evaluation, since interest holder groups may vary in how they view or value different types of information. If walking into a situation where interest holders are primarily quant oriented or postpositivist in their worldview, then how you use and explain qual data in the evaluation is an important consideration. As an evaluator you may even choose to prioritize the quant data in your design in response to the interest holders' perceived worldview. Conversely, the evaluation could be transformative in nature, aiming at revealing inequities and supporting social justice within the program and community context. With this orientation it would be very important to express that stance and perspective with the various interest holders and prioritize the information (whether it be qual or quant) that highlights the adopted social justice orientation. Even though these worldviews may appear abstract, an evaluator needs to remember that they represent the roots of how people fundamentally view the nature of reality, how it can be understood, and how relevant different types of knowledge and information is. Without this awareness a mixed methods evaluation can fall apart due to interest holder rejection of the quality and relevance of the data collected. Therefore, it is important for the evaluator to consider the alignment between the purpose for the evaluation, evaluation questions, and orientation to the methods used.

MIXED METHODS TOOLS AND FUTURE DIRECTIONS

During the past several years there have been many technological developments that can aid in the conduct and analysis of mixed method evaluation studies. These developments include the creation of software that supports the integration of qual and quant findings. The software has reached a level that allows users to directly compare quant data with the corresponding qual data. For example, assume that you are conducting a convergent design and collecting survey and interview data on the program's ability to increase team-building skills. Software such as MaxQDA[3] (which is custom-built for mixed methods) allows you to thematically code each interview for the mentions of team-building skills by participants, and also includes subcodes that show whether this experience was positive or negative. In addition, each interview can be linked to the participants' survey response. This allows for the direct comparison of survey responses (quant) and interview responses (qual) about the topic of team-building skills. This comparison is a form of joint data display that can also be used to disaggregate the quant or qual findings by any relevant characteristic that is collected. This can allow the evaluator to see the qual and quant data by gender, ethnicity, age, or by qual themes (positive/negative team-building experiences), or quant ratings (high/low ratings).

The software capabilities can also be used in explanatory and exploratory mixed methods designs. When conducting an explanatory design, the quant data can be mapped on to the qual data to help explain the quant findings. So if the evaluation needs to explain an unexpected quant finding (such as higher dropout rates for men), the qual data (interviews with men who have dropped out) can be linked to the quant data and the coded themes from the interviews could be used to help identify common factors contributing to the decision to drop out (academic, health, financial reasons). Similarly, in an exploratory sequential mixed method design the qual data can be coded and thematically organized, and then these themes can be used in the development of quant items or measures. Each qual theme could be linked to a specific set of quant items to ensure that they are represented in the quant phase of the study. This would improve the links between the qual and quant phase of the mixed method study. In addition, different types of qual data can be integrated into many of these software packages, including direct audio (without transcripts), video clips, and scanned document images (e.g., advertisements), and also linked (through the program or explicit coding) to quant information and data.[4]

These abilities help to reduce the complexity of organizing and tracking data and information from qual and quant sources, which in reality can be very challenging without some form of structure or framework. However, the software does not eliminate the need to think carefully about what analysis to conduct, or subgroups to examine in depth. Ideally, you need to initially consider the important variables that are directly relevant to answering the evaluation questions and focus the qual and qual data analysis on them. This is true for convergent, explanatory, and to a slightly lesser extent in the exploratory. For example, in a convergent design you have to think about the quality of the qual and quant data and how they each capture or operationalize the outcome. In the explanatory design you need to consider the important or relevant quant patterns (e.g., the average case, or outliers) that would be most useful for the evaluation to explain before delving into the qual phase. Similarly, the qual phase in the exploratory design needs to be thoroughly analyzed, and the relevant themes that emerge should be selected before starting the quant phase. These decisions will aid in focusing and structuring the analysis, and help you avoid sinking in too much data and information.

---

[3] *www.maxqda.com*

[4] There are other software packages that have similar capabilities, including:
- Dedoose: *www.dedoose.com*
- ATLAS.ti: *https://atlasti.com*
- NVIVO: *www.qsrinternational.com/nvivo/nvivo-products*

CONCLUSION

The information deluge will continue as there are more recent advances in the accessibility of data for use in evaluation. This becomes even more apparent since the passage of the Foundations for Evidence-Based Policymaking Act of 2018 (*Congress.gov*; 2019), where a mandate was delivered to make government-collected data and information more accessible through the development of standardized data management systems. This is noteworthy because it provides opportunities for evaluators to access additional information (primarily quant in nature) about the contexts that the programs are in. For example, community characteristic information in the form of geographic information system (GIS) data allows evaluators to create interactive maps that can describe a specific location or general area, including levels of education, walkability, and distance to various community resources (health, education), along with a myriad of other variables. In a mixed methods evaluation this information can be used convergently, or sequentially to help show changes in outcomes, offer additional explanations to program effects, or to help identify and select a sample to interview. This capability has the potential to reduce some of the most challenging aspects of mixed methods design, mainly time and money. With accessible quant data it may be possible to complete or supplement the quant phase of a mixed methods design, without the need to directly collect the data. This was discussed in an article (Kamstra et al., 2023) that explores the potential integration of GIS data with qual data to better understand the connection between mental health experiences and geographic location. This trend of integrating available databases in mixed methods will most likely continue to grow in the future due to improved software capabilities, demand for contextual- or systems-level understanding of program and policies, and heightened concerns about the time and money needed to conduct a mixed method study.

Even though this trend may grow, it will be challenging to optimally use the various new forms of qual and quant data. This is why the future of mixed methods should also see the development of new and creative techniques and procedures. The use of GIS to integrate quant and qual data is a relatively new development that can offer a way to represent the complexity of the environment in which the mixed method evaluation is being conducted, and balance that with high-level findings and insights that can inform the decision-making process. There are still many new development opportunities within this methodology. This is an exciting time to design and implement a mixed method evaluation, because through its practice one can still discover and share new approaches to integration, interpretation, and use within mixed methods. Even though not everything is completely agreed upon within this literature, there is more than enough room to innovate and create something truly impactful through the use of this approach.

REFERENCES

Alkin, M. C., & Vo, A. T. (2017). *Evaluation essentials: From A to Z*. Guilford Press.

Azzam, T. (2011). Evaluator characteristics and methodological choice. *American Journal of Evaluation, 32*(3), 376–391.

Bryman, A. (1988). Quantitative and qualitative research strategies in knowing the social world. In T. May & M. Williams (Eds.), *Knowing the social world* (pp. 138–156). Open University Press.

Creswell, J. W., & Plano Clark, V. L. (2017). *Designing and conducting mixed methods research*. SAGE.

Feldon, D. F., & Kafai, Y. B. (2008). Mixed methods for mixed reality: Understanding users' avatar activities in virtual worlds. *Educational Technology Research and Development, 56*(5–6), 575–593.

Fetters, M. D., Curry, L. A., & Creswell, J. W. (2013). Achieving integration in mixed methods designs—Principles and practices. *Health Services Research, 48*(6, Pt. 2), 2134–2156.

Fielding, N. G. (2012). Triangulation and mixed methods designs: Data integration with new research technologies. *Journal of Mixed Methods Research, 6*(2), 124–136.

Foundations for Evidence-Based Policymaking Act of 2018. Public Law No. 115-435 (2019). Available at *www.congress.gov/bill/115th-congress/house-bill/4174*

Furlong, P., & Marsh, D. (2002). A skin not a sweater: Ontology and epistemology in political science. In D. Marsh & G. Stoker (Eds.), *Theory and methods in political science* (pp. 17–41). Palgrave Macmillan.

Guba, E. G., & Lincoln, Y. S. (1994). Competing paradigms in qualitative research. In N. K. Denzin & Y. S. Lincoln (Eds.), *Handbook of qualitative research* (pp. 105–117). SAGE.

Guest, G. (2013). Describing mixed methods research: An alternative to typologies. *Journal of Mixed Methods Research, 7*(2), 141–151.

Guetterman, T., Creswell, J. W., & Kuckartz, U. (2015). Using joint displays and MAXQDA software to represent the results of mixed methods research. In M. T. McCrudden, G. J. Schraw, & C. W. Buckendahl (Eds.), *Use of visual displays in research and testing: Coding, interpreting, and reporting data* (pp. 145–175). Information Age.

Guetterman, T. C., Molina-Azorin, J. F., & Fetters, M. D. (2020). Integration in mixed methods research [Special issue]. *Journal of Mixed Methods Research, 14*(4), 430–435.

Ivankova, N. V., & Stick, S. L. (2007). Students' persistence in a distributed doctoral program in educational leadership in higher education: A mixed methods study. *Research in Higher Education, 48*(1), 93–135.

Kamstra, P., Farmer, J., McCosker, A., Gardiner, F., Dalton, H., Perkins, D., . . . Bagheri, N. (2023). A novel mixed methods approach for integrating not-for-profit service data via qualitative geographic information system to explore authentic experiences of ill-health: A case study of rural mental health. *Journal of Mixed Methods Research, 17*(4), 419–442.

Kern, F. G. (2018). The trials and tribulations of applied triangulation: Weighing different data sources. *Journal of Mixed Methods Research, 12*(2), 166–181.

Mastenbroek, E., & Doorenspleet, R. (2007, September). *Mind the gap! On the possibilities and pitfalls of mixed methods research*. Paper presented at the 4th ECPR General Conference, Pisa, Italy.

Maxwell, J. A. (2016). Expanding the history and range of mixed methods research. *Journal of Mixed Methods Research, 10*(1), 12–27.

Maxwell, J. A., & Mittapalli, K. (2010). Realism as a stance for mixed methods research. In A. Tashakkori & C. Teddlie (Eds.), *Handbook of mixed methods in social and behavioral research* (pp. 145–168). SAGE.

Mills, E. J., Seely, D., Rachlis, B., Griffith, L., Wu, P., Wilson, K., . . . Wright, J. R. (2006). Barriers to participation in clinical trials of cancer: A meta-analysis and systematic review of patient-reported factors. *Lancet Oncology, 7*(2), 141–148.

Morgan, D. L. (2007). Paradigms lost and pragmatism regained: Methodological implications of combining qualitative and quantitative methods. *Journal of Mixed Methods Research, 1*(1), 48–76.

Onwuegbuzie, A. J., & Dickinson, W. B. (2008). Mixed methods analysis and information visualization: Graphical display for effective communication of research results. *Qualitative Report, 13*(2), 204–225.

Onwuegbuzie, A. J., & Teddlie, C. (2003). A framework for analyzing data in mixed methods research. In A. Tashakkori & C. Teddlie (Eds.), *Handbook of mixed methods in social and behavioral research* (pp. 351–383). Sage.

Reichardt, C. S., & Rallis, S. F. (Eds.). (1994). The qualitative–quantitative debate: New perspectives. *New Directions for Program Evaluation, 61*, 1–98.

Sandelowski, M., Voils, C. I., & Knafl, G. (2009). On quantitizing. *Journal of Mixed Methods Research, 3*(3), 208–222.

Sweetman, D., Badiee, M., & Creswell, J. W. (2010). Use of the transformative framework in mixed methods studies. *Qualitative Inquiry, 16*(6), 441–454.

Tashakkori, A., & Creswell, J. W. (2007). The new era of mixed methods [Editorial]. *Journal of Mixed Methods Research, 1*(1), 3–7.

Tashakkori, A., & Teddlie, C. (1998). *Mixed methodology: Combining qualitative and quantitative approaches*. SAGE.

Tashakkori, A., & Teddlie, C. (Eds.). (2010). *Sage handbook of mixed methods in social and behavioral research*. SAGE.

Turner, S. F., Cardinal, L. B., & Burton, R. M. (2017). Research design for mixed methods: A triangulation-based framework and roadmap. *Organizational Research Methods, 20*(2), 243–267.

Wittink, M. N., Barg, F. K., & Gallo, J. J. (2006). Unwritten rules of talking to doctors about depression: Integrating qualitative and quantitative methods. *The Annals of Family Medicine, 4*(4), 302–309.

Part IV
PLANNING, MANAGING, AND IMPLEMENTING EVALUATIONS

Chapter 19

Designing and Planning an Evaluation
Beyond Methods

Darlene F. Russ-Eft

CHAPTER OVERVIEW

Planning an evaluation effort is a neglected activity that is rarely if ever covered as part of a graduate student's or even a young professional's development. Unfortunately, it represents an activity that can lead to success or failure in an evaluation. The present chapter discusses various aspects of such planning. It includes planning related to the (1) scope of the project, (2) data collection and data analysis, (3) work and schedule, (4) people, (5) budget, and (6) potential risks.

As part of my graduate education, I took courses in different aspects and theories, as well as courses, in quantitative and qualitative methods. When I joined a nonprofit research organization, I found that I was able to use some of that knowledge. What I lacked, however, was knowledge and experience in planning a research study or evaluation project. How did one decide how much time to allocate to a specific data collection effort? In fact, what exactly was involved in that data collection? How much should be budgeted for the various steps? After all, one's success in this organization involved not only being able to secure funding but also to complete a funded project on time and within budget (see Bickman, Chapter 21, and Bamberger, Chapter 24, this volume, for a detailed treatment on how to budget for an evaluation).

Recently some colleagues and I were reminiscing about these early experiences. Furthermore, one of my colleagues decried the fact that so many of the projects that their organization funded did not complete the expected activities on time or on budget. As a result, we decided to collaborate on the development of a book that tries to provide some tips and tools for those novices and more experienced evaluators who face issues related to planning an evaluation. That book is titled *Managing Applied Social Science Research* (Russ-Eft et al., 2017). This chapter draws heavily on the insights and suggestions provided in that text.

Before launching into any discussion of planning, it seems appropriate to describe what it is we might be planning. Since this is a text on program evaluation, it is safe to assume that program evaluation will be the focus of our planning. At this point, a novice may say, "Well, to plan this evaluation, I will need to create the online survey, then get it approved by the IRB [institutional review board], then analyze the data, and send in the final report." Yes, we can all agree that those are some of the steps in one type of evaluation but planning the evaluation requires more thought and attention and effort.

Indeed, the Russ-Eft et al. (2017) text on planning applied social science research and evaluation projects suggested three stages for such projects: (1) planning the study, (2) executing the study, and (3) closing out the study. Then, within the stage of the evaluation project that involves planning, there are several aspects to consider. These include planning the (1) scope of the evaluation effort, (2) data collection and the data analysis, (3) evaluation work and schedule, (4) people, (5) budget, and (6) risks. The remainder of this chapter discusses each of these aspects of planning and provides some tools that may be used. (For those interested in more details concerning project management in general, consider the Project Management Institute, 2021.)

PLANNING THE SCOPE OF THE EVALUATION EFFORT

When an evaluator is responding to a specific request for proposals (RFP), planning the scope of the evaluation may appear to be rather straightforward. We might note here that such RFPs can come from government agencies, state agencies, foundations, for-profit organizations, and nonprofit organizations. Those coming from government agencies tend to be more formal requests, while those from for-profit organizations may simply result from a meeting or even a telephone call. In any case, the evaluator would do well to read or listen to the request carefully in order to plan the scope of the evaluation. After all, the scope of the evaluation should mirror what appeared or was stated in the original request. But to win the project, the evaluator must be able to use previous ideas and work and present some adaptations and new ideas.

At the same time, however, it is important to keep in mind that circumstances change. For those employing a responsive or developmental evaluation or some qualitative methods (Creswell & Báez, 2021; Creswell & Creswell, 2023; Patton, 2011; Stake, 2004; Wallerstein et al., 2017), changes in the scope should be expected and, to the extent possible, anticipated. After all, with a developmental evaluation, new and different issues can arise. Even in a seemingly straightforward project involving the analysis of an existing database, there may be surprises. One recent experience involved the proposed use of a database available from a state agency. After several meetings with agency staff and repeated assurances of access, we learned that the database did not actually exist; the agency personnel had simply been hoping to be able to create that database. So the evaluation project had to undertake primary data collection with school districts throughout the state.

To plan the scope of an evaluation, one must (1) identify the expectations of all **interest holders**; (2) determine the focus, including potential accomplishments and importance; (3) identify potential issues, such as logistical concerns, timeframe issues, and ethical issues; and (4) write the proposal. By planning the scope, some of the details of the data collection, data analysis, schedule, budget, people, and risks should emerge.

Identify Expectations

The identification of expectations should begin with the evaluator determining their own expectations. What does the evaluator want to see happen in the evaluation? What is their **worldview** (Creswell & Creswell, 2023)? Indeed, the evaluator's worldview may determine whether the person will even consider responding to the request. We should, however, recognize that for some, particularly those with a pragmatic view of simply wanting to solve a problem, this consideration may not be important. In any case, having decided to respond to the RFP, the evaluator should be quite clear as to the outcomes that they want from the evaluation. If a team of evaluators is engaged in the work, it is imperative that the lead evaluator work with the entire team to define the expectations and to reconcile any differences.

The interest holders' expectations also need to be considered. Indeed, unlike a research project, the interest holders in an evaluation represent an important voice guiding decisions. Russ-Eft and Preskill (2009) identified three levels of interest holders. These include the primary, secondary, and tertiary interest holders, defined in the paragraphs to follow. During planning, the evaluator should attempt to consider the expectations of each of these levels as well as their input as to the design, logistics, and involvement in the evaluation.

Russ-Eft and Preskill (2009) suggested some questions that evaluators might ask themselves in order to identify the interest holders and their potential level as related to the evaluation:

- Who has a vested interest in what is being evaluated and the evaluation outcomes?
- Whose position could be affected by the evaluation's findings and the actions taken on the findings?
- Who cares about the program, process, or product being evaluated?
- How might the evaluation findings be used and by whom?
- What groups will be affected by the evaluation if recommendations are made and acted upon?
- Who are the clients or customers of the program, process, or product, and what stake might they have in the outcomes of the evaluation?
- Who has a "right to know" the evaluation results? (pp. 167–168)

It is likely that the evaluator will attend to the primary interest holders and their input, since that person or group provides the support and funding needed for the evaluation to occur. Presumably it is from the primary interest holders that the evaluator can determine what the outcomes are expected for the evaluation. At the same time, it is also very important to understand the history and context surrounding the proposed evaluation. Specifically, the primary interest holder or interest holders can clarify why the evaluation is being done at this particular time and what has been done in the past. The evaluator should clarify with the primary interest holder any concerns about the conduct of the evaluation. These may involve issues of design of the study, timing and schedule, and possibly even logistics. Most important is to determine the level of involvement of the primary interest holder and potentially of other interest holders in the evaluation effort. For example, if one of the expected outcomes is the building of interest holders' evaluation capacity, then the evaluator must plan for the appropriate involvement of interest holders (e.g., Preskill & Russ-Eft, 2016).

Less likely to be considered, however, may be the expectations of the secondary interest holders and the tertiary interest holders. Secondary interest holders are those who are somewhat removed from the direct funding and decision making but who may be impacted by the evaluation and may affect the evaluation's conduct and outcomes. Secondary interest holders may include middle managers and employees whether in a for profit, a nonprofit, or as part of the government agency staff. Identifying the expectations, concerns, constraints, and possible uses of the evaluation findings by the secondary interest holders may help to ensure not only the success of the evaluation but its future use within the organization.

Tertiary interest holders are those who are not necessarily affected by the evaluation but who may be interested in the process or the findings, such as other evaluators or other organizations or agencies. A savvy evaluator will want to identify potential tertiary interest holders. Communication with these interest holders during the evaluation may provide background information to help plan the evaluation as well as a possible way to expand the use of the evaluation findings.

Determine Focus

Unlike an applied social science research project, an evaluator may think that determining the focus of an evaluation project is not that important. Unlike a research project where the investigator must determine the guiding research question, the request or RFP presumably defines the focus. Some requests can be specific and detailed, and in these cases, the evaluator needs to have a response that is in compliance. Others can be wide open and require the evaluator to help refine the focus. In some cases, that may mean that the evaluator must meet with the client or primary interest holder to clarify the request. Thus, it is important for the evaluator to determine early in the process how much or whether to get involved in developing the focus of the evaluation.

Nevertheless, it is critical for the evaluator to use that request or RFP along with knowledge of the various expectations to clarify the exact focus of the evaluation in terms of what it will accomplish, why it is important, and how it will be undertaken. The evaluator must make a determination using the statement in the request as well as from interactions with the interest holders regarding the expectations for the evaluation. Such expectations may include the design, types of data collection and analysis, involvement of interest holders, logistical issues and constraints, timing, and reporting to interest holders and to others.

Considering what an evaluation will accomplish is a critical step. This may be determined by the primary interest holder—for example, that person or group may clearly indicate that the evaluation will help to determine whether the program is making a difference and for what groups. Such determination as to the outcomes and benefits of a program may lead interest holders to decide whether to continue funding the program. But, in most cases, the decision is focused on any needed changes to the funding in terms of what mechanisms might be used and to which groups. In this case, the evaluator may decide to plan for a **summative evaluation** (Rossi et al., 2019; Scriven, 1966, 1967a, 1967b).

In other cases, the interest holder may be interested in knowing what improvements are needed in the program. The focus here may not be simply on funding issues but on ways to improve the services provided, the processes used for these services, and the personnel providing these services. Questions that might be addressed in such evaluations can include:

- What is the quality of the services and their implementation?
- What are barriers to the services and their implementation?
- In what ways might the services be improved?
- To what other groups might the services be provided?

This focus suggests a **formative evaluation** (Black & William, 2009; George & Cowan, 1999; Scriven, 1967a). (See Powell et al., Chapter 12, this volume, on implementation evaluation.) In other cases, both types of information are of interest—that is, there is a concern about the funding and possible changes as well as the services and how they might be improved or expanded. With both a summative and formative focus becoming of greater interest, so too has grown a greater interest and use of **mixed methods** (Creswell, 2015; Creswell & Clark, 2018; Onwuegbuzie & Hitchcock, 2015); and a mixed methods design is appropriate in summative and formative work. (See also Azzam & Jones, Chapter 18, this volume, on mixed methods.)

Simply determining the expectations and proposed outcomes is not sufficient. The evaluator should also create a statement as to the importance of the evaluation. Unlike a research project, a thorough literature review is not a critical step in an evaluation. Nevertheless, an evaluation should have some knowledge of the topic in order to go beyond previous efforts and to avoid earlier mistakes (Bryman, 2016). Using that knowledge, the evaluator can make the case for why these outcomes are needed by the different levels of interest holders. Furthermore, a literature review may reveal previous similar work that can be used in the evaluation planning, such as possible instruments that could be applied in data collection, useful data collection approaches, and potential data analysis methods. Such a review might also identify colleagues who would be interested in the evaluation and who might be able to provide some advice or even some consulting.

Finally, the evaluator should also begin to decide on the approaches and methods to be used in the evaluation. Although specific planning of the data collection and data analysis is discussed in a future step, it is wise to begin early to discuss the methods, as well as the evaluation key questions and any questionnaire or interview questions with the primary and secondary interest holders. After all, it may be that one or more interest holders either have a preference for certain types of data collection and analysis approaches or hold a clear objection to some approach or to certain questions.

As an example, I met with a client who had a clear preference for a specific data collection approach and analysis concerning a proposed evaluation of a training program for employees. A colleague had made the initial contacts, and I came to the meeting to gather information to help guide the data collection effort. Given that the organization hired mostly recent immigrants, I set up the meeting primarily to determine what would be the best ways to gather data from these employees. What I quickly learned, however, was that the primary decision maker (or the primary interest holder), who was an engineer by training, was most concerned, and almost agitated, about the approach to data analysis. Specifically, he wanted to know what statistical methods we would be using. When I discussed issues related to undertaking a multiple analysis of variance with repeated measures, he suddenly seemed quite calm. At that point, we were able to discuss the approaches to data collection, which were to include surveys, interviews, and some observation. Even though the purpose of the meeting was to discuss the data collection issues, it was important to address possible data analysis methods with the primary interest holder and then discuss data collection.

Table 19.1 may help to clarify what might be expected from the various interest holders.

Identify Issues

As part of the planning process, the evaluator should attempt to identify any possible issues, particularly with regard to logistics, timeframe, and ethics that could affect the planning, design, or implementation of the evaluation. The following paragraphs discuss some of the typical issues that can be expected.

Logistical Issues

Almost any evaluation project requires the evaluator to think about logistical issues as part of the planning process. Basically, the questions involve some of the following:

- What data need to be collected? How will the data be collected? Where will the data be collected?
- Who will be involved in data collection? And to what extent will the data collection personnel need to be trained?
- How will the data be analyzed?
- Who will be involved in data analysis? To what extent will data analysis personnel need to be trained?

Not only should the evaluator include such decisions as part of the planning process but these issues also need to be discussed with the primary interest holder(s). It may be, for example, that the client wants to have their own staff participating in data collection or in data analysis or both. It is especially important to involve individuals with lived experiences and where there is a focus on participatory methods. Indeed, even when the evaluator may prefer to involve the interest holders, that decision should be discussed with the client in advance.

Timeframe Issues

Another major issue involves that of the timeframe. In most cases, the client or primary interest holder indicates when interim or final reports are needed. But in addition to such **milestones**, there may be timing issues that need to be decided and addressed. For example, typical times to avoid collecting data from individuals would involve vacation times, such as July or August or December. But there may be specific times when major staff meetings have been planned. Depending upon the circumstances, these may be good times to gather data from staff, or alternatively, these may be times that the client would prefer that staff not be contacted.

One evaluation project involved data collection from museum directors. It turned out that these individuals were holding a special 3-day gathering to discuss certain issues and challenges. This meeting provided a good opportunity to meet with and interview a sampling of these directors. In addition, listening to and observing the discussions provided some important

TABLE 19.1. Using Interest Holder Preferences to Guide the Evaluation

Interest holder	Questions/ information needs	Data preferences	Timing issues	Logistical issues	Ethical concerns	Cultural issues	Access issues (primary and secondary data)
Primary							
Secondary							
Tertiary							

background knowledge to guide the evaluation effort.

Ethical Issues

Monette et al. (2014) stated that "ethics involves the responsibilities that researchers bear toward those who participate in research, those who sponsor research, and those who are potential beneficiaries of research" (p. 50). Although these authors were discussing social research, the same holds for any program evaluation effort. The reader may also want to refer to the chapter by Morris (see Chapter 7, this volume).

As adapted from Russ-Eft et al. (2017), the evaluator should consider the following questions during the planning stage:

- Who will have access to the findings?
- Should participants be informed about the purpose of the evaluation before collecting data?
- How can participants in a control group be treated fairly?
- What additional actions and safeguards are required when collecting data from protected populations (e.g., children, prisoners)? (With children, there is a need to obtain the permission of a parent or guardian. With prisoners or other protected groups, one may need to obtain special permissions, apply for a **Certificate of Confidentiality** [Office for Human Research Protection, 2003], or undertake other methods to protect those individuals.)

Upon reviewing these questions, it should be clear that ethical concerns must be considered from the inception of the evaluation, throughout the data collection, analysis, and reporting, and even following the evaluation effort. Although the evaluator may be aware of such ethical concerns during data collection, analysis, and reporting, there may be a need to house the materials for a specified period following the conclusion of the evaluation as well as to dispose of the data in a way that ensures confidentiality to the participants. The website (*www.hhs.gov/ohrp/regulations-and-policy/belmont-report/#xethical*) contains valuable information on some basic ethical principles as well as some guidance on addressing specific issues. When planning an evaluation of a federal program, it is also important to consider the guidelines from the Office of Management and Budget (2002).

Evaluators should also refer to the American Evaluation Association *Guiding Principles for Evaluators* (2018) as well as the *Program Evaluation Standards* (Yarbrough et al., 2011). In addition, Morris (see Chapter 8, this volume) provides some useful guidance on ethical challenges.

Write the Proposal

The last, but perhaps the most important step in planning the scope of the evaluation, involves writing the proposal. This document summarizes the evaluator's understanding of the expectations, the focus, and the ethical issues. Furthermore, it includes a description of the proposed work, the deliverables, a schedule, and a budget. As stated by Russ-Eft et al. (2017), "the written proposal, once approved, often serves as the contract for the work" (p. 38). This is particularly the case when working with for-profit organizations. The reader may want to refer to the chapter on "The RFP: Writing One and Responding to One" in Russ-Eft et al.

PLANNING THE DATA COLLECTION AND DATA ANALYSIS

Bauer and Gaskell (2000) described four different dimensions related to data collection and analysis, specifically (1) design principles, (2) data elicitation, (3) data analysis, and (4) knowledge interests. Since the design principles can be closely aligned to the knowledge interests, I combine those two dimensions; and since the data elicitation tends to dictate the data analysis, I combine those two dimensions as well:

1. Design principles (e.g., case study, experiment, ethnography) and knowledge interests (control and prediction, consensus building, empowerment).
2. Data elicitation (e.g., focus group, individual interview, questionnaire, document review) and data analysis (e.g., inferential statistics, content analysis).

Each of these is discussed separately below.

Design Principles and Knowledge Interests

The decision on the research design to be used will affect and possibly determine what happens in the remaining two dimensions. Furthermore, as is true with any research project (which tends to have either hypotheses or focus questions), the key questions for the evaluation will suggest the appropriate design. So, for example, a key question that asks about the results or outcomes of a program would tend to suggest an experimental or quasi-experimental approach or at least the gathering of quantitative data. (An overview of both experimental and quasi-experimental designs can be found in Russ-Eft & Hoover, 2005, and in Harbatkin et al., Chapter 16, and Peck & Snyder, Chapter 13, this volume.). On the other hand, a key question that asks about perceptions of or experiences with the program or suggestions about needed improvements would tend to indicate more of a qualitative approach. Data collection would typically then ask for opinions and suggestions from staff or participants, typically using some form of interviewing, whether with individuals or through a focus-group process.

In addition to the key questions, another factor that can influence the design may be the worldview that the evaluator holds, as that worldview relates to the knowledge interests. Various researchers and theorists have suggested different frameworks for these worldviews (e.g., Creswell & Creswell, 2023; Creswell & Poth, 2018; Neuman, 2014; Yin, 2016). Rather than try to summarize all of these I simply use the framework suggested by Carr and Kemmis (1986) and Creswell and Creswell—these are positivism and postpositivism, interpretivism, critical social science, and pragmatism. The positivist or postpositivist focuses efforts on trying to determine the truth or falsity of a proposition. The evaluator in this case attempts to confirm some hypothesis or to predict some behaviors. In contrast, the interpretivist attempts to examine some activities of "people in natural settings" in order to understand how "people create and maintain their social world" (Neuman, 2014, p. 104). Critical social science focuses on critique, challenge, transformation, and empowerment. Thus, the critical approach seeks to change the program, organization, or society.

Those holding a pragmatic worldview attempt to solve real-world problems, in some ways similar to those with the critical view. They are, however, not necessarily concerned with inequities but rather with solving a problem or issue. Rather than focusing on the context, these evaluators concentrate on the consequences or outcomes. Their concern is with the practicality of the approach and the results.

Data Elicitation and Data Analysis

After a decision about the design, the evaluator will need to consider issues involved in data collection. As stated above, the design, knowledge interests, and focus of the evaluation tend to influence the choices concerning data collection. Furthermore, how the data will be gathered can affect the schedule, the people to be involved in data collection, the budget, and the risks.

Evaluators with a postpositive view and a concern about control and prediction tend to use quantitative data from available records, archives, and databases or data gathered through large-scale surveys. With available records, archives, and databases, the evaluator needs to be concerned about (1) how to gain access to the data, (2) how and from whom those data were gathered, and (3) in what form the data currently exist. If planning to undertake some large-scale survey, the evaluator should also determine what sampling will be undertaken and what procedures will be used to contact potential respondents and encourage their participation. Furthermore, the evaluator needs to decide what survey tool will be used and how the **reliability** and **validity** of that tool will be determined. Another issue involves what approaches will be used to reduce the level of nonresponse and what will be done to examine the level of **nonresponse bias**. Some sources on this issue include Hendra and Hill (2019), National Research Council (2013), Singer (2006), and Standish and Umbach (2019).

Typically, the data that are gathered from a database or a large-scale survey are quantitative or numeric in form. The evaluator needs to determine which quantitative or statistical methods will best answer the key questions of the evaluation. The reader may want to consult Pham et al. (see Chapter 17, this volume) for more details on conducting a quantitative analysis.

Those with an interpretivist and potentially a critical perspective tend to gather data from individual interviews or focus group interviews. As with the quantitative data collection, the evaluator needs to decide on the sampling and the procedures for contacting potential respondents and obtaining their willingness to participate. The data collector should consider recording the interviews in order to (1) capture what the person says and (2) stay focused on the conversation and the person rather than on writing down exactly what the person says. But there are situations when people do not want to be recorded and when note taking is needed. In such cases, two people are needed so that one person can facilitate the group interview while the other person writes down the responses.

When recording the interview, whether it is in person, on the telephone, with one person, or with a focus group, the evaluator needs to obtain informed consent and to follow procedures as approved by the IRB. Another consideration involves whether to have two recording devices or a colleague taking notes in case of equipment failure. Depending upon the sample, the evaluator may need to consider cultural and language issues with any primary data collection. In any case, whether gathering quantitative or qualitative data, the reader may want to examine Donaldson (see Chapter 27, this volume), with respect to ensuring that evaluation is culturally sensitive.

Having gathered individual interviews or focus group interviews and having recorded them, the evaluator must decide whether to transcribe the recordings or to have someone else do the transcription—recognizing that it will probably take some 3–4 hours to transcribe a 1-hour interview. Transcription services are very reasonable, and there are both low-cost as well as free software that can undertake such transcriptions; and now even Microsoft Word can do reasonably well in transcribing.

Another issue that should be of concern involves using methods that ensure the trustworthiness of the qualitative analysis. Some typical procedures involve **member checking, interest holder involvement, peer review,** and **triangulation.** Member checking involves having the respondents or the interviewees review and approve the transcription and the resulting analysis. Also, as noted earlier, having people with lived expertise as part of the research process is a growing element in some areas of evaluation.

Peer review consists of having a colleague or colleagues undertake the analysis independently, and then there would be a comparison of the results. This may result in some reconciliation of the differences. Alternatively, the peer review may simply involve a review and approval of the analysis by a colleague. Triangulation refers to the comparison with some other data. For example, the results of some interviews with employees may be compared with a previously conducted employee survey. The reader may want to consult Chapter 15, "Evaluation as Storytelling: Using a Qualitative Design" for more details. Another resource would be Chapter 4 "Plan the Data Collection and the Data Analysis" from Russ-Eft et al. (2017).

PLANNING THE WORK AND SCHEDULE

Having determined the scope of the project and identified some aspects of the data collection and data analysis, the evaluator is now ready to dive into the planning of the work and the schedule. This section briefly introduces two tools that can be used: (1) the **work breakdown structure** (WBS) and (2) milestones for scheduling. An approach similar to the description here is provided by Bickman (see Chapter 21, this volume).

Work Breakdown Structure

A WBS is a visual picture of the work needed to complete the evaluation effort. It provides a detailed listing of the tasks needed for the work. Figure 19.1 is an example of WBS for a specific part of an evaluation of a training program in an organization—namely, the development of a system for assessing leadership skills and sales skills.

This WBS shows some of the steps needed to design and test the assessments. As such, a WBS can provide a means for monitoring the work, determining the schedule, and calculating the costs. Furthermore, it represents one method for communicating the work to each of the interest holders. There are a number of online software tools that can help you create the WBS.

The following steps suggested by Dionisio (2017) and Russ-Eft et al. (2017) can be used to

Designing and Planning an Evaluation

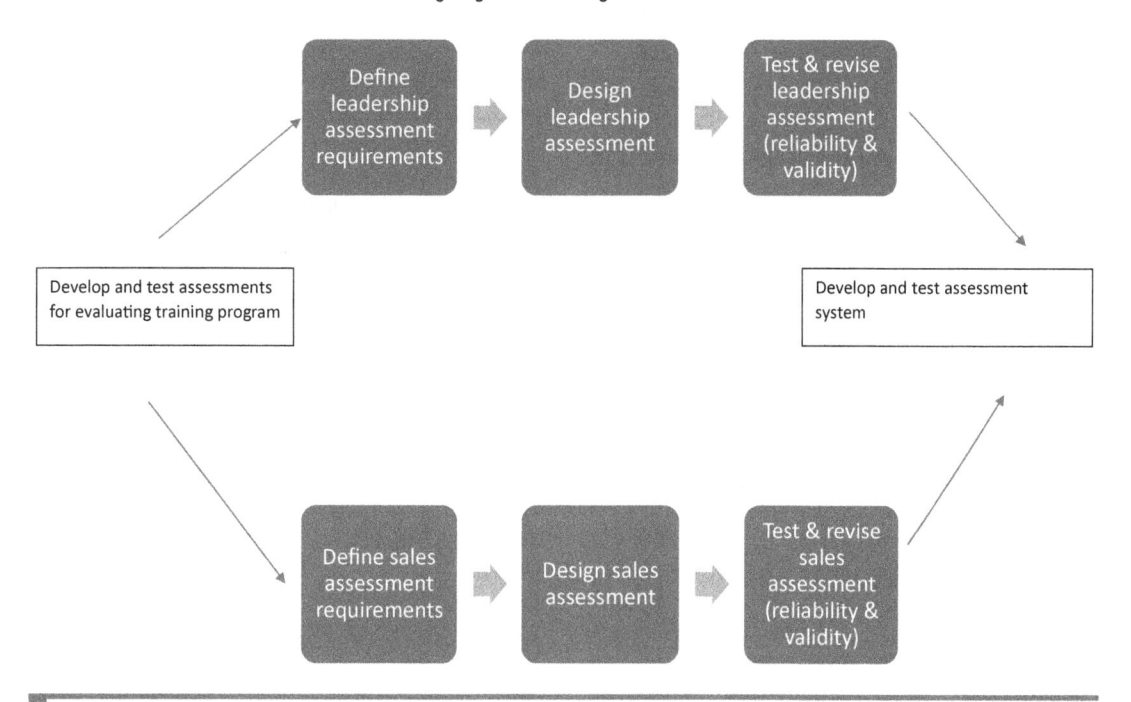

```
                    ┌─────────────┐      ┌─────────────┐      ┌─────────────┐
                    │   Define    │      │   Design    │      │Test & revise│
                    │ leadership  │  →   │ leadership  │  →   │ leadership  │
                    │ assessment  │      │ assessment  │      │ assessment  │
                    │requirements │      │             │      │(reliability │
                    └─────────────┘      └─────────────┘      │ & validity) │
                           ↑                                   └─────────────┘
┌──────────────────────────┐                                          ↘
│ Develop and test assess- │                                    ┌──────────────────────────┐
│ ments for evaluating     │                                    │ Develop and test         │
│ training program         │                                    │ assessment system        │
└──────────────────────────┘                                    └──────────────────────────┘
                           ↓                                          ↗
                    ┌─────────────┐      ┌─────────────┐      ┌─────────────┐
                    │   Define    │      │   Design    │      │Test & revise│
                    │   sales     │  →   │   sales     │  →   │   sales     │
                    │ assessment  │      │ assessment  │      │ assessment  │
                    │requirements │      │             │      │(reliability │
                    └─────────────┘      └─────────────┘      │ & validity) │
                                                              └─────────────┘
```

FIGURE 19.1. Work breakdown structure (WBS) for developing an assessment system as part of an evaluation.

create the WBS, whether done individually by the evaluator or by the team:

1. Identify the major deliverables or milestones. (In the example, the major deliverables are the assessment tools, which will then be used as part of the assessment system.)
2. Determine the work needed to create those deliverables. These are called "work packages." (In the example, one of the work packages is "define leadership assessment requirements.")
3. Draw the dependencies between the work packages. (In the example, there is an arrow between "define leadership assessment requirements" and "design leadership assessment.")

This represents a very basic WBS. In addition, using the WBS, the evaluator or evaluation team can also decide for each task:

- Who will be responsible?
- How much time will be needed?
- How much effort and what type of resources will be needed?
- What is the completion date?
- What risks might exist?

As can be seen, the WBS provides the basis for determining the schedule, the people, the budget, and the risks. The next section discusses approaches to scheduling: that of using milestones.

Milestones for Scheduling

The WBS enables the evaluator or the evaluation team to identify the specific tasks and their dependencies. It does not, however, indicate exactly when those tasks will be undertaken. Thus, the next step in the planning process involves developing the schedule for the work, based on what was determined from the creation of the WBS.

Milestones represent significant points in the project, typically requiring no time to complete. Thus, the interim or final report are examples of milestones (or products of the evaluation). Writing these reports takes significant amounts of time but the reports in and of themselves do not require any time. To create the schedule, the following steps can be used, which are similar to the development of the WBS:

1. Identify all of the milestones or products.
2. Determine the work needed to create each milestone.
3. Decide on the dependencies between each milestone.
4. Based on those dependencies and working backward from the end of the project, determine when each work package must start and end.
5. Reexamine the dependencies, both in terms of the work packages as well as the people involved.

Table 19.2 illustrates the milestones for a simple evaluation project as an example.

Using the information from the WBS and the milestones, the evaluator can create either a Gantt or a **program evaluation and review technique (PERT)** chart. Both provide a graphical representation of the project and its schedule. A Gantt chart uses horizontal bars to show the start date and the end date of a work package. Thus, it can show work that can be done at the same time, as well as tasks that cannot be undertaken until some other task has been completed. Various online tools, as well as Excel, can be used to create a Gantt chart. A PERT chart is an alternative approach to presenting the projects schedule with the start and end dates, the milestones, and the dependencies or which tasks depend upon some other task. In this case, circles or rectangles represent project milestones, and lines represent the tasks. According to Kopp (2022), "The PERT chart is often preferred to Gantt charts because it identifies task dependencies. However, a PERT can be more difficult to interpret" (para. 2). Table 19.3 presents a Gantt chart, and Figure 19.2 provides that same information in a PERT chart. Both of these tools also can be developmental in terms of helping to plan the scope of the study. Seeing overlapping tasks and the staff time needed, for example, may indicate the need for more staff or a reduction in the tasks. (But neither the Gantt chart nor the PERT chart include staffing details.)

PLANNING THE PEOPLE

In some cases, the evaluation project involves one person: the evaluator. In other cases, particularly for large-scale and complex evaluations, the project involves a team or group working together. This team may consist of employees within the same organization or a team with subcontractors or consultants. In some cases now, especially with work and personnel in remote locations, the organization is a set of loosely tied consultants that may need even more structures. In both cases, however, there will be interest holders who may influence the evaluation work as well as others who may support the evaluation. Thus, in every evaluation

TABLE 19.2. Planning Milestones and Schedule for Simple Program Evaluation Project

Milestone	Start date (for beginning work on milestone/product)	End date (or due date)	Contingent on prior activity or other person?
Meeting with client			
Meeting with interest holders			
Data collection instruments			
OMB clearance			
IRB approval			
Data collection completed			
Data analysis completed			
Data interpretation completed			
Final report			

Note. OMB, Office of Management and Budget; IRB, institutional review board.

TABLE 19.3. Example of Gantt Chart for a Simple Evaluation Project

	September		October		November		December	
	1–15	15–30	1–15	15–31	1–15	15–30	1–15	15–31
Meet with client	■							
Meet with interest holders		■						
Complete data collection instruments		■	■					
Complete data collection				■	■			
Complete data analysis					■	■	■	
Submit final report								■

effort, it is important to plan for the people. The following is described below: (1) developing a matrix of people and tasks, (2) recruiting and hiring project staff, (3) providing needed training, and (4) planning for communication.

Matrix of People and Tasks

Russ-Eft et al. (2017) recommended that the evaluator create a matrix that includes the interest holders, the people involved in the evaluation, the tasks that need to be accomplished, and the skills needed for those tasks. This may need to be an iterative procedure in which the evaluator may first need to identify the task and then determine who would be the best person to complete the task. Table 19.4 provides a simple example.

Even if the evaluator can possibly do the work alone, there may be times when it makes sense to have others do the work. The evaluator may need to engage a statistician to conduct some analyses or a person to transcribe interview recordings or a colleague to undertake a peer review of a qualitative analysis. A consideration may be that there is more to do during a particular time period than can be done by one person or that having multiple people engaged in a particular task would be more efficient. There may also be issues of cost effectiveness—thus, having someone else who is stronger in a particular analysis technique may be more cost-effective than struggling through a new process. Language or cultural concerns may suggest hiring others to undertake interviews as well.

Even if the evaluator plans to conduct the project alone, that person may need to engage interest holders in various aspects of the work, such as helping to determine the key questions, provide access to respondents and encourage

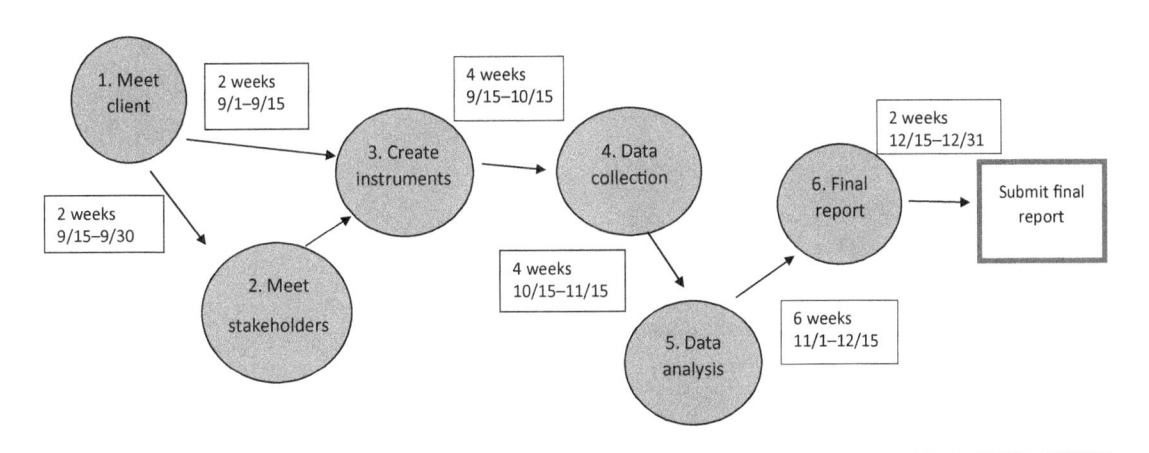

FIGURE 19.2. Example of a PERT chart for a simple evaluation project.

TABLE 19.4. Matrix of Tasks, Skills Needed, and Project Staff

Tasks	Knowledge and skills	Staff
Literature review		
Locate articles and write abstracts	Familiarity with literature search process; access to library and interlibrary loan service; ability to write concise abstracts	Graduate research assistant
Read abstracts and prepare literature review	Familiarity with topic and literature; good writing skills	Denise and Samuel
Review literature review for insights	Familiarity with topic; ability to identify information and possible approaches for the evaluation	Melinda and David

participation, and review and reflect on the results. If the evaluator is working with a team, then decisions need to be made concerning what role interest holders will play versus that of the staff. Thus, even with the solo evaluator, it is important to develop the matrix of people and tasks.

Recruitment and Hiring

As stated above, the evaluator may work in an organizational setting with staff available to support the project. In other cases, the evaluator may be a solo, independent consultant. In either case, the evaluator will have created a matrix of tasks and identified the people involved, such as particular staff members or even specific interest holders. There may be certain tasks that do not have an assigned person or there may be a need to recruit and select an internal person or hire an external person for the particular task. To do so the evaluation should create a job description for the position. Such a job description should include:

- A summary of the position.
- Specific job duties.
- Minimal qualifications.
- Preferred qualifications.

This job description can, then, be posted internally, or it can be posted externally through newsletters or relevant professional websites, such as *www.eval.org*, *www.ahrd.org*, or *www.psyccareers.com/employer-offers#events*.

Typically, more people apply than are needed for the position. In such cases, the evaluator or the evaluation team may want to interview the applicant or applicants. Such interviews can be done by phone, online conferencing, or in person. The evaluator or team members involved in the interviewing process should have copies of the job description and the interviewee's résumé or curriculum vitae. The interview team should be familiar with prohibited questions regarding race, color, religion, sex, national origin, age, and disabilities. Furthermore, it is highly recommended to use a behavioral event interviewing approach. Rather than ask a more general question, such as "How good are you at working in a team?" the interviewer would ask, "Tell me about a time when you experienced a problem working in a team. What actions did you take to deal with that problem? What was the response; what happened?"

In some cases, it may be important to have the potential candidate involved in a simulation. For a clerical position, there may be a keyboarding test. For a statistical analyst position, there may be a requirement to run some analyses or to interpret the results of some analyses. If such simulations or tests are used for hiring purposes, they must be shown to be reliable and valid.

Training

In some cases, the evaluator may need to provide training to someone on the evaluation team. It may be that the schedule is such that the evaluator is unable to undertake all of the data collection.

The evaluation effort focused on an examination of team-related efforts taking place in 10 different organizations located throughout the

United States. Data collection required two people to undertake observational sessions, individual interviews, focus group interviews, and survey data collection with both managers and employees at each location. Since data collection had to take place during a 1-month period, the evaluator had to provide data collection training to other staff. This training involved the development of a brief workbook, data collection instruments, and simulations of the data collection, along with feedback from the evaluator.

The need for such training appeared obvious in the above example, given the schedule. In other cases, the evaluator may want to consider undertaking a needs assessment using a knowledge and skills approach, or a job-task analysis, or a competency-based assessment (Sleezer et al., 2014). Having identified a developmental need, the evaluator should consider not only training but also coaching and mentoring.

Communication

Another aspect related to the people working on the project involves communication among the team members and the interest holders. Some of this communication may be related to "(a) decision making concerning some aspect of the process, (b) information about upcoming activities and progress . . . , (c) presentation of draft or final . . . reports, and (d) presentation of manuscripts for publication" (Russ-Eft et al., 2017, p. 90). Typical formats for communication involve working sessions, meetings—in person, by videoconference, or by phone, memos, reports, and newsletters. Furthermore, particularly with in-person, videoconference, or phone meetings, it is important to identify a procedure and communication method to document decisions.

It may be helpful to prepare a table with some of the details on the people involved, the format, and the schedule. Table 19.5 presents an example of such a planning device. Further ideas concerning communications can be found in Torres et al. (2004), Russ-Eft and Preskill (2009), and in O'Neil (see Chapter 25, this volume).

PLANNING THE BUDGET

An important part of planning involves determining what resources will be needed to complete the evaluation. Thus, the budget will necessarily be a part of the proposal to the client or the agency. Two important concepts are full-time equivalent (FTE) and projecting unit costs. One FTE indicates the equivalent of one person working full-time or presumably 40 hours in 1 week. Projecting unit costs refers to an indication of the costs for completing one portion or unit of a task, so for example, the costs for completing one interview transcription. In addition to this brief section, the reader may want to examine Chapter 21 by Leonard Bickman, "Resource Planning," and Chapter 24 by Michael Bamberger, "Conducting Evaluations under Budget, Time, and Data Constraints: An International Perspective."

The typical expenses for an evaluation include (1) personnel (involving not only staff but also consultants), (2) materials and supplies, (3) equipment, (4) communications, (5) travel, (6) facilities, (7) participant incentives, and (8) transcription costs. In addition, depending

TABLE 19.5. Example of a Portion of a Communication Plan for an Evaluation

Participants	Purpose	Format	Timing/schedule
Team members	Refine evaluation focus	Working session	Mid to end January
	Review and revise schedule	Weekly meeting	Mid to end January
	Decide on data collection sites and instruments	Working session	Early February
Client/primary interest holder(s)	Review and refine evaluation focus and schedule	In-person meeting	Mid-February
	Inform about data collection progress	Email	End March
Midlevel managers	Inform about data collection progress	Email	End March
Employees	Inform about data collection progress	Newsletter	April

upon the organization and the funder, there may be (9) overhead costs, and (10) an additional fee.

In most cases, the major category of expenses involves the personnel, which includes salaries and fringe benefits. In some cases, a specific person is identified for the project, perhaps the lead evaluator. In this case, the person's actual salary and benefits for the specified period are used. In other cases, a specific person may not be named but rather a category of personnel, such as a statistician or a clerical assistant. In all cases, the percentage of time or the number of hours for the work needs to be determined in order to calculate the salary and fringe benefits for the person. When calculating the number of person hours in a year, most organizations use 2,080 hours, though some use a number that removes vacation time.

Materials and supplies comprise items that can be considered disposable, such as pens, paper, and software. The evaluation effort may require the purchase of a database or a specific assessment tool. Typically, such a database or assessment tool, or even a software package may not be available following the conclusion of the project.

Equipment, on the other hand, refers to items that will remain available following the project. This would include computer and printer hardware and videoconferencing and recording equipment. With larger organizations, the costs for existing equipment are simply included as part of overhead. If, however, such equipment needs to be acquired, it is important to decide whether it is cost-effective to purchase such equipment for future use or to lease the equipment for a specified time period. Furthermore, if the equipment is purchased, a decision needs to be made as to whether the costs should be depreciated over time.

Communication costs refer to the costs involved in communicating with the client and interest holders, the participants, and possibly even the evaluation team members (particularly those in distant locations). These communications costs may involve videoconferencing costs, as well as the costs associated with producing and distributing project reports. It should be noted that more graphics tend to be needed and used in project reports. Furthermore, these reports may need to adhere to **508 compliance**, and such compliance involves not only reports but websites. Section 508 of the Rehabilitation Act (29 U.S.C. § 794d) requires that information and communication technology be accessible to people with disabilities. And that requirement is applicable not only to those who work for the federal government.

Some projects require travel, not only for meetings with the client and other interest holders but also for data collection purposes. The budget, then, would need to include the costs for transportation, hotel, and meals.

Participant incentives may need to be included in the budget. There may be individual incentives, such as a gift card for responding to a survey, or the offer of participation in a raffle for some larger reward, such as a computer. It may be important to examine the type of gift card being offered in different communities. For example, Target gift cards are not often valued as highly as Walmart because the money can go further in Walmart. Dillman et al. (2014) provide good suggestions on the use of such incentives in survey research. (At the same time, however, be sure to check on the organization's policies, since some do not allow such incentives to be given.)

In the case of focus groups, there may be some individual incentives or the focus group may be planned during a mealtime, with participants offered food and beverage for their participation. For vulnerable populations, you may need to offer/provide transportation and day care. Other arrangements and expenses with the use of a focus group may involve the hiring of a person trained to handle focus groups, someone to take notes, and a location that includes a two-way mirror. More details on conducting focus groups can be found in Krueger and Casey (2015).

Finally, we should recognize that different client organizations require different amounts of detail in the budget as part of the proposal. Typically, a government agency requires detailed information and justification for the budgeted items. In contrast, a private, for-profit organization may simply want to know the total amount for the project. In other cases, though, it behooves the evaluator to plan the budget in as much detail as possible. That budget detail can later be used for monitoring the project expenses. Powell et al. (see Chapter 12, this volume) should provide some detail on monitoring program implementation. More information on developing budgets can be found in Bickman (Chapter 21, this volume) and Bamberger (Chapter 24, this volume).

PLANNING THE RISKS

Undertaking any evaluation project entails some form of risk, since the specific project at that specific time with the specific team members and participants has never been undertaken previously. As defined in Russ-Eft et al. (2017), "A risk that could lead to falling short of an established target is a threat; a risk that could lead to exceeding an established target is an opportunity" (p. 110). An example of a threat would be when participants fail to respond to an online survey. An example of an opportunity would be when the budgeted funds for data analyses exceed the actual costs.

In order to plan for the risks, the evaluator needs to identify all of the possible risks to the project. These risks may exist throughout the life of the project or may be related specifically to the planning phase, the execution phase, or the close-out phase. An example of a risk/threat would be the departure or change in the primary interest holder. Indeed, the departure of any interest holder or staff member may create a risk for the project. Having identified a risk, the next step is to try to determine the likelihood of that risk occurring. For example, there can be a risk of being unable to recruit enough participants or of having a specific data collection site refuse to participate. In some cases, it may be useful to indicate a specific probability of that threat, while in other cases, the evaluator could simply indicate "high," "medium," or "low" likelihood. Next, the evaluator should try to imagine the possible impact of that risk. For example, the departure of the primary interest holder may lead to a major change or even cancellation in the project. The inability to recruit enough participants or to have a site withdraw from participation may lead to needing to recruit other participants or other sites.

A final step in the process involves determining the response to each of the risks. Portney (2013) suggested the following responses:

- The ostrich approach: Ignoring all risks or pretending they don't exist.
- The prayer approach: Looking to a higher being to solve all your problems or to make them disappear.
- The denial approach: Recognizing that certain situations may cause problems for your project but refusing to accept these situations may occur. (p. 192)

Unfortunately, these responses cannot solve the problems that may arise when the risks do occur. Instead, it will be more productive to undertake the following responses:

Responses to Threats

- Avoid the risk by taking different action.
- Reduce the likelihood or impact of the risk. (In the example of failing to recruit enough participants or losing a site, the evaluator may decide to provide a higher level of incentive; alternatively, it may require undertaking the data collection using different methods, or in the case of the loss of a site, it may mean identifying alternative sites upfront.)
- Fallback by waiting for the risk to occur before taking previously planned actions.
- Transfer or spread the risk so that the consequences are less serious. (If concerns exist, for example, regarding the recruitment of a sufficient number of participants, the evaluator may transfer the risk by hiring a firm to do the work.)
- Accept the risk (i.e., decide to live with it and proceed).

Responses to Opportunities

- Exploit by ensuring that the opportunity will happen . . .
- Enhance by increasing the likelihood that the opportunity will happen . . .
- Reject by deliberately deciding to not take advantage of the opportunity . . .

Table 19.6 presents a portion of a risk matrix for an evaluation project. A more complete risk matrix can be found in Russ-Eft et al. (2017, pp. 112–114).

TABLE 19.6. Portion of a Risk Matrix for an Evaluation Project

Possible risk	Likelihood (high, medium, low)	Impact	Response to threat (avoid, reduce, fallback, transfer, accept)	Response to opportunity (exploit, enhance, reject, share)
Possible risk throughout project				
Lead evaluator leaves project				
Client/primary interest holder leaves organization or agency				
Changes in team members				
Conflicts arise among team members				
Possible risks during planning				
Information about client or interest holders is unknown				
Interest holder expectations are unknown				
Budget lacks sufficient detail				
Possible risks during executing				
Assignment not completed on time				
Respondents fail to participate				
Possible risks during closeout				
Client/interest holders become involved in other activities and lose interest				
Team members transferred to new assignments				

By attending to the risks as part of the planning process, the evaluator may be able to avoid disasters with the threats and to capitalize on the opportunities.

CONCLUSIONS

Planning an evaluation may not be a top-of-the-mind issue for an evaluator. But it is a critical process for ensuring the success of the evaluation effort. Beginning this planning as part of the proposal process can help to clarify the proposal itself. Not only should the evaluator plan the focus, the data collection, the data analysis, the schedule, and the budget but also the participants and the risks. The following is a brief vignette describing the first part of an evaluation project.

Sally was a faculty member at a university, and she also undertook some consulting work as an independent consultant separate from the university. With each project, she had to work with the university to decide whether the project should be undertaken through the university or as an independent consultant.

One day a colleague contacted her concerning a potential evaluation project. The colleague worked for a training organization, and he was heading the development of a training program for a technology firm. The client at the technology firm was interested in the development of an assessment instrument that would later be used as part of an evaluation of the training program. The colleague asked Sally whether she was interested in working on developing the assessment instrument to be followed by an evaluation of the training.

Sally asked her colleague about any requirements concerning the (1) schedule, (2) budget, (3) locations, and (4) meetings with the client. The colleague gave his opinions but he suggested that Sally contact the client directly. Sally called the client and obtained some information to help with the proposal. She thought about what would be needed to complete the project, and she decided that the project would benefit from support from a university colleague as well as some specialized statistical work, potentially from a graduate student. For those reasons, she decided to develop the proposal through the university, and she confirmed that decision with the university research staff.

As part of the proposal process, Sally contacted her colleague to make sure that he was available and interested in the work. Also, she obtained his suggestions as to his FTE and the salary that would be required for the work. Based on the information that she had gathered from the client and her colleague, she developed the proposal, which included the focus, the schedule, and the budget. At the same time, Sally created a risk matrix to help her ensure the successful progress of the project.

A day following submission of the proposal, Sally received the good news that the client approved of the project. Sally immediately began more detailed planning. She notified the university research office to make arrangements for the budgeting. She developed a WBS, which she shared with her colleague and made revisions based on his comments. She created a position description and announcement and distributed it to graduate students in the college's doctoral programs.

During the first week of the project, Sally traveled to the client's location to meet with the primary interest holders and some of the organization's managers. As part of that visit, she provided more details on the focus of the evaluation, the data collection and analysis plans, the proposed communications, and the proposed schedule. Based on feedback from the interest holders, Sally revised each of the plans and shared those revisions with the interest holders and her colleague.

Upon her return, Sally and her colleague interviewed several doctoral students, and they decided upon a third-year student. The student had completed his preliminary oral examinations and was working on his dissertation proposal. Sally and her colleague met with the student, and the three reviewed the proposal and most particularly, the focus of the project, the WBS, the data collection and analysis plans, the communication plan, schedule, budget, and the risk matrix. The doctoral student suggested some additional analysis approaches, and Sally informed the primary interest holder of these suggestions.

Everything seemed to be proceeding according to plan, when her colleague announced that he had accepted a position at another institution. Furthermore, given his new commitments, he could not continue with the project. As part of the risk matrix, Sally had identified that as a potential threat, and in the earlier meetings with her colleague and the doctoral student, they had identified another faculty member who might be able to work on the project. Sally approached that person, and she agreed enthusiastically. Both Sally and the doctoral student did, however, have to spend some time reviewing the completed work and the ongoing plans.

Throughout the project, Sally and the team referred to the various plans and made revisions where necessary. Any such revisions were communicated to the primary interest holder. All of the planning helped to keep the project on task, on schedule, and on budget. As a result of the success of the first phase of the project, Sally and the team were asked to undertake the second phase.

REFERENCES

American Evaluation Association. (2018). *Guiding principles for evaluators*. Author.

Bauer, M. W., & Gaskell, G. (2000). Quality, quantity, and knowledge interests: Avoiding confusion. In P. Atkinson, M. W. Bauer, & G. Gaskell (Eds.), *Qualitative researching with text, image and sound: A practical handbook* (pp. 3–18). Sage.

Black, P., & William, D. (2009). Developing the theory of formative assessment. *Educational Assessment, Evaluation and Accountability, 21*(1), 5–31.

Bryman, A. (2016). *Social research methods* (5th ed.). Oxford University Press.

Carr, W., & Kemmis, S. (1986). *Becoming critical: Education, knowledge, and action research*. Falmer Press.

Creswell, J. W. (2015). Revisiting mixed methods and advancing scientific practices. In S. Hesse-Biber & R. B. Johnson (Eds.), *The Oxford handbook of multimethod and mixed methods research inquiry* (pp. 57–90). Oxford University Press.

Creswell, J. W., & Báez, J. C. (2021). *30 essential skills for the qualitative researcher* (2nd ed.). Sage.

Creswell, J. W., & Clark, V. L. P. (2018). *Designing and conducting mixed methods research*. Sage.

Creswell, J. W., & Creswell, J. D. (2023). *Research design: Qualitative, quantitative, and mixed methods approaches* (6th ed.). Sage.

Creswell, J. W., & Poth, C. N. (2018). *Qualitative inquiry and research design: Choosing among five approaches* (4th ed.). Sage.

Dillman, D. A., Smyth, J. D., & Christian, L. M. (2014). *Internet, phone, mail, and mixed-mode surveys: The tailored design method* (4th ed.). Wiley.

Dionisio, C. S. (2017). *A project manager's book of forms: A companion to the PMBOK guide* (3rd ed.). Wiley.

George, J., & Cowan, J. (1999). *Handbook of techniques for formative evaluation: Mapping the student's learning experience*. Routledge.

Hendra, R., & Hill, A. (2019). Rethinking response rates: New evidence of little relationship between survey response rates and nonresponse bias. *Evaluation Review, 43*(5), 307–330.

Kopp, C. M. (2022, October 9). Program evaluation review technique—PERT chart definition. *Investopia*. www.investopedia.com/terms/p/pert-chart.asp

Krueger, R. A., & Casey, M. A. (2015). *Focus groups: A practical guide for applied research* (5th ed.). Sage.

Monette, D. R., Sullivan, T. J., & DeJong, C. R. (2014). *Applied social research: A tool for human services* (9th ed.). Brook/Cole Cengage Learning.

National Research Council. (2013). *Nonresponse in social science surveys: A research agenda*. National Academies Press.

Neuman, W. L. (2014). *Social research methods: Qualitative and quantitative approaches* (7th ed). Pearson Education.

Office for Human Research Protection. (2003, February 25). *Certificates of confidentiality—privacy protection for research subjects: OHRP guidance (2003)*. U.S. Department of Health and Human Services. www.hhs.gov/ohrp/regulations-and-policy/guidance/certificates-of-confidentiality/index.html

Office of Management and Budget. (2002). Guidelines for ensuring and maximizing the quality, objectivity, utility, and integrity of information disseminated by federal agencies: Republication 2002. Originally at 67 FR 369-378; corrected (February 5, 2002) at 67 FR 5365, pp. 8451–8460. www.federalregister.gov/documents/2002/02/22/R2-59/guidelines-for-ensuring-and-maximizing-the-quality-objectivity-utility-and-integrity-of-information

Onwuegbuzie, A. J., & Hitchcock, J. H. (2015). Advanced mixed analysis approaches. In S. Hesse-Biber & R. B. Johnson (Eds.). *The Oxford handbook of multimethod and mixed methods research inquiry* (pp. 275–295). Oxford University Press.

Patton, M. Q. (2011). *Developmental evaluation: Applying complexity concepts to enhance innovation and use*. Guilford Press.

Portney, S. E. (2013). *Project management for dummies* (4th ed.). Wiley.

Preskill, H., & Russ-Eft, D. (2016). *Building evaluation capacity: Activities for teaching and training* (2nd ed.). Sage.

Project Management Institute. (2021). *A guide to the project management body of knowledge* (7th ed.). Author.

Rossi, P. H., Lipsey, M. W., & Henry, G. T. (2019). *Evaluation: A systematic approach* (8th ed.). Sage.

Russ-Eft, D., & Hoover, A. (2005). The joys and challenges of experimental and quasi-experimental designs. In R. A. Swanson & E. F. Holton, III (Eds.), *Research in organizations: Foundational principles, processes, and methods of inquiry* (pp. 75–95). Berrett-Koehler.

Russ-Eft, D., & Preskill, H. (2009). *Evaluation in organizations: A systematic approach to enhancing learning, performance, and change*. Basic Books.

Russ-Eft, D. F., Sleezer, C. M., Sampson, G., & Leviton, L. (2017). *Managing applied social science research*. Jossey-Bass.

Scriven, M. (1966). The methodology of evaluation. *Social Science Education Consortium, Publication 110*. Purdue University.

Scriven, M. (1967a). The methodology of evaluation. In R. E. Stake (Ed.), *Curriculum evaluation* (American Educational Research Association Monograph Series on Evaluation, No. 1, pp. 39–83). Rand McNally.

Scriven, M. (1967b). The methodology of evaluation. In R. W. Tyler, R. M. Gagne, & M. Scriven (Eds.), *Perspectives of curriculum evaluation* (pp. 39–83). Rand McNally.

Singer, E. (Ed.). (2006). Nonresponse bias in household surveys [Special issue]. *Public Opinion Quarterly, 70*(5), 637–809.

Sleezer, C. M., Russ-Eft, D. F., & Gupta, K. (2014). *A practical guide to needs assessment* (3rd ed.). Wiley.

Standish, T., & Umbach, P. D. (2019). Should we be concerned about nonresponse bias in college student surveys? Evidence of bias from a validation study. *Research in Higher Education, 60*, 338–357.

Stake, R. E. (2004). *Standards-based and responsive evaluation*. Sage.

Torres, R. T., Preskill, H., & Piontek, M. E. (2004). *Evaluation strategies for communicating and reporting: Enhancing learning in organizations* (2nd ed.). Sage.

Wallerstein, N., Duran, B., Oetzel, J., & Minkler, M. (Eds.). (2017). *Community-based participatory research for health: Advancing social and health equity* (3rd ed.). Jossey-Bass.

Yarbrough, D. B., Shulha, L. M., Hopson, R. K., & Caruthers, F. A. (2011). *The program evaluation standards: A guide for evaluators and evaluation users* (3rd ed.). Sage.

Yin, R. K. (2016). *Qualitative research from start to finish*. Guilford Press.

Chapter 20

Logic Models and Program Theory

Joy Frechtling

CHAPTER OVERVIEW

This chapter discusses logic models and the value they add to an evaluation. I discuss how logic models relate to theories of change and other approaches to conceptual mapping, as well as how they work to enhance understanding of why things work or don't work. I also discuss the components of a logic model and provide illustrations of what such a model might look like in different situations. The chapter presents an overview of the logic model development process and how program and evaluation staff can work together to create a shared understanding of the work, its steps, and what is expected to be learned. Finally, I suggest additional ways that logic models can be used that go beyond evaluation.

The purpose of this chapter is to introduce readers to two critical tools in evaluation: **logic models** and **program theory**. These tools assist evaluators in conducting work that provides not only the assessment of whether a program is meeting its goals but a deeper understanding of why or why not this may be happening. Together they define evaluation as a **"theory-driven"** enterprise, one that goes beyond tracking the linkages between activities and outcomes (an approach might be described as *input/output*) to clearly defining the steps along the path to change and the rationales for expecting them.

Logic models and program theory are not designs or methodologies but rather they are ways of framing an evaluation and guiding the evaluation questions. They are tools to support and expand evaluation thinking (see Archibald et al., Chapter 3, this volume). While we frequently associate the idea of a theory with the idea of disciplinary theory, such as social science theory, in the context I am discussing a theory can be derived from various sources, such as practitioner beliefs and experiences, as well as disciplinary investigation (Chen, 1990; Frechtling, 2007; McLaughlin & Jordan, 2010).

Although incorporating theory-driven work in evaluation has become more commonplace today with request for proposals from federal agencies and other funders routinely including a logic model or the request for a logic model (Coldwell & Maxwell, 2018), this approach has not always been an expected part of the evaluators' toolkit. Bickman (1989) states, "Casual reading of the evaluation literature should be enough to convince the reader that the use of theory in evaluations is infrequent" (p. 387).

Historians (Rogers et al., 2000; James, 2011) credit Suchman (1967) with introducing the idea behind theory-driven work, Weiss (1995, 1997) with promoting it early on (in 1972) and into several decades, and Bickman (1987), Wholey (1987), Chen (1990), Schon (1997), and Funnell (1997) with developing it and bringing it into prominence in discussion (see also Mark, Chapter 4, this volume). A major contributor and promoter of this approach was Joseph Wholey and his work on evaluability assessment—an approach developed to assess a program's "readiness" to be evaluated against its outcomes. Patton (2008) credits Wholey's work in evaluability assessment as playing a major role promoting the use of logic models and theories of change in evaluation work. Tools depicting causal relationships, such as logic models, were also being promoted by the nonprofit sector—specifically the United Way of America (1996), and the W. K. Kellogg Foundation (2004). McLaughlin and Jordan (2010) also credit the emphasis on managing for results and measuring performance as leading to the expanded use of program theory and logic models (also see Rog, Chapter 11, this volume).

Today the idea of attending to the theory underlying an effort and creating visualizations to express them is seen as critical. Increasingly, federal agencies such as the Substance Abuse and Mental Health Services Administration, Centers for Disease Control and Prevention (2018), Department of Education, and National Science Foundation have required the inclusion of a logic model in program and evaluation plans and many different technical assistance efforts have been devoted to helping grantees develop and use program theory and logic models as part of their program development (Frechtling, 2007, 2010). Families of tools have been developed to describe and portray causal relationships, including *log frames*, *causal pathways*, *concept maps*, *results frameworks*, *outcome maps*, and *balanced scorecards*. Lemire et al. (2023) identify 10 different approaches to visualizing program theories, each with related benefits and limitations.

> **BOX 20.1. Key Terms in Theory-Driven Evaluation**
>
> - Program theory
>   - Theory of change
>   - Theory of action
> - Logic model

Perhaps an indicator of the extent to which these tools have become accepted is the fact that discussions of program theory and logic models have a strong focus on "how to" create and use them, with relatively less attention being directed toward providing an argument for their utility.

WHAT IS PROGRAM THEORY? WHAT IS A LOGIC MODEL? HOW DO THEY DIFFER? HOW DO THEY CONVERGE?

There is no single accepted definition of the terms *program theory* or *logic model*, although underlying the various alternatives is the concept of describing *what leads to what from program inception to program outcome*. For the purpose of our discussion, I believe that program theory and logic models are ways of describing a program or activity that make it clear how a program is expected to work.

According to Funnell and Rogers (2011, p. 31), "A program theory is an explicit theory or model of how an intervention, such as a program, an initiative, or a policy, contributes to a chain of intermediate results and finally to the intended or observed outcomes." Rogers (2011, p. 24) suggests that program theory can be divided into two subcomponents: (1) "a theory of change—the process by which change comes about," and (2) "a theory of action—how the intervention is constructed to activate the theory of change."

A logic model is a popular tool that translates the theory into visual form. Knowlton and Phillips (2013, p. 4) offer the following description of a logic model:

> Logic models are a graphic way to organize information and display thinking. They are a visual approach to the implicit maps we all carry in our minds about how the world does or should work. Logic models describe the planned action and its expected results.

There is some debate as to whether logic models and program theory are simply different approaches to conveying a program's underlying structure or whether they are different in some fundamental ways. Wilder Research (2005) simply, "Program theory explains why a program is expected to work and a logic model illustrates a program theory" (p. 1).

Those who believe there are some important differences between the two suggest that logic models focus in a more simplistic and linear way on what leads to what in a particular intervention, while program theory more broadly addresses connections and alternative connections, as well as the endogenous and exogenous factors that affect them (Clark & Anderson, 2004). It may be that for simple interventions the information they provide is virtually identical, whereas in more complicated situations, the logic model is a reduced presentation of the broader theoretical thinking. The key takeaway, however, is their common focus on describing how and why an intervention leads (or is expected to lead) to a particular set of outcomes and clarifying the intermediate steps in the process of change. Critical here is understanding that evaluation, at its best, is not just an evaluation of a specific program but rather the exploration of a theory or alternative theories underlying an effort. It is not just a thumbs-up or a thumbs-down on a particular program but a contribution to the knowledge base and an extension of our conceptual understanding of a problem or approach. The logic model facilitates enhancing this conceptual understanding and provides views of both the design and the implementation.

With this background in place, in the remainder of this chapter, I focus on logic models and how logic models can scaffold a theory-driven approach to evaluation.

WHAT DOES A LOGIC MODEL LOOK LIKE?

While there are variations in how logic models are presented, at a minimum a logic model includes a set of components—inputs, activities, outputs, outcomes, impacts, and context—and connections between the components (W. K. Kellogg Foundation, 2004; Frechtling, 2007). Figure 20.1 presents a simple, generic logic model.

The components are defined as follows:

- **Inputs** are the resources brought to a program, typically funding sources or the experiences and knowledge of the individuals and institutions involved.

- **Activities** are the components that describe what the treatments or services a program is providing. They are the actions taken to move toward the program's goals and outcomes.

- **Outputs** are the products of the activities. Outputs document the implementation of an activity in simple, itemized ways. They document whether an activity has been carried out, frequently through simple counts, or other quantitative data on products, participants, and events.

- **Outcomes** are results or changes in behaviors or learning. Outcomes identify the goals and objectives of the program. Outcomes are typically specified in the short and longer term. How to differentiate short- and long-term out-

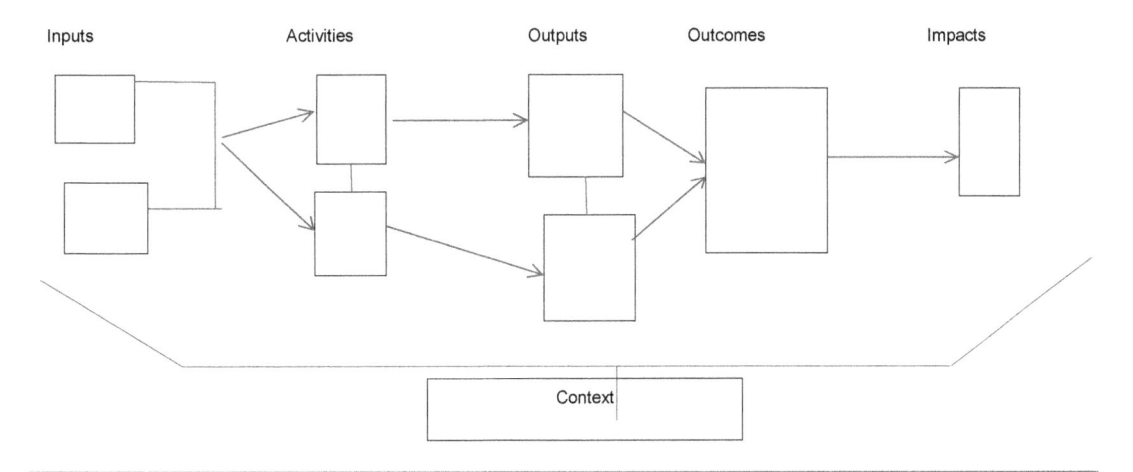

FIGURE 20.1. Generic logic model.

comes is program specific and determined in large part by the complexity of the changes that are being made.

- **Impacts** are broader changes at the systems level that are expected to occur if the program is successful. The difference between an outcome and an impact is that the outcome describes what results from a specific program, whereas the impact addresses more far-reaching changes within the system that includes the program.[1]

- **Contextual factors** are factors that are out of control of the program but may help or hinder achievement of the outcomes. Context can include both current context and historical context, as previous experiences may color how participants perceive a current experience. Context can refer to features of the organization, sociocultural, technological, and/or policy variables that may influence outcomes and potential success in different situations and with different populations. Understanding of context helps inform where approaches and findings might and might not be generalizable.[2]

A common error in the development of a logic model is confusing outputs with outcomes. Take, for example, the following scenario for a professional development program (see Figure 20.2). In this model, the desired outcome is a change in skills and knowledge. However, in reporting on attainment of program goals, frequently the output variable (in this case, number of attendees) is reported on as evidence of success and the actual change in skills and knowledge is not addressed. While attendance would certainly be considered an important step to document in exploring the theory of change underlying the work and provides information on program implementation, it is not in and of itself evidence for a positive outcome. Attending a professional development session and changing in some way because of that attendance are quite different things.

Connecting the components within a logic model and showing relationships between and among them are a series of arrows and lines that show expected interdependences or consequences. These arrows may show connections within a component or between components. The arrows are a critical part of the logic model, showing specifically what is hypothesized to lead to what. The arrows are also important in that they clarify how earlier parts of the work may influence later parts, showing, for example, how activities and outputs are expected to lead to short-term outcomes. We return to this distinction below.

---

[1] Frequently, evaluators have come to use the term *impact* to refer to changes that occur in comparison to a counterfactual. The logic model does not assume the presence of a counterfactual in using this language but focuses more on the distinction between the project and systems levels.

[2] Unfortunately, context does not typically receive adequate attention in many evaluations and there seems to be an implicit assumption that the outcomes/impacts of interventions are context neutral.

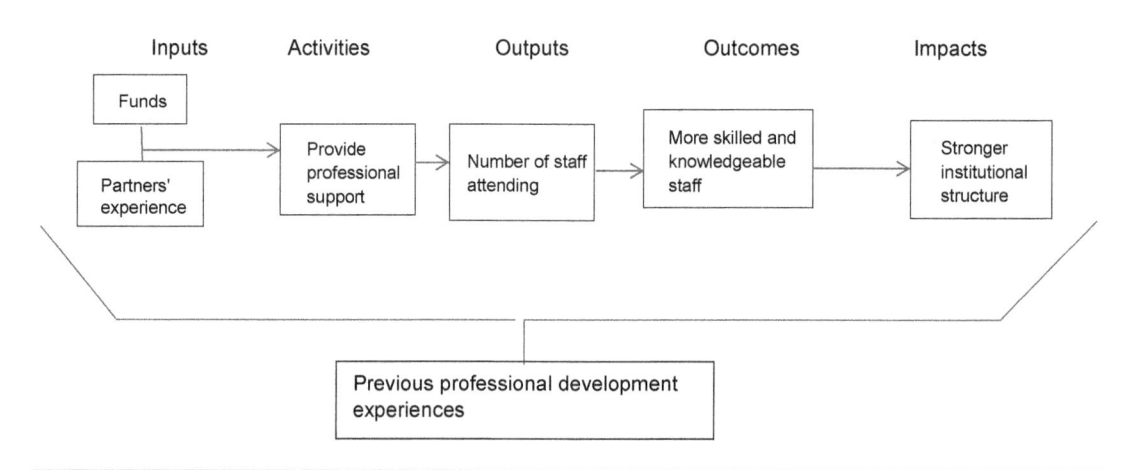

FIGURE 20.2. Logic model for a professional development program.

In developing this logic model, we have adopted the format developed by the W. K. Kellogg Foundation (2004), showing a horizontal progression starting with inputs on the left and moving toward outcomes and impacts on the right. While this is the most commonly used format for a logic model, others exist and may also be useful. For example, another format that is frequently used tells the story vertically. Circular diagrams can also be useful (see Figures 20.3 and 20.4).

Which model is the best model to use is probably a matter of personal preference. The authors of the Community Tool Box (*https://ctb.ku.edu/en*) do suggest, however, that the linear model may be better in portraying cause and effect, whereas the circular model better shows the interdependencies among the components expected to produce that effect.

Regardless of format, critical in using a logic model is clearly identifying what each of the components includes and the connections within and across components that are expected to occur. Moreover, in all but the most basic situations the logic model shows some differentiation, with not all activities, for example, leading to the same outputs or outcomes. While it is not uncommon to see a visual such as that portrayed in Figure 20.5 called a logic model, such a depiction would describe the underlying theory of change in a limited way due to the lack of differentiation in the connections among the elements of each component.

Let's take an example of an intervention and develop a logic model for it. As the description above shows, the goals for this digital learning program are defined on several levels. Ultimately, the goal is to make system change and

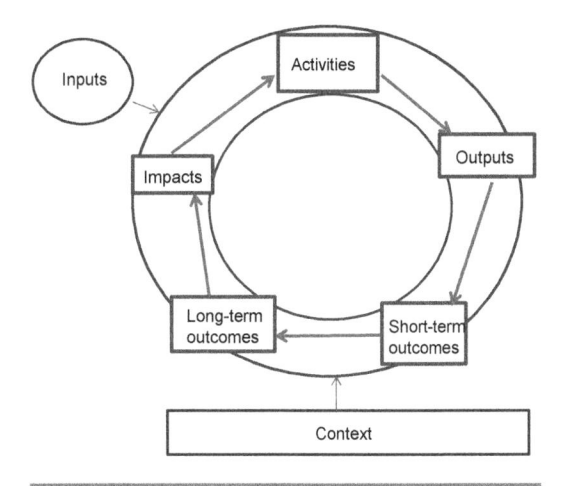

FIGURE 20.4. A circular depiction of a theory of change.

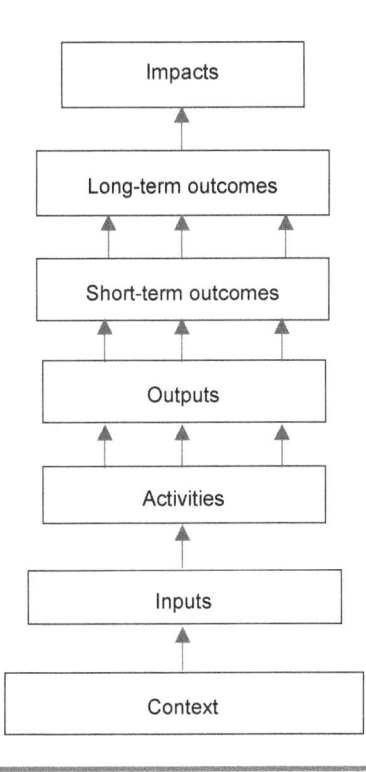

FIGURE 20.3. A vertical depiction of a theory of change.

BOX 20.2. Example of an Intervention: New Digital Learning Curriculum

Recognizing the importance of digital literacy for postsecondary and career success, XYZ Inc. is developing a new digital learning curriculum for middle school. The curriculum is built on the hypothesis that promoting digital literacy requires experiences that (1) provide students with needed skills in the use of digital technology, (2) allow students to explore a real-life problem, (3) allow students to identify their own solutions to solving the problem, and (4) provide recognition for successful execution of the solution. Other program features believed to contribute to potential effectiveness of the intervention include (1) allowing students to problem solve using a team approach, and (2) giving students the opportunity to comment on and analyze one another's solutions.

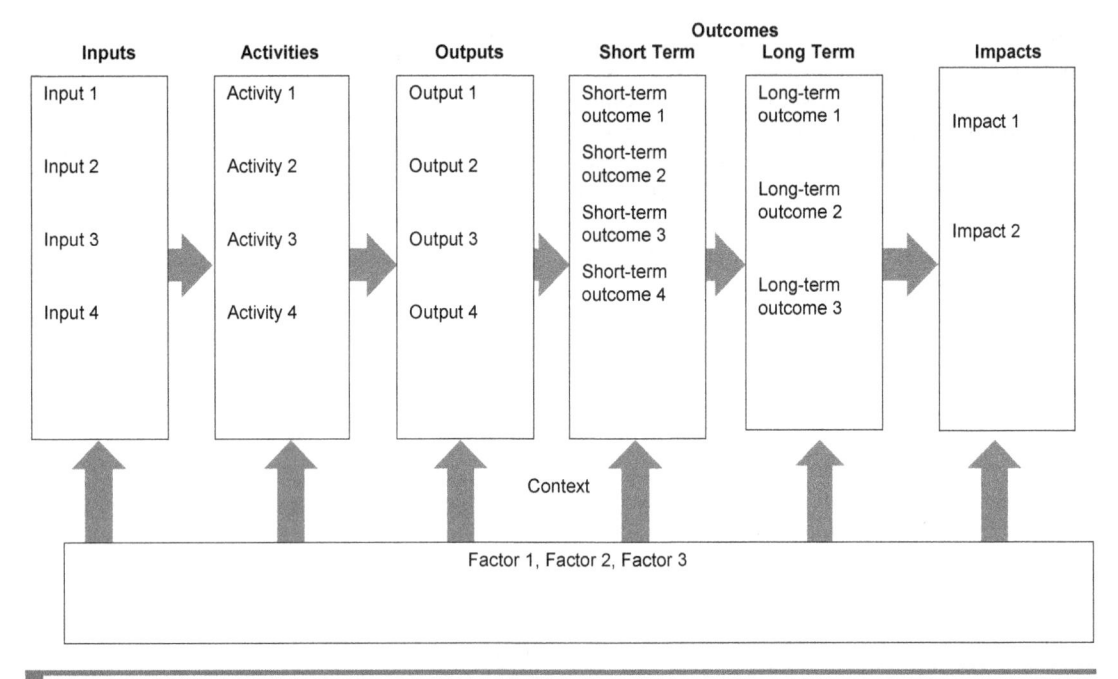

Inputs	Activities	Outputs	Outcomes Short Term	Outcomes Long Term	Impacts
Input 1	Activity 1	Output 1	Short-term outcome 1	Long-term outcome 1	Impact 1
Input 2	Activity 2	Output 2	Short-term outcome 2	Long-term outcome 2	
Input 3	Activity 3	Output 3	Short-term outcome 3		Impact 2
Input 4	Activity 4	Output 4	Short-term outcome 4	Long-term outcome 3	

Context: Factor 1, Factor 2, Factor 3

FIGURE 20.5. Logic model with limited differentiation.

influence how digital literacy is incorporated into the educational process. There are also goals for participants in the system, principally students. The developers believe that participation in these activities will have positive impacts on students' learning and engagement, which, in turn, will lead to higher graduation rates and continuing into postsecondary education. The theory of change also posits that to reach these goals, teachers not only have to acquire the skills and knowledge provided through the training but also transfer these skills to creating new learning experiences for students.

The program developers want to test this theory of change, comparing the academic outcomes of students who participate in the digital literacy course with similar students who do not participate.

Figure 20.6 presents the logic model for this intervention using the Kellogg format. How does creating this logic model help in developing a successful evaluation? It helps on multiple levels. First, it helps by providing a clear picture of what the program is trying to accomplish, the steps that are hypothesized to lead to the outcomes, and the contingencies among them. On the right-hand side, we see outcomes specified for three levels of the system: teachers, students, and the educational program overall. On the left-hand side of the logic model, three activities are highlighted that are foundational to the work being undertaken: developing the curriculum, training the teachers, and delivering the program to students. The middle columns provide a more fine-grained look at the consequences of these activities. The outputs column provides a series of indicators that an activity did take place. Note that this set of items says nothing about the quality of the activity, only that it occurred. The next column provides an enumeration of the short-term results from the

---

BOX 20.3. Value Added of a Logic Model to an Evaluation

- Makes expectations explicit.
- Clarifies timeline and sequencing.
- Identifies critical junctures for formative assessment.
- Creates an opportunity to prioritize questions and research priorities.

activities. There are results called out in separate boxes for teachers and students. And within this set of short-term outcomes, there are also arrows that show relationships among them. For example, the student outcomes are shown as a result of teachers providing instruction aligned with the program's theory of change. The long-term outcomes repeat this approach of tracking change for the two key participant groups: teachers and students. Finally, under the impact column earlier outcomes converge, leading to a system-level impact.

The logic model also clarifies the timeline for the steps, helping to identify when different types of questions might be asked. Related to this, it lays out opportunities for formative assessment for checking on implementation and early outcomes that can be assessed well before longer-term outcomes might be expected to emerge. Assessing these outcomes in a timely manner can provide the opportunity for midcourse corrections and reexamination of the implementation processes, instead of waiting for the full intervention to run its course. (Of course, it might be that the underlying theory of change is incorrect, allowing developers to reexamine their assumptions.) Finally, by showing all of the components and connections that are relevant to the theory, it challenges the evaluator to prioritize evaluation opportunities and make some hard decisions about what to measure and when, at the beginning of the evaluation process. Even in a relatively simple evaluation such as the one described here, there are often more aspects that could be evaluated than time or money can typically support.

Critics of logic models point to the linear nature of the change theory depicted, suggesting that it is a misrepresentation of how interventions actually develop. For anything but the simplest intervention, it is likely that the theory of change will evolve, with initial learnings about short-term outcomes (on the right) feeding back into the components presented earlier

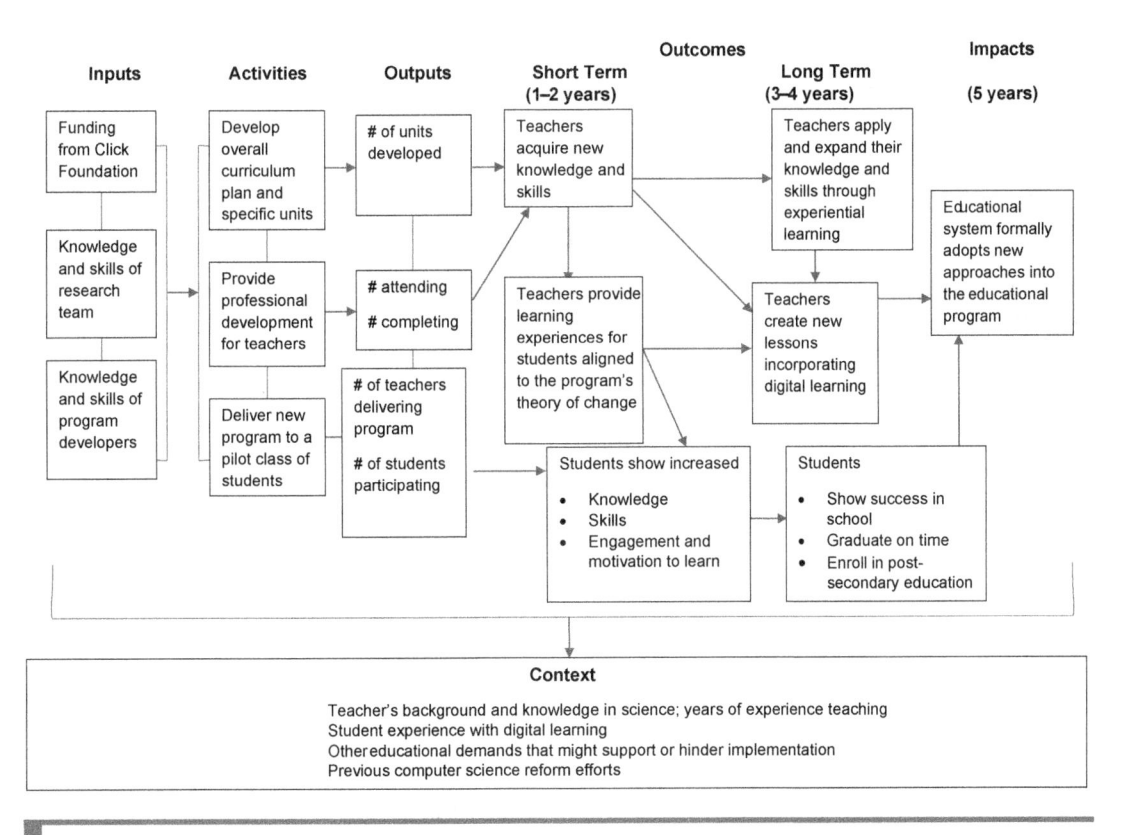

FIGURE 20.6. Logic model for a new digital literacy program.

in the diagram (on the left), such as activities. This is a fair criticism but not a fatal one. There is nothing to stop an evaluator from creating a logic model that accounts for this feedback by showing arrows that indicate where such inputs might occur. Additionally, there is nothing that says that the program itself and the logic model, once created, will not evolve. Indeed, it would be surprising if the initial logic model developed for an intervention did not evolve as the program is implemented and more information emerges through data collection and testing of hypotheses. In fact, in work I have done, we have used the logic model precisely as a tool for documenting our evolving understanding of the underlying theory and the factors along the path of change that really make a difference.

It is important to recognize that creating a logic model provides a strong scaffolding for the work of designing and implementing an evaluation but it is only a first step. In addition to establishing priorities among the components and connections described in the logic model, the evaluator needs to determine how to measure the prioritized pieces and establish criteria for success. Typically other interest holders have a role in this process (see discussion below on developing a logic model) but the evaluator still is responsible for the final decisions that are made.

Frequently it is useful to spell out additional details regarding measures, either in documents linked to the logic model or in the logic model itself. Returning to the example above, consider the short-term outcome: Teachers provide learning experiences for students aligned to the program's theory of change. An accompanying document would refer to the features of instruction described earlier and provide information on the indicators that will be used to measure them and how the data will be collected.

DEVELOPING LOGIC MODELS

Developing a logic model can be a challenging process, especially when an intervention is complicated or complex. Further, in situations where a **developmental evaluation** is appropriate, the lack of a complete underlying theory of change may require piecemeal development of the logic model itself or even the development of multiple alternative models that align with the emergent understanding of the nature of the program.

While a single person or group may lead the development of a logic model or create an initial draft, in the long run the most benefit is gained when key interest holders who play different roles and may have different perspectives engage in the process, at least to some extent. Of course, when logic model development is approached through a participatory lens, it may be necessary to first develop a joint understanding of what a logic model is and is not. Partners need to understand the definitions of key components—inputs, activities, outputs, outcomes, impacts, and contexts—as well as the importance of tracing specific linkages within and among components.

While developing a logic model is possible and useful at any point in a program's evolution, it can be maximally useful if logic model development starts at the planning stage and continues throughout the program's life cycle. There is no single prescription for how this should be done and the need for revision depends on the program and how it evolves. For some programs, it is sufficient to simply visit the logic model at the beginning and end of the program; for others it is important to review the logic model each time new data come in, when changes in the program are made, or when a reporting event is looming. The important point is recognizing that a logic model should be expected to be a "living" and developmental depiction. As stated above, information gathered from outputs may well lead to suggestions for changes in activities; examination of actual short-term outcomes against the originally posited short-term outcomes can also lead to changes in program design, timeline, or level of anticipated outcomes. Modifications are to be expected and even celebrated as the evaluation provides new information.

Like any other participatory activity, who is involved in the development of a logic model will differ depending on the program and who is a key interest holder. In some cases, it is sufficient to have program leadership and the researcher/evaluator at the table. In other cases, it may be necessary to include participants and other key interest holders, such as representatives from the broader community, in the process. If the logic model is to be part of a participatory evaluation, then the evaluation participants should also be represented at the logic modeling phase. Including representation from a broad range of groups can have a significant payoff in the long run, if ownership and engagement are established. Decisions about the value or worth of an activity can be facilitated when groups with varied roles and initial understandings have been given the opportunity to create a shared vision. However, the more diverse the groups engaged in logic model development, the more challenging the process and the greater the demands on time and resources, as reaching agreement may require several meetings and revisions to create such a consensus document. One strategy to obtain diverse inputs without overloading this phase of the evaluation work would be to concentrate the interest holder engagement efforts on gathering inputs on priorities and questions of interest but not requiring that consensus be reached on the final contents and format of the logic model itself. Indeed, the exercise and discussion of the factors can benefit interest holders, open doors to new discussions, and be a positive end in and of itself.

Sometimes it is useful for the researcher/evaluator to draft an initial version of the logic model and use this model to kick off broader discussion. If the participants have a general understanding of what a logic model is, they can be asked to create their own logic models and bring them for sharing and discussion. In other cases, a meeting might start with a clean slate, allowing the development to occur as a group activity. Each strategy has strengths and weaknesses and may work well or badly depending on the particular nature of the individuals involved. If time is limited, the first approach—starting with a logic model generated by the researcher/evaluator—is likely to be the most cost-effective.

Although the traditional logic model has a linear appearance, starting with inputs and ending in impacts, the development of a logic model rarely starts with inputs and moves successively through the various components, ending with impacts. Especially when the program is in its planning or early implementation stages, it may be more productive to start with what a program is trying to achieve—desired outcomes or impacts—and work backward, identifying more proximate outcomes and assessing their linkages to the activities proposed to accomplish them (taking into account the inputs or resources available). It can be helpful to pose a series of questions, such as what are you trying ultimately to achieve. Who or what are you targeting to bring about these changes? Do the activities appear likely to lead to these outcomes? If not, what else do you need to do to bring these changes about? How long will it take these changes to occur? What factors in your specific environment influence the course and speed of change? Can you do what you need to do with the resources you have available? If not, what are the alternatives? In essence, the discussion needs to bounce back and forth or toggle among the components to assess the extent to which they hang together and work as an integrated whole.

Part of the development of a logic model is also clarifying what is meant by achieving a goal and the value of different types of evidence for documenting goal attainment. Especially when a goal is stated at a high level of abstraction, interest holders may hold different perceptions of how "success" should be defined. If, for example, a program goal is to improve student learning, participants may define learning in vastly different ways, including solving complex problems, generating new and innovative ideas, performing well on tests, or acquiring new habits of mind. Each of these has value but would, in all likelihood, require different strategies or activities to be undertaken. Activities that might be judged appropriate for increasing test score performance might be quite different from those for generating new and innovative ideas.

Table 20.1 provides a step-by step summary of one approach to structuring interest holder engagement.

Development of a logic model and clarifying the meaning of terms can help interest holders develop a shared vision of what the program is trying to accomplish and how desired goals are to be reached. At the same time, the discussions can unearth differences in perceptions and understandings that in the short run, at least, may cause anxiety and tensions to emerge among groups. Sometimes an accord has been reached among different interest holders only by deliberately allowing some terms to remain fuzzy—a potentially dangerous but sometime necessary tactic. Logic model developers need to be aware of this potential for creating disequilibrium and be prepared to take the time to hear out the

TABLE 20.1. Steps in Interest Holder Engagement for Logic Model Development

Step 1: Premeeting

Activities:
- Develop preliminary logic model based on existing information
- Identify gaps or inconsistencies in the model
  - Outcomes not logically linked to precursors
  - Activities that are not connected to outcomes
- Identify potential formative and summative questions
- Determine timeline for addressing the questions

Participants:
- Evaluator/evaluation team

Product:
- Initial logic model
- Questions for participants
- Interest holder meeting agenda

Step 2: Interest holder engagement meeting 1

Activities:
- Present initial logic model
- Ask for feedback and comments on accuracy and completeness
- Clarify what the program is trying to accomplish
- Describe how the program proposes to attain these accomplishments
- Engage interest holders in discussion and strive to ensure that power relationships don't stifle discussion
- Identify shared understandings and divergent opinions, explore and, to the extent possible, resolve differences
- Address previously identified gaps and inconsistencies (if not addressed in discussion)

Participants:
- Evaluator/evaluation team
- Interest holder group representatives[a]

Product:
- Annotated logic model
- Meeting notes

Step 3: Postmeeting 1

Activities:
- Update logic model based on interest holder meeting 1
- Identify remaining issues to be resolved

Product:
- Revised logic model
- List of remaining issues
- Interest holder meeting agenda

Participants:
- Evaluator/evaluation team

Step 4: Interest holder engagement meeting 2

Activities:
- Summarize takeaways from interest holder meeting 1
- Present revised logic model
- Address remaining gaps and inconsistencies
- Present potential formative and summative evaluation questions and discuss priorities

Participants:
- Evaluator/evaluation team
- Interest holder group representatives

Product:
- Annotated logic model
- Meeting notes

Step 5: Postmeeting 1[b]

Activities:
- Summarize conclusions from interest holder engagement meeting 2
- Create a working logic model based on meeting 2

Participants:
- Evaluator/evaluation team

Product:
- Memo to interest holder engagement participants with working logic mode

[a]Although program developers are typically included as interest holder, who else falls into this category may vary by problem and audience for the work. [b]May also include asking leadership for a final sign off.

different voices and work with participants to reach and understand the different viewpoints and help create a solution. Even if there is agreement, however, it is possible that the discussion that goes hand in hand with logic model development will unearth gaps in the program's theory of change that no one has recognized. For example, it is not atypical for the development of a set of activities to take on a life of their own, with the connection to program goals getting lost in the process. There may be both activities that do not seem to have any necessary connections to desired outcomes and outcomes that do not link back reasonably to activities once the theory of change is systematically examined. In such cases, it may be useful to rethink why such activities were included, what research and past experience have to say about what works and what doesn't, and whether some program redesign is needed. Several sessions of discussion separated by time for reflection and regrouping may be needed before consensus can be achieved.

That said, it might be that in some cases consensus cannot be achieved and after considerable discussion, differences remain in important areas. What happens then and what is the appropriate role for the evaluator? In a world of unlimited resources, the solution could be to move forward with the alternative logic models (and program variations) and design the evaluation to test these different logic models and underlying theories of change. For example, in the New Digital Literacy Program described in Box 20.2, it might be that strong differences are found in interest holders' opinions regarding the importance of collaborative activities or teamwork in achieving goals for students. In such a case, it might be possible to modify the design for the program (and the evaluation) to examine directly the role that collaborative learning and teamwork play. In other cases, this may not be possible, and the program director will ultimately have to make some hard decisions regarding the underlying program theory and what outcomes are to be evaluated.

OTHER USES OF LOGIC MODELS IN EVALUATION

Our discussion of logic models above focuses on developing and using a logic model to describe the theory of change underlying a single program. It is also important to note that logic models can be used in similar ways to describe families of programs, all of which are part of a broader initiative. A logic model can be developed to describe the theory underlying the portfolio overall and then separate logic models created to describe the individual programs funded through it.

Figure 20.7 shows a portfolio logic model. This model depicts the theory of change for a grant program designed to increase the percentage of underrepresented minorities in tenured positions at doctoral universities—very high research institutions. The theory of change presented here is the theory of change for the funders' investment—the logic model shows the funder's expectations for impacts, starting with the award of individual grants and resulting in bigger system changes.

In our discussion heretofore, we have situated the use of the logic model as a tool for clarifying a program *after* the decision has been made to evaluate it. However, another important use of the logic model is in helping to determine *whether a program can/should be evaluated*. This is called **evaluability assessment** (see Rog, Chapter 11, this volume).

According to Wholey (1987):

Evaluability assessment clarifies program intents from the points of view of key actors in and around the program; explores program reality to clarify the plausibility of program objectives and the feasibility of performance measurements; and identifies opportunities to change program, resources, activities, objectives and uses of information in ways likely to improve program performance. (p. 78)

Evaluability assessment is usually conducted before an evaluation or when an evaluation is being considered to determine whether (1) the program and its purposes are clearly enough defined, (2) there is a clear logic underlying the program, (3) there is agreement on evaluation priorities and how the data will be used, and, finally, (4) there is a willingness to act on the basis of what is learned from the evaluation.

Evaluability assessment can be very useful as it identifies both situations where "there is no there there" and where additional development is needed before an evaluation should take

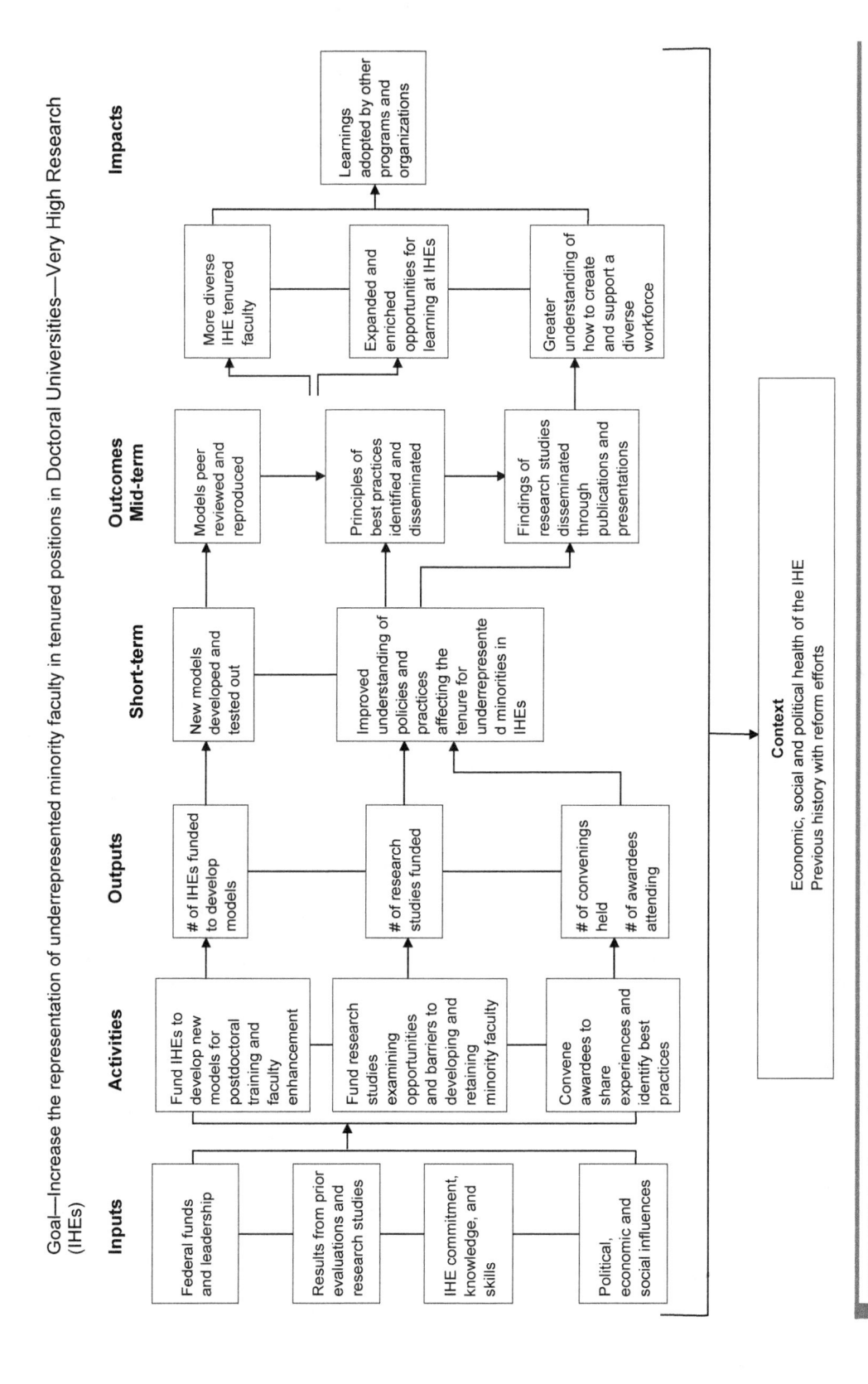

FIGURE 20.7. Logic model for the Initiative for Faculty Transformation.

place. It can help to eliminate wasted investments in evaluation when a program is found to be too poorly or inconsistently defined to make evaluation worthwhile.

WHAT ARE THE BENEFITS INCORPORATING PROGRAM THEORY AND LOGIC MODELS INTO AN EVALUATION? WHAT ARE THE DRAWBACKS?

Incorporating program theory and logic models into an evaluation can have many benefits. That said, it is important to recognize that there are also drawbacks (Frechtling, 2015; Bickman, 1989). On the plus side, incorporation of a logic model in an evaluation can:

- Provide a context in theory and research.
- Contribute to social science research knowledge.
- Scaffold the design and metrics.
- Identify critical junctures for measurement.
- Clarify beliefs and misunderstanding.
- Support ongoing program improvement.

On the minus side, developing and using logic models can:

- Be time- and resource consuming, especially if multiple interest holder groups are involved.
- Require greater theoretical and content knowledge on the part of the evaluator.
- Cause additional confusion in complex or complicated situations.
- Give the appearance of a conflict of interest for the evaluator, if the activity leads to reshaping and/or modifying the program.

Bickman (1989, citing Chen & Rossi, 1987) also raises the possibility that working from a program theory can to some extent reduce challenges to internal validity, even without using a rigorous experimental design, such as the randomized treatment control approach. The logic model is treated as a form of methodology that can be interpreted as supporting causality. The argument here is that having and confirming an a priori theory of change mitigates the threat of not having an appropriate counterfactual. In other words, it supports the idea of contribution, if not going so far as to support attribution. (See Peck & Snyder, Chapter 13, this volume, for further discussion of this issue.)

As the field of evaluation has moved toward incorporating logic modeling into the evaluators' toolkit, there have emerged a range of guides and other supporting documents to assist evaluators in developing and using logic models. These tools include checklists, rubrics, and even software that can facilitate logic model development. Largely the conversation has shifted from discussing whether program theory and logic models should be used, to discussing how best to develop and use them in different situations (see Lemire et al., 2023). A number of these tools are included in the references.

USES OF LOGIC MODELS BEYOND EVALUATION

I have discussed the value of logic models for evaluability assessment as well as scaffolding the evaluation process itself. The utility of logic models (and program theory) is not, however, limited to evaluation and can serve the needs of a range of leaders, including both program developers and program managers. Having a clear understanding of how and why specific activities are expected to lead to an outcome is important for both designing and managing/monitoring a plan or program as well as doing formal evaluation work. Logic models are useful throughout the life cycle of an activity: before—for planning and assessing the feasibility of a plan; during—for developing understanding, determining priorities, monitoring workflow, and supporting continuous improvement; and after—for documenting what was learned. McLaughlin and Jordan (2010) cite using logic models to describe management functions, websites, and the performance management process itself.

PROGRAM THEORY, LOGIC MODELS, AND EVALUATOR COMPETENCIES

King (see Chapter 2, this volume) discusses the 2018 American Evaluation Association's Evaluator Competencies, laying out competencies in five domains: professional practice, methodology, context, planning and management, and interpersonal. The principles discussed in this chapter on the use of program theory and development of logic models call upon competencies in each of the five domains. While the strongest alignment is in the methodological domain (i.e., identifies evaluation purposes and needs, uses program logic and program theory, as appropriate, identifies assumptions that underlie methodologies and program logic, etc.), competencies called out in other domains—especially those addressing interest holder engagement and respect for different perspectives—are also critical to the successful and ethical use of these tools. Being a strong evaluator and implementing the work described in this chapter are clearly aligned.

CONCLUSIONS

Logic models and program theory are useful tools for scaffolding evaluations. Theory-driven evaluations go beyond addressing the questions of whether "X leads to Y" to explore why the connections may or may not occur. Developing a logic model can also help ensure that evaluators, program developers, and other interest holders have a shared vision for the program and a shared understanding of the questions that the evaluation can and will explore. There are many benefits to incorporating the theory-driven approach. At the same time, it takes resources, time, and skills to use these tools effectively.

REFERENCES

Bickman, L. (Ed.). (1987). Using program theory in evaluation. *New Directions for Program Evaluation*, No. 33.

Bickman, L. (1989). Barriers to the use of program theory. *Evaluation and Program Planning*, 12(4), 387–390.

Centers for Disease Control and Prevention Program Evaluation Framework. Step 2. Retrieved December 27, 2018, from *www.cdc.gov/eval/steps/step2/index.htm*

Chen, H. (1990). *Theory driven evaluation*. SAGE.

Clark, H., & Anderson, A. A. (2004). *Theories of change and logic models: Telling them apart*. Paper presented at the meeting of the American Evaluation Association, Atlanta, GA.

Coldwell, M., & Maxwell, B. (2018). Using evidence-informed logic models to bridge methods in educational evaluation. *Review of Education*, 6(3), 267–300.

Community Tool Box. *http://ctb.ke.edu/tools/en/sub_section-main-1877.htm*

Frechtling, J. (2007). *Logic modeling methods in program evaluation*. Wiley.

Frechtling, J. (Ed.). (2010). *The 2010 user-friendly handbook for project evaluation*. National Science Foundation.

Frechtling, J. A. (2015). Logic models. In *International encyclopedia of the social and behavioral sciences* (2nd ed., pp. 299–305). Elsevier.

Funnell, S. C. (1997). Program logic: An adaptable tool. *Evaluation News and Comment*, 6(1), 5–17.

Funnell, S. C., & Rogers, P. J. (2011). *Purposeful program theory: Effective use of theories of change and logic models*. Wiley.

James, C. (2011). Theory of change review: A report commissioned by Comic Relief. Available at *www.theoryofchange.org/pdf/James_ToC.pdf*

Knowlton, L. W., & Phillips, C. C. (2013). *The logic model guidebook*. SAGE.

W. K. Kellogg Foundation. (2004). *Logic model development guide*. Author.

Lemire, S., Porowski, A., & Mumma, K. (2023). *How we model matters—visualizing program theories*. ABT Associates.

McLaughlin, J. A., & Jordan, G. B. (2010). Using logic models. In J. Wholey, H. Hatry, & K. Newcomer (Eds.), *Handbook of practical program evaluation* (2nd ed.). Jossey-Bass.

Patton, M. Q. (2008). *Utilization-focused evaluation*. SAGE.

Rogers, P. (2011, January 25–26). *Program theory and logic models for systemic evaluation*. Paper

---

BOX 20.4. Lessons on Logic Models and Program Theory

- Logic models and program theory provide the evaluator with tools to enhance the value of the evaluation process.
- They assist the evaluator in going beyond *what happened* to *why it happened*.
- There are standard sets of descriptors—components and connections—that evaluators can use to develop a logic model. A number of tools have been developed to facilitate the process.
- A logic model clarifies what needs to be measured and provides the scaffolding for identifying indicators ad measures.
- Development of a logic model is a participatory process that involves both evaluators and other interest holders.
- Theory-driven evaluation has many benefits but also may pose challenges in terms of time, resources, and skills needed.

presented at the International Conference on Systemic Approaches in Evaluation, Eschborn, Germany.

Rogers, P., Petrosino, A., Huebner, T., & Hacsi, T. (2000). Program theory evaluation: Practice, promise, and problems. *New Directions for Evaluation*, No. 87.

Schon, D. A. (1997, April). *Theory of action evaluation*. Paper presented to the Havard Evaluation Task Force.

Suchman, E. A. (1967). *Evaluative research: Principles and practice in public service and social action programs*. Russell Sage Foundation.

United Way of America. (1996). *Measuring program outcomes: A practical approach*. Author.

Weiss, C. H. (1995). Nothing as practical as good theory: Exploring theory-based evaluation for comprehensive initiatives for children and families. In J. P. Connell, A. C. Kubisch, L. B. Schorr, & C. H. Weiss (Eds.), *New approaches in evaluating community initiatives: Concepts, methods, and contexts* (pp. 65–92). Aspen Institute.

Weiss, C. H. (1997). Theory-based evaluation: Past, present, and future. In D. Rog & D. Fournier (Eds.), *Progress and future directions in evaluation: Perspectives on theory, practice, and methods. New Directions for Program Evaluation*, No. 76.

Wholey, J. S. (1987). Evaluability assessment: Developing program theory. In L. Bickman. (Ed.), Using program theory in evaluation. *New Directions for Program Evaluation, 33*, 41–55.

Wilder Research. (2005). *What's your theory? Tips for conducting program evaluation*. Amherst H. Wilder Foundation.

Chapter 21

Resource Planning

Leonard Bickman

CHAPTER OVERVIEW

Before making decisions about the specific design to use and the type of data collection procedures to employ, the evaluator must consider the resources available and the limitations of these resources. I highlight four types of resources that impact evaluations that need to be considered in planning.

Data. What are the sources of information needed and how will they be obtained? This includes primary data collection where the evaluator will be collecting new data. In planning the new data collections, the evaluator has to consider issues of external validity or generalizability in selecting sites, statistical power, authorization to access sites, confidentiality and privacy, and the data collection processes. In particular, what care needs to be taken in selecting participants. This chapter reviews relevant research on recruitment and retention, the consideration of logistics, and the practical considerations of issues such as accessibility and supports needed for data collection. The evaluator may also consider the use of secondary data or data that already exist. The chapter describes special considerations that need to be considered in using secondary data. Finally, the chapter describes recent in innovations in data collection, such as artificial intelligence and "big data."

Time. How much time is required and planned to conduct the entire evaluation and each major aspect of the evaluation? These considerations include what I call calendar and clock time, data collection time, and planning for reviews such as the institutional review board (IRB) and the creation of a time budget. To produce such a budget the evaluator needs to describe each major task to be accomplished, including the description of the stages of research planning, pilot and feasibility studies, data collection planning and analysis, and the reporting of results.

Personnel. How many people are needed to conduct the evaluation and what are their skills? The chapter shows how to produce a skills inventory, how to assign each person to each task, and how to illustrate this using Gantt charts.

Money. How much money is needed to plan and implement the evaluation and in what categories? The chapter shows how to assign costs to each task, how to monitor implementation expenses, and how to use management software to plan and manage the evaluation.

This chapter focuses on the resources needed to conduct evaluations, a topic not usually covered in courses on research or evaluation methods or in textbooks. Program evaluation, however, requires the careful consideration of the realistic constraints on the planning and implementation of an evaluation, many beyond the control of the evaluator. Before making decisions about the specific design to use and the type of data collection procedures to employ, the evaluator must consider the resources available and the limitations of these resources. Planning and care in implementing the evaluation can be as important as the evaluation questions asked and the data collected. This chapter details the steps that evaluators need to take to help ensure that they have sufficient resources to complete the evaluation.

A distinctive emphasis on resource planning is provided by Bamberger (see Chapter 24, this volume). His chapter is an excellent complement to this chapter for it emphasizes evaluations that are subject to conditions that are often found in evaluations outside of industrialized nations. However, the constraints he describes are frequently found in all evaluations. Client biases, politics, unexpected budget cuts, unrealistic client expectations, shortened time frames, and denial of access to data or participants can occur in any evaluation. The trade-offs he suggests in dealing with very real constraints make his chapter a valuable companion to the current chapter.

In addition to Bamberger's chapter (Chapter 24), the chapter by Russ-Eft (Chapter 19, this volume) on designing and planning an evaluation provides some additional information on planning that is not covered in this chapter. Russ-Eft considers planning issues beyond resources, which is the focus of this chapter. Her chapter includes advice on planning the scope of the evaluation, identifying ethical issues, planning for risks, and writing proposals for funding. Both chapters present additional complementary information on work schedules, budgets, and staffing.

At the outset of an evaluation, the evaluator needs to consider the resources available before finalizing the evaluation questions to be addressed. The evaluator can at times be faced with trying to reconcile a gap between the resources available and the resources ultimately needed to adequately address the evaluation questions. Caught between a rock (resources) and a hard place (evaluation questions and design), the evaluator may have no choice but to renegotiate the questions if additional resources cannot be allocated. I focus on realigning the evaluation questions as the price of the evaluation is usually more difficult to change.

This chapter describes how to assess and consider resources before making "final" design and data collection decisions. Note that I put the word *final* in quotation marks. Balancing resources and evaluation tasks are dynamic and constantly changing as the environment is ever-changing. Even very careful planning cannot consider the myriad of unanticipated events that will occur in the real world. The evaluator therefore has to continually balance resources and the evaluation plan. Over the course of an evaluation, these two critical areas of evaluation questions and resources likely will have to be reconsidered multiple times because both are subject to change as the program and the evaluation are implemented. While contractual obligations need to be followed, the evaluator should appreciate the dynamic nature of these two factors.

In this chapter, I highlight four types of resources that impact evaluation and need to be considered in planning:

1. *Data.* What are the sources of information needed and how will they be obtained?
2. *Time.* How much time is required and planned to conduct the entire evaluation and each major aspect of the evaluation?
3. *Personnel.* How many people are needed and what are their skills?
4. *Money.* How much money is needed to plan and implement the evaluation and in what categories?

DATA AS A RESOURCE

One of the most important resources for any evaluation are the data used to answer the evaluation questions. Data for an evaluation can usually be obtained in two ways: from original data collected by the evaluator, and from existing data. The issues of **primary data** collection are discussed first, followed by **secondary data** analysis.

Primary Data Collection

Planning for primary data collection includes several main issues: site selection, authorization, the data collection process, accessibility, and other support needed.

Site Selection

Program evaluation and basic research differ among several dimensions but probably the most salient difference is the location of the work (Bickman, 1981). In most cases, basic research takes place in a site that is controlled by the researcher, often a psychological laboratory or a college classroom. Program evaluation can occur in any setting. Sometimes the site is specified by the evaluation question, as when the evaluator is asked to assess the functioning of a particular program in a particular site or sites. In other cases, the evaluator has the option of choosing among various sites in which the program is or will be operating.

When multiple sites exist, the selection of which site to include in the evaluation is of utmost importance to the success of the project. For example, the setting will have a clear impact on the evaluation not only in defining the population studied but also in formulating the evaluation question to be addressed, the evaluation design implemented, the measures used, and the inferences that can be drawn from the evaluation results. Choosing settings can also determine whether there are a sufficient number of appropriate evaluation participants available to successfully conduct the evaluation. It is thus important to realize that site selection not only determines the data available about sites, and how they may differ, but also on the variability of participants that can vary by site. An evaluator, for example, would usually not want to select a health club to evaluate a new smoking cessation program, because most of the members of the club probably do not smoke. Olsen and Orr (2016) note that the representativeness of the setting and participants is critical to survey research but often ignored in program evaluation. By not formally sampling representative sites of programs, the evaluator may be reporting on a biased sample of sites, program recipients, and personnel implementing the program. Also often overlooked in selecting sites is the degree of maturity of the program, which may differ widely among sites. It could be expected that more mature sites, where a program may have been in operation for a considerable amount of time, will differ in quality of implementation compared to sites just starting off. Moreover, we know that the characteristics of a site and its organization can affect the success of a program in important ways. For example, a mental health intervention implemented at a well-organized site was successful while a similar site with poor leadership and poor organization failed to implement the program (Bickman et al., 2016). An important way to gain information about sites is through evaluability assessments as described by Rog (see Chapter 11, this volume). An evaluability assessment is conducted before committing to a full-scale evaluation and provides important information including whether the site is ready to undertake an evaluation.

External validity or *generalizability* are issues that relate to the ability to generalize the results of a study to other settings, persons, treatments, outcomes, and times (Degtiar & Rose, 2023; Findley et al., 2021). While the sponsor may indicate that the focus of the evaluation is on a specific program implemented in a specific place, implicit in the evaluation is the issue of generalizability. Underlying most evaluations is the question of whether similar results will occur if the program is implemented in the future with clearly different individuals and expected planned or unplanned variations in treatment. Thus, the consideration of external validity should be part of every evaluation plan even if not specified by the sponsor (Galiani & Quistorff, 2023). Lack of consideration of the factors that limit generalizability can lead to the misapplication of the results of an evaluation to settings in which the results of the original evaluation cannot be replicated because some critical element or elements that produced the original results are not found in the new situation (Peck, 2022). This is especially the case when the findings of an evaluation are used to move from a small-scale evaluation to a much larger scale, such as moving from a single school to multiple schools or school districts (Gennnetian, 2021; Olsson et al., 2023).

Olsen and Orr (2016) recommend a traditional survey sampling approach to site selection in which random selection is used to obtain a representative sample of sites. However, in most evaluations I would not expect such a sampling approach to be feasible because it is expensive, and most sponsors are not typically concerned with external validity. Olsen and Orr suggest that the second way to deal with biased site selection is through what Bell and Stuart (2016) describe as analytical methods that can reduce the bias in unrepresentative samples through, for example, weighting the contributions of sites according to how well they match the population of interest. It is important to note that site selection is not just an issue for quantitative evaluations but also impact the validity of qualitative approaches (Willoughby, 2016).

Recent advances in research on the conduct of clinical trials, or what in the medical literature are called pragmatic trials, has led to some helpful tools that assist researchers and evaluators in planning trials in routine clinical practice. The GetReal Trial Tool is a helpful decision support tool that considers seven domains with 43 questions that the planner should answer before conducting the trial (Boateng et al., 2023). These include (1) participant selection, recruitment, and attrition; (2) site selection and recruitment; (3) outcome selection and measurement; (4) randomization, comparator choice, and treatment strategies; (5) data collection; (6) safety monitoring; and (7) monitoring of trial conduct and data quality.

In contrast to more formal methods of dealing with generalizability, evaluators have developed rules of thumb that are useful to consider when more formal methods are not feasible. Because these are fallible there is typically no single correct choice in selecting sites. Is it best to choose "typical" sites, a "range" of sites, "representative" sites, the "best" sites, or the "worst" sites? There are always more variables that can be used for site selection than resources for implementing the evaluation. Moreover, no matter what criteria are used, evaluation critics will claim that other *more* important variables were omitted. For this reason, it is recommended that the site selection decision be done in close coordination with the evaluation client and/or advisory group. In general, it is also better to concentrate on as few sites as are required, rather than stretching the time and management efforts of the evaluation team across many locations that are difficult to manage. Not considering the complexity, financial cost, and time of using multiple sites is a major hazard that inexperienced evaluators often underestimate. Because of the importance and the preciseness of **statistical power** estimates (see Harbatkin et al., Chapter 16, this volume), the power issue may be preeminent and overshadow both the foreseen and unforeseen risks involved in managing multiple evaluation sites. Site, however, is not always the unit of analysis that is considered in computing power. The appropriate unit depends on how the intervention is implemented. It could be site, if for example, sites are randomly assigned to treatment or control conditions. Or it might be a smaller unit where the experimental conditions are assigned. For example, schools are the unit if the conditions are randomly assigned to whole schools, or classrooms could be the unit if the conditions are assigned at the class level. In the latter case, classes are considered nested within schools in what is considered a two-level **nested design**.

Another example of an emphasis on settings is provided by Jorgensen (2015) on participant observation. Jorgensen characterizes settings as differing in visibility and openness. A visible setting is one that is available to the public. Some of these settings, such as universities and hospitals, may have a very visible presence on the web. Other visible settings may be less public but still accessible, such as areas that involve drugs or prostitution that police know about. Invisible settings are hidden and concealed from outsiders. These settings include both legal and illegal activities. In most organizations, there are groups of individuals whose activities are kept secret from nonmembers and, in some cases, even from members. A setting's openness depends upon the degree of negotiation that is required for access, but visibility and openness are not the same. A private university is a visible institution, but the deliberations in the provost's office concerning faculty salaries are usually not open to the faculty, let alone the general public. Highly visible settings may also contain less visible activities—for example, public parks can be a location for illicit activities.

A distinction of "front stage" and "backstage" made by Goffman (1959) also helps distinguish settings. Front-stage activities are available to anyone, whereas backstage entrance is limited. Thus, the courtroom in a trial is the front-stage activity that is open to anyone who can obtain a seat. Entrance to the judge's chamber is more limited, presence during lawyer–client conferences is even more restricted, and presence as an observer during jury deliberations is practically impossible. The evaluator needs to assess the openness of the setting before taking the next step: seeking authorization to access a site for the evaluation. The concept of front stage and backstage has been applied to understanding how customers evaluate services (Liu et al., 2017).

Authorization

Even totally open and visible settings usually require some degree of authorization for data collection. Even when the evaluation is mandated by an authority, access to all aspects of the organization may be limited by others. Public space may not be as totally available to the evaluator as it may seem.

If the setting is a closed one, the evaluator will be required to obtain the permission of the individuals who control or believe they control access. If several sites are eligible for participation and they are within one organization, it behooves the evaluator to explore the independence of these sites from the parent organization. In planning a study in a supermarket, we had the choice of contacting the headquarters of the company or approaching each supermarket manager for permission to conduct the evaluation. If the main office was approached first and we were refused permission, then the project could not be implemented. If one local manager refused, however, another one could be approached. In this case, we first approached a local manager, who informed us that he could not participate without headquarter's approval. The manager, however, was persuaded to provide a supporting letter to accompany our request for permission. A personal visit to the head of security helped obtain the necessary cooperation.

Not only does the evaluation planner need to know at which level of the organization to negotiate but also which individuals to approach. Again, this takes some intelligence gathering. Personal contacts help because authorities are usually more likely to meet and to be cooperative if the evaluator is recommended by someone they know and trust. Thus, the evaluator should search for some connection to the organization. For example, if the planner is at a university, then it is possible that someone on the board of trustees is an officer of the organization. If so, contacting the university's development office is advisable. The idea is to obtain advance recommendations from credible sources and hence to avoid approaching an organization cold.

Permission from a central authority does not necessarily imply cooperation from the sites needed for data collection. Nowhere is this more evident than in state/county working relationships. Often central approval is required to approach local sites. The evaluator should not believe, however, that central approval guarantees cooperation from those lower down on the organization's hierarchy, as this can lead the evaluator into behaving in an insensitive manner. Those at the upper levels of an organization tend to believe they have more power than they actually wield. A wise evaluator puts a great deal of effort into obtaining cooperation at the local level. At this level are the individuals who feel they control that environment and with whom the evaluator will be interacting during the data collection phase. The persons in this environment include not only management but the workers and their representatives (e.g., unions). Keeping them informed of the purpose and progress of the evaluation and what is happening to and in *their* environment should be a high priority.

This organizational perspective is especially important in dealing with schools in a school system. Most school districts maintain a central approval mechanism to conduct any research or evaluation in schools. Some also may insist

---

BOX 21.1. Notify Relevant Authorities If There Is Fieldwork

It is a good idea to notify the authorities if the evaluation team will be present in some public setting for an extended period of time. Though the evaluator's presence is certainly not illegal and does not require permission to conduct observations or interviews, residents of the area may become suspicious and call the police. For example, in one of my studies, interviews were conducted in a rural area. The interviewers, being unfamiliar with the area (which lacked street signs), drove through the same stretch of road repeatedly looking for particular houses. Residents, not accustomed to seeing unfamiliar cars, called the sheriff. The interviewers were stopped and taken to the sheriff's station for questioning. Calls were made to the university to verify the interviewers' legitimacy. A simple letter or call to each local law enforcement office could have prevented this problem.

> **BOX 21.2. Be More Cautious If They Are Armed**
>
> I had a contract from the state criminal justice authorities to conduct an evaluation of the citizen involvement program that was being conducted by a large municipal police department. I contacted the proper police liaison and arranged to interview police commanders using a written structured interview. I showed up at headquarters to conduct the interviews and was met by a police lieutenant who asked the purpose of all the papers I was carrying. Those were the structured interviews I was going to follow. The lieutenant expected to be present for all of the interviews. I did not object to that and even suggested that he make copies of the interview so that he could fill it in as we did. He excused himself, I thought to copy extra questionnaires, but actually to consult with higher -ups. When he returned, he told me to leave the building, which of course I did. A call to the state agency director got me another meeting but not before they vetted the structured interview. But even then, cooperation was minimal since they had scheduled all the police commanders at the same time, which meant some had to wait several hours. As you might imagine, this did not lead to a very pleasant interview. The point of this example is my lack of understanding about how to deal with a police agency cost the project several months of delay and ate up financial resources that I did not anticipate.

that central approval must be accompanied by approval at the school (principal) or even class (teacher) level as well as parents and students. Many school systems have specific schedules during the year when application for approval has to be submitted. Missing a scheduled date can substantially delay an evaluation.

Confidentiality and informed consent are usually significant issues with any organization. Will participants be identified or identifiable? How will the data be protected from unauthorized access? Will competitors learn something about the organization from this evaluation that will put it at a disadvantage? Will individuals in the organization be put in any jeopardy by the project? These issues need to be resolved before approaching an organization for an evaluation. Many organizations will not allow an evaluator to directly contact the people that organization serves because of confidentiality issues. The evaluator usually has to go through a time-consuming multiple-step process in which the organization first obtains a consent to contact before evaluators can directly deal with clients. The sponsor or the hosting organization also might require the approval of an IRB to proceed. The rules governing evaluations are different from typical research and under some circumstances an evaluation may not be considered research and thus need not be submitted to an IRB (*https://irbo.nih.gov/confluence/display/ohsrp/Step+1*). Program improvement evaluations may fall into this category. However, some institutions require that this be an IRB determination and not one made by the evaluator. This determination of whether the evaluation is not considered research is different from the standard IRB—exempt from review research categories in the federal rules (*www.hhs.gov/ohrp/regulations-and-policy/regulations/45-cfr-46/common-rule-subpart-a-46104/index.html*).

Confidentiality issues can be very complex in an evaluation. In conducting an evaluation of a welfare program, for example, an evaluator found that it was a violation of Massachusetts state law if field interviewers, in seeking to locate former Aid to Families with Dependent Children recipients, let it be known to any other persons that the individual they were seeking was or ever had been a recipient of public welfare monies. The state sent periodic reminders that the project director could be fined if there was any evidence that such disclosures had been made. Needless to say, training of interviewers heavily emphasized the confidentiality issue, and interviewers were not allowed to discuss with anyone other than the respondent the purpose of their survey.

Collecting health information has special rules that must be followed to protect the privacy of individuals. These are usually termed Health Insurance Portability and Accountability Act regulations (*www.hhs.gov/hipaa/index.html*). Privacy rules are not uniform worldwide. Currently European rules are more protective than those in the United States. The rules are also subject to change so that keeping current on regulations is important.

Organizations that have experience with evaluation usually have standard procedures that they follow with evaluators. For example, school systems typically have standard forms to complete and deadlines by which these forms must be submitted. These organizations understand the importance of program evaluation and are accustomed to dealing with evaluators. In contrast, other organizations may not be familiar with evaluation—most for-profit corporations fall into this category. In dealing with these groups, the evaluator first has to convince the authorities that the evaluation, in general, is a good idea and that their organization will gain something from their participation. Most important, the organization has to be convinced that it will not be taking a significant risk in participating in the evaluation.

Finally, any agreement between the evaluator and the organization should be in writing. This may be an informal letter addressed to the organization's project liaison (there should be one) for the evaluation. The letter should describe the procedures that will take place and indicate the dates that the evaluator will be on-site. The agreement should be detailed and include how the organization will cooperate with the evaluation. This written agreement may avoid misunderstandings that are based on past in-person or telephone discussions (i.e., "I thought you meant . . . ").

Data Collection Process

Gaining access for primary data collection is just the start of the planning process. Careful attention then needs to be paid to the details of the evaluation. These include recruiting the participants, what resources are needed to get the information from them, and the logistics required at the site.

RECRUITMENT: SELECTING PARTICIPANTS

In a quantitative study, the primary purpose of obtaining access to a site is typically to be able to collect data from or about people. The evaluator should *not* assume that having access ensures that everyone agrees to participate in the evaluation. Moreover, skepticism is warranted in accepting the assurances from management concerning others' willingness to participate in the evaluation. Some evaluations may require that certain categories of people participate in the evaluation. For example, evaluations confront logistical challenges in including people with disabilities, people experiencing homelessness, and people with addictions. In some cultures, it may be difficult to involve women or children in an evaluation. The evaluator needs to conduct a contextual or cultural analysis of the participant requirements to understand how best to approach recruitment and the challenges that may be faced, and secure sufficient resources to avoid or meet the challenges if the evaluation is going to be implemented. Special attention needs to be paid to ensure that recruitment strategies are not biased to specific races, ages, or other characteristics and backgrounds, and that they are designed to engage those most affected by the programs and issues under study. Research, for example, has firmly established big disparities in minority representation in research and evaluation (especially clinical trials) and little improvement in representation in the last decade (Buffenstein et al., 2023).

More than 30 years ago we were aware of problems in not recruiting the number of participants needed to ensure sufficient statistical power to conduct a valid evaluation. In a review of 30 randomized studies in drug abuse, Dennis (1990) found that 54% seriously underestimated the client flow, by an average of 37%. Realistic and accurate participant estimates are necessary to allocate resources and to ensure sufficient statistical power. This latter point often has been ignored in the past, however. Lipsey et al. (1985) found that 90% of the 122 evaluation studies reviewed had insufficient statistical power to detect small effect sizes, and 60% did not reliably find a medium-size effect if it was present. Lipsey et al. expressed similar concerns about the low power of studies in their review of 221 articles published in three psychological journals. They concluded that low power contributes to the difficulties many evaluators experience in replicating other's work. The role of low power continues to be a problem associated with poor replication 30 years later (Dreber & Johannesson, 2020). In addition, although the number of participants needed to be recruited is a salient number for both the evaluators and sponsors, it is important not only to hit that number but to be careful not to use recruitment strategies that introduce participant biases and can distort the results. For example, paying people large sums of money to participate could result in recruiting "professional" participants who make a living from participating in studies, a problem noted by Abadie (2019) with the evaluation of drug programs. Moreover, because participation in almost all evaluation is voluntary, paying people large sums of money to participate may be seen as coercive and thus unethical. Unfortunately, there is little consensus on what is considered too large, and this is often left to IRBs to decide. There are many ways biases can be introduced in addition to payment for participation. These include that the language used in recruitment materials may not be at the right literacy level, the materials may not be translated in the languages needed, location of recruitment sites, and who is conducting the recruitment.

Most funding agencies now insist that a statistical power analysis be conducted when submitting proposals. Moreover, these power analyses should be supported by evidence that the number of cases one hopes to recruit in these analyses are valid estimates and not wishful thinking. The recruitment issue has become a national priority in health care evaluation where expensive clinical trials are often discontinued because of recruitment failure. Parallel to this problem recognition has been the identification of researchers' sense of denial or overly optimistic perception that the number of participants to be recruited will be successfully obtained. This perception has been labeled as "Lasagna's Law," which is "the number of patients who are actually available for a trial is about 1/10 to 1/3 of what was originally estimated" or "Muench's Third Law," which is "In order to be realistic, the number of cases must be divided by a factor of at least 10" (Bogin, 2022, p. 1; Cooper et al., 2015, p. 347). Evaluations should consider different approaches to measuring and increasing the statistical power of an evaluation; I discuss several more fully in the next section on recruitment and retention.

In cases where potential participants enter into some program or institution over time, the evaluator should verify the actual subject flow (e.g., number per week). For example, if the evaluation requires participation of subjects who are receiving psychotherapy, then it is critical to know how many *new* patients enter the program each week and whether this number is typical of the program. In addition, the rate with which new patients entering therapy volunteer to participate in the evaluation needs to be estimated. Finally, in addition to the recruitment and volunteer rates, the attrition rate, which is the rate at which participants drop out of the program, will need to be estimated. These three rates contribute to estimating the final number of cases needed for a competent statistical analysis and the time it will take to accrue that number. If that total time proves too long, the planner will know that additional sites need to be recruited.

Related to the number of participants is the assurance that the evaluation design can be implemented successfully. Randomized designs are especially vulnerable to implementation problems. It is easy to promise that there will be no new taxes, that the check is in the mail, and that a randomized experiment will be conducted. It is often difficult to deliver on these promises. The evaluator should obtain agreement from authorities *in writing* that they will cooperate in the conduct of the evaluation. This agreement must be detailed, be procedurally oriented, and clearly specify the responsibilities of the evaluator and those who control the setting. A big expense can be the funds to retain people in studies, especially vulnerable, hard-to-reach persons. The evaluator may need to spend a lot of resources to keep track of participants and then also pay them for additional waves of data collection, often increasing the amounts.

> **BOX 21.3. Are Those Numbers Really Valid?**
>
> In an evaluation of a nutrition program for older adults, cooperation was obtained from the federal agency that funded the program and from each local project manager to implement and evaluate the program. Each local manager furnished the number of older adults in their site and estimated the percentage that they thought would participate in the evaluation. Random assignment of sites to treatment and control conditions proceeded based on these estimates. During the recruitment phase of the data collection, it was clear that the evaluation would fall far short of the required number of participants based on the faulty numbers provided by each project manager. The design of the evaluation was jeopardized when new sites had to be recruited to increase the sample size. Chapters in this volume by Bamberger (Chapter 24), Harbatkin et al. (Chapter 16), and Pham et al. (Chapter 17), each provide extended discussion on the importance of sample size, budgets, and statistical power.

RECRUITMENT AND RETENTION

Numbers have a particular salience. For example, the start and end dates of an evaluation are not only important descriptors but are used to judge whether an evaluation was efficient and started and completed on time. Dollar figures are also critical numerical values. Was the evaluation completed within the budget allocated? These numbers, and the judgments that accompany them, are easily recalled in judging the adequacy of the evaluation but there are not many concrete actions that the evaluator can do to affect those numbers. There are two other numbers that are also salient. These are the number of eligible participants recruited to take part in the evaluation and the number of recruited participants who are included in the analyses (i.e., the number retained in the evaluation). These numbers are critical to the evaluation as noted several times in this chapter. There is not an extensive program evaluation literature on recruitment and retention (R&R) so I borrow from the clinical trials literature.

WHY THE NUMBER OF PARTICIPANTS IS IMPORTANT

The most critical concern for quantitative evaluations is whether the number of participants provides sufficient statistical power to be able to conduct an adequate analysis. The second major reason to focus on R&R is the issue of external validity or generalizability of the evaluation. While the number of participants recruited and retained is important, it is also important to realize that it is not a simple numbers game. The characteristics of the participants in an evaluation are also critical.

There are two factors that should be considered in targeting recruitment. First is the need to identify to whom the evaluation should generalize. Second is the identification of important moderators of the effects of the intervention. Identification of important moderators of the treatment effect is important because it can affect the chances of finding a significant impact. If the intervention is not aimed at the right target, then it is unlikely to have an effect. One simple example is whether the group that is recruited into the evaluation has the problem that the intervention is trying to ameliorate. Obviously if the program is designed to stop smoking, then the evaluation has to target to smokers. Less obviously, the intervention has to target a group that also has a factor that is causally connected to the outcome. Thus, in this example the recruits are all smokers, but if they all have high self-esteem and the program is designed to improve self-esteem, then it is unlikely that the program will be shown to be effective. In this case self-esteem will not change sufficiently in the target group to impact smoking even if the program is effective with low-self-esteem participants. To be able to be specific about the causal linkage between the program intervention and recruitment can be critical to correctly identifying a program as effective or ineffective and usually requires a **program theory** (Bickman, 1987; Olsson et al., 2023). Tipton and Matlen (2019) describe a four-step process they have used to improve the generalizability of their randomized trial that could be adopted by evaluators.

Selection of participants is also important in meeting societal demands for participation of underrepresented groups in evaluation and research. It is well documented that there has not been equitable participation of many groups in research, especially health-related research for decades (Buffenstein et al., 2023). While this problem may appear less acute for program evaluation, since the target group is often selected by the program developers, it is still the responsibility of the evaluator to question the appropriateness of the target group selected. Kelsey et al. (2022) provide techniques to increase the diversity of research and evaluation participants that they believe will lead to lasting change in how recruitment should occur.

One more aspect of recruitment that evaluators should be aware of is the tension between improving the chances of finding an effect and the generalizability of the outcomes. The traditional priority of evaluations (and much research) is on demonstrating if there is an effect and not on the generalizability of the results. Again, I believe number salience is partially responsible for this orientation. In traditional significance testing there is typically one number that is critical—that is whether the probability level set (e.g., $p < .05$) is met. There is no comparable number for generalizability—it is a judgment. Given the priority of finding a statistically significant effect, the evaluator can use recruitment in ways to enhance the probability of finding that effect. The most general approach is to reduce the variability of the target group by limiting the heterogeneity of the participants. Of course, the danger is that without sufficient information it may be difficult to target a specific target group that has characteristics that are both targeted by the intervention and causally connected to the outcome (Saxe et al., 2022).

WHAT DOES RESEARCH INDICATE ABOUT HOW TO AFFECT R&R?

Previous research can usually be a helpful source of techniques and procedures to deal with problems in the design of evaluations. In the case of R&R there are several review articles that I summarize about what has been learned about how to improve R&R. Next, I describe in more detail specific research studies that might be helpful to the planner. Finally, we are fortunate given the dynamic nature of research in this area and the rapidly improving research base—I describe two online sources that can be used to search for specific techniques and studies in this area.

Research Reviews. Treweek et al. (2013) conducted an early review and meta-analysis of controlled trials examining recruitment. They identified 45 trials with over 43,000 participants. Some interventions were effective in increasing recruitment in a few studies: telephone reminders to nonrespondents, financial incentives, and use of opt-out rather than opt-in procedures for contacting possible participants. However, the influence of many other approaches was ambiguous. Bower et al. (2014) conducted a survey and a workshop on this topic. Responses were received from 23 individuals representing 18 clinical trials units. Although the respondents identified approaches they thought were effective, the authors concluded that there were significant gaps in knowing what works. They were hopeful about a new approach to funding the needed research, called study within a trial (SWAT). Conducting what seems to be rather mundane research on how to improve R&R is not very attractive to investigators or funders. Thus, the amount of research is small. Clarke et al. (2015) describe an approach to embed R&R trials in larger studies by providing resources, a framework for conducting such studies, and a way to disseminate the results. Treweek et al. (2018) and Ahmed et al. (2022) provide more recent details on this innovative approach.

The next group of reviews are from publications 7–10 years later. Has SWAT made a difference? First, has there been an increase in the number of SWATs? While I don't have access to overall numbers, the Prometheus project recruited interventions by offering financial and other support to projects that would include a SWAT. They funded 42 trials that added 18% and 79% more SWATs to the Cochrane systematic review of recruitment strategies and the Cochrane review of retention strategies, respectively (Doherty et al., 2023). Thus, there is some evidence that we should expect an increase in the number of R&R trials, although we do not expect this increase to have a big impact on new reviews of R&R since it takes several years for the research to be published.

Coffey et al. (2022) included in their review in 31 articles. A range of behavioral approaches were applied to R&R trials. Almost three-quarters of the studies were exploratory but those that evaluated interventions often did so within underserved populations. Most of the studies did not specify their behaviors with enough information needed for replication. The most-used approaches were based on broad theories including social cognitive theory, the theory of planned behavior, and the theoretical domains framework. This review primarily identified gaps in research in contrast to locating successful interventions.

Elfeky et al. (2020) looked at retention in 10 nonrandomized trials and their systematic review provides low or very low certainty evidence on the effectiveness of retention strategies. Gaunt et al. (2023) examined retention in 94 randomized pediatric trials and found some evidence to support the use of financial incentives and text reminders but concluded that they could not recommend any specific engagement methods due to the limited reporting of methods to improve retention. Gillies et al. (2021) identified 81 retention studies involving more than 100,000 participants that had studied different methods to encourage randomized trial participants to provide data and stay in the trial. They could not recommend with confidence any of the retention interventions they found because of plausible alternative factors, such as flaws with the design of the studies. Kilicel et al. (2023) investigated 13 studies that enrolled a total of 14,452 participants. They reported that there were benefits to using multiple recruitment methods, including monetary incentives, but in their sample of child and adolescent psychiatry trials, once participants were in the trial they stayed and completed it.

Without claiming that this summary is exhaustive of all the recent literature, it does not appear that there is yet an adequate body of knowledge that is sufficiently generalizable to recommend specific R&R techniques in planning an evaluation. However, there are some specific studies that I describe next that may be helpful.

Individual Studies. Determining appropriate incentive amounts is also an area with relatively limited evidence and significant uncertainty. Bickman and colleagues (2021) developed and tested a framework for assessment of financial incentives related to the amount of risk/burden of the respondents that could affect willingness to participate in a study. This framework can be used to gather information directly from potential participants to design study-specific approaches to the use of financial incentives based on the risk and burden that participants might experience in participating in a planned study. Cascini et al. (2022) provide an interesting discussion concerning the potential use of artificial intelligence (AI) to assist in recruitment but note that there is currently little use of AI. Kavalci and Harshorn (2023) provide an application of AI to enhance recruitment efforts. They successfully predicted early termination of participation using various machine learning modeling. Tsaltskan et al. (2022) compared web-based advertising and a social media advertisement. They found that Facebook was superior to web advertisements for participant recruitment especially for Spanish speakers. Although Facebook was more expensive, it was more cost-effective than web campaigns.

Conclusion. Previous individual studies provide some valuable information about what interventions might help evaluators optimize their R&R. The reviews, however, were rarely able to provide definitive recommendations about which interventions would work best given the context planning a specific study. In particular, the effectiveness of any R&R intervention is likely dependent on the characteristics of the population. For example, it is unlikely that there are incentives that equally apply to all persons. Nevertheless, efforts like SWAT are adding to our knowledge. However, we are fortunate that there are current efforts to help plan studies based on accumulating ongoing research. The two sites that I recommend are:

- Cochrane Library strategies to improve retention in randomized trials (*www.cochranelibrary.com/cdsr/doi/10.1002/14651858.MR000032.pub3/full*).
- The ORRCA project (Online Resource for Research in Clinical triAls) brings together published and ongoing work in the field of R&R research into searchable databases (*www.orrca.org.uk*)

LOGISTICS IN DATA COLLECTION

The ability to implement the evaluation depends on the ability of the evaluator to carry out the planned data collection procedures. A written plan for data collection is critical to success but it does not guarantee effective implementation. A pilot or "walk-through" of the procedure is necessary to determine whether it is feasible. In this procedure, the evaluator needs to consider the following:

Accessibility

There are a large number of seemingly unimportant details that can damage an evaluation project if they are ignored. Will the evaluation participants have the means to travel to the site? Is childcare needed? Is there sufficient public transportation? If not, will the evaluator arrange for transportation? If the evaluation is going to use an organization's space for data collection, will the evaluator need a key? Is there anyone else who may use the space? Who controls scheduling and room assignment? Have they been notified? When using someone else's space, it is important to make certain that the evaluator is able to control it during the time it is promised. For example, an evaluator about to collect posttest data in a classroom should ensure that they will not be asked to vacate the space before data collection is completed. In addition, there may be variations among the participants about which types of environments they are most comfortable with. Other factors such as the need for privacy, whether in the home or elsewhere, also need to be considered.

Other Support Needed for Data Collection

Are the light and sound sufficient for the evaluation? If the evaluation requires the use of electrical equipment, will there be sufficient electrical outlets? Will the equipment reach the outlets, or should extension cords be brought? Do the participants need food or drink? How will these be provided? Are there restroom facilities available? Are the surroundings quiet enough to conduct the evaluation? Can necessary modifications be made in the environment to conduct the evaluation? Is the environment safe? Is there enough space, chairs, computers, forms, and assistants available to collect the data? If Wi-Fi is needed, is it available and are passwords needed? If the data collectors are in the field, do they have proper identification? Are the appropriate persons in the home organization aware of the evaluation and the identity of the data collectors? Are those persons prepared to vouch for the legitimacy of the evaluation? Is there sufficient space not only to collect the data but to house the evaluation team, assemble the data collection instruments, and analyze and store the data? Is childcare needed? Space is a precious commodity in many institutions—do not assume that the evaluation project will have sufficient space. A checklist of needs might be a good way to organize the evaluation requirements for safe and efficient data collection.

Secondary Data

Another approach to conducting an evaluation is to use existing data. Existing data have the advantage of lower costs and time savings but may also entail managing a large amount of flawed and/or inappropriate data. Only in rare cases will these data exist in a format that is designed for evaluation purposes. A number of secondary data sources are available, developed by university consortia, and federal sources such as the U.S. Census Bureau. In some evaluations, the data exist as administrative records that were *not* designed to answer evaluation questions.

In the planning process, the evaluator must ensure that the records contain the information that is required for the evaluation. Assurances from authorities are helpful, but the evaluator should conduct a direct examination of a representative sample of records. Sampling records will provide the evaluator with an indication not only of the content of the records but also of their quality. It is frequently the case that clinical or administrative records are *not* suitable for evaluation purposes. First, the records may be stored in a way that makes them inaccessible for evaluation purposes. For example, there may not be a central collection point for all records, thus increasing the costs of collecting data. Second, if the records are all digitized, this will be of tremendous advantage to the evaluator. But some of the information may have been collected on paper may not have been transferred to a digital database. The evaluator needs to confirm the availability and content of records needed for the evaluation.

The planner must also have some confidence in the quality of the records. Are the records complete? Why were the data collected originally? The database may serve some hidden political purpose that could induce systematic distortions. What procedures are used to deal with

---

BOX 21.4. Quality Is Relative

In one state-level study on a diversion program for nonviolent offenders, we were informed that the program had a very high-quality management information system that could be used for the evaluation. In meeting with the program director, we asked a number of questions about the quality of the data and reviewed printouts of the data. The director was proud of the system and that they took great efforts to ensure that the background information, program participation, and outcomes were complete and recorded. However, in asking whether anyone could be missing from the data system, they noted that no—not as long as they participated for at least 3 months. Given that we were interested in all people who had been assigned to the program and not just those who elected to stay 3 or more months, we discovered that the system could not be used as is and needed supplementing.

missing data? Do the digital records bear a close resemblance to the paper original records? Are some data items updated or purged periodically from the data file? How were the data collected and entered, and by whom? To have a good idea of quality, the planner should interview the data collectors, observe the data entry process, and if written records were used, they should be compared to the digital version. Conducting an analysis of administrative records, as was noted earlier, only seems easy if it is not done carefully. There is ongoing research on the use of existing administrative records that should be consulted (e.g., Groves & Schoeffel, 2018; Green et al., 2015; Soneson et al., 2023).

To gain access to a record system, the evaluator also must demonstrate how the confidentiality of the records will be protected. If the records contain client names, then there is a significant risk associated with providing those records to an evaluator. If individual names are not necessary, the organization may be willing (often at a cost) to provide de-identified records with personally identifying information removed. In cases where the names are not important to the evaluator but it is important to link individuals to the database or to data collected later, then a computerized linking file should be established that the providing organization can use to link names with evaluator-established identification numbers. Special care needs to be taken if the records are considered protected health information and are governed by complex federal government rules (*www.hhs.gov/answers/hipaa/what-is-phi/index.html*). It is also important that the evaluator understand the differences between **anonymous, de-identified,** and **limited datasets.**

> **BOX 21.5. Creating Multisite Datasets**
>
> Often there is a desire to merge data across different program sites. The challenge can be reduced if the programs use the same system, such as homeless program sites that use the Homeless Management Information System, a system supported by the U.S. Department of Housing and Urban Development. However, even when using the same data elements and standards, creating a merged system can be complicated by the different platforms sites use to store the data.

> **BOX 21.6. Measurement Challenges**
>
> Reviewing existing administrative data takes great care in ensuring that not only the elements meet your needs but how they are stored in the database. In several studies we have conducted of services received by individuals across multiple service systems in a state, we discovered that the data were available in monthly arrays—that is, whether a service was received at least once in that month. The database developers believed that this level of measurement was the most reliable and valid method—having more detailed data were not viewed as reliable due to missing data. Having only monthly receipts of service data, however, restricted the types of analyses that could be conducted and the sensitivity of analyses to see differences across program and comparison groups.

Finally, the investigation should not assume that the level of effort needed to process extant data will be small or even moderate. Datasets may be exceedingly complex, with changes occurring in data fields and documentation over time. Specific expertise may be necessary in certain programming languages, and the time necessary to check, clean, and merge data and create working analysis files can be enormous. A good summary of secondary analysis issues can be found in Logan (2019).

Planning for Innovations in Data Collection and Analyses

There is a revolution going on in the area of data collection and analysis that program evaluation must be part of. This is the use of **big data** and AI to deal with many of society's problems, especially in the area of precision medicine. The use of these approaches has important implications for resource planning for program evaluations. Evaluators need to develop strong competencies in these areas in order to properly use these new approaches and tools in their work. In many cases the use of existing big data can save an evaluation money. In the primary data collection, there is a whole new universe of new data that are available to evaluators. Social media, geospatial analyses, smartphones, **natural language models** (print and audio), **ecological momentary assessments,** and the **internet of things** are just some of the innovative sources of data that are available to evaluators. The reader is referred to several sources that can better explain the characteristics of these sources and how they can be used in evaluations (Bamberger, 2020; Bickman, 2020; York & Bamberger, 2020).

TIME AS A RESOURCE

In 1748 Benjamin Franklin said, "Time is money." That is still true today. That aphorism applies to figuring out resources needed for an evaluation. Time takes on two important dimensions in planning applied evaluation: **calendar** and **clock time**. Calendar time is the total amount of time that is available for the project. Calendar time varies across projects: It may be a semester for a course-related evaluation project, 3 years for an externally funded evaluation grant, or 2 weeks for a local evaluation contract. The calendar time can substantially influence the scope of an evaluation project. Clock time is typically the number of hours, days, weeks, or years allocated to a task regardless of the calendar. For example, a task may have the calendar time of May–August and a clock time of 3 weeks, usually expressed in person hours. This means that the task needs to be accomplished within that calendar period and requires 40 person hours. Those person hours may be one person working 40 hours or 4 people working 10 hours each depending on the requirements of the task and the availability of personnel.

Calendar Time and the Evaluation Question

The calendar time allowed in an evaluation should be related to the evaluation questions. Is the phenomenon under evaluation something that lasts a long period of time, or does it only exist for a brief period? Does the phenomenon under evaluation occur in cycles? Is the time allocated to data collection sufficient?

The first consideration of time, therefore, is to examine its relationship to the **evaluand** that is being studied. For example, if the event to be studied occurs infrequently for a short period of time, and if it is somewhat unpredictable, then a long period of calendar time may be needed to capture enough occurrences of this event. If the evaluation deals with a program designed to prevent physical aggression on the streets, for example, and if the evaluator wants to measure changes in physical aggression by observing it, then under most circumstances a long period of observation would be needed. In fact, the nature of this infrequent and unpredictable event would probably rule against using observation as a data collection technique. Other times, the effects of a program or evaluand may take a long period of time to unfold and manifest themselves. For example, a drug treatment program that takes a lengthy period for its effects to materialize would require a long period of evaluation if the evaluator wanted to document an impact. If the phenomenon is cyclical in nature, then the evaluator should plan the length of the data collection period to include the various cycles to obtain an accurate representation of the phenomenon. To complicate matters even more, it is likely that different outcomes have different time trajectories associated with them. Some may emerge quickly and others slowly, while others may have linear growth and others may be discontinuous, appearing as a sudden change. In addition, if it is a newly implemented program, the evaluator may need to wait for the program to stabilize before collecting data. Until this initial stage is completed, the program may be highly variable in its operation. Calendar time needs to be allocated in the evaluation for this aspect of program development. All of these points argue that in planning an evaluation project, the evaluator must have some familiarity with the phenomenon under evaluation. The evaluator may fail to implement a good evaluation if the relationship between time and the program studied is not considered.

Time and Data Collection

The second way in which time should be considered is in terms of the actual or real *clock time* needed to accomplish a task. The event that is being studied might exist infrequently and only for a short period of time—thus, we might need a long period of calendar time devoted to the project but only a short period of clock time for data collection. As noted in subsequent parts of this chapter, estimating time is related to many other estimates made during the planning of evaluation. Once having established the time estimates, the evaluator needs to estimate how long it will take for actual data collection. In computing this estimate, the evaluator should consider questions of recruitment, access, and cooperation. For example, if an evaluation is being conducted in a hospital setting using patients, the planner should determine the criteria for inclusion in the evaluation, calculate how many patients would meet those criteria, and estimate the percentage of the patients that would volunteer to participate in the evaluation. An estimate of attrition or dropout rates from the evaluation is also needed. If high attrition is predicted, then more time is needed for data collection to have sufficient statistical power. Thus, in computing time, the evaluator should have an accurate and comprehensive picture of the environment in which the evaluation will be conducted. Subtle, but important factors can have a major impact on recruitment time.

Of special note is accounting for time to obtain Office of Management and Budget (OMB) clearance for surveys that ask identical questions to 10 or more people. This clearance is required under the Paperwork Reduction Act (PRA) if you are operating under a U.S. federal contract (not a grant). A contractual relationship with the federal government means you are collecting information at their request, which is not the same relationship under a grant. This is a complex process and can take several months to complete. Each federal agency appears to have its own time estimates so the amount of time to obtain clearance is variable. A federal guide is provided to help researchers judge whether their project is exempt from the PRA (*https://pra.digital.gov*). Program evaluations are specifically listed as having to comply with the PRA. Not building sufficient time to prepare the application, respond to questions from the OMB, and obtain their approval may mean the premature termination of the project. See this site for more information of clearance process: *www.usability.gov/how-to-and-tools/guidance/traditional-clearance-process.html#Steps%20For%20Preparing%20and%20Submitting%20Requests*.

Another approval process that was described in more detail earlier is the IRB. All institutions that receive federal funds (i.e., almost all universities and institutions that conduct research, especially health care organizations) require the approval of a review board if the activity is both research and involves human subjects. Program evaluation, under some conditions, may not be considered research and thus may not need IRB approval. Each IRB can have its own rules about what is considered research and what is considered human subjects. In most cases the IRB requires the evaluator/researcher to submit some application to them so they can decide whether the activity is exempt from their review because it is not research or does not involve human subjects. If the relevant organization does not have a standing IRB, then there are commercial IRBs that review the evaluation for a fee.

Time Budget

Both *calendar* and *clock time* need to be budgeted. To budget calendar time the duration of the entire project must be known. In program evaluation the duration typically is set at the start of the project and the evaluator then tailors the evaluation to fit the length of time available. There may be little flexibility in total calendar time on some projects. A report may be needed for a legislative decision, or the contract may specify a product at a certain time.

Funded evaluation projects usually operate on a calendar basis—that is, the project will be funded for a specific amount of time. This sets the upper limit of the time budget. The evaluators then plans what they believe can be accomplished within that period of time. Students usually operate with semester or quarter dead-

---

BOX 21.7. A. Pipeline Study Can Be Critical

In the evaluation of a community-based mental health program for children, I did a pipeline study to examine the flow of youth through the program. I based the time I needed to conduct the evaluation on those estimates but careful monitoring of recruitment showed a major shortfall. Two factors were responsible for this problem. First, I did not include the eligibility requirement that only one sibling from a family would be included in the evaluation. The large percentage of siblings receiving services at the site was depressing recruitment. While there was little I could do to change that since I did not want to change eligibility requirements, the second factor was an employee who did not agree with the random assignment process and did her best to not follow the random assignment process by assigning few potential participants to the control group. She was replaced by the CEO of the program.

lines. Again, the project needs to be tailored to the amount of time available. Regardless, the work often expands to fit the time available. Evaluators must be able to specify the project scope and approach to fit a limited timeframe. A mistake many evaluators make in estimating the time budget is to underestimate the time needed, often resulting in the late delivery of their products, or not having sufficient financial resources to complete the evaluation.

The second time budget refers to clock time. How many hours or days will it take to develop a questionnaire or to interview all of the participants? It is important to decide what unit of time will be used in the budget. In other words, what is the smallest unit of analysis of the evaluation process that will be useful in calculating how much time it takes to complete the evaluation project? To answer this question, we now turn to the concept of tasks.

Tasks and Time

To "task out" an evaluation project, the planner is required to list all of the significant activities (tasks) that must be performed to complete the project. The tasks in a project time budget are similar to the expense categories needed in planning a personal financial budget. The financial budget is calculated on various categories such as rent, utilities, food, and so on—when listing all of these expense items, a decision must be made concerning the level of refinement that will be used. For example, under the food budget, it is rare for a family to categorize their food budget into vegetables, meat, fruit, and milk products. On the other hand, a family might decide to divide the food budget into eating in restaurants versus the purchasing of food for home consumption. In a similar vein, the evaluator needs to decide what categories will be used to plan the evaluation.

Table 21.1 shows an example of an abbreviated task outline for an evaluation project. It shows the major tasks proceeded by an action verb. These major tasks usually are divided into finer subtasks; the degree of refinement depends on how carefully the evaluator needs to budget and how complicated the tasks might be (e.g., the task "Develop design and instruments" might include several design components and multiple instruments and it may be more accurate to de-

TABLE 21.1. Major Tasks of a Typical Evaluation Project

Task 1	Conduct literature review and develop conceptual framework.
Task 2	Develop design and instruments.
Task 3	Construct sample frame and select sample.
Task 4	Collect data.
Task 5	Analyze data.
Task 6	Write report.

velop time budgets for each of these tasks rather than guess them altogether). The evaluation sponsor may also require a budget that includes specific categories. When the estimates need to be precise, tasks should be divided more finely. A more refined task outline, however, can serve as a useful tool in determining the staffing needs of a project and in guiding the actual implementation of the project. In addition, these details might provide guidance on how to modify plans when the evaluation has implementation problems, as most evaluations do.

Conceptual Development

The first category in Table 21.1 usually encompasses conceptual development that should form the foundation of a well-designed evaluation. This includes literature reviews and thinking and talking about the problem to be investigated. Time needs to be allocated for consulting with experts in areas where evaluators need additional advice. Interviews with interest holders are also a critical element to consider in planning an evaluation. The literature reviews could be categorized into several steps ranging from computerized searches to writing a summary of the findings. This is also the opportunity to develop or refine the program theory that underlies the intervention.

Pilot and Feasibility Testing

It should *not* be assumed that either the intervention being studied or the evaluation are feasible to be conducted in the planned setting. It is advisable to build into the evaluation plan a pilot or feasibility study in advance of full implementation to get information and feedback of potential participants about problems that may occur in the actual evaluation. Also, part of pilot testing is instrument selection, development, and refinement. Regardless of whether the evaluator plans to do intensive face-to-face interviewing, self-administered questionnaires, or observation, time needs to be allocated to identify, adapt, or develop relevant instruments used to collect data. Time also needs to be allocated for pilot testing the instruments. In pilot testing, preliminary drafts of instruments are used in the field with persons similar to the participants in the evaluation. Some purposes of pilot testing are to ascertain the length of time needed to administer the instrument, check on ease of administration, practice coding of information, and determine whether there are ambiguities in how respondents interpret the instrument. At this point the evaluator should also be able to identify any costs associated with the use of any measures since many are copyrighted and may charge for use.

Pilot testing therefore should usually be part of planning any project. Typically, there will be "new" problems that were not noted by members of the evaluation team in previous applications of the instrument. Respondents often interpret instruments differently from evaluators and from previous users of the instrument. Widespread use of an instrument does not ensure that participants in your evaluation project will interpret the instrument in the same way earlier users have interpreted it. Reliability and validity are not characteristics of the instrument alone but a combined interaction of the instrument, the actual use of the instrument, and the characteristics of the sample of participants for which it was used. In addition, pilot tests should involve testing procedures (training procedures, contact procedures, etc.) as well as testing the instruments. However, it should be recognized that the evaluator is typically operating in someone else's organization and usually not in a research-oriented environment. While pilot testing is usually critical in a research project, it just may not be feasible in an evaluation where pilot testing can be seen as disruptive to an organization. To some it also may convey a sense of a lack of an evaluator's confidence in their evaluation because it communicates a degree of uncertainty, which may be valid but may not be acceptable to the host organization.

If the study being planned is expensive and important (they are not the same) and the facts underlying the planning are guesses, then a pilot study or studies might be the most appropriate action. There are several sources that offer a concise guide on the conduct of pilot studies (Teresi et al., 2022; Bond et al., 2023; Morin, 2023), as well as a journal that is devoted to this topic (*Pilot and Feasibility Studies*).

The reasons for conducting a pilot include (1) assessing the feasibility of key processes, which includes recruitment and retention rates and feasibility of data collection; (2) assessing time and resource problems that can occur, such as time taken to conduct interviews and capacity of sites; (3) exploring different management approaches, including personnel and data management; and (4) conducting scientific tests that include an estimate of treatment effects (sample size), although this estimation can be misleading in a small pilot (Leon et al., 2011; Gruijters & Peters, 2022). Before conducting a pilot there has to be clear criteria for success, such as the minimum number of participants that need to be recruited per month. Thabane and Lancaster (2019) have updated their widely cited 2010 article to include guidelines for reporting protocols in the journal *Pilot and Feasibility Studies*.

If the data collection approach involves extracting information from administrative records, pilot testing must take a different form. The evaluator should pilot test the training planned for data extractors and test the data-coding process. Checks should be included for accuracy and consistency across coders.

As discussed earlier, when external validity or generalizability may be a major concern, the evaluator needs to plan especially carefully the construction of the participant sample. The sampling procedure describes the potential participants and how they will be selected for the evaluation. This procedure may be complex, depending upon the type of sampling plan adopted. The issue of generalizability is discussed in more depth in several places earlier in this chapter.

Data Collection

The next phase of evaluation is usually the data collection. Data collection can include many activities. For example, the evaluation may involve reviewing previous records. The evaluator needs to determine how long it will take to gain access to those records, as well as how long it will take to extract the data from the records. It is important to ascertain not only how long it will take to collect the data from the records but whether information the evaluator assumes is on those records is there. Records kept for administrative purposes often do not match evaluation needs. Careful sampling and inspection of those records in planning the project are necessary steps to avoid the embarrassment of inability to complete the project because of a lack of data. In planning evaluation, assumptions about data need to be recognized, questioned, and then checked carefully. Records can include paper but more frequently records come from data systems that require extraction and interpretation to be useful in an evaluation.

If the evaluator is planning to conduct a survey, the procedures for estimating the length of time needed for this process are often complex. The steps needed in conducting a survey include developing or refining the instrument, recruiting and training interviewers, sampling, and the actual collection of the data. Telephone interviews require some additional planning as well as conducting surveys over the internet. This chapter cannot go into depth about these and other data collection methods other than to indicate that time estimates need to be attached to each task associated with data collection.

An important issue for any data collection procedure is the issue of sampling from a population. If the evaluation requires a representative sample to help ensure that the results are generalizable to a population (be it individuals, sites, or types of programs), then the technical requirements of such an evaluation may require the expertise of a sampling consultant, which could be expensive. If such representativeness is not required, which is the case for most evaluations, then the task is a lot simpler but not without challenges. Many evaluations sample from existing lists, which takes fewer resources than creating a sampling frame, but lists can be biased depending on how they were developed. Ensuring that existing lists are not biased can take additional resources.

Data Analysis

The next phase usually associated with any evaluation project is data analysis. Whether the evaluator is using qualitative or quantitative methods, time must be allocated for the analysis of data. Analysis not only includes statistical testing but also the preparation of the data for computer analysis. If the data are in paper form, which is becoming thankfully rare, steps included in this process are cleaning of the data (i.e., making certain that the responses are readable and are not ambiguous for data entry personnel if the data were originally written), physically entering the data, and checking for the internal consistency of the data. For example, if a participant said no in response to a question about whether they eat meals out of the home, there should be no answers recorded for that person about the types of restaurants that they frequent. Other procedures typically included in quantitative analysis are the production of descriptive statistics (i.e., frequencies, means, standard deviations, and measures of skewness). Many tedious and error-prone steps are eliminated if the data are collected electronically. If the data can be collected on smartphones, which most people possess, then this cost is reduced. More complex studies may require conducting inferential statistical tests. The reader is referred to Chapters 13, 16, and 17, this volume. Analytic procedures for qualitative data collection procedures need to be tailored for the specific project.

Reporting Results

Finally, time needs to be allocated for communicating the results. Evaluation projects typically require a final report—this report is usually a lengthy and detailed analysis. Because most people do not read the entire report, it is critical to include a two- or three-page executive summary that succinctly and clearly summarizes the main findings. In evaluation projects, the lay audience typically is not concerned with statistical tests, methodology, or literature reviews. These individuals just want to know what was found. The quality of the findings cannot be interpreted, however, without an understanding of the methodology and analysis. The executive summary should focus on the findings and present these as the highlights of the evaluation. The evaluation plan may also include or require the review of multiple drafts of the final report by different interest holders. This can be a lengthy and time-consuming process that should be included in the budget.

No matter how much effort and innovation went into data collection, the procedures are of interest primarily to other evaluators and not to typical sponsors of evaluation. The best the evaluator can hope to accomplish with the latter audience is to educate them about the limitations of the findings based on specific methods used. The report must include a discussion of any limitations of the results and conclusions based on the methods and analyses used. Finally, the evaluator may have no control over when a report is released since the evaluation may be embedded in a sensitive political context.

The evaluator should allocate time not just for producing a report but also for verbally communicating this information to sponsors and other interest holders. Before committing to a final report, the evaluator may want to consult with various interest holders to learn how they perceive the data and to help identify and hopefully resolve any inconsistencies. Verbal communications may include briefings as well as testimony to legislative bodies. Moreover, if the evaluator desires to have the results of the evaluation utilized, it is likely that time needs to be allocated to work with the sponsor and other organizations in interpreting and applying the findings of the evaluation. Specific expertise may be needed to provide professional graphics for presentations. This last utilization-oriented perspective often is not included in planning a time budget. The chapters by O'Neil (see Chapter 25) and by Azzam and Jones (see Chapter 18, this volume) are particularly helpful here.

Time Estimates

Once the evaluator has described all the major tasks and subtasks, the next part of the planning process is to estimate how long it will take to complete each task. This is a difficult process unless there are previous data upon which to base these estimates. One way to approach this problem is to reduce each task to its smallest unit. For example, in the data collection phase, an estimate of the total amount of interviewing time is needed. The simplest way to estimate this total is to calculate how long each interview should take. Pilot data are critical to developing accurate estimates. If pilot interviews took an average of 2 hours each to complete, and if the evaluation calls for 100 interviews, then simple arithmetic indicates that 200 hours need to be allocated for this task. Does this estimate, however, include everything that is important? Is travel time included? Are callbacks to respondents who are not home part of this estimate? Is the time required for editing the data and coding open-ended responses included?

Whatever estimate the evaluator derives, it is likely to be just that: an estimate. There will be a margin of error associated with this estimate. Whether the estimate is too conservative or too generous depends in part on the context in which the planning needs to occur. For example, if the evaluator is planning to compete for an evaluation contract, then it may be the case that an underestimate will occur, as competition may place pressure on the planner to keep the costs of conducting the evaluation as low as possible. However, honesty is critical here as in all aspects of program evaluation, for "lowballing" or purposively underestimating the cost of a bid on a federal proposal may be illegal. On the other hand, inexperienced individuals operating under no particular time pressure (e.g., graduate students) may overestimate time required for conducting an evaluation project. As a rule of thumb, underestimates are more likely and more costly than overestimates. If the evaluation sponsor can afford the time and the money, it would be safe to add at least an extra 10–15% to any initial estimate. Clearly, this addition indicates a lack of certainty and precision. Project planning or management software can be very useful in estimating and adjusting budgets. Some examples of these software programs are MeisterTask, Basecamp, Nifty, and Zoho Projects. These software packages usually include the capacity to make task lists, schedules, and links between project documents and various reporting mechanisms to keep the process current.

The clock time budget simply indicates how long it will take to complete each task. What this budget does not tell you is the sequencing and the real calendar time needed for conducting the evaluation. Calendar time can be calculated from the above estimates but the evaluator needs to make certain other assumptions. For example, if the evaluation uses interviewers to collect data and 200 hours of interviewing time are required, the length of calendar time needed for this depends on a number of factors. Most clearly, the number of interviewers is a critical factor. One interviewer takes a minimum of 200 hours to complete the task, whereas 200 interviewers can do it in 1 hour. The larger number of interviewers, however, may create the need for other mechanisms to be put into place (e.g., interviewer supervision and monitoring), as well as create concerns regarding the quality of the data. Thus, one needs to specify the staffing levels and evaluation team skills for the project. This is the next kind of budget that needs to be developed.

PERSONNEL AS A RESOURCE

Skills Inventory

Once the evaluator has described the tasks that need to be accomplished, the second step is to decide what kinds of people are needed to conduct those tasks. What characteristics are needed for a trained observer or an interviewer? What are the requirements for a supervisor? What skills does a data analyst need? Who will be able to manage the project and write the reports? Evaluators need to consider these decisions in planning an evaluation project. To assist in answering these questions, the evaluator should complete a skills matrix. The matrix shown in Figure 21.1 describes the requisite skills needed for the tasks and attaches names or positions of the evaluation team to each cluster of skills. Typically, a single individual does not possess all the requisite skills, and so a team will need to be developed for the evaluation project. In that case, the labels are simply "economist," "statistician," and so on. The evaluator should be sensitive to the possibility of including local expertise among the evaluation human resources. Locals may have a unique and informative perspective on the program and the evaluation that should not be missed. Development of local capacity to conduct research and evaluation (institutional development) should also be considered a goal of evaluations if supported by sponsors.

In describing personnel as being labeled by specific titles we do not want to gloss over the need for interpersonal and leadership skills. A successful evaluation requires collaboration of many individuals as well as the ability to deal with sponsors, clients, and guardians of site access. Managerial support is necessary to coordinate activities and meet deadlines (Smith & Thew, 2017).

In addition to specific evaluation tasks, every evaluation project needs management. Someone needs to manage the various parts of the project to make sure that they are working together and that the schedule is being met. For example, a manager must decide about how to organize the administration of the interviews. It is not reasonable, unless the individual subjects are dispersed geographically, to use 200 interviewers for 1 hour each simply because of the excessive amount of time that would be needed to recruit, supervise, and train that many interviewers. The first consideration is how many individuals can be recruited, supervised, and trained to carry out certain tasks. Second, how finely can tasks be categorized so that more individuals can accomplish them? For example, it is sensible to use multiple interviewers but not to use multiple data analysts. One person might be best working full-time to conduct the data analysis.

Person	Evaluation design	Instrument development	Sampling	Institutional development	Cost analysis	Statistics	Interviewing
Director	X	X		X	X		X
Statistician	X		X		X	X	
Economist				X	X	X	
Evaluation assistant 1		X					X
Evaluation assistant 2	X		X	X	X	X	X

FIGURE 21.1. Skills matrix.

On the other hand, one person working full-time doing all of the interviews would not be recommended. Considerations of time available, skills, supervision, training, continuity of project staff, and burnout are all relevant in computing the next table: the number of hours per person to be allocated for each task.

Person Loading

Once the evaluator specifies the tasks and estimates the amount of time required to complete each task, they then need to assign these tasks to individuals. A person-loading chart (see Figure 21.2) describes the assignment plan. This table shows a more refined categorization of the tasks needed to develop instruments. The left-hand side of the table lists the tasks required for the project. The top of the table lists all the individuals, or categories of individuals, who will be needed to accomplish these tasks. The example shows that the specification of data needs will be conducted by the project director for 10 hours. Locating existing instruments will be done by the evaluation assistants working a total of 40 hours each. The interviews will be conducted by the evaluation assistants, with 10 hours of supervision by the project director, for a total of 40 hours each. The statistician will be involved in two tasks: specifying data needs (10 hours) and analyzing interviews (15 hours). This table allows the evaluator to know whether (1) the right mix of skills will be present in the evaluation team to accomplish the tasks, and (2) the amount of time allocated to each individual to conduct those tasks is reasonable. Both of these, the skills and the time, are necessary for the evaluator to develop the next planning tool. In large projects additional support personnel usually are also involved who do not appear in person-loading tables because their costs may not be able to be directly charged to the grant or contract. These costs are assumed under the category of overhead or indirect costs.

Gantt Charts

We need to return to real, or calendar, time at some point in the planning process, given that the project will be conducted under real-time constraints. Thus, the tasking chart needs to be superimposed on a calendar. The allocation of calendar time to each task and subtask is shown in Figure 21.3. The figure is called a **Gantt chart**. It simply shows the tasks on the left-hand side and months on the top of the chart. Each bar

		Director	Evaluation assistant 1	Economist	Statistician	Evaluation assistant 2
Task 2	Develop instruments					
2.1	Specify data needs	10	—	5	10	—
2.2	Review existing instruments					
2.21	Locate instruments	—	40	—	—	40
2.22	Evaluate instruments	20	20	—	—	20
2.3	Construct instrument-need matrix	20	20	—	—	20
2.4	Develop new instruments					
2.41	Develop interviews	20	20	—	—	30
2.42	Conduct interviews	10	40	—	—	40
2.43	Analyze interviews	10	40	—	15	40
2.44	Construct scales	20	50	—	—	50
2.45	Field test instruments	10	40	—	—	40
Total (hours)		120	270	5	25	280

FIGURE 21.2. Person loading chart for one task.

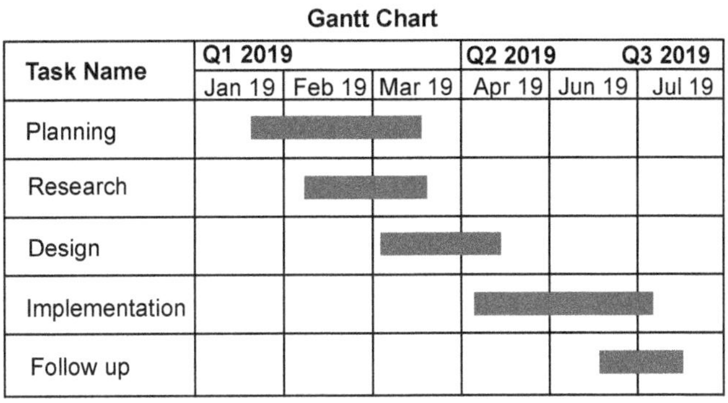

Gantt Chart

Task Name	Q1 2019			Q2 2019		Q3 2019
	Jan 19	Feb 19	Mar 19	Apr 19	Jun 19	Jul 19
Planning	▓▓▓▓▓▓▓▓▓▓					
Research		▓▓▓▓▓				
Design			▓▓▓▓▓▓▓			
Implementation				▓▓▓▓▓▓▓▓▓▓		
Follow up					▓▓▓▓▓	

FIGURE 21.3. Gantt chart example.

shows the length of calendar time allocated for the completion of specific subtasks. This does not mean that if a bar takes up 1 month, the task will actually take a whole month of clock time to complete. The task might only take 15 hours but need to be spread over a full month.

The Gantt chart shows not only how long each task takes but also the approximate relationship in calendar time between tasks. Although inexact, the chart can show the precedence of evaluation tasks. A more detailed and exacting procedure is to produce a **PERT chart** showing the dependency relationships between tasks. These charts typically are not needed for the types of evaluation projects used in social sciences.

One of the key relationships and assumptions made in producing a plan is that individuals will not work more than 40 hours a week. Thus, the person-loading chart needs to be checked against the Gantt chart to make sure that the task can be completed by those individuals assigned to it within the period specified in the Gantt chart. This task is more complex than it seems because individuals typically will be assigned to multiple tasks within a specified time. It is important to calculate, for each individual involved in the project, how much actual calendar time they will be working for all of the tasks to which they are assigned. Individuals should not be allocated to more tasks or time than can be handled. As noted earlier reasonably priced software programs are available to help the planner do these calculations and draw the appropriate charts. At this point in the planning process, the evaluator should have a very clear estimate of the time budget. Both the time budget and person-loading chart are needed to produce a financial budget, which is the next step in the planning process.

FINANCIAL RESOURCES

Budget and Work Plan

While it may appear to be obvious that the resource allocation must match the evaluation work plan, detailed planning is critical to provide evidence that the evaluator fully understands the resources needed to conduct the evaluation. For example, if the evaluator plans to pay participants, then the dollar amount in the budget must match the number of participants and the amount of payment. However, even this scenario is more complicated than it seems—for example, should the dollar amount match the expected number of participants based on attrition or the maximum that could be recruited? My advice is to use the maximum so there is no budget shortfall if you underestimate recruitment.

A more complex question to answer is whether the budget, be it time or money, is sufficient to conduct a successful evaluation. Reviewers may decide that your work plan may be too ambitious and thus not feasible if there is not a good match between the resources you are requesting and the work that is planned. A mismatch may indicate that you do not have a good grasp of the evaluation plan, or the resources needed.

Usually, the biggest part of any evaluation budget is personnel: evaluation staff. Most evaluations are very labor intensive. Moreover, the labor of some individuals can be very costly. To produce a budget based on predicted costs, the evaluator needs to follow a few simple steps. This section describes how to develop a financial budget for a grant or contract but the specific requirements of funding agencies in completing an application must also be followed.

Based on the person-loading chart, the evaluator can simply compute total personnel costs for the project by multiplying the hours allocated to each individual by their hourly cost. The evaluator should compute personnel costs by each task. In addition, if the project crosses different years, then the planner needs to provide for salary increases in the estimate. Hourly cost typically includes salary and fringe benefits—if the evaluator needs to break out costs by month, this procedure will allow that as well. Table 21.2 illustrates personnel costs for each task. The figures used in this table are for illustrative purposes only and are not meant to represent actual salaries for these individuals. Budgets for contracts usually follow this procedure. For grant applications from academic institutions, these calculations are not necessary—however, they are recommended to be able to plan and monitor a project adequately.

Table 21.2 illustrates how other items need to be allocated to the budget to include such cost items as servers, supplies, duplication, postage, telephone, and travel. In computing how much needs to be allocated in each one of these areas, the same type of analysis used for personnel should be applied.

Travel costs can be estimated in a similar fashion. If travel will be by air to a specific location, then the web can provide the cost of each trip. Given the complex fare structures available, the evaluator might want to use an average cost or, to be on the safe side, the maximum regular air fare (if allowed; not all funding sources allow the maximum to be proposed). If the evaluation team plans to visit a number of places across the country that cannot be specified until the project is funded, then a scenario needs to be developed. Such a scenario could include computing average fares to 10 or 12 likely places to visit. In computing the budget then, one simply takes the average cost of travel to these 10 places and multiplies it by the number of visits and number of persons making visits. The use of a personal car typically is reimbursed at a fixed rate per mile. To estimate meals and lodging, calculate the average cost of meals and hotel stays in that particular city at a cost per day. Some contracts may specify a per diem or the fixed amount that is allocated on food and lodging per day.

The evaluator needs to examine the tasks to determine whether there are any special costs associated with the project—for example, if a telephone survey is going to be conducted, then it is critical to compute this part of the budget accurately. If a mailed questionnaire is the method, then postage for initial mailings, return mail, follow-up reminders, and other correspondence must be computed. Web-based surveys should include any special software development that might be needed.

After computing personnel and other costs, institutions usually have an indirect or overhead cost added to the direct expenses of the project. This is the cost associated with conducting evaluation that cannot be allocated to each specific project. These typically include costs for space, utilities, and maintenance, as well as those associated with the university's or firm's management and accounting systems related to grants and contracts. Indirect costs vary from institution to institution and should be included as part of the budget. For-profit firms also will add a profit percentage to a contract. More details on budgeting for independent evaluators can be found in Barrington (see Chapter 23, this volume) on independent consultants.

In calculating a budget, the distinction between academic and nonacademic settings should be kept in mind. Evaluators in academic institutions are not accustomed to calculating personnel budgets as described. Instead, an estimate is made about how many people would be needed or what percentage of time a faculty

TABLE 21.2. Personnel Costs

	Director	Economist	Statistician	Evaluation assistant
Total (hours)	120	5	25	280
Hourly rates	$150	$120	$100	$25
Total costs	$18,800	$600	$500	$7,000

member is willing or able to devote to a project, and that is included as part of the budget. This often is a workable solution because the faculty time is fairly flexible. Thus, when the workload of one project is underestimated, the faculty member may just work harder or longer on that project and not spend as much time on other activities. To have an accurate estimate of personnel time required for a project, however, the procedure described above is recommended.

After the budget has been calculated, the evaluator may be faced with a total cost that is not reasonable for the project, either because the sponsor does not have those funds available or because the bidding for the project is very competitive. If this occurs, the evaluator has a number of alternatives available. The most reasonable alternative is to eliminate some tasks or to reduce their scope. For example, instead of interviewing 200 persons, interview 100. Alternatively, keep the number of persons interviewed the same, but cut back on the length of each interview to reduce costs. There is, of course, a limit to how far the project can be cut back. For example, a series of tasks that grossly underestimate the amount of time required will not be evaluated favorably by knowledgeable reviewers. The underestimate will simply indicate to the reviewers that the evaluator does not have the capability of conducting the evaluation because they are not realistic about the amount of time or resources required. Another alternative to reducing the size of the budget is to use less expensive staff. The trade-off is that a more expensive staff usually is more experienced and may be able to accomplish a task in less time. Using less experienced staff, however, should result in an increase in the amount of time allocated to conduct that task. The evaluator might also want to look for more efficient methods of conducting the evaluation. For example, the use of **matrix sampling** (where individuals receive different parts of questionnaires) may reduce costs. If a randomized design is possible, it may be feasible but often very risky, to collect only posttest data and eliminate all pretest data collection. The evaluator needs to use ingenuity to try to devise not only a valid, reliable, and sensitive project but one that is efficient as well. Bamberger (see Chapter 24) and Barrington (see Chapter 23, this volume) have numerous suggestions for cutting the costs of an evaluation.

The financial budget, as well as the time budget, should force the evaluator to realize the trade-offs that are involved in program evaluation. Should the evaluator use a longer instrument at a higher cost, or collect less data from more subjects? Should the subscales on an instrument be longer and thus more reliable, or should more domains be covered with each domain composed of fewer items and thus less reliable? Should an emphasis be placed on **representative sampling** as opposed to a **purposive sampling** procedure? Should the evaluator use multiple data collection techniques, such as observation and interviewing, or should the evaluation plan include only one technique, with more data collected by that procedure? These and other questions are ones that any evaluation planner faces. When under strict time and cost limitations, however, the saliency of these alternatives is very high. In order to be able to test different budget scenarios, at a minimum, budgets should be developed in Excel or other software used for project development and planning.

In addition to requiring a budget that identifies items and their cost, evaluation sponsors usually require the evaluator to provide a budget justification for each of these items. For example, while the budget may identify travel as costing several thousand dollars, the justification for this amount must be provided. This would entail describing the purpose of the travel (e.g., site visit, attend a conference) and the costs associated with that travel. For example, travel to a site may include air and ground transportation, meals, and hotels. The justification would provide the cost of the air fare, the cost of ground transportation, the daily cost of hotels, and the number of days and the costs of meals (which usually is limited). Some funders provide a per diem, which is a fixed a fixed amount of money to cover daily living expenses, including lodging, meals, and incidental expenses.

The Good News/Bad News

The good news is that your evaluation was funded. The bad news is that your budget was cut. How can you do the same work for less money (this assumes that calendar time was also not reduced)? This outcome is a usual occurrence in most grant funding. Thus, the good planner will include in the work plan aspects of the evaluation that can be "sacrificed" in case the budget is cut without endangering the key aims of the evaluation. In addition, within ethical constraints the budget may include activities that include some cushion, such as using the maximum number of subjects instead of some estimated guess that could be wrong. I have added some additional suggestions to the list provided by Rice et al. (2006) about what to do when a budget is cut. Bamberger (see Chapter 24, this volume) is also helpful to deal with this problem. However, these actions usually require negotiations among the funder, the organization conducting the evaluation, and the evaluation leaders. These actions include reducing:

- Effort of expensive personnel and consultants.
- Travel by combining meetings or using the internet.
- The number of study sites.
- The number of data collection points if it is a longitudinal evaluation.
- The amount of data collected or using less expensive alternatives, such as phone interviews instead of in-person interviews.
- Sample size by considering other ways to increase statistical power, such as new analytic techniques.
- Direct costs by cost sharing with organization doing the evaluation on such items as dissemination and salaries.
- The number of full-time persons and replacing them with part-time persons who do not get fringe benefits.
- The number of deliverables.
- Subcontracting to less expensive organizations.

Monitoring Project Implementation Expenses

Finally, the evaluator should be sure to include in the planning phase a procedure for monitoring the project's tasks so that action can be taken to keep the project on schedule. Budgetary responsibility requires at least monthly accounting of the expenses. The detailed Gantt chart can be very helpful in determining whether the project is slipping behind schedule. It is often the case that what is implemented in the field does not follow what was planned. The purpose of the planning is not to force a rigid structure on the field operations but to anticipate and minimize difficulties. Unless some standard is developed and applied, the evaluator cannot be sure that the project is tracking correctly. The use of these planning tools as management tools can help the evaluator obtain the goal of a competently conducted project. Powell et al. (see Chapter 12, this volume) provide more detailed information on how to monitor an evaluation.

PROJECT PLANNING AND MANAGEMENT SOFTWARE

All of the processes I have described in this chapter can be accomplished more efficiently using software. For complex projects the use of these software packages is practically mandatory especially when it comes to pricing out the total cost of a project. There are many variables that affect the price of a proposal. Deciding which aspects of the proposal should be adjusted to meet a total price target or range is not possible without software programs. Each software suite has its own advantages and disadvantages. Although I mentioned some specific software packages earlier, because of the volatility of the software market, I do not provide recommendations for specific software packages but encourage you to seek out objective reviews. There are many websites that claim to provide objective software reviews but it is difficult to judge the veracity of these claims. In addition, recent development in AI has provided an additional approach to improving these software programs either through development provided by the software developers themselves or as add-ons to existing planning programs (Teslia et al., 2023). Project management software is also critical in successfully managing project implementation.

CONCLUSION

Planning and implementing an evaluation can be very complex as I hope this chapter has illustrated. There are many aspects of the evaluation that must be carefully planned if the evaluation is going to be successfully implemented.

Careful planning can help avoid major mistakes but because evaluation takes place in the messy real world, unexpected problems are bound to occur. The best way to plan for the unexpected is to have done careful planning for the expected problems.

REFERENCES

Abadie, R. (2019). The exploitation of professional "guinea pigs" in the gig economy: The difficult road from consent to justice. *American Journal of Bioethics, 19*(9), 37–39.

Ahmed, S., Airlie, J., Clegg, A., Copsey, B., Cundill, B., Forster, A., . . . Farrin, A. J. (2022). A new opportunity for enhancing trial efficiency: Can we investigate intervention implementation processes within trials using SWAT (study within a trial) methodology? *Research Methods in Medicine and Health Sciences, 3*(3), 66–73.

Bamberger, M. (2020). Evaluation in the age of big data. In M. Bamberger & L. Mabry (Eds.), *Real-World evaluation: Working under budget, time, data and political constraints*. SAGE.

Bell, S. H., & Stuart, E. A. (2016). On the "where" of social experiments: The nature and extent of the generalizability problem. In L. R. Peck (Ed.), *Social experiments in practice: What, why, when, where, and how of experimental design & analysis* (pp. 47–59). New Directions for Evaluation, 152.

Bickman, L. (Ed.). (1981). Some distinctions between basic and applied social psychology. In *Applied social psychology annual 2* (pp. 23–44). SAGE.

Bickman, L. (1987). The functions of program theory. *New Directions for Evaluation, 3*, 5–18.

Bickman, L. (2020). Improving mental health services: A 50-year journey from randomized experiments to artificial intelligence and precision mental health. *Administration and Policy in Mental Health, 47*(5), 795–843.

Bickman, L., Domenico, H. J., Byrne, D. W., Jerome, R. N., Edwards, T. L., Stroud, M., . . . Harris, P. A. (2021). Effects of financial incentives on volunteering for clinical trials: A randomized vignette experiment. *Contemporary Clinical Trials, 110*, 106584.

Bickman, L., Douglas, S. R., De Andrade, A. R. V., Tomlinson, M., Gleacher, A., Olin, S., & Hoagwood, K. (2016). Implementing a measurement feedback system: A tale of two sites. *Administration and Policy in Mental Health, 43*, 410–425.

Boateng, D., Kumke, T., Vernooij, R., Goetz, I., Meinecke, A.-K., Steenhuis, C., . . . GetReal Initiative. (2023). Validation of the GetReal trial tool—facilitating discussion and understanding more pragmatic design choices and their implications. *Contemporary Clinical Trials, 125*, 107054.

Bogin V. (2022). Lasagna's law: A dish best served early. *Contemporary Clinical Trials Communications, 26*, 100900.

Bond, C., Lancaster, G. A., Campbell, M., Chan, C., Saskia, E., Hopewell, S., . . . Eldridge, S. (2023). Pilot and feasibility studies: Extending the conceptual framework. *Pilot and Feasibility Studies, 9*(1), 24.

Bower, P., Brueton, V., Gamble, C., Treweek, S., Smith, C. T., Young, B., & Williamson, P. (2014). Interventions to improve recruitment and retention in clinical trials: A survey and workshop to assess current practice and future priorities. *Trials, 15*(1), 1–9.

Buffenstein, I., Kaneakua, B., Taylor, E., Matsunaga, M., Yung Choi, S., Carrazana, E., . . . Ghaffari-Rafi, A. (2023). Demographic recruitment bias of adults in United States randomized clinical trials by disease categories between 2008 to 2019: A systematic review and meta-analysis. *Scientific Reports, 13*(1), 42.

Cascini, F., Beccia, F., Causio, F. A., Melnyk, A., Zaino, A., & Ricciardi, W. (2022). Scoping review of the current landscape of AI-based applications in clinical trials. *Frontiers in Public Health, 10*, 949377.

Clarke, M., Savage, G., Maguire, L., & McAneney, H. (2015). The SWAT (study within a trial) programme: Embedding trials to improve the methodological design and conduct of future research. *Trials, 16*(Suppl. 2), 209.

Coffey, T., Duncan, E. M., Morgan, H., Lawrie, L., & Gillies, K. (2022). Behavioural approaches to recruitment and retention in clinical trials: A systematic mapping review. *BMJ Open, 12*(3), e054854.

Cooper, C. L., Hind, D., Duncan, R., Walters, S., Lartey, A., Lee, E., & Bradburn, M. (2015). A rapid review indicated higher recruitment rates in treatment trials than in prevention trials. *Journal of Clinical Epidemiology, 68*(3), 347–354.

Degtiar, I., & Rose, S. (2023). A review of generalizability and transportability. *Annual Review of Statistics and Its Application, 10*(1), 501–524.

Dennis, M. L. (1990). Assessing the validity of randomized field experiments: An example from drug treatment research. *Evaluation Review, 14*, 347–373.

Doherty, L., Parker, A., Arundel, C., Clark, L., Coleman, E., Hewitt, C., . . . Torgerson, D. (2023). PROMoting the use of studies within a trial (PROMETHEUS): Results and experiences from a large programme to evaluate the routine embedding of recruitment and retention strategies within randomised controlled trials routinely. *Research Methods in Medicine and Health Sciences, 4*(3), 113–122.

Dreber, A., & Johannesson, M. (2020). Statistical significance and the replication crisis in the social sciences. In A. Dixit, S. Edwards, & K. Judd

(Eds.), *Oxford research encyclopedias: Economics and finance*. Oxford University Press.

Elfeky, A., Gillies, K., Gardner, H., Fraser, C., Ishaku, T., & Treweek, S. (2020). Non-randomised evaluations of strategies to increase participant retention in randomised controlled trials: A systematic review. *Systematic Reviews, 9*(1), 224.

Findley, M. G., Kikuta, K., & Denly, M. (2021). External validity. *Annual Review of Political Science, 24*, 365–393.

Galiani, S., & Quistorff, B. (2023). Assessing external validity in practice. *NBER Working Paper Series*, No. 30398.

Gaunt, D. M., Papastavrou Brooks, C., Pedder, H., Crawley, E., Horwood, J., & Metcalfe, C. (2023). Participant retention in paediatric randomised controlled trials published in six major journals 2015-2019: Systematic review and meta-analysis. *Trials, 24*(1), 403.

Gennetian, L. A. (2021). How a behavioral economic framework can support scaling of early childhood interventions. In J. List, D. Suskind, & L. Supplee (Eds.), *The scale-up effect in early childhood and public policy: Why interventions lose impact at scale and what we can do about it*. University of Chicago Press.

Gillies K., Kearney, A., Keenan, C., Treweek, S., Hudson, J., Brueton, V. C., . . . Aceves-Martins, M. (2021). Strategies to improve retention in randomised trials. *Cochrane Database of Systematic Reviews, 3*(3), MR000032.

Goffman, E. (1959). *The presentation of self in everyday life*. Doubleday.

Green, B. L., Ayoub, C., Bartlett, J. D., Furrer, C., Von Ende, A., Chazan-Cohen, R., . . . Nygren, P. (2015). It's not as simple as it sounds: Problems and solutions in accessing and using administrative child welfare data for evaluating the impact of early childhood interventions. *Children and Youth Services Review, 57*, 40–49.

Groves, R. M., & Schoeffel, G. J. (2018). Use of administrative records in evidence-based policymaking. *Annals of the American Academy of Political and Social Science, 678*(1), 71–80.

Gruijters, S. L. K., & Peters, G.-J. Y. (2022). Meaningful change definitions: Sample size planning for experimental intervention research. *Psychology and Health, 37*(1), 1–16.

Jorgensen, D. L. (2015). Participant observation. In R. A. Scott & S. M. Kosslyn (Eds.), *Emerging trends in the social and behavioral sciences*. Wiley.

Kavalci, E., & Hartshorn, A. (2023). Improving clinical trial design using interpretable machine learning based prediction of early trial termination. *Scientific Reports, 13*, 121.

Kelsey, M. D., Patrick-Lake, B., Abdulai, R., Broedl, U. C., Brown, A., Cohn, E., . . . Bloomfield, G. S. (2022). Inclusion and diversity in clinical trials: Actionable steps to drive lasting change. *Contemporary Clinical Trials, 116*, 106740.

Kilicel, D., De Crescenzo, F., Pontrelli, G., & Armando, M. (2023). Participant recruitment issues in child and adolescent psychiatry clinical trials with a focus on prevention programs: A meta-analytic review of the literature. *Journal of Clinical Medicine, 12*(6), 2307.

Leon, A. C., Davis, L. L., & Kraemer, H. C. (2011). The role and interpretation of pilot studies in clinical research. *Journal of Psychiatric Research, 45*(5), 626–629.

Lipsey, M. W., Crosse, S., Dunkle, J., Pollard, J., & Stobart, G. (1985). Evaluation: The state of the art and the sorry state of the science. *New Directions in Program Evaluation, 27*, 7–18.

Liu, Y., Xu, Y., & Ling, I. (2017). The impact of backstage cues on service evaluation. *International Journal of Quality and Service Sciences, 9*(2), 165–183.

Logan, T. (2019). A practical, iterative framework for secondary data analysis in educational research. *Australian Educational Researcher, 47*, 129–148.

Morin, K. H. (2023). Clarifying the importance of pilot studies. *Journal of Nursing Education, 62*, 9.

Olsen, R. B., & Orr, L. L. (2016). On the "where" of social experiments: Selecting more representative samples to inform policy. In L. R. Peck (Ed.), *Social experiments in practice: The what, why, when, where, and how of experimental design & analysis* (pp. 61–71). New Directions for Evaluation, 152.

Olsson, T. M., Kapetanovic, S., Hollertz, K., Starke, M., & Skoog, T. (2023). Advancing social intervention research through program theory reconstruction. *Research on Social Work Practice, 33*(6), 10497315221149976.

Peck, L. R. (2022). Insights into the generalizability of findings from experimental evaluations. *American Journal of Evaluation, 43*(1), 66–69.

Rice, M., Broome, M. E., Habermann, B., Kang, D. H., & Davis, L. L. (2006). Implementing the research budget. *Western Journal of Nursing Research, 28*(2), 234–241.

Saxe, G. N., Bickman, L., Ma, S., & Aliferis, C. (2022). Mental health progress requires causal diagnostic nosology and scalable causal discovery. *Frontiers in Psychiatry, 13*, 898789.

Smith, K. V., & Thew, G. R. (2017). Conducting research in clinical psychology practice: Barriers, facilitators, and recommendations. *British Journal of Clinical Psychology, 56*(3), 347–356.

Soneson, E., Das, S., Burn, A. M., van Melle, M., Anderson, J. K., Fazel, M., . . . Moore, A. (2023). Leveraging administrative data to better understand and address child maltreatment: A scoping review of data linkage studies. *Child Maltreatment, 28*(1), 176–195.

Teresi, J. A., Yu, X., Stewart, A. L., & Hays, R. D. (2022). Guidelines for designing and evaluating feasibility pilot studies. *Medical Care, 60*(1), 95–103.

Teslia, I., Yegorchenkov, O., Khlevna, J., Yegorchenkova, N., Kataeva, Y., Khlevny, A., & Klevanna, G. (2023). Development of the concept of intelligent add-on over project planning instruments. *Lecture Notes on Data Engineering and Communications Technologies, 178*, 149–161.

Thabane, L., & Lancaster, G. (2019). A guide to the reporting of protocols of pilot and feasibility trials. *Pilot and Feasibility Studies, 5*, 37.

Tipton, E., & Matlen, B. J. (2019). Improved generalizability through improved recruitment: Lessons learned from a large-scale randomized trial. *American Journal of Evaluation, 40*(3), 414–430.

Treweek, S., Bevan, S., Bower, P., Campbell, M., Christie, J., Clarke, M., . . . Williamson, P. R.,(2018). Trial forge guidance 1: What is a study within a trial (SWAT)? *Trials, 19*(1), 139.

Treweek, S., Lockhart, P., Pitkethly, M., Cook, J. A., Kjeldstrøm, M., Johansen, M., . . . Mitchell, E. D. (2013). Methods to improve recruitment to randomized controlled trials: Cochrane systematic review and meta-analysis. *BMJ Open, 3*, e002360.

Tsaltskan, V., Nguyen, K., Eaglin, C., Holers, V. M., Deane, K. D., & Firestein, G. S. (2022). Comparison of web-based advertising and a social media platform as recruitment tools for underserved and hard-to-reach populations in rheumatology clinical research. *ACR Open Rheumatology, 4*(7), 623–630.

Willoughby, L. (2016). This doesn't feel right: Selecting a site for school-based ethnography. In K. Taylor-Leech & D. Starkes (Eds.), *Doing research within communities: Stories* (pp. 22–29). Routledge.

York, P., & Bamberger, M. (2020). Measuring results and impact in the age of big data: The nexus of evaluation, analytics, and digital technology. Available at *www.rockefellerfoundation.org/wp-content/uploads/Measuring-results-and-impact-in-the-age-of-big-data-by-York-and-Bamberger-March-2020.pdf*

Chapter 22

The Role of an Internal Evaluator

Arnold Love

CHAPTER OVERVIEW

This chapter focuses on internal evaluation—that is, the use of internal staff to evaluate programs or problems of direct relevance to the organization's management. In the recovery from the pandemic, internal evaluation continues to grow rapidly, but there is a serious gap in knowledge about internal evaluation and how it may be best used. This chapter has three purposes: (1) briefly discuss nature of internal evaluation and its strengths and limitations; (2) outline the various roles of the internal evaluator; and (3) describe key models of internal evaluation that are responsive to specific organizational contexts, and identify key strategies for building internal evaluation capacity and managing internal evaluation resources effectively.

Internal evaluators are employees who report directly to an organization's management and evaluate programs or problems of direct relevance to the organization itself (Love, 1991, 2004). In contrast, external evaluators are independent of the organization's management and usually evaluate policies and programs on behalf of an outside entity (e.g., legislative, oversight, or funding body). Both types of evaluators have their unique strengths and potential shortcomings. It is increasingly common to find both internal and external evaluators working on relevant aspects of an evaluation.

In her review of the history and growth of internal evaluation, Mathison (2011) estimated that internal evaluators conduct 80% of the evaluations in Australia, 75% in Canada, 75% in France, 50% in the United States, and 50% the United Kingdom. In some parts of the world, such as Japan and Korea, internal evaluators conduct virtually all evaluations. Ironically, leaders in these cultures puzzle how external evaluations—conducted by outsiders, without deep knowledge of the organization's values, goals, culture, and lacking strong relationships with managers and staff—can produce any meaningful and enduring results.

The number of internal evaluators in the professional evaluation associations also reflects the demand for internal evaluation. In Canada, fully half of the Canadian Evaluation Society members are internal evaluators (Love, 2015; Volkov, 2011b). When the American Evaluation Association (AEA; 2014) inaugurated the new internal evaluation Topical Interest Group (TIG), it ranked six out of 51 TIGs. In addition, the AEA also reported that four of the five largest TIGs—Non-Profits and Foundations,

International and Cross Cultural, Government Evaluation, and Evaluation Managers and Supervisors—had a large proportion of members who were either internal evaluators or who managed evaluation units within their organizations. As a final point, there is evidence (Lam et al., 2023) that the COVID-19 pandemic greatly increased the demand for internal evaluators to help organizations navigate the challenges and adapt their production and delivery models.

On a personal note, I trace my interest in internal evaluation to the influence of the late Aaron Wildavsky, better known as the "Dean of American Public Policy," who was an exemplary evaluator and author of his landmark book *Speaking Truth to Power* (Wildavsky, 1979), which helped define the evaluation field worldwide. Although Wildavsky strongly believed that *external evaluations were important*, he was convinced that *internal evaluations were essential* for ongoing policy and program improvement. For Wildavsky, it followed that internal evaluation was *essential for every organization* and especially those in the public sector.

This chapter reflects my views about internal evaluation forged over four decades of practice both as an internal and external evaluator. A description of my own journey as an internal evaluator appears in Volkov (2011b). I have a deep commitment to "practical wisdom" for evaluators (Love, 2022) and it is my fervent hope that the timeless lessons learned from my experience in this chapter will give you useful guidance. Although I have been informed by scholarship, research, and conversations with my clients and colleagues, any shortcomings are mine alone.

UNDERSTANDING INTERNAL EVALUATION

Internal evaluators are usually employees who report directly to an organization's management and evaluate programs or problems of direct relevance to the organization (Love, 1991, 2004). External evaluators, in contrast, are independent of the organization's management and often evaluate policies and programs of concern to an outside entity (e.g., legislative, oversight, or funding). Each type has unique strengths and potential shortcomings, and it is increasingly common for both internal and external evaluators to evaluate aspects of the same program or project.

Is Internal Evaluation the Same as Internal Audit?

Regarding terminology, frequently there is confusion between internal evaluation and internal audit. *Internal evaluation* assesses the performance of a program or policy to help decision makers accurately assess its design, delivery, and/or effectiveness. On the other hand, an **internal audit** provides assurances about the organization's risk management strategy, management control framework and information, both financial and nonfinancial, used for decision making and reporting about the areas of risks and the systems of control. In some instances the same department will manage both the internal audit and internal evaluation functions. It is wise to ask and confirm the terms that an organization uses for internal audit and internal evaluation.

How Does Internal Evaluation Differ from Other Forms of Evaluation?

Internal evaluation is an action-oriented, applied research process that takes place within the organizational context and supports organizational improvement and change.

At first glance, internal evaluation may appear to resemble other forms of evaluation, but the *context of internal evaluation* is what makes it unique. It is important to recognize that internal evaluation differs substantially in its assumptions, values, mission, sponsors, audiences, relationships between evaluators and other members of the organization, and ethical concerns—all of these are altered by the fact that internal evaluation takes place *within* the organizational context.

Taking place within an organization, the mission of internal evaluation is twofold: it has both an **informational function** and a **behavioral function** (Love, 1991). The *informational function* of internal evaluation is to provide accurate information on the performance of programs for validating results, improving program quality and delivery, and for organizational learning. Accordingly, internal evaluation addresses not only program design and process but also factors in the *organizational context* that affects performance, such as a program's structure, supervisory relationships, staffing, and operations, as well as relevant influencers in the broader organizational environment, known as the PESTEL factors—that is, political, economic, social, technological, environmental, and legal factors.

The *behavioral function*, however, derives from the position of internal evaluation as evaluation *within* the organizational context. The key message is that when evaluation takes place within an organization, the process of evaluation has a strong effect on the behavior of those in the organization (Love, 1991). As a result, internal evaluation is not only a powerful tool for change—as captured in the mantra, "What gets measured, gets done"—but it also increases the influence and use of evaluation information, and thereby shapes the behavior of the organization and its members.

Above all, as Wildavsky (1979) noted, internal evaluation is an essential tool for managers and an integral part of the management process. A major conceptual shift is the realization that instead of having evaluation *done to them* by external evaluators, managers and staff are *doing evaluation together* with internal evaluators. They are partners in the evaluation process and active users of evaluation information. In this way, internal evaluation becomes an integral part of organizational design and organizational development that focuses on the issues and concerns of its members. After you have read the example in Box 22.1, ask yourself how you and your students, and perhaps your fellow teachers, parents, school administrators, and union representatives might genuinely work on the evaluation and improvement process together in a fair and honest way.

CHARACTERISTICS OF INTERNAL EVALUATION

There are four major characteristics that distinguish internal evaluations from external evaluations (Love, 1993). Each one is explained briefly below:

1. *Primary responsibility for evaluation.* The primary responsibility for internal evaluation resides within the organization—that is, with the board, executives, managers, and team leaders of the organization, rather than with those outside the organization, such as government, funders, grant makers, or oversight bodies.

2. *Focus of the evaluation.* The focus of internal evaluation is on the issues and concerns of the organization itself, as guided by its policies, priorities, and needs. In contrast, the focus of external evaluation is usually the interests of those outside the organization being evaluated, such as funders, policymakers, or regulators.

3. *Accountability of evaluators.* Internal evaluators are directly accountable to the organization they are evaluating and are under its authority. On the other hand, external evaluators are independent of the program or organization they are evaluating. They are accountable to the body that funded or commissioned the evaluation and not the program or organization that is being evaluated.

4. *Internal evaluation is an organizational intervention.* Internal evaluation is a form of **action research** that supports organizational development and intentional change. Internal evaluation is an **organizational intervention**, focused on practical concerns, and shaped by political and organizational constraints.

Strengths and Limitations of Internal Evaluation

The Achilles heel of the external evaluator is trying to scramble up a steep learning curve to understand the organizational context in very little

---

BOX 22.1. Example 1: The Effect of Evaluation on Behavior

Imagine that you are teaching in a middle school that has a reputation for nurturing each student's talents through a student-centered approach to learning. You learned from the director of education that students in your school achieved only mediocre ratings on the last set of standardized tests and, as a result, your school's funding and number of educational assistants may be reduced.

Your principal takes you aside and informs you that the school district's school improvement team will be reviewing student performance for the next 3 months and that your class has been selected for the study. The school improvement team has been tasked to find the reasons for your school's mediocre performance and improve it.

How might the presence of this internal evaluation team affect you? What you teach? The way you teach? Why?

time. On the other hand, Table 22.1 shows that the major strength of the internal evaluator is the depth of their knowledge about the organization and its members. As staff members of an organization, internal evaluators tend have a deep understanding about the organization's programs, organizational context, and political processes. Internal evaluators know the resources, both technical and human, that are available to collect or access data for evaluations and the organization's policies, procedures, and timelines required. This knowledge allows them to select evaluation strategies that fit the unique characteristics of their situation, cut through red tape, and promote evaluation findings more effectively. The relationships they build over time reduce the anxiety and fear often associated with external evaluation. Perhaps most importantly, internal evaluators become a valued corporate resource by communicating relevant evaluation findings in a timely fashion to various levels of the organization and by being available to offer crucial evaluation information at the right time for strategic planning and policy decisions.

Internal evaluation also has limitations to overcome. Table 22.1 indicates that the major limitation of internal evaluation is a greater perception of bias. Although bias can affect external evaluation, nonetheless, external evaluators are usually perceived as being more objective because they are independent from management and not subjected to the pressures from the web of relationships that constitute life within an organization. The most common limitations of internal evaluation, however, are practical ones, such as difficulty in balancing the demands for evaluation and available time. Another practical limitation may be the lack of specific expertise, sufficient staff, or specialized evaluation tools to conduct a particular evaluation. Rather than place additional workloads and technical demands on internal evaluators, in some situations it is clearly more cost-effective to hire external evaluators with the know-how, staff, and the right tools. For example, if an evaluation requires face-to-face community surveys with complex sampling frames, assessing innovative new media programs, or evaluating the implementation of a basket of programs delivered in different geographic regions, then evaluation firms specializing in this type of work may be the better choice. As a final point, internal evaluators have a variety of roles both as evaluators and as members of their organization. For example, an internal evaluator is expected to report fair and honest findings, including negative results, while at the same time being seen as a member of the team and supportive of its members. It is obvious that some roles conflict with other roles—this clash can produce role confusion and cause considerable stress. The various roles of internal evaluators is an important topic and is discussed later in this chapter.

Guidelines for Selecting Internal or External Evaluation

A careful review of the known strengths and limitations of internal and external evaluation leads us to a number of typical situations in which external evaluation is either required or strongly recommended. Table 22.2 summarizes these common situations.

Table 22.2 shows that *external evaluation is mandatory* if there is a specific legal requirement for external evaluators—that is, if legislation or the regulations that accompany legislation require evaluators to be fully independent of the program. External evaluation is also necessary when circumstances demand the highest levels of *both real and perceived* credibility, impartiality, and or outside perspective. In other words, even if internal evaluators are capable of a highly credible evaluation, the optics of the situation demands using external evaluators because of potential risks.

High-risk evaluation situations are led by those with financial concerns, which may range

---

TABLE 22.1. Strengths and Limitations of Internal Evaluation

Strengths of internal evaluation
- Understanding of organizational culture
- Better matched to the organization's needs
- Rapid access to evaluation resources
- Results more readily accepted by staff
- Data better understood by staff
- Lower costs

Limitations of internal evaluation
- Greater perceived potential for bias
- Not independent of the organization and management
- Difficult to balance demands for evaluation and available time
- May lack special expertise required for some evaluations
- Potential for role confusion

TABLE 22.2. When External Evaluation Is Strongly Recommended

- Legal requirement for external evaluation
- Specialized knowledge is necessary
- Credibility, impartiality, and/or outside perspective are required by regulations or legislation
- Relevance, alternative program designs, and comparative worth or merit must be assessed
- Financial issues or concerns
- Shortage of evaluation staff resources

from suspected malfeasance to heated competition for scarce funding; evaluation of the mandate for a program; evaluation of the continued relevance of a program and whether the program can be better delivered by another arrangement (e.g., private sector delivers a pubic sector program); evaluations that render an evaluative judgment to terminate or continue a program; evaluations that assess the merit or worth of a program in comparison with alternative choices; and circumstances where the program sponsors demand an objective, outside perspective to ensure the credibility of the evaluation findings.

Table 22.2 also summarizes a number of conditions where an *external evaluation is strongly recommended*, usually for practical reasons. When an organization has limited internal evaluation staff, it can be a wise choice to meet its evaluation needs by seeking external evaluators who have sufficient expertise and human resources. This solution works well when the evaluation requires a fresh perspective, special evaluation proficiency or technology, subject matter expertise, broad experience with evaluating similar programs in other organizations, or has a tight timeline. It is also a wise option when the scope of the evaluation spans multiple sites, geographic locations, or levels of government. If some of these conditions exist and external evaluators with the right skills and experience are hired, there also can be efficiencies that result in lower costs.

Who Should Evaluate?

In keeping with the *AEA Guiding Principles for Evaluators* (2018), in my own professional practice I follow a systematic process for deciding whether an external or internal evaluator should evaluate a specific program.

My position on this point is clear:

> . . . the choice of whether an evaluator should be external or internal depends on the purpose of the evaluation and a careful consideration of who is in the best position to conduct the evaluation. In some cases it is internal evaluators, but in other cases it is external evaluators. (interview with Arnold Love, in Volkov, 2011b, p. 6)

The highly respected textbook *Program Evaluation: Alternative Approaches and Practical Guidelines* (Fitzpatrick et al., 2010) describes in detail the systematic steps professional evaluators use for designing program evaluations. Selecting whether the evaluator should be internal or external is the *second step* in the process. The first step is obtaining background information about the program, learning the purposes and use of the evaluation, understanding the program's major evaluation information needs and evaluation questions from the interest holders' perspective, clarifying the resources and time available for the evaluation, and discussing the program and organizational context. This leads to the second step in planning an evaluation: Who should evaluate, an external evaluator or an internal evaluator?

For several decades, the evaluation field has been using a general guideline to maximize the

BOX 22.2. Example 2: External Evaluators Augment Internal Evaluators

A medium-size agency that assists immigrant families wanted to gain a better understanding of the social needs of immigrant youth who were 12–18 years old. The agency needed this information quickly to meet grant submission deadlines. The agency had two internal evaluators who were able to do a literature scan, speak with key informants from other settlement agencies, and analyze a wide variety of quantitative data about the youth in this target group. To provide an in-depth qualitative view of the needs of the immigrant youth within a 3-week timeframe, the agency hired external evaluators with sufficient skilled staff and current technology to collect valid and reliable data using computer-assisted telephone surveys, online panel sessions, and youth-moderated online conversation groups.

benefit and minimize the risk associated with the decision to use internal or external evaluators. The guideline has its genesis in Edward Suchman's (1967) classic distinction between **formative evaluation** and **summative evaluation**. According to Suchman, formative evaluation serves to shape the direction of a program and help it to "form" or "develop" into a program capable of producing its intended outcomes. In contrast, summative evaluation "adds up" or "sums together" the overall results of a program in terms of its outcomes, and perhaps also its longer-term impacts and cost benefit.

The distinction between formative and summative evaluation is easier to picture by looking at a diagram of the program life cycle in Figure 22.1. This diagram is based on the notion that there is a sequence of events during the life cycle of a program. At Stage 1 the evaluator affirms that there is a genuine need for the program and the need is not already being met by existing services or supports. Through a review of the evidence-based literature and evaluator discussions with expert advisors, the evaluator verifies that a new *program*, rather than another strategy, is a reasonable response to reduce or eliminate the need.

If these conditions are met, in Stage 2 the evaluator assists in the design of the program by assessing the organizational and program contexts, clarifying the longer-term outcomes of the program, specifying the shorter-term outcomes that must be attained to achieve the longer-term outcomes, and then identifying the right activities to attain those shorter-term outcomes. The evaluator checks a draft **logic model** for evidence of its efficacy to produce the desired outcomes and then supplements the logic model with a durable and testable **theory of change**. At this point, the evaluator works with the program to specify accurately the resources (fiscal, human, intellectual) needed to implement the program and drafts operational plans together with suitable performance indicators (e.g., number of persons served, number of staff, locations, intensity of services).

Now that the need for the program has been established and the design and operational plan assessed, in Stage 3 the evaluator assesses the actual implementation of the program. This stage usually takes place in at least two parts: (1) conducting an initial pilot test of the design of the program, including its draft logic model and theory of change, the cogency of the opera-

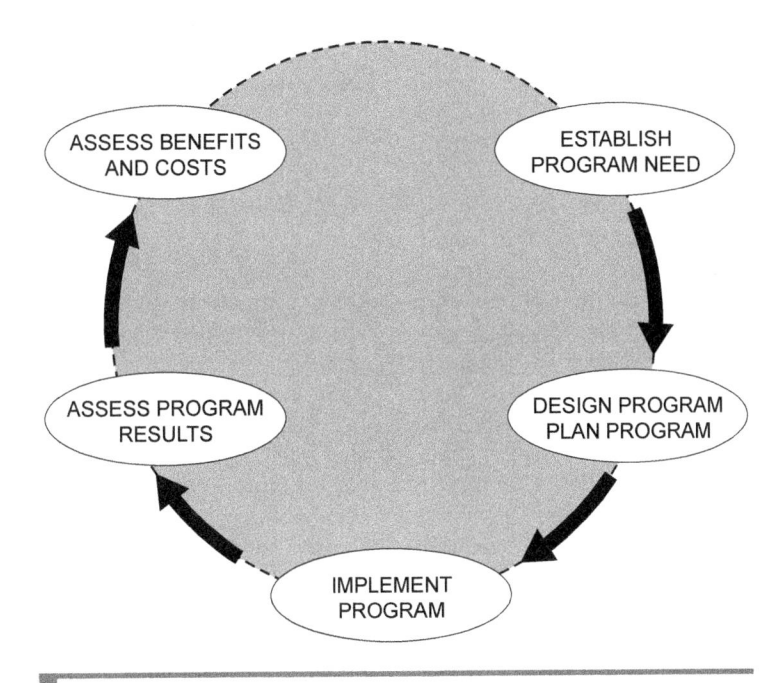

FIGURE 22.1. Diagram of program life cycle. From Arnold Love, PhD, Research and Evaluation Strategy Keynote, 2013.

tional plan, influences of the organizational and program contexts, and, after the initial bugs are corrected; (2) establishing ongoing monitoring of the implementation of the program.

As the program is being pilot tested and then implemented, in Stage 4 the evaluator appraises the effectiveness of the program to achieve the short-term outcomes in terms of its effects on program participants, both intended effects and unintended consequences. The shortest-term outcomes are "immediate" outcomes—for example, whether a skill was learned during a training session—whereas other short-term outcomes may take weeks or months to achieve, depending on the design of the program. Finally, after the program has been implemented fully and judged capable of producing results, in Stage 5 the evaluator assesses the longer-term outcomes, perhaps months or even years after the program is completed. For example, the evaluation of the comparative effectiveness of university education delivered via recorded lectures and online group discussions on increasing the students' income level may take several years after graduation to discern conclusively. After a period of time, a decision may be taken to repeat the program life cycle by reverting to Stage 1 and verifying the continued need for the program and the whether the mandate for the program should be extended in its current form or modified.

We have seen that formative evaluation shapes the direction of a program and helps it to develop into a program capable of producing its intended longer-term outcomes and that summative evaluation "adds up" the overall results of a program with respect to its longer-term outcomes. With this in mind and looking again at Figure 22.1, we see that Stages 1–4 are formative evaluation and Stage 5 is summative evaluation.

The general guideline applied in the evaluation field is that internal evaluators have unique strengths and very few limitations when conducting formative evaluations. Formative evaluations give guidance to those delivering the program by monitoring performance indicators to ensure that the program is on track and providing timely feedback for program improvement. In contrast, *the general guideline is that external evaluators are seen as having more credibility, and perhaps more robust knowledge and capability, when conducting summative evaluations* to inform legislators, funders, and others accountable for results about the comparative worth or merit of a program.

Choosing whether to use internal or external evaluators is an important decision that must be made early in the program evaluation planning process. Understanding the comparative strengths of internal and external evaluation and carefully considering the program's place in the program life cycle provides useful guidelines for making this decision.

> **BOX 22.3. Example 3: Internal Evaluators "Tasting the Soup"**
>
> This general guideline is captured nicely in Robert Stake's well-known analogy: "When the cook tastes the soup, that's formative evaluation; when the guest tastes it, that's summative evaluation" (cited by Scriven, 1991, p. 19). In this case, *internal evaluators* help the program managers and staff to "taste the soup" as it's being cooked so they can make timely adjustments to the recipe. *External evaluators*, such as food critics, can help potential customers know how well the soup compares to a culinary standard or to competitors' offerings. This combination of internal and external evaluation helps the chef to improve the recipe and then provide critical information to customers and owners about the comparative quality of the soup.

ROLES OF INTERNAL EVALUATORS

The early history of internal evaluation was often characterized by friction between managers and evaluators caused by lack of recognition that *both* managers and evaluators have complementary roles and responsibilities throughout the internal evaluation process (Love, 1991; Mathison, 1991). The "new vision of evaluation" that emerged in the early 2000s conceptualized internal evaluation as an *ongoing process* within organizations, a process that fosters program improvement, accountability, and learning. In this vision, internal evaluators do evaluation *with* program managers and staff rather doing evaluation *to* managers and staff. In other words, the "new vision" sees successful internal evaluators as working closely with managers and program delivery staff to provide the feedback essential for staying on track, correcting problems, and achieving success.

Portrait of the Internal Evaluator

The roles of internal evaluators is arguably the theme that receives the most attention in the internal evaluation literature and remains a perennial discussion topic at evaluation conferences. This includes understanding the range of roles internal evaluators play, identifying successful and unsuccessful roles, and managing role conflicts. In the quote below, Aaron Wildavsky (1979) vividly depicts the challenging and often conflicting roles that internal evaluators play:

> Evaluators must become agents of change in favor of programs as yet unborn and clienteles still unknown. Prepared to impose change on others, evaluators must have stability to stick with their own work. They must hang on to their own organization while preparing to abandon it. They must combine political feasibility with analytic purity. Only a brave individual would predict that these qualities can be found in one and the same person and organization. (p. 213)

Both supporters and critics of internal evaluation agree on the same thing: It is not easy to be an internal evaluator. It is vital that internal evaluators avoid roles that are known to be unsuccessful and to assume roles more likely to be successful. Table 22.3 presents some typical roles for internal evaluators, both the successful roles and the unsuccessful ones.

Successful Roles of Internal Evaluators

In order for internal evaluation to achieve its potential within organizations, internal evaluators must assume proactive and challenging roles. Some roles may not be relevant or possible to implement in a specific setting. The roles all demand that internal evaluators have a well-balanced set of interpersonal and technical skills, together with a strong moral and ethical compass. Table 22.3 presents a number of successful roles of internal evaluators that are valued by organizations and rewarding for the evaluators themselves.

Honest Broker

Arguably at no time in recent history are honest brokers more needed than now. A reliable compass is needed to navigate an organization in a climate that promotes conflicting views about the nature of truth, sanctions division and the dominance of powerful interest groups, and questions findings based on evidence while promoting partisan views. As championed by Wildavsky (1972), internal evaluators have the important role of *speaking truth to power* and steadily challenging the notion that *power determines the truth.*

Navigator

A number of years ago in Hawaii I gave a workshop about internal evaluation to diverse nonprofit and community organizations. After listening for a while, some Native Hawaiians told the group that in their tradition, the *kilo hōkū*, or navigators, guided their ancestors as they struggled to find their way across the Pacific Ocean. They saw the similarities—the internal evaluator was like a navigator who accompanied each voyage. The internal evaluator used evaluation data points to guide programs and the organization, just as traditional navigators used cues from the stars, winds, and seas to safely guide the captain and crew on their dangerous journey across the vast ocean from one small island to another.

TABLE 22.3. Typical Successful and Unsuccessful Roles of Internal Evaluators

Successful roles
• Honest broker
• Navigator
• Management consultant
• Change agent
• Information specialist
• Evaluation facilitator

Unsuccessful roles
• Spy
• Number cruncher
• Archaeologist
• Publicity agent
• Quibbler
• Terminator

Management Consultant

Acting as a management consultant is a positive role for internal evaluators who have formal training in management (or a related area) and field experience in managing several areas of their organization. Internal evaluators with management and field experience, together with a reputation for integrity and access to senior managers, have the credibility needed to diagnose problems and recommend solutions. These internal evaluators consult with managers on the use of data-based evaluation approaches for setting strategic goals and performance indicators, monitoring and improving program performance, and assessing outcomes. In the management consultant's role, the internal evaluator acts as a leader who contributes actively to the organization's current operations and helps to create its future successes.

Change Agent

In this positive role, internal evaluators are change agents who use their evaluation skills to foster organizational learning and promote change. Internal evaluators play an active role in assessing the outcomes of major change initiatives and the organizational development efforts that comprise those initiatives. For example, evaluation may be used to assess and improve a pilot test of cross-functional team building that is part of a longer-term initiative to develop stronger teams that are capable of working together seamlessly on complex projects.

Information Specialist

Internal evaluators support managers and staff by providing information they need to avoid pitfalls, ensure that programs and projects are on track, and make the best use of information systems to improve overall results. They are able to employ the latest technology and methods for analyzing and synthesizing data about the organization's internal and external environment to develop alternate futures for deliberation by management. Internal evaluators in this role are expert at analyzing the organization's information needs, designing data systems, ensuring data integrity, using technology to support the evaluation process, providing actionable evaluative information, and helping to mobilize evaluation findings into action.

Evaluation Facilitator

In the facilitator role, the internal evaluator supports project planning and implementation as a member of a project team. The evaluator educates the members of the team about evaluation, integrates evaluation into the project life cycle, and demonstrates how evaluation data provides guidance for project management. The internal evaluator advocates for data-oriented decision making and facilitates the evaluation capacity building in the members of the group.

Unsuccessful Roles of Internal Evaluators

Table 22.3 also lists some well-known but unsuccessful roles of internal evaluators. I have given each role a tongue-in-cheek descriptor to make it more memorable: spy, number cruncher, archaeologist, publicity agent, quibbler, and terminator. Unfortunately, these negative roles are not rare and I have seen each more than once in my professional career.

Spy

Instead of evaluating the program, the internal evaluator collects information about the job performance of individuals and relays this information to management. This role violates evaluation's ethical principles, perverts its purposes, and creates enduring resistance to the evaluation process.

Number Cruncher

The number cruncher presents the caricature of an isolated technician who avoids interaction with others in the organization. By relying exclusively on analyses from data systems, without validating and balancing them with direct feedback from staff and clients, the number cruncher often draws wrong or irrelevant conclusions. As a result, the number cruncher builds resentment while contributing little information of value for decision making or program improvement.

Archaeologist

In the role of archaeologist the internal evaluator rummages through legacy databases containing archived data. With great effort the evaluator tries to assemble these "bones" and interpret the findings. Rarely do managers or staff use this outdated information for decision making. At worst, the internal evaluator is irrelevant. At best, the internal evaluator is relegated to the role of a data archaeologist, rather than as a guide for the present and a builder of the future.

Publicity Agent

In the role of publicity agent, the internal evaluator succumbs to political pressure from management by focusing only on program successes and ignoring gaps, shortcomings, or failures. In some cases, the evaluator deliberately covers up problems. This is an egregious example of pseudoevaluation masquerading as genuine evaluation. Rather than acting as an evaluation professional rendering a fair assessment of a program, the internal evaluator is merely a publicity agent or cheerleader for the program or organization.

Quibbler

Whereas the "publicity agent" looks for success alone, internal evaluators in the "quibbler" role do their best to catch a program making trivial mistakes, while avoiding the important findings. The quibbler appears to have little empathy with the pressures that the real world places on managers and staff. As a result, the quibbler lacks perspective and presents slanted evaluation reports that "stone the program to death with popcorn." This undermines both the confidence in the program and the integrity of the evaluation process.

Terminator

The internal evaluator in a terminator role demonstrates bias against a program. This is another form of pseudoevaluation. Instead of a data-based approach to the evaluation, the internal evaluator deliberately collects negative information to support a *predetermined conclusion* that the program, manager, or staff are performing poorly and should be terminated.

Complementary Roles of Managers and Internal Evaluators

In the "new vision" of evaluation, managers and internal evaluators have complementary responsibilities for evaluation (Love, 2004). Managers carry the organizational responsibility for evaluation, as part of their manager's role. In turn, internal evaluators have the responsibility for assessing evaluation information needs, determining the feasibility of meeting needs with existing information, and creating alternative designs. Both managers and internal evaluators together have the responsibility for deciding what data are needed and ensuring the integrity of the data. Internal evaluators have the responsibility for creating alternative evaluation designs, assessing the usefulness of information (timeliness, value, cost), collecting dependable data in an ethical way, analyzing the data, and communicating evaluation findings. Managers in turn hold the primary responsibility for weighing the evaluation findings, considering the political and organizational implications of implementing changes, and deciding on a course of action. Internal evaluators have the responsibility for establishing monitoring indicators and monitoring the implementation of action plans that are faithful to the evaluation findings.

Understanding and successfully managing the roles of the internal evaluator is a perennial topic of discussion and debate. Get the roles right and life is good; get the roles wrong, then not so much. For the interested reader, Boris Volkov (2011a) offers an insightful review of the multiplicity of roles of the internal evaluator.

MAJOR MODELS OF INTERNAL EVALUATION

This section examines some of the common models of the internal evaluation function. The term *model* refers to the way internal evaluation is structured within an organization. The expression **"internal evaluation function"** is a generic term that covers the full range of internal evaluation models, ranging from a mom-and-pop shop with a couple of part-time evalu-

TABLE 22.4. Major Models of Internal Evaluation

- Part-time internal evaluator
- Independent internal evaluation unit
- Embedded internal evaluator
- Hybrid internal evaluation model
- Nonspecialist internal evaluators
- Closely bound contractors

ators, to independent evaluation units, and even to self-evaluating organizations with internal evaluators embedded into program teams—and everything in between. Space doesn't permit addressing the infinite variety of models, so this section concentrates on the models used most often (see Table 22.4): part-time internal evaluator, independent internal evaluator unit, embedded internal evaluator, hybrid internal evaluation model, and the use of trained nonspecialist internal evaluators. It also discusses the use of closely bound contractors as internal evaluators across all internal evaluation models.

Part-Time Internal Evaluator

The simplest model of internal evaluation is that of the *part-time internal evaluator*. It is often the only model possible for organizations with limited resources for evaluation. Usually the internal evaluator is a full-time employee but carries only part-time evaluation responsibilities, typically 2 or 3 days per week. For the rest of the time, the part-time evaluator usually holds the position of a program manager, team leader, or similar management responsibility. In terms of responsibilities, part-time internal evaluators usually work cooperatively with service delivery managers and the organization's support staff (e.g., information system staff, records clerks, customer support workers) to develop an evaluation system that supplies a steady stream of the data needed for monitoring program implementation and basic evaluation information, such as client satisfaction data; achievement of performance indicators; strengths and weaknesses of programs; attainment of shorter-term outcomes; and specific data needed for annual reports, audits, and funding applications.

The part-time model is practical, efficient, supplies essential evaluation information, and positions the internal evaluator as part of the organization's management team, rather than as a technical specialist who operates in isolation from the organization's managers. Being a member of the management team allows the part-time internal evaluator to assume *successful internal evaluation roles* that are highly valued by the organization.

Embedded Internal Evaluator Model

Since the 1990s, a variety of internal evaluation models have emerged in response to the new evaluation approaches designed for ongoing program improvement, organizational learning, and enhancing community outcomes. Some examples of the newer approaches to evaluation include participatory, empowerment, developmental, community-oriented, and deliberative democratic evaluation. A popular internal evaluation model for implementing these approaches is known as the "embedded evaluator" model. In this model the internal evaluator is said to be a member of a project team, or in evaluation lingo, the internal evaluator is *embedded* in the team.

If an internal evaluator is part of the team that designs and implements a project or program, isn't the objectivity of the evaluator compromised? As we saw earlier, an internal evaluator ordinarily is not an impediment when the evaluation is *formative* and used for improving programs and enhancing organizational learning and development, rather than for accountability. In fact, there often is a distinct preference for an internal evaluator because of the internal evaluator's knowledge and understanding of the organizational context, subject matter expertise, and field experience.

> **BOX 22.4. Example 4: Part-Time Internal Evaluation in a Small Nonprofit**
>
> A small nonprofit agency with few staff and limited budget found it essential to have evaluation information for grant and funding applications and to meet new reporting requirements for nonprofits. The agency uses a part-time internal evaluator to obtain feedback from clients, collaborate better with its partners, and assess the difference it is making for its clients and the community.

> **BOX 22.5. Example 5: Embedded Internal Evaluator**
>
> The Board of Directors of a large charity that funds new projects run by local groups needs evaluation data to prove to donors that their money is producing real results in areas of prime community concern. The CEO decides to embed an internal evaluator in each project team. The evaluator builds the capacity of the team to assess and continuously improve the projects, while supplying feedback to the charity that will improve its strategic grant-making ability.

As a member of a project team, the internal evaluator first educates the other team members about the role of the evaluation process in project management and program development. Next, the embedded evaluator works together with the team to assess their evaluation information needs and then design and implement the evaluation. Throughout the evaluation process the internal evaluator acts as an *evaluation facilitator* by working with the team to interpret the evaluation results in actionable terms, and empowering them to apply the findings for data-based decision making. Over time, through this coaching process, the project team builds its capacity for evaluation. Within a year or so, the project team is empowered to conduct basic evaluations: assess clients' needs, validate program theory, improve program performance by monitoring key performance indicators, and apply their findings to organizational learning and change.

This is a flexible model that allows internal evaluators to be embedded in a number of teams, yet it is highly efficient, so the internal evaluator has time available for evaluations of strategic value to the entire organization. This model is an excellent fit with organizations that have a distributed or network management model that is organized around project teams, rather than having a hierarchical or departmental structure. As the project teams build evaluation capacity over time, the embedded evaluator switches to a mentor or consultant role as other team members take the evaluation lead. As a result, after learning the basics of evaluative thinking and practical evaluation skills from an experienced evaluator, those team members can serve as the evaluation lead in other project teams, thus further integrating evaluation into the entire organization.

Internal Evaluation Unit

The *internal departmental model* tends to be found in larger organizations that have one or more *evaluation units*. The actual number of internal evaluators working in the unit may be small, sometimes only two or three full-time evaluators, perhaps with a few part-time special supports (e.g., project managers, data analysts). In my experience, the average number of internal evaluators is about five, but large government departments or agencies may have 20 or more internal evaluators, plus several supporting specialists (quantitative and qualitative data analysts, database managers, survey specialists, online metrics specialists, data presentation specialists).

Over the decades, there has been much controversy concerning the nature of evaluation units and how one defines whether they are really external or internal (see Alkin & Vo, 2018, for a recent discussion). Currently, the term *independent evaluation unit* is being used to stress the separation and objectivity of the evaluation function.

Because the traditional focus of independent evaluation units is *accountability for outcomes or longer-term impact*, this perceived objectivity is important. To emphasize its objectivity, an independent evaluation unit usually occupies a separate position on the organizational chart (or organogram), has its own director or head, and reports directly to the highest levels in the organization or to the body that has oversight responsibility.

In their comprehensive book, *Enhancing Evaluation Use: Insights from Internal Evalu-*

> **BOX 22.6. Example 6: Independent Internal Evaluation Unit**
>
> The U.S. General Accountability Office (GAO) reports on federal programs and services. To make plain the independence of its evaluation function, the mission statement of the GAO states clearly that it serves Congress and the American people. To reinforce this independence, the GAO is led by the comptroller general of the United States.

ation Units, Loud and Mayne (2014) provide an insider's glimpse into the latest efforts of organizations in a number of countries to develop effective independent internal evaluation units that are relevant and systematic, while struggling to manage the complex interplay of power, red tape, rituals, rigidity, and inveterate self-interest inherent in organizational life. This web of structures and interactions raises the fundamental issue of whether an independent internal evaluation unit can be truly independent.

For nearly a half-century, critics have expressed concern that the complete "independence" of an independent evaluation unit is an illusion. Some benign critics offer the analogy of "fish swimming in an aquarium" that are not aware of their surrounding environment (assumptions, values, scope). Without a way to examine and challenge their basic assumptions, the fish mistake the narrow confines of the aquarium as the freedom of open waters. Less forgiving critics have voiced concerns that independent evaluation units can mirror the "fort-within-a-fort" mentality of an isolated and defensive evaluation unit within an isolated and defensive organization—one that is inward looking and captive to its own narrow assumptions, values, and mandates.

Internal evaluation expert Bastiaan de Laat (2014) has come to the conclusion that the classic dichotomy in the evaluation literature between external and internal evaluator is false. This dichotomy equates the external evaluator with independent evaluation and associates the internal evaluator with biased evaluation. In his view, valid evaluation depends not so much on whether the evaluator is external or internal but on the *arrangements built into the different organizational settings to safeguard the independence of the evaluator, even if the evaluation is internal*. It is particularly important that the roles of the person who commissions the evaluation (commissioner) and the person who manages the program being evaluated (evaluand) be separated (Bastiaan de Laat, personal communication, October 10, 2013).

Loud and Mayne (2014) note that the independence of internal evaluation units can be greatly enhanced by additional measures, such as keeping the evaluation unit independent from line management, involving *advisory committees* to review methodologies and find-

> **BOX 22.7. Example 7: Multiple Internal Evaluation Units**
>
> An international development aid organization has an evaluation unit at headquarters that sets evaluation standards and guidelines, digests high-level evaluation findings, and reports its findings to the executive directors and major interest holders of the organization. The organization also has regional evaluation units and country-level evaluation units, and sector-specific evaluation units (e.g., education sector, agricultural sector, health sector) that cut across regions and countries, as well as project-level evaluation units.

ings, and introducing *reporting mechanisms* to identify pressures or obstructions during the evaluation process. Complicating the situation, larger organizations often have more than one type of internal evaluation unit. These multiple evaluation units can appear like Matryoshka (nesting) dolls, where you open one and another appears inside, or like recursive reflections in an infinite mirror, each generally similar but with a different mission and level of independence.

Hybrid Internal Evaluation Model

We have learned earlier that both internal and external evaluation have their strengths and limitations, and the same is true for the various models of structuring the internal evaluation function. In recent years, the search for a more adequate structure that takes advantage of the strengths of both internal and external evaluation has led to the *hybrid internal evaluation model*. In this model, external evaluators concentrate on the assessment of outcomes and other requirements that demand greater independence and/or specialized skills. They work together with internal evaluators to obtain the access to data they need to evaluate and interpret program outcomes accurately. Internal evaluators, for their part, concentrate on the formative aspects of the program, such as conducting needs assessments, drafting and testing logic models and theories of change, creating performance measures, providing feedback about program activities, and pilot testing early program implementation for coherence with the program plan and its ability to generate immediate and shorter-term outcomes.

Mathison (2011) has noted that the hybrid approach creates a functional partnership that actively engages internal evaluators and interest holders and the external evaluators in the design and implementation of the evaluation. Le Menestrel et al. (2014) identify several factors that need to be considered when deciding whether to use a hybrid approach. The first factor is the purpose of the evaluation. A major benefit of the hybrid model is that it brings "outsider" expertise, broad experience, and an independent viewpoint at the time in the program cycle where those attributes are most valuable—namely, at the summative phase (i.e., Stage 5 in the program life cycle discussed earlier). An organization with a strong culture of internal evaluation is likely to make good use of the hybrid approach. Collaboration between internal and external evaluators can increase the external evaluators' understanding of the organizational context and "open the black box," thereby facilitating improvements in the evaluation design and implementation. Finally, even when the evaluation is focused on outcomes, Volkov (2011b) observed that the increased emphasis on internal accountability and performance measurement by organizations encourages both external and internal evaluators to work together to assess outcomes.

Closely Bound Internal Evaluation Contractors

Both external evaluators and **closely bound internal evaluators** work under contract, except for one major distinguishing feature: these internal evaluators do not have the independence from the organization usually found with external evaluators. Before you begin flipping through your legal dictionary, let me clarify the distinction. These internal evaluators may be full- or part-time evaluators, or they may be embedded in a project team or a member of an internal evaluation unit. In any scenario, the key is that they are not employees of the organization. Instead they work *within* an organization and are "closely bound" to the organization through reporting relationships and contractual obligations. In contrast, although external evaluators also work under contract, their reporting relationships and source of remuneration is with a body (e.g., funding, regulative, legislative) that is at arm's length from the organization they are evaluating.

Closely bound internal evaluators have distinct benefits for both the organization and the evaluators. As discussed earlier, the main reason organizations hire external evaluators is because they have specialized skills and a wide range of evaluation experience. An organization can offer a skilled and experienced external evaluator a long-term assignment, usually for a specific number of days per week at an affordable rate, and have them work directly with the organization's managers and staff, as if they were part of the team. This desirable arrangement provides the closely bound evaluator with a stable base income together with the flexibility to accept other evaluation assignments. Once closely bound contractors are hired, they become part of the organization's team, acquire a firsthand understanding of the organization and how to work effectively with its members and culture, and become a valuable asset to the organization.

Nonspecialist Internal Evaluators

The COVID-19 pandemic accelerated the need for internal evaluators to help organizations respond to new challenges and make adaptive changes. Given a finite supply of professional evaluators, whether they are internal evaluators or external evaluators hired at contract, there is a now growing trend to expand internal evaluation resources by training **nonspecialist evaluators**. The specialist evaluator is a professional evaluator with evaluation as the core function. While the specialist internal evaluator may be expected to be able to design and lead a complete evaluation, no such expectation exists for the nonspecialist. Nonspecialists may include senior managers, team leaders, and professionals from other fields who are systematically educated to acquire evaluative thinking and evaluation skills, and then to apply evaluation to enhance their own work. In other words, nonspecialists initiate and support internal evaluation and its use, while retaining their principal roles and continuing their respective professional work. A recent article by Lam et al. (2023) presents a variety of key considerations and illustrative case examples for educating and using nonspecialist internal evaluators in a wide range of settings.

DEVELOPING EFFECTIVE INTERNAL EVALUATION CAPABILITY

In previous sections we have seen that there are a variety of models for structuring internal evaluation and successful roles for internal evaluators to play. Irrespective of the structure of internal evaluation or the number of positive roles evaluators play, internal evaluation *must become an integral part of organizational culture* to be truly useful and valued. Elsewhere I have described how the internal evaluation becomes a substantial asset once it is applied *systematically* across all program areas (Love, 1991). The benefits from systematic internal evaluation can be fully accrued only after the organization has built sufficient *evaluation capability*. Organizations face the difficult task of continuously developing evaluation capability across the entire organization while cultivating the relevance and credibility of ongoing internal evaluations.

Key Factors in Developing Internal Evaluation Capability

The sections below outline the *key factors* that are essential for developing effective internal evaluation capability (see also Table 22.5). The key factors are clustered into three areas: (1) organizational support for evaluation, (2) organizational structure, and (3) organizational culture.

Organizational Support

Organizational support is the foundation for effective internal evaluation. In order to engage managers and staff in evaluation, the Board of Directors and senior management (CEO and executive managers) must provide tangible and unequivocal proof of their commitment to internal evaluation. Senior management demonstrates this commitment through a clearly stated evaluation policy, sufficient and stable funding for internal evaluation, adequate staffing by skilled evaluation staff, and a suitable timeframe that allows internal evaluation to systematically build evaluation capability while operating in sync with the organization's planning and budget cycle.

Organizational Structure

The structure of an organization has repeatedly been identified as fundamental to the successful development and implementation of internal evaluation. Although a thorough discussion is beyond the scope of this chapter, two factors have already been identified—that is, role definitions and the location of the internal evaluation unit.

We have already examined positive and negative role definitions for internal evaluators. One common thread is that an internal evaluator usually has several roles in the organization and that the effectiveness of these roles is closely linked to the structural connections between evaluators and other members of the organization. Another important finding is that internal evaluators who have had frontline and/or management experience in the organization are more likely to be seen as having positive roles and their judgment as being credible, independent, and realistic.

The independence and influence of the internal evaluation function correlates with the level of reporting relationship. For an evaluation function to have the greatest independence and influence if its purpose includes accountability for results, then the head of the internal evaluation function should report to the Board of Directors of the organization. If that is not possible, then the head of evaluation should report to the CEO or a senior vice president of the organization. As a general rule, as the internal evaluation function reports to successively lower levels in the management hierarchy, not only is the independence and influence of the evaluation function diminished but also a tipping point can be reached where the fundamental credibility of the entire internal evaluation function evaporates completely.

Organizational Culture

Achieving the full potential of internal evaluation benefits from a strong evaluation culture

TABLE 22.5. Key Factors in Building Internal Evaluation Capacity

- Organizational support
- Organizational structure
- Organizational culture

throughout the organization. Evaluation capacity building (ECB) is an important tool for growing an evaluation culture for internal evaluation. For example, *The Art, Craft, and Science of Evaluation Capacity Building* (Baizerman et al., 2002) illustrates ECB applied within diverse organizations, such as the Centers for Disease Control and Prevention, American Cancer Society, World Bank, and in school districts. Case studies show that organizations implement ECB in a number of ways, such as offering basic evaluation courses, mentoring, internships and placements, specialized evaluation workshops, and undertaking evaluations in collaboration with staff and clients. The education of nonspecialist evaluators is emerging as another important tool for building an evaluative culture (Lam et al., 2023). Of special value to internal evaluators, Boris Volkov and Jean King (2007) have written a "checklist for building evaluation capacity," designed specifically for using ECB to support internal evaluation.

In summary, organizations with an effective internal evaluation capability tend to have adequate organizational support, strong organizational structure, and an organizational culture that nurtures internal evaluation. Such organizations evidence top management support for evaluation, positive leadership by the head of the internal evaluation function, adequate resources and skilled evaluators, clear evaluation policies and lines of authority and accountability, an organizational culture that supports continual learning, integration of evaluation into the culture of the organization, and a highly visible presence of internal evaluation as an integral part of the organization and its commitment to results.

MANAGING THE INTERNAL EVALUATION RESOURCE

Effective internal evaluation resource management has the goal of improving the availability, accessibility, and use of evaluative information within the organization, while simultaneously supporting individual evaluators or project teams so they can respond to evaluation requests in a timely manner. This section offers some practical suggestions that will help you avoid or correct common failings that seriously impair the management of internal evaluation as a corporate resource.

Formal Process

If I were allowed to offer only one practical suggestion to internal evaluators, it would be this: *Follow a formal process* for managing your evaluation work and avoid the temptation to be informal. A formal process achieves at least two important objectives. First of all, it helps avoid the debilitating effects of *role confusion* caused by the ambiguity of the multiple roles of the internal evaluator (Mathison, 1991; Volkov, 2011b; Rogers et al., 2019). Without a formal process for receiving evaluation requests and assessing the requests carefully, it is common for internal evaluators to be inundated and then overwhelmed by routine or informal requests. Not only is any sense of priority abandoned, internal evaluators find that they don't have sufficient time for strategic and emergency evaluations. The sections below highlight some important aspects of managing the internal evaluation function that require a formal process.

Receive an Evaluation Request

The internal evaluation planning sequence begins by receiving a *letter* or *memo of request* for an evaluation. The request triggers an initial meeting to clarify the purposes of the evaluation, identify evaluation users, obtain background information, and assess the feasibility of the request.

Letter of Confirmation

If the evaluation is feasible, then a *letter* or *memo of confirmation* from internal evaluation follows. It confirms the understanding about the evaluation information needs, major evaluation issues, purposes and scope of the evaluation, timeframe, estimated resources from internal evaluation and from those requesting the evaluation, and agreement regarding evaluation authority and approval steps.

Terms of Reference

Once the request is confirmed, internal evaluation drafts a formal *terms of reference* (TOR). The TOR states the objectives of the evaluation, primary and secondary users of evaluation information, scope of the work, potential evaluation/ethical issues and how they will be addressed, internal evaluator(s) assigned to the evaluation, reporting relationships, mutual responsibilities of the internal evaluators and those requesting the evaluation, overall design of the evaluation and overview of methodology, procedures for amending the evaluation plan, and the main deliverables with a timeline for their completion.

Within an organization, the signed and dated TOR serves as a contract for the internal evaluation. To emphasize the importance of the TOR: Although one wouldn't expect an external evaluation without a contract being negotiated and signed, in my experience it is still rare to find internal evaluation shops that have a signed TOR. Many of the persistent problems faced by internal evaluators could be avoided by taking the step of including a signed TOR in the evaluation planning process (see Table 22.6).

Evaluation Work Plan

Whereas the *evaluation TOR* is the contract between the internal evaluators and their clients in the organization, the *evaluation work plan* is the management plan for each evaluation. The evaluation work plan usually includes a synopsis of reasons for the evaluation, purposes and scope, specific tasks and evaluation approaches used to achieve the study purpose, methodology and a list of tasks with due dates and person(s) responsible for each task (internal evaluators and others), overall completion date of the evaluation, methods for communicating evaluation findings (e.g., written reports, briefings, presentations) and timeline for reporting (e.g., monthly, interim report, final report), audience(s) for reporting evaluation findings and type of information required (e.g., one-page talking points, **webinar** summary, detailed findings), travel and resources required, and budget with breakdown and expenditure limits. The initial evaluation work plan should be as detailed as possible and revised quarterly as the evaluation is implemented and the situation evolves.

Evaluation Methods

In my experience, it is possible for internal evaluators to use any evaluation methodology. The choice of methods is usually limited only by the purposes of the evaluation, the organizational context, and available resources. High-tech social media companies, for example, have internal evaluators run sophisticated experimental evaluations that test each proposed change in their services. A small community organization may use more basic descriptive methods, such as feedback questionnaires and focus groups with parents and youth to assess satisfaction with a summer camp program and possible improvements. Many organizations of all sizes, however, have switched to online or hybrid service delivery as a result of the COVID-19 pandemic. It is now common for the person responsible for online resources, website, and social media to work closely with internal evaluators and incorporate their metrics and analytics data into monitoring and evaluation efforts.

Data Integrity

A persistent problem for internal evaluation has been and continues to be the integrity (validity and dependability) of the data used for internal evaluation. I see this as a shared responsibility—both internal evaluators and managers and supervisors within the organization must work together to ensure data integrity. They both must confirm that policies and procedures are in place to verify the validity and dependability of the data. Evaluators have a special responsibility to test the data for accuracy by pulling samples from databases and comparing them with the original data entry forms. Although I have encountered instances where data tampering is deliberate, in my experience, poor supervision and inadequate monitoring of data entry cause most inaccuracies. Managers bear responsibility for correcting the situation. For example, with increased workloads for frontline staff, it is not unusual to find them entering a month's worth

---

TABLE 22.6. Internal Evaluation Terms of Reference

An internal evaluation terms of reference (TOR) contains:

- Statement of evaluation objectives
- List of potential evaluation issues
- Description of the evaluation project team
- Evaluation scope (e.g., major evaluation questions, data required, sources of data, staff resources needed, timeline, ways of sharing findings)
- Procedures for amending the evaluation overview
- Authority to undertake the evaluation
- Resources committed to the evaluation
- Main deliverables and due dates

of client contact data in the last day or two of the month from memory alone.

Knowledge Mobilization and Organizational Learning

As part of the internal evaluation planning process, internal evaluators are expected to develop a communications plan that addresses the evaluation issues and questions outlined in the TOR and tailors the findings and recommendations to the key audiences and major direct users of evaluation information. One of the key positive roles for internal evaluators is that of *evaluation facilitator*. In the facilitator's role, the evaluator not only presents evaluation findings and recommendations but also facilitates discussion about the implication of the findings for program improvement. The internal evaluator also facilitates the development of an action plan that describes actionable steps toward change. The responsibility for the action plan rests with management, but the internal evaluator develops indicators for monitoring the implementation of the action plan. The internal evaluator expedites organizational learning by leading a discussion about the relevance of the evaluation findings on other aspects of the organization, including strategic implications for the organization and policy implications for the organization and its partners.

Closing Procedures

The final step in the formal process for managing an internal evaluation relates to closing procedures. Although this varies somewhat, it usually involves a *letter* or *memo of closing* that summarizes the evaluation, specifies the key findings and elements of the action plan, appends a single page with key talking points and a three-page executive summary to the letter or memo, and is signed by the parties that signed the initial letter of confirmation and the TOR.

EXEMPLARY INTERNAL EVALUATION

As an example of an outstanding internal evaluation effort, I have selected the following summary for two reasons: (1) it illustrates the masterful application of many of the key principles, tips, and lessons presented in this chapter; and (2) the details of this case are available as a book

> **BOX 22.8. Example 8: Ontario School Improvement Project Internal Evaluation**
>
> The case presents a multiyear project to improve the Ontario public education system—the largest public education system in Canada. Dr. Keiko Kuji-Shikatani and her colleagues faced the challenge of designing an evaluation approach that met the demands for accountability while fostering the innovation, learning, and continuous adaptation required for system improvement. Improving the education system so it can achieve sustainable education outcomes, however, is a complex and long-term *learning* process that requires experimentation, testing of emergent strategies, and ongoing evaluation embedded into the system change efforts.

chapter (Kuji-Shikatani et al., 2016) for study by the interested reader.

Kuji-Shikatani and her colleagues applied a developmental evaluation approach that fostered evaluative thinking by using logic modeling to guide the process. Applying experiential learning methods, specialist internal evaluators educated formal and informal leaders about evaluation tools and methods at all system levels. These nonspecialist internal evaluators received tailored instructions on integrating evaluation tools and results into their professional roles. In turn, these nonspecialist evaluators infused evaluative thinking and promoted learning and system improvement.

As the leaders experienced the benefits of evaluative thinking, they began applying it throughout program planning and implementation cycles. Over time, nonspecialist internal evaluators collaborated to make evaluation education available across the public sector. As a result, evaluative thinking, evaluation education, and system innovation for nonspecialists developed strong roots and have flourished, as evidenced by tangible student outcomes (e.g., graduation rates, standardized test results, the closing of achievement gaps). Public response also has been positive.

CONCLUSIONS

In conclusion, I hope that this chapter gives you greater insight about internal evaluation and encourages you to delve more deeply into internal evaluation, either as a rewarding career path or as a component of your evaluation practice. Remember that you will learn a great deal from taking field notes about your internal evaluation experiences and discussing your thoughts with your evaluation clients and colleagues. This process will raise many questions. By considering the questions carefully, reading evaluation journals and books, experimenting with solutions, joining AEA's internal evaluation TIG, and sharing your experiences more broadly at local and national conferences and online, you will continue to expand your competency in internal evaluation and have interesting conversations at the same time.

REFERENCES

Alkin, M. C., & Vo, T. V. (2018). *Evaluation essentials: From A to Z* (2nd ed.). Guilford Press.

American Evaluation Association. (2014). Message from President Beverly Parsons AEA 2014 president: Reflect on your TIG memberships, share your thoughts. *AEA Newsletter, 14*(3), 1.

American Evaluation Association. (2018). *AEA guiding principles for evaluators*. Author.

Baizerman, M., Compton, D. W., & Stockdill, S. H. (Eds.). (2002). The art, craft, and science of evaluation capacity building. *New Directions for Evaluation*, 93.

de Laat, B. (2014). Evaluator, evaluand, evaluation commissioner. In M. L. Loud & J. Mayne (Eds.), *Enhancing evaluation use: Insights from internal evaluation units* (pp. 15–35). SAGE.

Fitzpatrick, J. L., Sanders, J. R., & Worthen, B. R. (2010). *Program evaluation: Alternative approaches and practical guidelines* (4th ed.). Pearson.

Kuji-Shikatani, K., Gallagher, M. J., Franz, R., & Börner, M. (2016). Leadership's role in building the education sector's capacity to use evaluative thinking: The example of the Ontario Ministry of Education. In M. Patton, K. McKegg, & N. Wehipeihana (Eds.), *Developmental evaluation exemplars: Principles in practice* (pp. 252–270). Guilford Press.

Lam, C. Y., Kuji-Shikatani, K., & Love, A. (2023). Meeting the challenges of educating internal evaluators. *New Directions for Evaluation*, 95–103.

Le Menestrel, S. M., Walahoski, J. S., & Mielke, M. B. (2014). A partnership model for evaluation: Considering an alternate approach to the internal–external evaluation debate. *American Journal of Evaluation, 35*(1), 61–72.

Loud, M. L., & Mayne, J. (Eds.). (2014). *Enhancing evaluation use: Insights from internal evaluation units*. SAGE.

Love, A. J. (1991). *Internal evaluation: Building organizations from within*. SAGE.

Love, A. J. (Ed.). (1993). Special issue on internal evaluation. *Canadian Journal of Program Evaluation, 8*(2).

Love, A. J. (2004). Internal evaluation. In S. Mathison (Ed.), *Encyclopedia of evaluation* (pp. 206–208). SAGE.

Love, A. (2015). Building the foundation of the CES professional designation program [Special issue]. *Canadian Journal of Program Evaluation, 29*(3), 1–20.

Love, A. (2022). Practical wisdom for evaluators: What it is and how to achieve it. In M. Hurteau & T. Archibald. (Eds.), *Practical wisdom for an ethical evaluation practice* (pp. 11–24). Information Age.

Mathison, S. (1991). Role conflicts for internal evaluators. *Evaluation and Program Planning, 14*(3), 173–179.

Mathison, S. (2011). Internal evaluation, historically speaking. *New Directions for Evaluation, 132*, 13–23.

Rogers, A., McCoy, A., & Kelly, L. M. (2019). Evaluation literacy: Perspectives of internal evaluators in non-government organizations. *Canadian Journal of Program Evaluation, 34*(1), 1–20.

Scriven, M. (1991). *Evaluation thesaurus* (4th ed.). SAGE.

Suchman, E. A. (1967). *Evaluative research*. SAGE.

Volkov, B. B. (2011a). Beyond being an evaluator: The multiplicity of roles of the internal evaluator. In B. B. Volkov & M. E. Baron (Eds.), *Internal evaluation in the 21st century* (pp. 25–42). *New Directions for Evaluation*, 132.

Volkov, B. B. (2011b). Internal evaluation a quarter-century later: A conversation with Arnold J. Love. In B. B. Volkov & M. E. Baron (Eds.), *Internal evaluation in the 21st century* (pp. 5–12). *New Directions for Evaluation*, 132.

Volkov, B. B., & King, J. A. (2007). *A checklist for building organizational evaluation capacity*. The Evaluation Center, Western Michigan University.

Wildavsky A. (1972). The self-evaluating organization. *Public Administration Review, 32*(5), 509–520.

Wildavsky, A. (1979). *Speaking truth to power: The art and craft of policy analysis*. Little, Brown.

Chapter 23

The Independent Consultant
An Insider's Guide to a Consulting Career

Gail Vallance Barrington

CHAPTER OVERVIEW

Independent consulting sounds attractive to many evaluators, but they must be willing to overcome start-up challenges and the changing demands of the field. This chapter describes the consulting landscape and focuses on evaluation services. The personality traits and ethics needed to be successful are described. Key requirements for start-up are explored, including financial stability, a sound business plan, and essential business systems and processes. The chapter examines marketing strategies and both formal and informal ways to get work. Templates for proposal writing are provided. To prevent burnout in this challenging career, several strategies are offered to foster mental health and personal growth. The chapter concludes by describing some of the advantages to independent consulting that have been identified by new consultants.

Everyone thinks they can be a consultant. It's a fallback position if "things don't work out." It reminds me of the apocryphal story of Margaret Atwood and the brain surgeon. Meeting her at a cocktail party, he said, "I'm going to be a writer when I retire." She replied, "And I'm going to be a brain surgeon when *I* retire." It seems there is a lot more to becoming either a writer or a consultant than appears on the surface, so what is a consultant and why consider becoming one?

THE CONSULTING LANDSCAPE

The definition in Box 23.1 provides an overview of the role of an evaluation consultant (Barrington, 2005). Consultants are categorized in the North American Industry Classification System (NAICS) in Sector 541, Management, Scientific and Technical Consulting Services, an industry group primarily engaged in providing expert advice by selling their expertise, knowledge, and skills (U.S. Census Bureau, 2022).

While the term *program evaluator* does not appear in NAICS, a similar occupation, *management analyst*, is provided. It is a promising area, slated to grow 11% from 2021 to 2031, faster than the average for all occupations, because of the need for organizations to improve efficiency (U.S. Bureau of Labor Statistics, 2023). Program evaluation can certainly contribute to achieving these results. In 2017, the total amount of federal contract funding labeled

> **BOX 23.1. Definition of an Evaluation Consultant**
>
> Consultants provide independent, objective information and advice to clients in a variety of organizational settings to assist them in achieving their objectives. . . . [They] provide their professional expertise on a temporary basis and have no authority to implement the changes they recommend. They have both academic and practical experience and have strong communication and instructional skills. In their independent capacity, it is critical that they model ethical business and research practice.

"program evaluation, review, or development" was $651 million (Lemire et al., 2018).

Consulting firms that offer program evaluation services tend to be either very large or very small. A few large-scale firms capture the bulk of government spending in the United States. As Lemire et al. (2018) found, the biggest spender was the U.S. Department of Health and Human Services, which awarded $217 million in contracts related to evaluation services in 2017. Most of the contract dollars were awarded to five firms: Mathematica Policy Research, ICF, MDRC, Research Triangle Institute, and Abt Associates.

These giants may dominate the market in terms of actual money spent but most evaluation contracts are found elsewhere, and this is where independent practitioners find their consulting opportunities. That's because most consulting firms, 75% in all, are very small and employ fewer than five employees (Barrington, 2012b). They are often run by a sole practitioner who either provides specialized services, focuses on a specific industry, specializes in a specific practice area, operates in a single geographic region, or serves a single client. Their operating costs are much lower than those of larger firms, which means, according to Hwalek and Straub (2018), that clients can get more for their money by hiring them.

A survey of 187 members of the American Evaluation Association's (AEA) Independent Consulting Topical Interest Group (TIG), representing roughly 20% of TIG membership, reported that 82% of their respondents were White, 5% Black, and 13% other ethnic groups or unspecified (Hwalek & Straub, 2018). Women dominated the group at 83%. Respondents' median age was 53 and ranged from age 28 to 78. The majority held doctorates in social sciences or education. The median size of their largest contract was $86,400 and the median length of their contracts was 3 years. Revenues came mainly from government agencies (48%) and foundations (23%), while the remainder came from nonprofits and other organizations. The median income for independent consultants with 5–9 years' experience was $122,500 (Independent Consulting Topical Interest Group Committee, 2015).

KEY TRAITS AND ETHICS

While the landscape may look promising, independent consulting is not for everyone. In fact, management consulting gurus Greiner and Metzger (1983) described it as "the most damnable profession in the world." It can be lonely, frustrating, and unpredictable. One could legitimately ask, therefore, why consider consulting at all? There is one broadly held answer: It is because consultants feel in control of their own destiny. This sense of freedom outweighs the angst and insecurity associated with going out on one's own. However, certain personality traits are more likely to foster success.

Intellectual Capacity

Consultants need to be quick studies. They enter a new organization, find out what is needed, provide the appropriate service, and leave gracefully, all within budget and on time. Competition is often keen, and those with the best educational credentials and specialized training have a decided edge. Mature consultants bring their wisdom, expertise, and broad networks to the table. Younger consultants also shine, especially with their state-of-the-art skills in data analytics, data visualization, and software knowledge, as well as their social media savvy.

Along with a strong knowledge of evaluation theory and methods, consultants need excellent research skills to interpret and synthesize information quickly. They tend to be agile thinkers who can problem solve, reframe situations, see patterns, and make connections. Their varied field experience makes it easy to relate to clients.

It also gives them an intuitive understanding of the complex relationships and processes so often found in organizations.

Self-Confidence

A skilled consultant can walk into a room of strangers and sell them on an idea. A strong professional identity, presence, and personal style give them an edge. They are good evaluators, good listeners, and good leaders in an unassuming way, gently nudging clients toward solutions they might not have reached on their own. They are lifelong learners and continually incorporate best practices into their work.

Courage

Because they often find themselves operating outside of their comfort zone, consultants need courage, energy, and vision. They have the capacity to go against the common view and can make an evidence-based, persuasive case to consider even difficult study findings. They can land in a strange town at midnight, scrape the ice off of their rental car, and find their hotel without the benefit of GPS. They can get up the day after they lost the best proposal they have ever written and start all over again (Barrington, 2012b).

Adaptability

One of the ironies of consulting is that the parameters of terms of reference, proposals, and contracts tend to be rigid and fixed, yet the reality they will encounter in these engagements is unpredictable and complex. Several adaptive strategies are needed to help mitigate this role conflict: pragmatism, innovation, critical thinking, and collaboration.

Resilience

A resilient consultant can recover from the stress of ambiguity. A reflexive stance, healthy lifestyle, supportive network, and holistic perspective provide the psychological strength needed to deal with adversity and change. As new consultant Marcela Gutierrez said (Barrington, 2019), "I don't see a distinction now between how I work and how I live. It's seamless."

Ethics

Ethics are essential to the trust relationship that exists between evaluator and client. It is predicated on the moral accountability of doing "the right thing." However, as Morris (2008) reminds us, "what one evaluator views as an ethical issue may be perceived as simply a political problem, a philosophical disagreement, or a methodological concern by another." Ethical dilemmas can arise rapidly and without warning, often allowing little time for consultation. In this pressure-cooker situation, the consultant needs to step away to think through the problem. Four different perspectives lenses can be used to view the issue at hand (Barrington, 2012c):

- The values perspective, a foundational viewpoint, is crafted by family, race, religion, geography, politics, and economics. As Melvin Hall (personal communication, 2018) suggests, this world view shapes our implicit theories about how things work. It defines the consultant's personal bottom line.

- The methods perspective offers a way of seeing that is crafted by the consultant's training in research and evaluation. The Program Evaluation Standards (Yarbrough et al., 2011) can be used to categorize potential solutions in terms of utility, feasibility, propriety, accuracy, or accountability. Once a relevant standard is identified, useful tips and case examples are provided to assist with problem solving.

- The conduct perspective looks at behavior on the job. Evaluators are well supported by the AEA's Guiding Principles (2018), which provide advice about systematic inquiry, competence, integrity, respect for people, and the common good/equity. Other useful resources can be found in the well-described set of case studies in *Evaluation Ethics for Best Practice* (Morris, 2008) and Morris's chapter (see Chapter 7, this volume).

- The business perspective examines how the consulting practice is managed. Despite the number of evaluation consultants operating as small businesses today, there are no specific guidelines to assist with business management. While accountable money management and transparent billing practices may seem self-evident, a surprising number of consultants have been tempted to conceal information or engage in fraudulent or shady practice. For example, two wide-ranging scandals involving Enron in the United States and the Sponsorship Program in Canada, involved consultants at the heart of the malfeasance. In both countries, business and government suffered serious consequences, consulting firms went bankrupt, and several consultants found themselves in prison.

- The Institute of Management Consultants (2018) and the Canadian Association of Management Consultants (2017) provide codes of conduct that outline consultants' professional obligations to the public, the client, themselves, and the consulting profession. Key topics include:
  ○ Understanding duty of care to the client.
  ○ Determining what constitutes conflict of interest.
  ○ Reaching a mutual understanding with the client about project objectives, scope, work plan, costs, and fee arrangements before accepting the assignment—in writing and prior to beginning work.
  ○ Avoiding financial gain from an assignment in addition to the agreed-upon fees.
  ○ Not using colleagues' or clients' proprietary information or methodologies without their permission.
  ○ Not stealing a client's employee or encouraging them to work elsewhere.
  ○ Not advertising services in a deceptive manner and not misrepresenting or denigrating individual consulting practitioners, consulting firms, or the consulting profession.

Ultimately, consultants need to confront each ethical dilemma with integrity to ensure the best possible outcome for both the clients and themselves. Their future careers depend upon it.

STARTING UP

A lot of the success experienced by the new consultants I interviewed (Barrington, 2019) can be attributed to planning and preparation. Foundational elements include:

- Financial sustainability.
- A business plan.
- Business systems and processes.

Financial Sustainability

Financial sustainability is the key to success. Without it, small businesses fail—over and over. Poor cash flow management and inadequate cash reserves are frequently cited as the main causes for failure. The would-be consultant must explore the financial viability of their venture closely. Once in business, financial management must be a daily activity.

Critical questions to ask are (Barrington, 2017):

- Can I support myself for 3 months while I check out the market?
- Can I support myself for another 3 months to land my first contract?
- Can I then wait for up to 2 more months until my invoice is paid?
- What other financial resources can I rely on while getting up to speed?
- Will there be enough work to support my business in the future?

The rule of thumb for a start-up is the equivalent of 6 months' current salary plus additional cash reserves for emergencies. Many start-up consultants don't have this luxury. Instead, they establish a transition strategy like the following examples (Barrington, 2019):

- Worked part-time at their former job.
- Took projects from their former job to their new business (with permission).
- Got an interim job, knowing it was time-limited in nature.
- Worked on a subcontract basis for a larger consulting firm.
- Knew their upcoming retirement would provide a good pension.
- Negotiated a good severance package.

In each case, these individuals had already made the strategic decision to become consultants but they did most of their planning while working somewhere else. This gave them the financial security and time they needed to read, research, network, plan, and prepare for their new businesses. A few others had neither time nor choice, finding themselves without a job unexpectedly. Some of these individuals also launched their businesses successfully but a few are still hoping it will happen "someday."

A Business Plan

Consulting is a business venture and as such it needs serious planning. Jotting a quick list on a cocktail napkin will not suffice because, as Yogi Berra said, "You've got to be very careful if you don't know where you are going, because you might not get there."[1]

If consultants don't define their business goals, markets, clients, and services, their results are likely to be mixed at best. The act of preparing the business plan is also an opportunity for some soul-searching and personal development. The plan demonstrates the consultant's capacities as an evaluator, researcher, and entrepreneur. It's a road map and a financial plan as well as a marketing tool and it has long-term utility because it provides both an accountability framework and benchmarks.

Preparing the plan generally takes at least 2 months, if the consultant dedicates about 10 hours per week for research, interviews, and writing (Barrington, 2012b). To begin, a solitary weekend retreat can provide the impetus needed. In this protected space, the consultant can craft their vision and mission statements; assess potential business strengths, weaknesses, opportunities, and threats; and identify key goals. With these essentials in place, additional research and planning can be completed over the next couple of months. The business plan can become the hallmark document that demonstrates the consultant's professionalism. Box 23.2 provides a list of suggested topics for the business plan (Barrington, 2017).

---

[1] https://ftw.usatoday.com/2015/09/the-50-greatest-yogi-berra-quotes

Business Systems and Processes

As the consultant completes the business plan, it quickly becomes clear that a variety of business decisions are needed to make the dream a reality. These include the business name, ownership structure, location, fee structure, cashflow management, staffing, and insurance.

The Business Name

A business name has far-reaching implications. It is worth the effort to select a name that is easy to remember, has positive connotations, and describes the services planned. For example, using the consultant's name, such as *Mary Smith*, or *Mary Smith Consulting*, is not informative enough. The potential client asks, "Consulting about what?" Likewise, *Mary Smith and Associates* is problematic because it disregards the role of future staff. Clients will want to speak only to Mary. Despite the importance of the business name, however, Hwalek and Straub (2018) warn that, in the end, the consultant's reputation is even more critical in the marketplace.

Ownership Structure

A critical start-up decision is how the business ownership will be structured. This has financial, tax, and legal ramifications. Small business is a well-established field and resources abound, including federal government websites like the U.S. Small Business Administration, and also books, blogs, websites, Chambers of Commerce resources, continuing education courses, and small business fairs. Table 23.1 outlines the pros and cons of five common ownership structures (Barrington, 2017).

The selected structure can also have an impact on professional identity. As new consultant David MacDonald commented regarding his incorporation (David McDonald, personal communication, August 6, 2018), " . . . it was one of the best things I did. It really made me feel quite different in terms of status (personal and professional status) and it changed the way I presented myself as a professional person."

BOX 23.2. Business Plan Template

1. Title Page, Table of Contents, and Executive Summary
   - Similar to proposal cover: name of company, contact information, purpose of document
   - Executive Summary prepared last but presented first (one page with vision or mission, uniqueness of services, identification of target market, key financial information)
2. Industry Overview
   - Definition of consulting industry
   - Summary of national, regional, and local trends
   - Economic outlook
   - Market niche of your business
   - Specialties or characteristics that differentiate your firm from others
3. Business Services and Prospective Clients
   - Specific nature of consulting services
   - Types of clients anticipated
   - Vision, mission, values, overview of goals and plans
   - Relevant expertise and unique skills
4. Market Analysis
   - Target market research and analysis of findings
   - Information interviews with 5 to 7 potential clients (their research needs, views on current market needs). Additional contact names obtained if possible.
   - Description of competitive advantage
   - Market niche definition
5. Marketing Plan
   - Realistic marketing objectives
   - List of organizations that can use proposed services, contact method, similar past projects
   - Pricing strategy
   - Marketing strategy: next month in detail, next 3 months and Year 1 in less detail, thumbnail plans for Years 2 to 3 to be updated monthly until adequate work is obtained; then updated on a quarterly basis or as needed
6. Management Plan
   - Business name
   - Ownership structure. Provide any of the following if appropriate:
     - Names of owners, officers, corporate directors
     - Partnership agreement
     - Articles of incorporation
     - Shareholder agreements
     - Management contracts
     - Service contracts
     - Leases
   - Licenses (e.g., due to business zoning [if needed]). Copies attached in appendix.
7. Operating Plan
   - Physical description of building and office site
   - Security considerations
   - Renovations needed
   - Planned staff/subcontractors and their location
   - Flowchart to highlight main business development events over next year
8. Financial Plan
   - Start-up costs related to facilities, materials, equipment, marketing
   - Opening balance sheet (current assets and liabilities, owner's equity)
   - Forecast of income and expenses or a profit-and-loss statement of revenue and expenses anticipated for the first year
   - Cash flow forecast on a monthly basis
   - Break-even analysis showing at what sales volume the business will break even
9. References and Advisors
   - Bank manager (to help navigate cash flow)
   - Accountant (to prepare financial year-end statements)
   - Attorney (to review contracts and help with incorporation)
   - Insurance broker (to find appropriate coverage for general liability insurance, errors and omissions insurance, vehicle insurance if needed)
   - Letters of reference from three past clients/employers
10. Appendices
    - Two-page CV
    - Business photo
    - List of relevant past projects
    - Other materials to support credibility

TABLE 23.1. Five Ownership Structures

Ownership structure	Pros	Cons
1. Sole proprietorship	• Easy to create or terminate • Cheap • Controlled solely by owner	• Unlimited liability • No difference between the individual and the business • Tax issues • Hard to borrow money • Depends on owner's needs
2. Partnership	• Relationship based • Profits shared • Easy to create • More resources available • Limited red tape and regulation	• Unlimited liability (both for the partner and the firm) • Each partner is "jointly and severally" liable—for their share of the partnership debts and for all the debts • A partnership agreement is needed • Potential for conflict • Stable only as long as partners continue; when a partner leaves or dies, a new partnership agreement is needed
3. Limited liability company (LLC; United States only)	• Hybrid of corporation and partnership or sole proprietorship • Owners not personally liable for company's debts or liabilities • Flow-through taxation similar to partnerships • Articles of incorporation are registered with the state	• Profits and losses are listed on personal tax return of owner and are not paid by the LLC • Registration at the federal level is required to obtain an employer identification number (EIN) • Dissolution is possible upon death or bankruptcy of one member • A business continuation agreement is required when one member leaves or dies or the LLC is dissolved
4. Incorporation	• A separate legal entity • In the United States, an LLC often used • Some tax advantages • Liability protection • More flexibility • Greater credibility	• Incorporation documents are required • Legal, tax, and administrative costs • Ongoing paperwork and minor costs
5. Nonprofit corporation	• Social mission • Not focused on profit • Separate legal status • Limited liability • Easier to work with foundations	• Complex paperwork, may need a special designation from the IRS, can be costly • Audits • Surplus funds go to support the organization's goals • A board of directors is required; management does not have the final say

Business Location

Where will the work happen? Table 23.2 summarizes the most common options for the start-up consulting office (Barrington, 2017). For most start-ups, the home office may be the logical choice but the consultant must be able to set clear boundaries for space, time, and availability.

Setting Fees

A big concern for new consultants is determining what to charge for their services. Table 23.3 identifies some common price-setting approaches (Barrington, 2016). The consultant may choose to use more than one pricing structure, depending on the nature of the engagement but first, a benchmark must be established. What is 1 day of the consultant's work worth? To find the answer, several calculations are required:

1. *Billable time.* The amount of time the consultant has available in a year to work on clients' projects.
2. *Overhead.* The yearly cost of running the business (e.g., rent, insurance, communications, marketing) but excluding the consultant's salary.
3. *Salary.* A realistic annual salary for the consultant, often related to the most recent employment salary received.
4. *Profit.* While thinking about profit may seem

premature, the ongoing health of a business demands that it operate in a profitable way. Typically, 10–15% of business income should be retained for business development, professional development, and contingencies.

Table 23.4 provides a sample of the calculation process (Barrington & Murray, 2024).

Time Tracking

Time is the currency of a consultant's work and tracking time is the best way to be accountable to the client. If questions arise about the consultant's activities, a time-tracking system can generate a detailed report of time on task. Many software programs are available and data can be stored on the cloud so it is accessible by mobile phone and computer. When preparing an invoice at the end of the month, the consultant can simply multiply the total days worked on the project by their daily rate. Even when a different price structure is used (e.g., fixed fee), the consultant can compare actual hours expended with the fee offered to determine whether it is profitable to take on this type of work. Time tracking offers confidence to the client and allows the consultant to assess the efficiency of their time use (Barrington, 2015).

Accounting Processes

Everyone loves money, but we love it more when it is flowing in rather than when it is flowing out. While the consultant is the heart and brain of their small business, money is the oxygen that keeps it alive. Reasons for business failure generally include lack of working capital, inability to manage cash flow, failure to budget, poor financial controls, and inadequate financial monitoring. Integrated accounting software allows a consultant to manage bills, create invoices, reconcile bank accounts, create financial reports, track cash flow, develop profit-and-loss statements, and manage taxes. To succeed, money must be managed every day.

TABLE 23.2. Five Suggested Locations for the Consultant's First Office

Office location	Pros	Cons
1. The home office	• Economical • Flexible • Control	• Impact on home life and family • Business image • Lack of meeting space • Infrastructure requirements
2. The client's office	• A good temporary solution • Close to the action • Can use client's infrastructure	• The tax department may deem consultant an employee • Employees may perceive the consultant as just another employee • May breed resentment
3. Shared space	• Pool or prorate expenses • Networking • Moral support • Common among freelancers, especially in the arts	• Depends on compatibility with office mates • Need good will, positive chemistry
4. Small business incubator	• Provides a graduated list of services • Can start with a professional identity package • Can rent space, often short term and flexible • Can meet other professionals • May provide training • The consultant is the incubator's client	• May not have enough identity • Can't stay too long (when no longer a start-up) • May be difficult to expand
5. Leased space	• Logical next choice after outgrowing other options • Business image is positive • Perceived stability in community	• Ongoing financial commitment and risk (3–5 years) • Legal documents required • More complex arrangements • Hard to downsize

TABLE 23.3. Ten Price-Setting Methods

Price-setting method	Characteristics
1. Daily rate	• Traditional price-setting method for consultants. • Based on time proposed and expended. • See Table 23.4 for calculation.
2. Fixed fee	• For small projects with a quick turnaround. • For workshop honoraria. • For evaluation designs to be included in a client's grant proposal.
3. Contingency fee	• A contentious alternative if the consultant will benefit from the advice given to the client, thus providing the consultant with a financial stake related to the outcome and incenting them to provide advice that will garner the greatest personal advantage. • Many independent consultants write funding proposals for free hoping to get the evaluation component of the resulting project if the client's proposal is successful. • Experienced consultants suggest that the consultant set up a small contract with the client to prepare the grant or evaluation component, thus being compensated regardless of whether the client is successful in obtaining the grant.
4. Standing offer	• The consultant provides an offer to the potential client to provide services at prearranged rates using preapproved staff, under set terms and conditions. Often used by government to call up a short list of consultants for a quick response to a request for proposal. • Similar to writing a proposal, the consultant submits an extensive description of skills, research methods, past projects with budgets and references, team members, and daily rates for the government department to keep on file, often for up to 3 years. • When a consultant is needed, the department sends a short description of needs to a small selection from the list; the consultant quickly prepares a brief proposal detailing design and price. • It's nice if the consultant is invited; no guarantees that any requests will be received.
5. Retainer	• Historically popular; some consultants still use this today. • Fee calculated on typical days/month at the agreed-upon daily rate. • The consultant is paid a set fee every month regardless of how much work is done for the client.
6. Value-based pricing	• Fees based on client's perceived value of the consultant's services. • While used by management consultants, particularly in business, it does not pass scrutiny with evaluation clients who tend to be cost conscious.
7. Benchmarking competitors	• Setting fees based on what other consultants charge without making sure that the consultant's own costs, desired salary, and profit margin are covered is a recipe for failure. • It is useful to know what others charge but this should not be the deciding factor in any consulting context.
8. Different fee structures for different markets	• The belief that "big fish" should help "little fish" by charging smaller, less solvent clients a cheaper rate, and recouping any losses through contracts with larger and wealthier clients is popular with some consultants. It is seen as a type of social justice. • It is not a good business model because it is difficult to predict how many big fish will come along.
9. Pro bono work	• When the consultant is committed to a cause, can offer to do consulting work for free. • There is usually an expectation that this will help to build the consultant's reputation. • There is a possibility of getting a tax receipt for the value of the work donated.
10. Celebrity status	• What do Bill Clinton and Oprah charge for speaking engagements? Very-high-profile consultants may be able to charge what they think they are worth—see number 6 above.

TABLE 23.4. Daily and Hourly Rate Calculation

Step	Calculation	Estimated Amount
Step 1	Determine desired salary	$90,000
Step 2	Determine operational costs	$30,000
Step 3	Total costs	$90,000 + $30,000 = $120,000/year
Step 4	Cost for 160 billable days	$120,000/160 = $750.00 base daily rate
Step 5	Profit @ 10%	$750.00 × 0.10 = $75.00
Step 6	Final daily rate	$750.00 + $75.00 = $825.00 (8-hour day)
Step 7	Hourly rate	$825.00/8 hours = $103.12/hour
		Round it up to $125.00/hour

From Barrington and Murray (2024).

Staffing

Once the practice gets underway, the scene can shift from not having enough work to having too much. Should the consultant hire staff or subcontract for specific skills? Table 23.5 describes some key considerations and questions to ask (Barrington, 2014).

For the sole practitioner, hiring is a big step because the decision has an impact on the entire business. Assessing needs can answer these questions. Are the needs administrative or project related? What level of competencies and skills are required? Who is likely to have what is needed—a student, recent graduate, young professional, or seasoned expert? Does current infrastructure support an additional individual? Can this be a virtual relationship? Is there enough work to support someone for a full year or is the need project specific? Finally, is the cash flow adequate and predictable enough to cover someone else's paycheck every month (Barrington, 2012b)?

For short-term needs, a subcontractor may be more appropriate. This individual is self-employed and only works on specific tasks for a defined period. To clarify the relationship, a subcontract is needed that clearly states the name of the project assigned, date of the engagement, tasks, expected number of days, daily rate, and expense reimbursement.

What may not be apparent is that no matter what staffing arrangement is established, staff management takes time—to supervise, coach, and assess performance and to intervene if difficulties are encountered. As the consultant is responsible to the client for the quality of all work done, the hiring decision is critical to the future success of the firm.

TABLE 23.5. Staffing Considerations and Questions to Ask

Key considerations	Questions
1 Biggest need	• Is it administration—answering the phone, running the office, bookkeeping? • Research support—collecting or analyzing data? • Senior tasks—more of the same work the consultant does?
2 How much? How long?	• How many hours per week? • Is it full-time or part-time? • One project or several? • How long will the work last?
3 Work site	In the consultant's office: • Office space? • Furniture? • Equipment? • Supplies? In the staff member's home office: • Telephone and computer compatibility? • Access to needed software and databases? • Document and file sharing? • Required security clearances?
4 Management tasks	• How long will it take to define tasks and make sure they are accomplished? • To supervise progress and communicate feedback? • To ensure project quality, completeness, and timeliness?
5 Costs	• Are there enough confirmed contracts to afford this person? • Is the firm's cashflow predictable enough to pay staff regularly? • What are taxes, benefits, and other payroll expenses? • What does government require of employers?

Cashflow Management

Of all the challenges I have faced as a consultant, cash flow management has been, and continues to be, the most challenging. Cash flow is the cycle of cash that comes into and goes out of the business every month. How it is managed can affect the consultant's bottom line, and more than that, it can make or break the success of the business.

As soon as the consultant has completed the agreed-upon work, they are starting to extend credit to the client, and that extension continues until the invoice is paid, the check is received, and the money is deposited in the consultant's bank. The potential for error among these various factors is large, uncertain, and difficult to control. A business convention enables clients to wait 30 days before paying the consultant's invoice (i.e., net 30) but during that period, they are holding the consultant's money (and receiving the benefit of it).

Meanwhile, the consultant is facing a series of financial obligations, such as subcontracts, rent, and marketing costs, that could be addressed if that money had already been received. The situation can be even more tenuous if the consultant has few contracts on the go, if the client tends to pay late, or if an unexpected glitch slows the client's accounting processes. Box 23.3 outlines some strategies to manage cashflow.

Insurance

Who wants to think about the many disasters that are out there waiting to happen: damage, injury, liability, loss, natural catastrophe? Insurance is often seen as too complex, time-consuming, expensive, and boring to worry about. I often see panicky posts online from independent consultants who are about to sign a contract that requires insurance. Sadly, they have never bothered to get any. Now their new contract hangs in the balance. Ironically, it is often the client who forces the consultant to face reality.

There are several ways to mitigate risk even before insurance is purchased. They relate to good business practice and a sense of professionalism (Barrington, 2012b). This means that the

---

BOX 23.3. Managing Cashflow: The Biggest Challenge

Accounts Receivable

- Bill in monthly installments, making sure to have a small deliverable to offer, such as a status report.
- Generate monthly cashflow statements and identify overdue invoices. Follow up immediately.
- Understand the client's accounting approval process and get to know the players involved. Email them if needed to track a slow payment.
- Ask to set up a direct deposit arrangement.
- Make sure projects are at different stages of development (new, midpoint, about to end). The cash generated by projects with late-stage predictable payments can help support the costs of projects in hesitant, start-up mode.
- Bill clients on time. Each day of delay has an impact on the length of time before payment.

Accounts Payable

- Monitor due dates closely and pay bills 1 day before they are due.
- Postdate payables online.
- Never start a project without a contract.
- Keep track of expended time for every project, even if the client does not ask for it.
- Keep the business lean, limit inventory, buy secondhand furniture.
- Manage vendors closely. Costs tend to rise from year to year. Renegotiate as needed.

Money Management

- Develop financial systems and keep them up to date or hire someone for this purpose. A shoebox approach is doomed to failure.
- Save 10% of each incoming check in a separate account for a rainy day or for registration costs at the next conference.
- Set goals for desired revenue each year and measure success.
- Focus on productivity and doing things smarter, faster, better.
- Get a line of credit to manage cashflow gaps.

Remember that no matter how interesting the project is, taking care of business comes first—every day.

consultant's responsibility to the client comes first. Well-organized systems, such as the use of written contracts and a clear understanding of legal requirements; careful selection of staff and subcontractors; effective record keeping, billing, data security, and other office procedures; effective quality-control systems; and good internal and external communications, all promote efficiency. Once these basics are attended to, the consultant is better prepared to face any potential risk and is ready to purchase insurance. Table 23.6 outlines the five main types of risk and offers some insurance options.

Unlike our panicked colleague above, the consultant should plan carefully, understand their level of exposure, and take the time to explore options. Clifford Carr, an independent consultant, who sometimes acts as an expert witness in consultants' lawsuits, sees insurance as an important deterrent. Regarding one case, he commented, ". . . they never would have brought it to trial if the evaluator had had insurance. They were quite clear that the cost would have been prohibitive . . ." (Barrington, 2012a, p. 192).

FINDING A MARKET NICHE

Assess Market Needs

To find work, the consultant's first step is assessing market needs. Watching evaluation trends, government funding decisions, and developments and innovations in the news becomes a spectator sport. Consultants often comment on X, LinkedIn, Instagram, Facebook, and other discussion platforms. Trends at evaluation conferences are followed closely. Requests for proposals (RFPs) are studied to see what clients are looking for. It is important to find out who is funding projects, what kind of projects are being funded, and what firms are getting the contracts.

TABLE 23.6. Five Business Risks and Related Insurance Options

Risk	Examples of risk	Insurance options
1 Running a business	• Overhead costs are unpredictable. • Revenue forecasts are not met. • Receivables cannot be collected. • Business is interrupted. • Vehicle used for business purposes is in an accident.	• Business interruption insurance • Vehicle insurance • Business loan insurance
2 Business property	• Catastrophic natural events destroy office property. • Vandalism, hacking, and criminal activity inflict damage.	• Property insurance • Homeowner's insurance (may cover part of losses if it is a home office)
3 Negligence of duty	• A duty to protect the client and the public by exercising reasonable care—what a "reasonable" person would do in any given circumstance. • A duty to protect employees and subcontractors.	• Group benefits plan • General liability insurance (covers negligence causing injury to clients, employees, and the general public)
4 Quality of work	• Human error. • Advice has unexpected negative impacts. • Contract provisions are violated. • Employees or subcontractors are unqualified or irresponsible.	• Errors and omissions insurance/professional liability insurance (N.B. Interchangeable terms)
5 Consultant's health	• Owner or partner has serious illness, disability, or dies. • Loss of major shareholder has impact on business decisions. • Absence of key employee has serious short-term effect.	• Health insurance (United States) • Travel insurance • Personal disability insurance • Overhead expense insurance • Partners' or shareholders' insurance • Key person insurance • Term life insurance

Note. For a more detailed discussion, see Barrington (2012b, Chapter 14).

Develop a Skills Inventory

The next step in identifying a market niche is to assess personal competencies by developing a skills inventory (Barrington, 2018b). After reviewing the full spectrum of evaluation activities, the consultant can select the areas that capture their imagination and match their skill set. Then it is a matter of reviewing past experiences for greatest successes, favorite projects, innovative designs, or particularly effective methods. Such deep thinking may reveal that unacknowledged expertise lies buried in past experiences. For example, volunteer work, training, hobbies, parenting, coaching, and lifelong learning can all reveal hidden strengths. Based on this reflective exercise, the consultant can develop a skills inventory that helps to narrow the market niche.

Meet the Competition

The next step is to discover who is doing the work that the new consultant wants to do. It is time to get to know competitors socially by meeting them for coffee or lunch. Joining a professional organization is a great way to get to know colleagues, as working together on activities and projects fosters strong relationships. While they may be bidding against these competitors on one project, the next could find them working on the same team. By taking a collaborative rather than a cutthroat approach, the consultant begins to build a positive reputation that is priceless in the long run.

Differentiate Services

When the consultant knows the kind of work they want to do and what their competitors offer, it is then possible to distinguish themselves in the marketplace. This takes a reversal from the usual way of thinking—it's not about *what* the consultant can offer—it's about *why* the client needs them. Are the planned services the ones most valued by potential clients? Can they match the quality of the services provided by competitors? Is there one specific area in which it is possible to excel beyond anything competitors can offer? To stand out, the consultant's services need to be memorable and innovative as well as solid and rigorous.

Use Plain Language

While new consultants may have a clear mental picture of the services they want to offer, it can be difficult to verbalize them. One can easily get tongue-tied or lost in terminology. Two strategies that counteract this problem are the elevator pitch and the value proposition.

The elevator pitch describes the consultant's services in 25 simple words that can be spoken in the time it takes to ride an elevator to the top of a tall building (Barrington, 2018a). It describes the consultant's expertise, specialized skills, most successful products, and reasons why clients like working with them.

The value proposition is a brief written statement that describes the tangible benefit the client will receive (Laja, 2017). It highlights the primary reason why a client should hire them and focuses on the outcomes their services will produce.

By organizing their thoughts into a couple of quick sentences or a small block of text, new consultants often gain clarity about their own services. They can then use their elevator pitch in marketing conversations and their value proposition in marketing materials.

GETTING WORK

The Informal Approach

One of the best-kept consulting secrets is that most independent consultants get most of their work informally. A recent marketing survey asked over 10,000 business consultants what type of marketing had the best result or brought in the most money (Mancha, 2015). Referrals had the greatest return for 36% of the consultants. Networking was next at 34%. Another strategy, building strategic alliances, was only chosen by 4% of business consultants in Mancha's survey but many evaluation consultants I have talked with say it is a great way to break into the market (Barrington, 2019). A final powerful strategy for those already working with clients is repeat business. Each of these strategies is described below.

Referrals

The magic of marketing is that the consultant can never plan for the way a connection will be made but it is possible to plant a few seeds. The simplest strategy is a direct request, letting an individual know that a referral would be welcomed. David Shorr, a new policy and evaluation consultant, got his first contract as a result of a luncheon between two friends and a consultant who worked with a large foundation—and he wasn't even there (Barrington, 2018c, with permission). Because his friends knew what he was looking for, when the appropriate topic arose, his name was mentioned. The result was his first consulting contract. This supports the belief held by many consultants that if their name is out there, work will come to them.

Networking

Everyone knows someone who is looking for what the consultant has to offer, or so the urban myth of six degrees of separation would have us believe. This makes networking an important marketing strategy. Many networks intersect in the consultant's life: work colleagues past and present; project interest holders; members of the evaluation community; adjunct fields like academia, government, and policy studies; and friends, relatives, and neighbors.

A spreadsheet or database can be set up to capture these and other categories. It is then a matter of remembering names, gathering contact details, email addresses, and social media links, and prioritizing the lists for potential linkages and availability. The consultant is now ready to begin contacting them, one at a time. It doesn't take very long before work opportunities start to appear.

Another strategy to raise a consultant's profile is to join a professional organization, volunteer to get involved, and attend events. As new evaluator Marcia Nation suggests, just showing up is important because sometimes it is enough to connect the consultant's services with someone's upcoming needs (Barrington, 2018c, with permission).

Strategic Alliances

Consultants benefit from collaborating with other independent consultants. Working together, each member contributes their specialized skills, creating a team designed for a specific project. Some of the benefits of these arrangements include (Barrington, 2009):

- Tailoring the skills of the team to the unique need of an individual project.
- Allowing independent consultants to pursue larger, more complex projects.
- Providing a role model for project management.
- Reducing competition through co-opting competitors.
- Offering competitive scheduling with more hands to do the work.
- Optimizing the budget by assigning tasks at appropriate skill levels.
- Offering different perspectives to strengthen the final analysis.

Another type of strategic alliance is to subcontract with a large firm (Hwalek & Straub, 2018). This can save time and effort for the independent consultant because the marketing has already been taken care of. The consultant can access more complex projects and an experienced team is ready to provide support. For those with specialized expertise, it is a risk-free way to start a consulting career. David McDonald began by subcontracting to firms that needed his expertise in criminal justice and substance abuse (Barrington, 2018b, with permission). While this proved to be a good transition, eventually he branched out on his own and now enjoys his direct relationship with grass-roots organizations.

Repeat Business

For start-up consultants, repeat business may not seem relevant but it is good to remember that work done now can affect future opportunities. In Hwalek and Straub's 2018 survey, respondents reported that, in the last 12 months, 51% of new projects had come from existing clients. Repeat business speaks to the quality of the consultant's work and the warmth of their relationship with the client (Barrington, 2009). Going into a project with knowledge of the context and the players is a distinct advantage. On the other hand, the consultant does not want to make the client dependent on their services. A long-term relationship can become so close that the consultant is perceived as an employee and thus may lose the credibility of an external advisor. This situation is also frowned upon by the tax department. The independent consultant must be able to prove there is no employer–employee relationship, so to remain at arm's length, the consultant should maintain a portfolio of clients and a diversity of projects. This strategy also enhances flexibility, promotes the cross-fertilization of ideas, and builds a broad client base.

Writing Proposals

The Letter Proposal

Many smaller organizations do not have a formal tendering process, and so a letter proposal is often used to secure a working relationship. While the letter format looks friendly, in terms of design, it requires nearly the same amount of preparation as an RFP. By preparing the budget first, the details related to scheduling, staffing, evaluation tasks, and costs can be scoped out. This permits the consultant to determine whether they can, indeed, afford to do this project (i.e., not lose money) and ensure that proposed activities will meet the client's needs. Box 23.4 provides a list of suggested topics for a letter proposal (Barrington, 2017).

The Formal Proposal

Responding to a formal RFP is often a thankless task for a new consultant. It is better to complete several successful consulting projects first before tackling an RFP. Writing a formal proposal is one of the most time-consuming of all marketing activities and statistically is the least likely to result in a contract—that is, unless the exact requirements are captured in such an attractive, comprehensive, yet parsimonious way that the potential client cannot say no. That's why support from other colleagues with different skill sets makes the chances of success just a little bit better. Moral support is also welcome during this daunting task. Eventually, with enough confidence, project success, and client recommendations, it may be time for the consultant to take up the challenge. Table 23.7 provides a quick checklist of proposal topics and strategies (Barrington, 2017).

BOX 23.4. Nine Topics for the Letter Proposal

1. Address the letter to the key decision maker or purchasing agent.
2. Thank the individual for the opportunity; provide an overview of the firm, mission statement, and a brief comment about similar work for similar clients.
3. Provide a rundown of special skills and experience relevant for this project.
4. Prepare a one-paragraph description of the study purpose, objectives, and planned methodology.
5. Present a brief task analysis with schedule (in chart form).
6. Add a couple of sentences about each team member and their key strengths in this project (attach their two-page résumés to the letter).
7. Provide a summary budget in chart form by inserting a minimized copy of the budget summary sheet from the budget workbook.
8. Review the total price and mention any tax considerations as well as invoicing procedures (e.g., monthly invoices accompanied by a status report).
9. Provide a final thank-you, contact information, and signature.

SURVIVAL SKILLS

If the consultant is to survive in this challenging landscape, mental health and personal growth must be addressed head on. The hours are long, the work is taxing, and the world is filled with complexity and conflict, so consultants can become depleted of energy. Unless survival skills are actively fostered, productivity and health can be affected. To reflect, refocus, experiment, and innovate, the consultant needs to think deeply and creatively. Here are a few suggestions.

Practicing Reflection

The habit of reflection can strengthen the consultant's response to daily challenge and uncertainty. One method is journal writing, especially in the morning when the mind is fresh. The "morning pages" technique involves producing three pages of longhand, stream-of-consciousness writing immediately upon waking in the morning (Cameron, 1992). It can be a piv-

TABLE 23.7. Thirteen Topics with Suggested Strategies for Formal Proposal Preparation

Proposal topic	Suggested strategies
1. Cover letter	• Write this section last. • Include key points about the consultant's track record and accomplishments. • Include firm's mission statement. • Provide proposal highlights. • Indicate reason for interest in this study.
2. Front pages	• Include title page with contact information, table of contents, and executive summary. • List the proposal evaluation criteria (if available) and identify page numbers for reviewers to find relevant information.
3. Introduction	• Demonstrate understanding of the issue with an overview of related literature. • Project size will determine how much effort is put into this section but be brief.
4. Study purpose, program theory, objectives	• Develop study objectives or clarify those provided in the terms of reference. • If appropriate, suggest a phased approach to the project and provide the focus and objectives for each phase. • Provide a draft logic model, research framework, or other visual model to guide the work. Indicate that this will be confirmed with interest holders once the contract is awarded.
5. Corporate background	• Introduce company, qualifications, number of years in business, and management structure. • Include relevant studies and experience, tailored to the requirements of this project. • Mention preferred approach to working with clients. • Refer to consultant's website for additional information.
6. Study team	• Introduce team members in decreasing order of responsibility for the project. • Provide one or two paragraphs per team member or subcontractor and describe their education, experience, and responsibilities in this project. • If required, include signed forms from the subcontractors, confirming their availability.
7. Study methodology	• Demonstrate understanding of the project. • Build a logical argument from problem to solution. • Describe proposed methodology carefully, matching the level of language to the client's interest in and knowledge of evaluation. • Ground the work in relevant literature but be brief; it is not an academic treatise. • Explain how each study method will be implemented; estimate sample sizes. • Discuss feasibility and degree of success expected. • Enumerate any limitations, risks, or anticipated problems and provide plans to mitigate them. • Identify strengths of the proposed research approach; include such topics as ethics, data security, and confidentiality. • Identify team member by task, indicating their level of effort or number of hours or days assigned for each. • Do not provide any financial information in this section.
8. Task schedule	• List the project tasks and critical dates for meetings and deliverables. • Use a Gantt chart or visual timeline of activities broken down by weeks or months.
9. Deliverables	• Include the deliverables as stated in the request for proposal (RFP) and describe each briefly. • Clarify whether recommendations will be included in the final report. • Indicate that the first deliverable is a detailed work plan even if not required; suggest monthly status reports. These may be "value-added" deliverables. • Provide a draft version of the table of contents for the final report. • Provide reporting options (e.g., full report, executive summary, short report with data tables in appendix, infographic, slide deck).
10. References	• Include references for three similar and/or recent studies providing dollar amount, timeframe, contact names, current phone numbers, and email addresses. • Remember to ask these individuals for permission each time their names are used.

(continued)

TABLE 23.7. *(continued)*

Proposal topic	Suggested strategies
11. Budget	• Include only the summary sheet from the budget workbook or use whatever budget format is required. • Provide a budget narrative at the level of detail required. • Be particularly clear about travel costs and cite the guidelines for travel and accommodations used by this agency. • Include only cost items that are identified in the RFP. • Identify any taxes.
12. Schedule of payments	• Specify expectations about payment (e.g., net 30 days). • Indicate that monthly invoices will be submitted along with a status report/milestone.
13. Résumés	• Provide brief résumés for each member of the team. These are not for academic purposes, so be brief (maximum length four pages). • Select projects of relevance to this study, as well as others that are notable or recent. • Add professional designations and volunteer experience of interest to the client.

otal tool to foster creativity and self-reflection, provide insight, and enhance a sense of self. By using emotional intelligence rather than logic, we can confront our technical errors, mistakes in judgment, and conflicted interactions, and can shift our frame of reference, thus deepening understanding of the substance, forms, and patterns of our experience (Barrington, 2018d). We can ask reflective questions that help let us refocus, experiment, and innovate, all within the nonjudgmental context of a personal and very private journal.

Another reflective strategy is meditation. It can reduce blood pressure and can also help to manage insomnia, depression, and anxiety (American Heart Association, 2014). As writer Richard Wagamese (2016) explains:

> I am constantly surrounded by noise: TV, texts, the internet, music, meaningless small talk, my thinking. All of it blocks my consciousness, my ability to hear the ME that exists beneath the cacophony. So I cultivate silence every morning. . . . Then wherever the day takes me, the people I meet are the beneficiaries of my having taken the time—they get the real me, not someone shaped and altered by the noise around me. Silence is the stuff of life.

For those who learn by talking, a different strategy is voice memoing. The smartphone offers a handy recording function and can be an effective way to mull over work-related issues and plan future actions (Miciak et al., 2020). Once the files are transferred to a computer, they can be coded for themes, categorized, and revisited over time.

Finally, the simplest and probably the oldest of reflection tools, walking, may also be the most profound. A 20-minute walk can be a way to find inner calm. Putting one foot after the other helps one become more in tune with one's surroundings. It can clear the head, focus thinking, and instigate breakthroughs (Cameron, 2003). By setting the question in advance, then forgetting about it and focusing on the sensory experience, a solution may arrive, unannounced.

Getting Feedback

Another survival strategy is getting client feedback. While it may seem a natural part of the evaluation process, it is easily forgotten due to the many pressures embedded in the consulting engagement. Sheer busyness, organizational changes, policy directives, political opposition, project lead turnover, lack of uptake, absence of longer-term outcomes, lingering concerns about the consultant–client relationship, and financial constraints can supersede the need for feedback. To counteract this omission, feedback must be a regular scheduled activity.

As Kubr (2002) reminds us, the way a consultant leaves a project is very significant. He comments, "it is of no benefit to anybody if the consultant is convinced of having done a good job while the client waits only for the consultant's departure in order to stop the project" (p. 245). It is in the interests of both the consultant and client to jointly determine whether the project can be termed a success, a failure, or something in between.

If the engagement has gone well it is a pleasure to reconnect with the client, but if there were difficulties, program flaws, conflict, or mismanagement, such conversations are ones that many would prefer to avoid. It is better to take a risk, be open, and ask, "What could we have done differently?" rather than to never find out what happened afterward. Creating a learning conversation can lead to less stress and more future success for both parties (Stone et al., 2010).

Professional Development

Annual evaluation conferences provide an opportunity to synthesize evaluation and consulting experiences. The act of presenting papers, participating on panels, and offering workshops allows time for reflection and adds new levels of meaning. Evaluators spend their working lives answering other people's questions but sometimes it is at the expense of their own curiosity. Gawande (2007) suggests that by researching something that we are curious about and then share the findings, professional growth is enhanced. Mentoring and teaching can also provide opportunities for personal learning.

Networking

Perhaps the most significant benefit offered by these professional meetings is the opportunity to network with colleagues. The consultants I interviewed stressed the value of professional evaluation organizations, such as the AEA and

---

BOX 23.5. Key Lessons

1. There is a market for independent consultants who offer services in program evaluation.
2. While a few large firms dominate the evaluation market in terms of contract size, most evaluation contracts are left to small firms or independent practitioners.
3. According to an AEA TIG survey of independent consultants, independent evaluators represent a wide range of ages, but their median age is 53. This study also found that the median size of their contracts was $86,000 and the median contract length was 3 years. Another similar TIG survey found that the median income for independent consultants with 5–9 years of experience was $122,500.
4. Important character traits for independent consultants include significant intellectual capacity, self-confidence, courage, adaptability, and resilience. Ethical practice is essential to support the trust relationship between consultant and client.
5. There are two foundational elements needed before considering a consulting career: these are financial sustainability and a sound business plan.
6. Deciding the business structure for a consulting practice is important both financially and legally. It also has a positive impact on the consultant's professional identity.
7. Several price-setting methods can be employed depending on the context of the consulting contract but independent consultants must also be able to calculate their daily rate based on real costs, including billable time, overhead, desired salary, and profit margin.
8. Time is the currency of consulting work and consultants who track their time have the evidence they need to support their billing practices and to plan great efficiencies for future contracts.
9. Risk management is essential for every consulting practice. It starts with professionalism, a sense of responsibility for the client, and good business systems but also includes appropriate insurance coverage.
10. Effective marketing strategies start with aligning the consultant's capabilities, strengths, and passions with market needs. Consultants must differentiate their services from those of their competitors. Preparing an effective elevator pitch and a value proposition will help focus the desired marketing messages.
11. Most consultants get most of their work informally. Strategies include obtaining referrals, networking, strategic alliances, and repeat business.
12. Consulting is a stressful career and so to survive, consultants must reflect on their work and their response to it. Strategies such as obtaining feedback on project outcomes, building capacity, sharing lessons learned, and enhancing one's professional life can lead to innovation and increased personal satisfaction.

the Canadian Evaluation Society because this is where they encounter their *community* or *tribe*. Networking fosters friendship and collaboration, new projects, marketing leads, and publishing opportunities. This is where independent consultants gain the professional contacts and peer support so needed in their busy but isolated lives (Barrington, 2006, 2019).

CONCLUSION

Becoming a successful independent consultant need not be overwhelming. Many topics and suggestions are provided in this chapter, but the good news is they don't have to be learned all at once. In fact, the development of consulting skills and strategies is a lifelong process, each one learned on the go as the need arises. Box 23.5 outlines some key lessons.

Just like a brain surgeon or famous novelist, the independent evaluation consultant faces a challenging career. There is much to learn, risks to face, and uncertainties to resolve, so why bother? The consultants I talked to were clear about the advantages of their new careers. They loved the sense of freedom and control not experienced in previous jobs. They had more choice in their projects and more meaningful connections with their clients. They scheduled their work to suit themselves and found more time for their families. They were energized, confident, and proud of their accomplishments, and looked forward to many productive years ahead.

Additional Resources

An overview of U.S. independent consultants:

Hwalek, M. A., & Straub, V. L. (2018, winter). The small sellers of program evaluation services in the United States. *New Directions for Evaluation, 160*, 125–143.

Government websites on business planning:
www.sba.gov/business-guide/launch-your-business/register-your-business
www.canada.ca/en/services/business/start.html

For information on how to prepare an elevator pitch:
www.barringtonresearchgrp.com/blog/108-cat-got-your-tongue-an-elevator-pitch-for-you.html

For information on how to write a value proposition:
https://conversionxl.com/blog/value-proposition-examples-how-to-create

A useful guide to community consulting:

Wolfe, S. M., & Price, A. W. (2023). *Guidebook to community consulting: A collaborative approach.* Cambridge University Press.

For an in-depth discussion of ownership structures, fee calculations, and insurance issues, as well as many other start-up topics:

Barrington, G. V. (2012). *Consulting start-up and management: A guide for evaluators and applied researchers.* SAGE.

REFERENCES

American Evaluation Association. (2018). *Guiding principles.* Author.
American Heart Association. (2014). Meditation to boost health and wellbeing. Available at *www.heart.org/en/healthy-living/healthy-lifestyle/mental-health-and-wellbeing/meditation-to-boost-health-and-wellbeing*
Barrington, G. V. (2005). Evaluation consultants. In S. Mathison (Ed.), *Encyclopedia of evaluation* (pp. 81–82). SAGE.
Barrington, G. V. (2006). The evaluation consultant's life cycle: Theory, practice, and implications for learning. *New Directions for Evaluation, 111,* 29–40.
Barrington, G. V. (2009). *Consulting skills for evaluators: Getting started, workshop workbook.* Workshop presented at the meeting of the American Evaluation Association, Orlando, FL.
Barrington, G. V. (2012a). *Consulting start-up and management: A guide for evaluators and applied researchers.* SAGE.
Barrington, G. V. (2012b). *Consulting start-up & management: A guide for evaluators & applied researchers.* SAGE.
Barrington, G. V. (2012c). *Ethics on the go: Which lens should we use?* Barrington Research Group. Available at *www.barringtonresearchgrp.com/blog/34-6-ethics-on-the-go-which-lens-should-we-use.html*
Barrington, G. V. (2014). *Hiring time.* Barrington Research Group. Available at *https://barringtonresearchgrp.com/blog/58-16-hiring-time.html*
Barrington, G. V. (2015). Days & hours: What should I use for billing? *Independent Consulting TIG Newsletter, 6*(3).
Barrington, G. V. (2016). *Getting started: Introductory consulting skills for evaluators, webinar series, day 2.* American Evaluation Association.

Barrington, G. V. (2017, December 5–14). *Introduction to consulting*. AEA eStudy 083 Webinar Series.

Barrington, G. V. (2018a, May 4). *Cat got your tongue? An elevator pitch for you*. Barrington Research Group. Available at *www.barringtonresearchgrp.com/blog/108-cat-got-your-tongue-an-elevator-pitch-for-you.html*

Barrington, G. V. (2018b). *Consulting after 50: Career transition issues*. Workshop presented at the meeting of the American Evaluation Association, Cleveland, OH.

Barrington, G. V. (2018c). *Market scoping for consultants: How to get work*. Barrington Research Group. Available at *www.barringtonresearchgrp.com/blog/114-market-scoping-for-consultants-how-to-get-work.html*

Barrington, G. V. (2018d). *The reflective practitioner: The road to innovation*. Paper presented at the 13th European Evaluation Association Biennial Conference, Thessaloniki, Greece.

Barrington, G. V. (2019, winter). Consulting after 50: Redirection and reinvention for career evaluators. *Independent Evaluation Consulting: Approaches and Practices from a Growing Field, 2019*(164), 155–167.

Barrington, G. V., & Murray, D. (2024). *Your daily rate: What's the magic formula? Day 2*. Webinar presented September 19, 2024, by the Independent Consulting Community of Interest (ICCI).

Cameron, J. (1992). *The artist's way: A spiritual path to higher creativity*. Tarcher/Penguin.

Cameron, J. (2003). *Walking in this world: The practical art of creativity*. Tarcher/Penguin.

Canadian Association of Management Consultants. (2017). *Code of professional conduct*. Available at *www.cmc-canada.ca/cmccacdesignation/codeofprofessionalconduct*

Gawande, A. (2007). *Better: A surgeon's notes on performance*. Metropolitan Books.

Greiner, L. E., & Metzger, R. O. (1983). *Consulting to management*. Prentice-Hall.

Hwalek, M. A., & Straub, V. L. (2018, winter). The small sellers of program evaluation services in the United States. *New Directions for Evaluation, 160*, 125–143.

Independent Consulting Topical Interest Group Committee. (2015). *Decennial Survey 2015: Unpublished data*. Author.

Institute of Management Consultants. (2018). *IMC USA code of ethics*. Available at *www.imcusa.org/ETHICSCODE*

Kubr, M. (2002). *Management consulting: A guide to the profession* (4th ed.). International Labour Office.

Laja, P. (2017). *Useful value proposition examples (and how to create a good one)*. Available at *https://conversionxl.com/blog/value-proposition-examples-how-to-create*

Lemire, S., Fierro, L. A., Kinarsky, A. R., Fujita-Conrads, E., & Christie, C. A. (2018, winter). The U.S. federal evaluation market. *New Directions for Evaluation, 160*, 63–79.

Mancha, A. (2015). *Marketing for consultants survey: Results* [infographic]. Consulting Success. Available at *www.dailyinfographic.com/marketing-for-consultants-survey-results-infographic*

Miciak, M., Barrington, G. V., & Lavoie, M. M. (2020). Reflective practice: Moving intention into action. *Canadian Journal of Program Evaluation*, 95–105.

Morris, M. (2008). *Evaluation ethics for best practice: Cases and commentaries*. Guilford Press.

Stone, D., Patton, B., & Heen, S. (2010). *Difficult conversations: How to discuss what matters most* (10th ed.). Penguin.

U.S. Bureau of Labor Statistics. (2023). *Occupational outlook handbook*. Available at *www.bls.gov/ooh/business-and-financial/management-analysts.htm*

U.S. Census Bureau. (2022). *North American industry classification system*. 2022 NAICS Definition, Sector 54. Available at *www.census.gov/naics/?input=54&year=2022&details=541*

Wagamese, R. (2016). *Embers: One Ojibway's meditations*. Douglas and McIntyre.

Yarbrough, D. B., Shulha, L. M., Hopson, R. K., & Caruthers, F. A. (2011). *The program evaluation standards: A guide for evaluators and evaluation users* (3rd ed.). SAGE.

Chapter 24

Conducting Evaluations under Budget, Time, and Data Constraints
An International Perspective

Michael Bamberger

CHAPTER OVERVIEW

There are many textbooks explaining how to design and implement evaluations of development programs when the required data can be easily accessed when necessary, funds and staff are available, there is sufficient time to collect and analyze the data, and there is a reasonable level of support from the key interest holders. However, it is very difficult to find guidance on how to conduct a methodologically sound evaluation when key data are not easily available, the evaluation budget is insufficient, the time available to conduct the evaluation is too short, and where some key interest holders do not support the evaluation and others may actively oppose. Furthermore, the client may decide to request additional information when the study is already underway or may announce that the report must be delivered earlier than planned, or that the budget must be cut but with no reduction in the information to be provided. This chapter summarizes the real-world evaluation approach designed to provide practical guidance on how to conduct evaluations under budget, time, data, and political constraints. The chapter discusses strategies to address each of these four kinds of constraints.

THE REAL-WORLD CONTEXT WITHIN WHICH EVALUATIONS ARE CONDUCTED

There are many evaluation texts that provide guidance on how to design and implement an evaluation when there are adequate financial and human resources and a reasonable timeline, and where required data are accessible, complete, and of good quality—where agencies are willing to cooperate with data collection. However, most of the literature does not prepare evaluators for the real-world contexts where budgets are insufficient and often unpredictable, deadlines for delivering key reports are unrealistic, key data are difficult to access, and agencies are reluctant to cooperate in making data available or actively obstruct data collection. A common scenario is when an agency only commissions retrospective evaluations (at the end of the project) and the evaluator has very limited access to baseline data. In these cases, the serious methodological limitations of retrospective evaluations tend to be underestimated (or ignored).

This chapter deals with the challenges of conducting evaluations when the available time and budget are less than what the evaluator considers necessary to conduct a methodologically sound evaluation. The chapter discusses two main scenarios: the first is when the evaluators are aware of the budget and/or time constraints before the evaluation proposal is submitted and approved, but where they decide to submit a proposal because they consider the evaluation is worth doing, and the second is where the constraints do not become apparent until after the evaluation contract has been approved. Under both scenarios the evaluator has the option to withdraw from the contract but there may be financial and other reasons why it is difficult to do so. The present chapter complements Bickman's chapter (see Chapter 21, this volume), which focuses on how to plan the budget for an evaluation under more normal conditions. In contrast to a number of the other chapters that focus on evaluation experience in the United States and other industrialized nations, I draw on my experience in conducting evaluations in developing countries. The term *real-world evaluation* is used to emphasize the fact that many of these evaluations must be conducted under budget, time, and data constraints—although these challenges are certainly not restricted to developing countries. We also discuss organizational and political factors that can be even more difficult to address but which receive less attention in the literature. Each section includes options for addressing the challenges. We also draw the reader's attention to the need to assess the threats to validity of evaluations conducted under these constraints. For example, while the client may be happy if the evaluator agrees to cut the sample size by 50% to reduce costs, this and other strategies raise questions about the validity of the evaluation findings and recommendations. Interested readers are referred to Bamberger and Mabry's (2019), *RealWorld Evaluation: Working under Budget, Time, Data, and Political Constraints*, where all of these issues are discussed in more detail.

THE FOUR TYPES OF REAL-WORLD EVALUATION CHALLENGES

There are three main types of constraints affecting the design and implementation of real-world evaluations discussed in this chapter:

1. Budget and resource constraints
2. Time constraints
3. Access to data

There are two additional constraints: organizational and political influences. However, both of these factors, which are often interlinked, play an important role at all stages of the evaluation. These can influence what questions are addressed, who is interviewed (and who is excluded), what kinds of data can be collected, and how findings are presented and disseminated. Box 24.1 summarizes the main political and organizational challenges for evaluations.

Table 24.1 illustrates the different ways in which these constraints are combined in the typical contexts in which evaluations are conducted. Sometimes the evaluator faces a single constraint but often evaluators find themselves simultaneously facing two or more of the constraints.

One kind of constraint often not discussed concerns the methodological preferences of clients. For example, while some clients have a preference for quantitative methods, others prefer qualitative or mixed method designs, and some prefer case studies, while others may favor qualitative and participatory approaches. Clients are also divided between those who believe that the purpose of evaluations is to promote social justice and to have clearly defined values, while others believe evaluations should be "objective" and avoid values. When these preferences are clearly defined in the evaluation terms of reference, the evaluator can address these in the proposal, or may even decide not to accept the contract if they disagree with the client preference. However, often these client preferences are implicit and only emerge once the evaluation has begun, often during the review of the inception report (if one is required). In these situations, the evaluators may find themselves pressured to make time-consuming and expensive

BOX 24.1. Organizational and Political Influences and Constraints Affecting Evaluations

Political Influences

There is a widespread recognition in the literature that evaluation is a political process and that there are likely to be political influences at all stages of the evaluation—from defining what should be evaluated, how the evaluation should be designed, what questions should and should not be asked, and how the findings are interpreted and disseminated (Wholey, 2010; Chelimsky, 1997; Schwandt, 2005). Space does not permit a review of this literature and the following observations are based on the author's experience, mainly working with international evaluation. Political influences and constraints refer not only to pressures from government agencies and politicians but also include the requirements of funding or regulatory agencies and pressures from interest holders. Evaluations are frequently conducted in contexts in which political and ethical issues affect design and use. All programs affect some portion of the public, and most programs consume scarce public funds. Decisions based on evaluation results may intensify competition for funding, expand or terminate programs needed by some and paid for by others, or advance the agenda of a politically oriented group. While evaluators can be quick to spot the political or ideological biases of their clients and interest holders, they may be less aware about their own ideological orientations.

Organizational Constraints

All evaluations must conform to, or at least adapt to, the organizational arrangements under which they are commissioned, and the administrative procedures of the different agencies involved in commissioning, financing, managing, and using the evaluations. Often there will be a number of different agencies involved in the evaluation, with different goals for the program and the evaluation. These may involve the kinds of information to be obtained, the preferred methodology, preferences for which interest holders to be involved and who is asked to comment on or approve the evaluation reports, the extent and form in which target populations are or are not involved, and how and to which audiences the evaluation will be disseminated. When more than one international agency is involved, the basic logistics of arranging joint missions to the country where the evaluation is being conducted can cause significant delays.

Balancing the preferences and operating styles of different agencies can be a major challenge for the evaluation team, particularly in cases where there may be differences of opinion among interest holders or lack of definition of their respective roles.

Even when only a single agency is involved, their administrative and operating procedures may provide further constraints and challenges for the evaluator. For example, when local counterparts have to be contracted, the procurement procedures of the funding agency or the host government may produce long delays or require the use of contractual procedures that do not work well for a particular evaluation. In other cases, the consultants are required to prepare an **inception report**, which must be submitted to the client after the consultants have completed their preparatory mission in which the proposed methodology on the evaluation design will be based. This may also include some proposed changes to the **terms of reference**, often proposing that the scope of the evaluation should be reduced based on issues relating to the feasibility of data collection within the time and budget. Often the terms of reference stipulate that evaluation fieldwork cannot begin until all of the involved departments have commented on this report, which can cause significant delays in the start of the evaluation—despite which the date for the completion of the evaluation often cannot be changed. Another common problem is that there is little flexibility in the time allowed for fieldwork in each country, despite the fact that it may be well-known that in some countries considerable numbers of days are likely to be lost arranging travel to difficult-to-reach regions. When consultants bring up these logistical problems, the evaluation manager may respond, "I entirely agree with you, but unfortunately, this is our administrative policy, so you will just have to do the best you can."

TABLE 24.1. Real-World Evaluation Scenarios: Time, Budget, Data, and Organizational/Political Constraints

\multicolumn{4}{c	}{The constraints under which the evaluation must be conducted}	
Time	Budget	Data	Organizational and political	Typical evaluation scenarios under each constraint
X				The evaluator is called in late in the project and told that the evaluation must be completed by a certain date so that it can be used in a decision-making process or contribute to a report. The budget may be adequate but it may be difficult to collect or analyze survey data within the timeframe.
	X			The evaluation is allocated only a small budget but there is not necessarily excessive time pressure. However, it will be difficult to collect sample survey data because of the limited budget.
		X		The evaluator is not called in until the project is well advanced. Consequently, no baseline survey has been conducted either on the project population or on a comparison group. The evaluation does have an adequate scope, either to analyze existing household survey data or to collect additional data. In some cases, the intended project impacts may also concern changes in sensitive areas, such as domestic violence, community conflict, women's empowerment, community leadership styles, or corruption, on which it is difficult to collect reliable data even when time and budget are not constraints.
			X	The funding agency or a government regulatory body has requirements concerning acceptable evaluation methods. For example, in the United States, the No Child Left Behind Act of 2001 included funding preference for certain types of research designs, particularly randomized controlled trials. In other cases, a client or funding agency may specifically request, for example, qualitative data, tests of statistical significance regarding measured program effects, or both. Often client preferences for a particular methodology can be a major constraint, either requiring more time or resources than originally planned, or affecting the validity of the findings.
			X	There is evidence that the evaluation is being commissioned for political purposes. For example, an evaluation of the effects of a conservation policy may be commissioned to deliberately delay the program's expansion.
			X	There is reason to suspect that the evaluation will be used for political purposes other than or contrary to those articulated in preliminary discussions. For example, an evaluator might suspect that an evaluation of charter schools might be used (and even misused) by a client with known advocacy for privatization of education.
X	X			The evaluator operates under time pressure and with a limited budget. Secondary survey data may be available, but there is little time or resources to analyze them.
X		X		The evaluator has little time and no access to baseline data or a comparison group. Funds are available to collect additional data but the survey design is constrained by the tight deadlines.
	X	X		The evaluator is called in late and has no access to baseline data or comparison groups. The budget is limited but time is not a constraint.
X	X	X		The evaluator is called in late, is given a limited budget, and has no access to baseline survey data, and no comparison group has been identified.

Note. To simplify the table, the possible combinations of political constraints with the other three factors have not been included.

changes to the evaluation methodology after the budget and the timeline have been finalized in the contract. Theoretically the evaluator could refuse to accept these changes, or in the extreme case refuse to continue. So, it is not uncommon for client methodological preferences to be a significant constraint in real-world evaluations.

ADDRESSING BUDGET CONSTRAINTS

The Challenges

Sometimes funds for the evaluation were not included in the original project budget, and the evaluation must be conducted with a much smaller budget than would normally be allocated. In other cases, funds were approved for the evaluation but the process of release may be so slow that only a part of the funds could be used within the fiscal year for which they were approved. As a result, it may not be possible to collect all the required data, including baseline or comparison group data. Lack of funds may also exacerbate time constraints because evaluators may not be able to spend as much time in the field as they consider necessary. Box 24.2 makes the point that it is important to understand whether the main constraint is budget or time (or both), because the best strategy will often be different in each case. Also, budget constraints often produce pressures to cut corners in the evaluation design—for example, spending less time on exploratory studies or pilot testing survey instruments, as well as cutting back on supervision and quality control during data collection.

> **BOX 24.2. Budget and Time Constraints Have Different Implications for the Evaluation Design**
>
> While budget and time constraints often have similar consequences for the evaluation design, they can require very different approaches. For example, if an evaluation must be completed by a certain date, the process of data collection can often be speeded up by bringing in consultants, hiring more experienced researchers, or increasing the number of interviewers. All of these measures may require significant budget increases. If, on the other hand, budget is the main constraint, the decision might be made to contract with a local university that would use cheaper though less experienced graduate students who might require more time for data collection because they cannot work full-time.

> **BOX 24.3. Six Options to Help Make the Budget Go Further**
>
> 1. Can we use a simpler and cheaper evaluation design?
> 2. Do we really need to collect all of this information?
> 3. Has someone already collected some of the information that we need?
> 4. Can we reduce the number of interviews, observations, cases, and so on without sacrificing the necessary precision?
> 5. Is there a cheaper way to collect the information?
> 6. Is it possible to utilize new information technologies to reduce costs of data collection and analysis?

Strategies for Addressing Budget and Other Resource Constraints

Box 24.3 presents options for addressing budget constraints, each of which is discussed below.

Option 1: Simplifying the Evaluation Design

When considering ways to simplify the evaluation design, it is important to keep in mind that there is no single evaluation design that will be appropriate in all situations, and the choice of design will be largely determined by the evaluation questions that are being asked. Stern et al. (2012) identify four common evaluation questions, each requiring different evaluation designs: (1) To what extent has the intervention contributed to the achievement of a specific impact or set of impacts?; (2) Did the intervention make a difference?; (3) How has the intervention made a difference?; and (4) Will the intervention work elsewhere? It is also important to keep in mind that in most cases there are several different approaches that could be considered for addressing any particular evaluation question (see Box 24.4). For example, Question 1, "Has the intervention contributed to achieving a specific impact?" could be addressed using an experimental (e.g., a randomized controlled trial [RCT]) or quasi-experimental (e.g., **pipeline**) design; a **qualitative comparative analysis**;

> **BOX 24.4. Alternative Approaches to the Evaluation of Impacts**
>
> The following are the most widely-used approaches for evaluating program impacts:
>
> - Experimental designs
> - Quasi-experimental designs
> - Participatory and qualitative evaluations (there are large numbers of different approaches)
> - Mixed methods designs
> - Theory-based designs (including theory of change)
> - Descriptive case studies
> - Qualitative comparative analysis case studies
> - Complexity-responsive evaluation designs
> - Gender-responsive evaluations
> - Econometric and statistical designs
> - Data science approaches
> - Systematic reviews
>
> Overviews of these approaches are available in Vaessen et al. (2016).

participatory consultations with intended beneficiaries; or the combination of several of these approaches in a mixed methods design).

One way to reduce the costs and time is to simplify the evaluation design. Any discussion on ways to simplify the evaluation design must take into consideration how different approaches will affect the ability of the evaluation to address the key evaluation questions of concern to interest holders, the kinds of decisions to which the evaluation will contribute, and the level of disaggregation of the findings. For example, small samples will likely only allow an estimate of the impact on total sample population. If separate estimates must be made for different geographical areas, types of economic activity, or ethnic groups, then a larger sample size would be needed and trimming down the sample to save money would not be prudent. It is important to keep in mind that while there are some general issues affecting all evaluations, the range of design options will be different for quantitative, qualitative, and mixed methods designs. Keeping these points in mind, the following are some of the possible options for simplifying the evaluation design:

- Reducing the number of observation points—for example, eliminating data collection during project implementation and only using a pretest–posttest design.

- Reducing the sample size (see "Option 4: Reducing Costs by Reducing Sample Size" below).

- Reducing the number of people to be interviewed in each household, community, or organization—for example, only interviewing a single household representative rather than interviewing both an adult male and female, or only interviewing the head teacher or administrators, rather than several teachers.

- Reducing the amount of information to be collected and the length of the survey instrument.

- Replacing a relatively large quantitative survey with a mixed methods design that combines a somewhat smaller sample survey with, for example, participant observation and/or focus groups. Bamberger and Mabry (2019, Chapter 14) argue that a mixed methods design can both reduce the cost of the evaluation while improving the quality of the data and the interpretation through triangulation. There is, however, a trade-off, as it is usually necessary to accept a lower level of statistical significance in order to free up resources for the qualitative studies.

- One practical design option to both reduce costs and increase access to a comparison group is the use of one of the variations of a wait-list or pipeline design. When projects are implemented in phases, the subjects selected for the subsequent phases can be used as the comparison group for Phase 1. These designs can produce significant cost reductions by using future project beneficiaries as the comparison group. These designs also make it more likely that the comparison group will be willing to be interviewed (as they are future project participants), which is a big advantage as it is hard to provide incentives to nonbeneficiaries to be interviewed.

- A final option involves the incorporation of big data and data analytics into the evaluation design. While big data sources and analytical techniques are not yet widely used in evaluation practice, a number of promising approaches are starting to be applied. For example, satellite data, drones, and remote sensors can be used to reduce the cost of certain kinds of data collection to strengthen sample design through propensity score matching, or through the economical generation of longitudinal data; social media analytics can be used to measure changes in behavior and attitudes; and mobile phones can estimate changes in income through air-time purchases (Bamberger, 2017). These and other big data techniques have become of increasing importance in recent years (see Bamberger & Mabry, 2019, Chapter 18, "Evaluation in the Age of Big Data").

Figure 24.1 illustrates how multiple sources of big data can sometimes be combined to permit the evaluation of a large program for a much lower cost than would be required for the use of analog (face-to-face) sample surveys and other conventional data collection methods. This project (the Sticky Rice Project) is designed to reach 1 million small rice farmers and to reduce carbon emissions and increase productivity. The big data sources that are being considered include satellite and drone images, remote sensors (to monitor farmer compliance with actions required to reduce carbon emissions and increase productivity), data from mobile phones, social media analysis, and block chain technology (to monitor performance and compliance and provide a secure financial platform that is independent of government regulations). While this design is obviously much more complicated than many of the other examples discussed in this chapter, it is in fact much simpler and cheaper than any of the other options that could be considered for trying to survey and generate continuous monitoring data on 500,000 farmers scattered across remote parts of Southeast Asia. The use of satellite and remote sensor data also requires expertise in the use of these specialized datasets. However, the agencies that use these kinds of data argue that it is no more expensive or difficult to contract and work with a big data analyst than it would be to hire a technical consultant in an area such as sample survey design.

For strategies that involve working with multiple datasets, it is important to check carefully to ensure that the different sources of information will be available, that they include the required kinds of information, covering the right target population and the appropriate time period, and that the quality and completeness of the data is satisfactory. Sometimes data are available but the costs of putting them into a usable format can be very high and time-consuming.

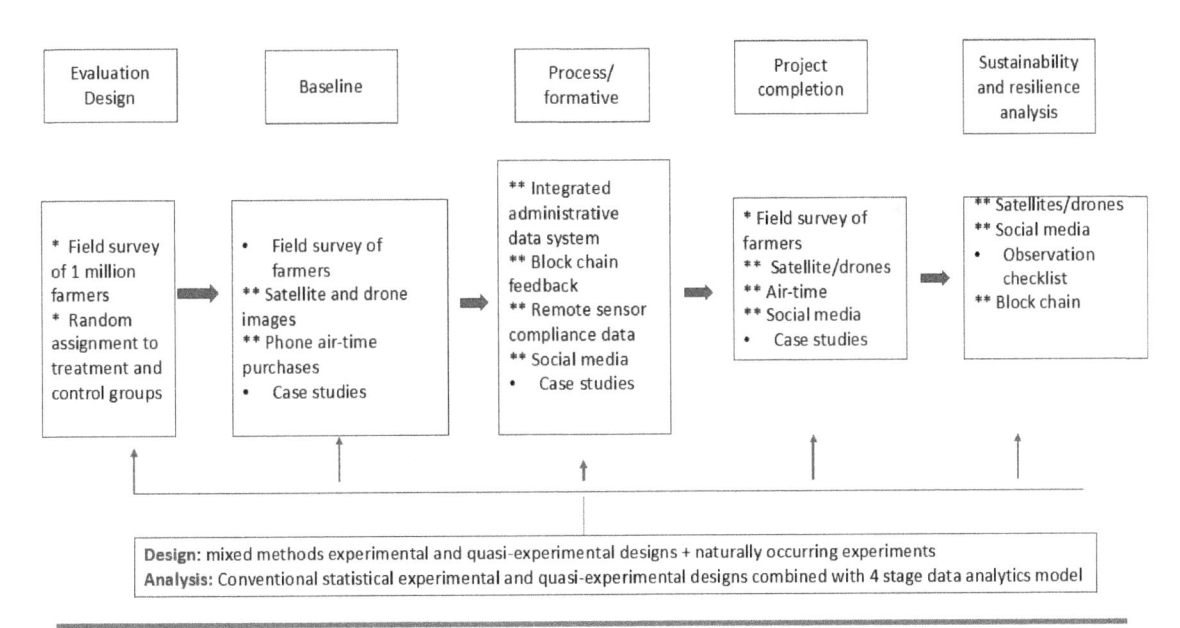

FIGURE 24.1. Example of the integration of big data into evaluation design: The Sticky Rice Project Carbon Emissions Reduction Project in Southeast Asia. ** = big data source.

UNDERSTANDING TRADE-OFFS AND COMPENSATING FOR WEAKER DESIGNS

While there are a few cases where it is possible to reduce costs and at the same time maintain the quality and coverage of the evaluation (e.g., using big data to reduce the costs and time of data collection and analysis, or eliminating questions that do not provide any useful information), in most cases cutting costs involves trade-offs. Sometimes these trade-offs reduce the ability to disaggregate the analysis to compare program impacts on different subgroups, while in other cases they may reduce the **statistical precision** of the findings as a result of sample size reduction, and in other cases the explanatory power of the analysis may be weakened if useful but expensive and time-consuming in-depth interviews and case studies have to be sacrificed.

Decisions on what trade-offs are possible must be made in close consultation with the client. I have been in situations where the client has complained, "What is the point of hiring an expert evaluator if you have to ask our advice on the best way to cut the budget?" The client must understand that these are strategic decisions based on knowledge of the political as well as the technical environment. What do government decision makers expect from the evaluation? What do they really need to know and how much detail is required?

So, when budgets are tight, the evaluator needs to strategize with the client on what cuts could be made and what kinds of information are critical. There are always a number of trade-offs to be assessed. Should the evaluation try to maximize sample size (making the study more credible to interest holders who believe in large numbers), or is it more important to provide in-depth insights on a smaller number of households, communities, or schools? How important is a longitudinal perspective? Is it sufficient to only interview the (frequently male) "household head," or is it important to understand the perspective of the partner and possibly other household members?

The main message is that while the evaluator can provide guidance on the methodological consequences of the different ways to reduce costs and time (e.g., the validity of the findings and conclusions about the risks of different kinds of bias, and the quality of the data), a decision on the consequences of the possible trade-offs must be based on the political judgment of the client. This involves an understanding of the expectations of the key interest holders. An important role for the evaluator is to advise the client on how well the evaluation methodology will stand up to scrutiny from an evaluation specialist if one is consulted. The evaluator should always prepare a short section discussing the limitations of the evaluation so that the report is transparent with respect to its strengths and limitations. The threats to the validity framework discussed in the "Taking into Account Threats to Validity When Addressing Real-World Constraints" section below can be a useful way to present the assessment of the evaluation methodology.

Throughout the chapter I discuss ways to compensate for these real-world constraints. Two of the methods that are frequently referred to are the use of mixed methods designs to effectively combine and triangulate among different quantitative and qualitative methods of data collection and analysis (see Azzam & Jones, Chapter 18, this volume), and constantly exploring opportunities to draw on big data and the new information technologies.

Option 2: Clarifying Client Information Needs

The costs and time required for data collection can sometimes be significantly reduced through a clearer definition of the information required by the client and the kinds of decisions to which the evaluation will contribute. Often clients request types of information that they think would be "interesting" but which are not essential for the evaluation. Working with clients to eliminate nonessential information can produce significant reductions in the amount of information to be collected. There are a number of approaches for assessing client information needs. One way is to conduct an interest holder survey electronically, or through individual interviews and focus groups. Another is to solicit comments on the draft data collection instruments. A useful but more time-consuming approach is to take advantage of workshops that many programs organize to plan the **theory of change** that is often used both as a program design tool and the framework for the evaluation. These workshops encourage all interest holders to express their ideas of program objectives and the implementation strategies required to achieve these objectives. The workshops also discuss the questions that each interest holder wishes the evaluation to address and the indicators that should be used to measure inputs, activities, outputs, outcomes, and impacts.

Option 3: Efficient Use of Existing Data

Often, secondary data can be identified that reduce the need for the collection of primary data:

- Census or survey data covering the project and comparison communities. Many governments conduct periodic national household surveys containing information on the socioeconomic conditions of households and communities and other information of interest to the evaluation. If the results can be disaggregated to the specific population and/or geographic area reached by a project, such secondary data can be helpful in a project evaluation.
- Data from project monitoring records (e.g., household income, type of housing, school attendance, microloans approved).
- Records from schools (e.g., enrollment, attendance, test scores), health centers (e.g., number of patients, types of illness), and other public service agencies (e.g., water supply and sanitation, public transport).
- Newspapers and other mass media often cover economic and social issues that projects address (e.g., schools, access to health and sanitation facilities, public transport).
- Records from community organizations (e.g., minutes of meetings, photographs, posters).
- Dissertations and other academic studies.
- The use of **big data** and **integrated data platforms** can open up many new sources of data that may be available free or at a relatively modest cost. While some of these data sources can be expensive, many are available free. Many social media platforms, such as Facebook and Twitter (now X), also provide powerful analytical tools free of charge. However, while individual data sources may be free and user-friendly, the creation of integrated data platforms that merge different datasets will usually be quite expensive and time-consuming to set up.

Also, when assessing integrated data platforms it is important to ask, "Expensive compared to what?" Combining big data and data integration software makes it possible to conduct sophisticated data collection and analysis, which previously was never done because of the complexity and cost. While these data platforms are clearly more expensive than conducting a single survey, they can vastly increase the kinds of data and the depth and breadth of the analysis—including, for example, accessing previously unavailable longitudinal datasets. It is important to be aware of problems and delays in getting access to and analyzing these kinds of information. Additional challenges are to ensure that the data cover the required population, provide the specific kinds of information required, and cover the correct time period. For example, the economic conditions of low-income households and their access to services can vary dramatically over time, so that data that are even 1 year different from the reference date can be very misleading.

Option 4: Reducing Costs by Reducing Sample Size

Often, sample sizes are defined by survey researchers without reference to the kinds of decisions to be made by clients and the level of **precision** actually required. Many clients assume that sample size is a purely technical question, and that the evaluator should tell the client what is the "right" sample size. However, the appropriate sample size depends on factors such as to what kinds of decisions will the findings contribute, and whether the results must be disaggregated (by geographical area, ethnicity, or economic activities; see Table 24.2 for a list of 10 factors that can influence sample size). When these factors are not taken into consideration, the sample may either be larger (and more expensive) than is actually required to answer the evaluation questions, or it may be too small to produce information that is useful to interest holders.

It is important to involve the client in decisions on the size and structure of the sample. It is critical to understand whether very precise statistical estimates are required or whether this is an exploratory study in which only the viabil-

TABLE 24.2. Factors Affecting the Sample Size

Factor	Explanation	Influence on sample size
1. The purpose of the evaluation	Is this an exploratory study, or are precise statistical estimates required?	The more precise the required results, the larger the sample.
2. Will a one- or two-tailed test be used?	In most cases a *two-tailed test* will be used to test whether the project has produced a significant change. However, if the purpose is only to determine whether the project has produced a significant improvement, then a *one-tailed test* can be considered.	The sample size can be reduced approximately 40% when a one-tailed test can be used.
3. Is only the project group interviewed?	In some evaluation designs, only subjects from the project group are interviewed. This is the case if information on the total population is available from previous studies or secondary data.	The sample size will be doubled if the same number of people must be interviewed in both the project and comparison groups.
4. Homogeneity of the group	If there is little variation among the population with respect to the outcome variable, then the standard deviation will be small. For example, if most farmers are growing a single crop and all have about the same area of land, it would be possible to estimate farming practices and production with a relatively small sample. However, if there are large variations in land and many different kinds of crops are produced, then a much larger sample would be required to obtain the same level of accuracy.	The smaller the standard deviation (i.e., variability), the smaller the required sample.
5. The effect size	Effect size is the amount of increase (change) the project is expected to produce. For example, if providing school meals to increase school attendance is expected to only produce a small increase in school attendance (small effect size), then a much larger sample would be required to determine whether the increase is statistically significant than would be required if a large increase in attendance is expected.	The smaller the effect size, the larger the required sample.
6. The efficiency with which the project is implemented	When project administration is poor, different individuals or groups may unintentionally receive different combinations of services. The quality of the services can also vary. This makes it difficult to determine whether lower-than-expected outcomes are due to poor project design or to the fact that many subjects are not receiving all intended services. There are other cases where the program design intentionally incorporates different combinations of services for different groups, or where beneficiaries can receive combinations of services. In these cases the evaluation design may address these variations (e.g., using factorial designs or case studies).	The poorer the quality and efficiency of the project, the larger the required sample.
7. The required level of disaggregation	In some cases, the client only requires estimates of impact for the total project population. In other cases, disaggregated results for different project sites are required.	The greater the required disaggregation, the larger the sample.
8. The sample design	Sampling procedures, such as stratification, can often reduce the variance of the estimates and increase **statistical precision**. If different subgroups can be identified, each with different characteristics likely to affect program outcomes, breaking the total sample down into strata can reduce the sample variance by controlling for the effect of differences between strata. Henry (1990, Chapter 4) presents four U.S. case studies of sample designs illustrating when stratification can be used. It was possible to stratify the sample in an evaluation of programs for families eligible for Social Security in North Carolina. The population was divided into three strata using lists of recipients of Aid to Families with Dependent Children, Supplemental Social Security, and the medically needy. However, in an evaluation of programs for institutionalized persons with mental illness in Virginia, available information did not make it possible to stratify the sample.	Well-designed stratification may reduce sample size.

(continued)

TABLE 24.2. *(continued)*

Factor	Explanation	Influence on sample size
9. The level of statistical precision	"Beyond a reasonable doubt" is usually defined as meaning there is less than a 1 in 20 possibility that an impact as large as this could have occurred by chance (defined as the ".05 confidence level"). If less precise results are acceptable, it is possible to reduce sample size by accepting a lower confidence level—for example, a 1 in 10 possibility that the result occurred by chance.	The higher the required confidence level, the larger the sample.
10. The power of the test	The statistical power of the test refers to the probability that when a project has a "real" effect, this will be rejected by the statistical significance test. The conventional power level is .8, meaning that there is only a 20% chance that a real effect would be rejected. The choice of the power of the test has a large impact on the required sample size. Typically, when testing for the statistical significance of change in the mean, increasing the required power of the test from .80 to .95 will increase the required sample size by around 75%. So, for example, when testing for a small expected effect size of only 0.20, it might be necessary to increase the required sample size from 618 to 1,078 (Bamberger & Mabry, 2019, Chapter 15). This is a simplified example as other factors can also affect the calculations, but it shows that the choice of sample size is critical when working under budget constraints.	The higher the required power level, the larger the required sample.

ity of the proposed model is being tested. The evaluator must also present the trade-offs between statistical credibility of the findings and the cost. In some cases, it is possible to reduce costs by cutting some information or analysis included in the initial terms of reference but the decision to do so should be made with the client. Dane (2011, Chapter 5) provides a useful explanation for clients who are not research specialists on the different kinds of samples and the benefits of each, which can be helpful when discussing trade-offs between cost and statistical rigor.

FACTORS AFFECTING SAMPLE SIZE FOR QUANTITATIVE EVALUATIONS

The required sample size for quantitative sample survey evaluations can vary greatly according to the characteristics of the population, the nature of the project intervention, and the purpose of the evaluation. Ten factors affecting sample size are described briefly in Table 24.2.

FACTORS AFFECTING THE SIZE AND COST OF QUALITATIVE SAMPLES

Qualitative evaluations have a different purpose from quantitative studies, and sample size is usually not the key factor in the study design. In some cases, an evaluation is based solely on qualitative methods, whereas in other cases a mixed methods design is used by combining quantitative and qualitative methods. When qualitative methods are used in conjunction with surveys and other quantitative methods, the purpose of the qualitative component is usually to explore situations in more depth so as to understand processes or behaviors, illustrate different typologies of subjects (individuals, families, schools, etc.), to triangulate survey data to increase validity, or to explore the broader context in which a program operates. When using mixed methods designs there are various ways that qualitative cases can be selected: to illustrate and explore in more depth each of the main groups identified in the quantitative analysis (in which case the qualitative cases are selected to be more or less representative of the different categories identified in the surveys), to identify and explain extreme or exceptional cases (outliers), or to focus on the most successful cases. Different sampling strategies would be required for each of these scenarios. In most evaluations the number of cases for the qualitative analysis are relatively small due to their cost and the amount of time that is often required for each case.

The cost of each case study is affected by at least four factors: (1) the number of subjects or units of observation (schools, families, drug dealers), (2) the number of physical locations in which observation takes place (the home, place of work, street, bar), (3) the period of time over which the observations take place (cases can be completed in one interview or they may continue over months or years), and (4) the frequency of observations (hourly, daily, weekly, etc.). Consequently, sample costs and time can be saved by reducing the number of subjects, reducing the number of physical locations (observe only in the street or only in the school), and the duration of the study or the number of time periods over which observations are made (every day for a week, every day for a month, once a week for a year).

The decision on the number of subjects, locations, duration of the study, or units of analysis usually depends on the professional judgment of the researcher. Some ethnographers argue that one should keep including more subjects until no new information is being collected.

Box 24.5 illustrates different ways to select case studies. At one extreme the cases are selected randomly, while at the other less-structured ethnographic methods are used.

Option 5: Reducing Costs of Data Collection and Analysis

The elimination of nonessential information can significantly reduce the length of the data collection instrument or the duration of the observation. Examples of areas where the amount of information could be reduced include (1) demographic information on each household member, (2) amount of information on agricultural production and food consumption in a community,

---

BOX 24.5. Examples of Two Methods for Selecting Qualitative Cases

Example 1: Studying crack cocaine addicts in New York City. This example illustrates a typical ethnographic approach in which there is no predetermined sampling plan and the goal is to include everyone who has an important influence on the lives of a number of crack cocaine dealers. New subjects are encountered at parties, on the street, and in the houses of the dealers and their families, friends, and customers.

> I spent hundreds of nights on the street and in crack houses observing dealers and addicts. . . . Perhaps more important, I also visited families, attending parties, and intimate reunions. . . . I interviewed, and in many cases befriended the spouses, lovers, siblings, mothers, grandmothers and—where possible—the fathers and stepfathers of the crack dealers. (Bourgois, 2002, p. 16)

Example 2: Two approaches to the selection of case studies in a study to help design rural health centers to make the services accessible to women. This hypothetical example illustrates how case studies can be selected in two different mixed methods approaches to the same question. In the first study option, cases are used to illustrate the findings of a quantitative survey. A national randomly selected sample of rural households is interviewed. The analysis identifies a typology of households and villages based on demographic characteristics of households (high and low educational levels, poor and less poor, different ethnic groups) and on different responses to the existing rural health centers (e.g., visits regularly, uses but with complaints, does not use). The case studies of villages and households within each village are selected to be broadly representative of the total sample population. The cases are used to illustrate and understand the findings of the quantitative survey. In the second option, the study is predominantly qualitative and data from the national household sampling frame is used to ensure that the case study villages are selected to be broadly representative of all villages. Case studies are then conducted in the selected villages but the households and household members are selected in a more open and less structured way as the study progresses. Many of the women were originally contacted in or near the health centers but follow-up meetings took place in their houses or in other parts of the community. Through the women the researchers met and came to know other household members as well as community leaders, local health workers, and so on. Important data were also collected through observation in the clinics and near the clinics but also observing discussion among family members on health-related topics. While the first option provides a more representative sample of respondents, the flexibility of the second option often makes it possible to dig deeper and identify patterns and behavior that might not emerge from the first option.

(3) information on urban or rural travel patterns, and (4) region of origin of each household member. As always, it is important to define information requirements with the client and not to arbitrarily eliminate information to produce a shorter data collection instrument. For many qualitative studies, the amount and type of information cannot be defined as easily as for quantitative surveys, and consequently, the list of questions or issues cannot be pruned quite so easily. While the original qualitative design—questions, issues, methods, instruments—is available for pruning from the start, the pruning process is more complicated. With emergent designs, issues and questions arise as the research progresses, and often, many of what prove to be the critical issues were not even included on the initial lists of questions. However, the following are examples of ways to reduce the amount of information to be collected:

- The range of topics can be reduced to those of greatest priority.
- The number of interviewees can be reduced.
- The number and types of documents to be analyzed can be reduced.
- The time period studied can be shortened.

A number of alternatives can significantly reduce the costs of data collection for both qualitative and quantitative evaluations:

- Collect information on community attitudes, time use, access to and use of services, and the like through **participatory rural appraisal (PRA)** group interview methods and focus groups. It is important to note, however, that well-designed focus groups are in themselves time-consuming. Focus groups require identifying appropriate interviewees, arranging times that all members of the group can get together, preparing and field testing the interview protocol, transcribing and validating the interview data, and conducting content analysis.
- Replace surveys with direct observation—for example, to study time use, travel patterns, and use of community facilities. It is again important to note that although some types of observation can be quite rapid and economical (e.g., observation of pedestrian and vehicular travel patterns in areas with relatively few roads), in other cases (e.g., household time-use surveys) it is not necessarily faster than a survey.

- Use key informants to obtain information on community behavior and use of services.

- Use self-administered instruments, such as surveys, self-evaluations, reflection or response forms, diaries, and journals, to collect data on income and expenditure, travel patterns, or time use.

- Make maximum use of preexisting data, including project records.

- Photography and videotaping can sometimes provide useful and economical documentary evidence on the changing quality of houses and roads, as well as on the use of public transport services (Heath, 2004; Kumar, 1993; Patton, 2002).

Option 6: Potential Applications of New Information Technology to Reduce the Costs and Time of Data Collection and Analysis

Over the past few years there has been a dramatic increase in the use of *new information technology*. This term includes both big data (e.g., satellite images and remote sensors; social media, such as Twitter [now X] and Facebook; and data from phone records and call-in radio programs), and information and communication technology data generated from mobile phones and other portable devices. New information technologies are described and their implications for evaluation are discussed in Bamberger and Mabry (2019, Chapter 18, "Evaluation in the Age of Big Data"). All of these technologies make it possible to collect survey data and other kinds of conventional evaluation data more economically and faster. Mobile phones, in particular, offer powerful new tools for conducting and analysis of surveys, mapping the location of services (e.g., the location of water supply and sanitation), identifying hot spots (e.g., danger spots for traffic accidents or gang violence), and for creating video and audio records.

Big data makes it possible to collect an enormous variety of data that even a few years ago often did not exist or was not accessible to evaluation. The characteristic of most kinds of big data is that they use data that were generated for some purpose other than evaluation (electronic financial transactions, social media and phone messages, satellite images collected for commercial or meteorological purposes, health data collected through wearable devices). Big data involve a fundamentally different approach to research and evaluation, using techniques such as predictive analytics and machine learning with which most evaluators are not familiar. These approaches greatly expand the range of tools and techniques that are becoming available to evaluators, and which can greatly reduce the costs of data collection and analysis. However, these techniques also raise a number of new challenges, which are also discussed in Bamberger and Mabry (2019).

ADDRESSING TIME CONSTRAINTS

The Challenges

The most common time constraint is when the evaluator is not called in until the project is already well advanced and the evaluation has to be conducted within a much shorter period of time than the evaluator considers necessary. Time constraints often make it impossible to conduct a pretest–posttest evaluation design with a baseline study that can be repeated after the project has been implemented. When operating under time constraints it is also unlikely that there is a control or comparison group, or that random assignment has been done. The time available for planning interest holder consultations, site visits and fieldwork, and data analysis may also have to be drastically reduced. These time pressures are particularly problematic for an evaluator who is not familiar with the area or even the country and who does not have time for familiarization and for building confidence with the communities and the agencies involved with the study. The combination of time and budget constraints frequently means that international evaluators (and out-of-town U.S. evaluators) can only be in the project location for a short period of time—often requiring them to use shortcuts that they recognize as methodologically weak.

Strategies to Address Time Constraints

It is important to distinguish between two different time constraints. The first concerns the duration of the evaluation and the delivery deadline, while the second refers to the level of effort (the number of allocated person/days). The solution to these two challenges may be different. If the challenge is to meet a deadline but where budget is not a constraint, it may be possible to bring in more consultants or staff to increase the level of effort. If, on the other hand, the problem concerns the level of effort, one of the options may be to replace an expensive international consultant with less costly national or local consultants. However, if local staff are less experienced, this approach may extend the time to complete the evaluation while reducing the cost.

Most of the strategies to reduce time are similar to those discussed in the previous section for reducing costs:

- Making more efficient use of expensive consultants. For example, hiring local consultants to conduct some of the preparatory work, such as selecting participants for focus groups or preparing briefing notes on the communities or agencies to be visited.
- Using videoconferences to prepare for consultant missions or to reduce time of the consultant visits.
- Hiring more data collectors.
- Coordinating with operations staff to include key information required for baseline and follow-up studies in the project monitoring system.
- Using new information technology to reduce time required for collection and analysis of data.
- Using rapid data collection methods (e.g., focus groups, key informants, using community groups to help with some kinds of data collection, exit surveys, observation checklists, audio–visual data collection and analysis, rapid ethnographic methods).

ADDRESSING DATA CONSTRAINTS

The Challenges

When the evaluation does not start until late in the project cycle, there is usually little comparable baseline information available on the conditions of the target group before the start of the project. Even if project records are available on program participants, they are often not organized in the form needed for comparative before-and-after analysis. Project records and other documentary data may suffer from reporting biases or poor record-keeping standards. Even when secondary data are available close to the project starting date, they usually do not fully match the project populations. For example, employment data may not cover the informal sector where many project families work, or school records may cover public schools but not religious and other private schools.

Many clients are only interested in collecting data on the groups or communities with which they are working and do not see the value of collecting data on a comparison group. They may also be concerned that collection of information on nonbeneficiaries might create expectations of financial compensation or other benefits, which further discourages the collection of data on a comparison group.

A challenge for many evaluations concerns the difficulties of identifying and/or capturing data on vulnerable groups, such as undocumented groups, the homeless, ethnic and other minorities, and groups or organizations that for some reason are not included in official statistics. In many countries, significant numbers of households or individuals are excluded from the sampling frames used for evaluation studies. Sometimes the existence of the missing groups is not acknowledged or in other cases it is considered too expensive to include them and some kind of statistical adjustment may be made to assume how they would compare with the mainstream population. Sometimes the existence of vulnerable groups is recognized but conventional data collection methods are not able to collect information on their particular situation. The lack of data on the differential impact of programs on women and men illustrate many of these challenges, and the issues are similar for collecting data on other groups. Many evaluations, partly for reasons of cost, only collect aggregate data on the household and not on the situation of individual household members such as women, young people, or older adults. Box 24.6 illustrates some of the problems in collecting information on women, their access to, and control over household resources, how they are

> **BOX 24.6. Problems Capturing Information from or about Women**
>
> - Many household surveys only interview the "household head," who is often considered to be the male. He often does not have all the information on female household members or gives low priority to their concerns. Many men, for example, say their wives are happy to spend several hours per day walking to collect water or fuel because they "sing and chat with their friends as they walk."
> - Women are often interviewed in the presence of other household members where they may not feel free to express their views.
> - Donor agencies often insist that women be invited to attend community meetings to discuss proposed projects. However, the women often do not feel free to speak in public, or they always say they agree with their husbands.
> - In many parts of the world, sexual harassment is one of the main reasons women do not use public transport. However, it is culturally impossible for women to mention this to an outside interviewer, so this major problem is often not captured in surveys.

affected by different programs, and some of the unintended negative consequences they may experience. The following section suggests ways to address these challenges within real-world budget and time constraints.

Strategies to Address Data Constraints

Reconstructing Baseline Data

When evaluations are not commissioned until toward the end of the project, it is common to find that no baseline study has been conducted. A number of techniques are available to reconstruct data on the situation of the project and comparison groups at the start of the project.

- *Using available administrative data.* Most agencies collect extensive data on the project population from monitoring, participant application forms, project visit reports, minutes of community meetings, and so on. Sometimes information is in a form that can be easily used but in other cases the organization of the data so that it can be analyzed can take much longer than anticipated. For example, the process of obtaining permission to use the data can take months. New information technologies make it possible to combine multiple information sources into an integrated data platform with a common metric so that different kinds of data (numerical, written, photograph, audio–visual, etc.) can be combined and compared.

- *Secondary survey data.* Government agencies, development agencies, and nongovernmental organizations (NGOs) have often conducted surveys and produced reports, often with information collected around the time needed for the baseline.

- *Retrospective surveys.* Retrospective surveys can be conducted in which respondents are asked to recall income, consumption, employment, travel, and other kinds of relevant data. However, with the exception of a few areas such as income and expenditure and fertility and contraceptive use, where large-scale longitudinal studies have been conducted that can be used to compare recall with real-time data, the problem with recall data is that no reliable source of information is available to correct for the magnitude or direction of recall bias. Time and cost considerations are similar to other kinds of surveys.

- *Key informants.* Key informants, such as community leaders, doctors, teachers, local government agencies, NGOs, and religious organizations, may be able to provide useful reference data on baseline conditions. However, these informants, like all sources, have potential biases and their own particular agendas. Consequently, the researcher should try to consult with people likely to have different sources of information and perspectives and never rely on a single source. For example, in the study of the sex trade (see Box 24.4) informants were selected to include people who know prostitutes in their family setting or community and as commercial associates or clients, as well as different perspectives (e.g., the police, neighborhood associations trying to force the prostitutes out of the community, religious leaders). It is also important not to assume that all informants should be in positions of authority. The perspective of a child, neighbor, or friend can be just as important as a local government official or the police chief. While the number of informants must be adjusted to the available time, this can be a major challenge as there are many situations in which some important informants can only be identified after the researcher has been in contact with the communities for some time and trust has been established. So the richness and depth of the information is often related to the period of time over which the researcher is in contact with the study population.

- *Participatory methods.* Over the past 30 years, a broad range of participatory research and evaluation techniques have become part of the evaluator's toolkit. These were a reaction against *top-down planning*, in which surveys were designed, conducted, and interpreted by outside experts. Participatory research methods, which have a number of different names, including PRA and participatory learning and action, are based on the principle of empowering the community to conduct its own analysis of its needs and priorities. All of the approaches work through community groups rather than individuals. Many techniques were developed for working with rural and urban communities with relatively low levels of literacy, and many approaches rely heavily on mapping and other graphical techniques. Participatory evaluation approaches are very useful for the present discussion as they have developed a wide range of techniques for reconstructing the history of the community and for the identification and analysis of critical events in the life of the community. While some of these techniques, such as PRA and other community participation techniques (see Kumar, 2002), can be conducted in a few days for each group, some of the participant observation methods can continue for weeks or much longer. While most of these techniques can be conducted within the framework of real-world time constraints, many kinds of information are discovered gradually as the confidence of the community is gained and as different stages of community life are observed. One danger is to reduce methods that ideally require significant amounts of time to a few days—without recognizing what is lost. One important consideration when using many of these techniques is to explore ways to extend the amount of time over which the participatory research can be conducted. For example, an anthropologist working with me spent more than a month living in a low-income community in

Cartagena, Colombia, to understand household structure and interhousehold patterns of transfers and support to families in times of need, before work began on the design of a quantitative survey. For a fuller description of the following participatory techniques, the reader is referred to Somesh Kumar's (2002) *Methods for Community Participation: A Complete Guide for Practitioners.*

- *Seasonal calendars.* These are often used in farming studies in which farmers report for each month factors such as rainfall, planting and harvesting of crops, labor demand, migration, market prices for agricultural products, and so on (Kumar, 2002; Theis & Grady, 1991). The group works together to prepare a chart marking the months. Participants are then asked to indicate the months with, for example, the highest incidence of famine, out-migration, or expenditures. Belli et al. (2009) describe the use of calendar and time diaries in the United States.

- *Time trends.* These can be used with any kind of population to study changes over time in farm yields, income, migration, malnutrition, and access to services. Often participants are asked to plot changes for each year but sometimes longer periods may be used (Kumar, 2002). In some cultures, the concept of a calendar year has no meaning, so reference points such as a major drought, the election of a new president, or the outbreak of a war may be used.

- *Historical profile.* This provides information on historical factors that are important for understanding the present situation in a community or region. This may cover, for example, building of infrastructure, introduction of new crops, epidemics, droughts and famines, foreign and civil war, and major political events (Kumar, 2002). Another approach is to give a recorder to different people in the community and ask them to narrate their version of community history. Triangulation is important to reconcile the major discrepancies of interpretation that are often found between the reports of different community members.

- *Critical incidents.* This is similar to the historical profile except that the analysis is focused on the stressful events or periods. Sometimes the analysis covers 1 year (looking at seasonal variations in stress), or it may cover a longer period.

- *Geographic information systems, (GIS), satellite images, and remote sensors.* GIS systems create electronic maps (Clemmer, 2010) that define the precise location of physical features (e.g., roads, rivers), services (e.g., hospitals, stores, public service facilities), populations classified by socioeconomic or other characteristics (e.g., income, ethnicity, number of children), or events (e.g., crime, high incidence of disease, infant mortality). In countries such as the United States, increasing amounts of electronic information are available, much of it free, and this can be used to construct a baseline or to measure change over time. GIS data are rapidly becoming available in many developing countries, although they are much less abundant. It is now possible for fieldworkers with GPS-enabled mobile phones to create GIS maps indicating the location of health and other services, roads and infrastructure, and hot spots with high crime rates or traffic accidents. Satellites can take repeat images of the same locations over time (e.g., number of dwellings, roads, irrigation systems in a particular village or larger area) making it possible to identify images taken around the time a project was launched and to compare these with the situation at the end of the project.

Satellite images and maps are now available free from a number of sources, including Google Maps among others, and more targeted information is available commercially. While the analysis of these images requires expertise, specialists say that hiring a geospatial analysis consultant is probably no more expensive than hiring a sampling design consultant.

TAKING INTO ACCOUNT THREATS TO VALIDITY WHEN ADDRESSING REAL-WORLD CONSTRAINTS

All of the constraints discussed in this chapter can weaken the rigor of the evaluation methodology and the validity of the findings based on the design. Budget constraints can reduce sample size and limit the ability to ensure quality control of data collection, time constraints make it difficult to devote sufficient time to developing and testing research instruments or to being able to follow-up on inconsistent or questionable findings, lack of access to key data

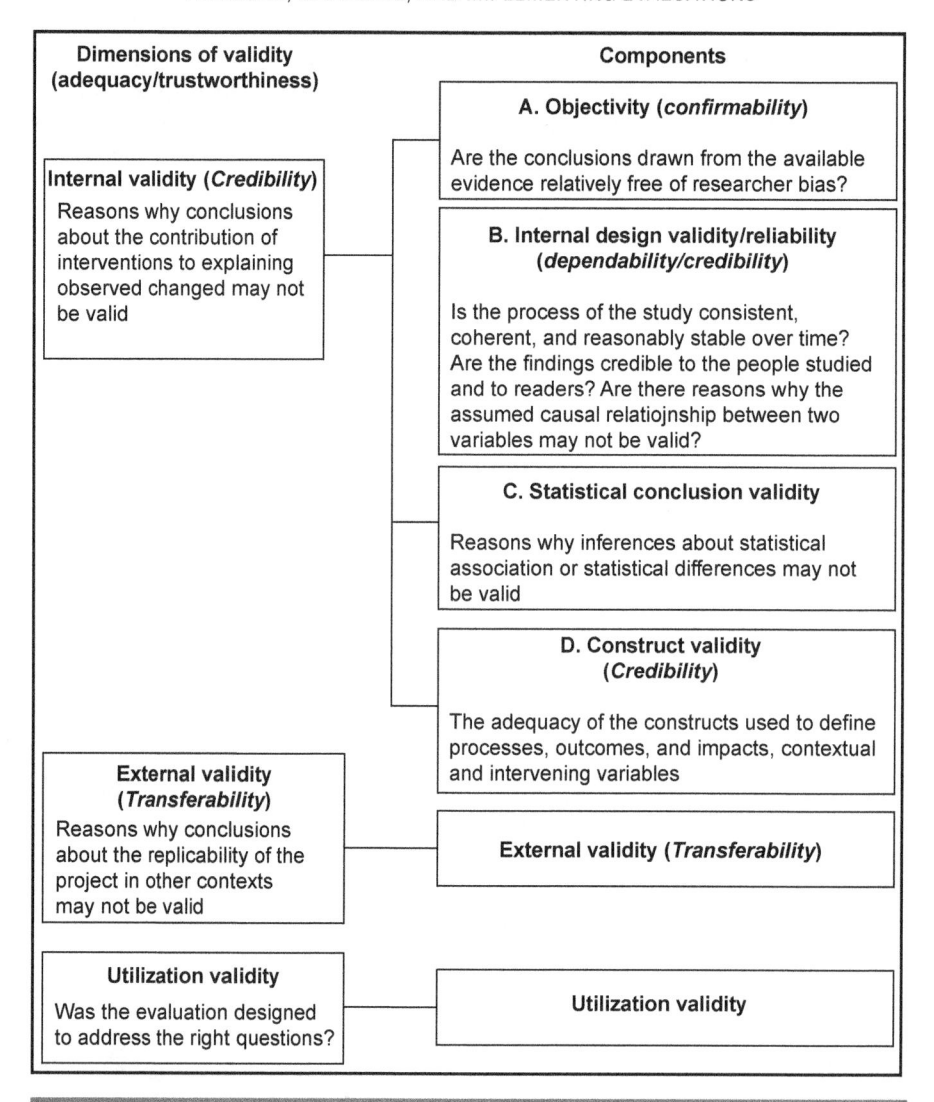

482 PLANNING, MANAGING, AND IMPLEMENTING EVALUATIONS

Dimensions of validity (adequacy/trustworthiness)	Components
Internal validity (*Credibility*) Reasons why conclusions about the contribution of interventions to explaining observed changed may not be valid	**A. Objectivity** (*confirmability*) Are the conclusions drawn from the available evidence relatively free of researcher bias?
	B. Internal design validity/reliability (*dependability/credibility*) Is the process of the study consistent, coherent, and reasonably stable over time? Are the findings credible to the people studied and to readers? Are there reasons why the assumed causal reliatiojnship between two variables may not be valid?
	C. Statistical conclusion validity Reasons why inferences about statistical association or statistical differences may not be valid
	D. Construct validity (*Credibility*) The adequacy of the constructs used to define processes, outcomes, and impacts, contextual and intervening variables
External validity (*Transferability*) Reasons why conclusions about the replicability of the project in other contexts may not be valid	**External validity** (*Transferability*)
Utilization validity Was the evaluation designed to address the right questions?	**Utilization validity**

FIGURE 24.2. Three dimensions of threats to validity in evaluation literature. Terms in **bold** indicate QUANT terminology and terms in ***bold italics*** indicate QUAL terminology.

makes it difficult to develop strong indicators or to reach all sectors of the target population, and organizational and political threats can make it difficult to interview nonproject beneficiaries or to ask certain questions. The framework presented in Figure 24.2 can be used to assess the effect of different kinds of threats on the validity of the research methods, the quality of the data, and the robustness of the data analysis.

Figure 24.2 identifies three dimensions of threats to validity that are discussed in the evaluation literature. The framework combines quantitative (e.g., Shadish et al., 2002) and qualitative (Lincoln & Guba, 1985) terminology, while the mixed methods evaluators (e.g., Teddlie & Tashakkori, 2009) combine elements from both approaches. The elements of the framework are presented below:

• Dimension 1: Threats to the internal validity of the evaluation. *Is the evaluation design, and how it was implemented, sufficiently robust to support the findings and conclusions included in the evaluation report?* This is categorized into four components: the objectivity of the findings, the internal validity of the design, the validity of the statistical conclusions, and how well the constructs used in the measurement capture the ideas they are intended to measure.

- Dimension 2: External validity. *How robust are the estimates of how successfully the program could be replicated in other contexts?*

- Dimension 3: Utilization validity. *Was the evaluation designed to address key interest holder questions, and was it designed, implemented, and disseminated to promote utilization?*

Each of these dimensions can be negatively affected by the trade-offs that have to be made when working on budget, time, and data constraints. For example, these constraints could affect each of the four components of internal validity. Objectivity could be affected if budget constraints meant that it was not possible to draw on all of the sources of evidence, and findings were only based on easily accessible data; design validity can be affected if resources do not permit the identification and use of an adequate comparison group; statistical conclusion validity is directly affected when sample size is reduced and the **statistical power** of the test is lowered; and construct validity is affected if the number of indicators used to measure complex constructs (such as poverty, wellness, or social inclusion) have to be reduced. The assessment of external validity and evaluation utilization can be similarly affected.

Bamberger and Mabry (2019) have developed checklists that can be used to assess the threats to validity of each of the three dimensions of an evaluation. This includes a set of indicators, each of which can be rated in terms of potential threats to the validity of the evaluation, together with reporting formats to present the assessment of validity, in a user-friendly format to managers and policy makers.

NEGOTIATING WITH CLIENTS WHEN CONDUCTING EVALUATIONS UNDER BUDGET AND TIME CONSTRAINTS

Scenarios under Which Discussions on the Evaluation Design Are Negotiated

Evaluators frequently find themselves conducting evaluations under significant budget and time constraints. Sometimes these constraints were clearly understood before the evaluation begins and the evaluators can factor them into their proposal and evaluation design. However, there are many instances in which some of the constraints occur, or only become apparent, after the evaluation contract has been approved, or even after the evaluation has started.

There are two main scenarios when the constraints are known before the evaluation begins. The first is when the evaluator is able to meet with the client to negotiate to reduce the scope of the evaluation, or to increase the budget or timeline. The second quite common scenario is where the contract procurement procedures do not allow the evaluator to discuss possible changes to the scope of work or the budget and timing.

There are also many real-world situations in which some of the constraints do not become apparent until after the contract has been signed. There are several reasons why this can happen. First, many clients have only limited experience with the logic and methods of evaluation, and concerns about rigor, causality, objectivity, and avoiding bias may seem purely academic. So, it may be assumed that it is quite easy for the evaluator to modify the design after the evaluation has started to include new questions, or to adapt to a reduced budget or shortened timeline. So, it is hard for the evaluator to explain, for example, why having to significantly reduce the sample size can seriously affect the validity of the findings.

A second reason is that evaluation offices often have little political influence in their agency, so when the board of directors or a country director decides that they need the report 2 weeks earlier than previously agreed, the evaluation office often does not feel they can argue with their superiors or change the contract. So, often the evaluator is simply told the evaluation must be completed earlier but the same high-quality product is expected.

A third reason is that the concept of impact and how it can be measured is often not well understood. Many programs are intended to produce a series of outcomes and impacts that will only occur over a period of years. For example, one of the intended impacts of a new road may be to gradually raise farmers' income over a period of years as easier access to markets allows farmers to gradually accumulate enough capital to invest in new equipment and seeds—a process that is not expected to show significant benefits for a number of years. While it will be clear to the consultant that it will not be possible to measure impacts within the stipulated evaluation time period, often the procurement procedures do not allow the evaluator to discuss or renegotiate the scope of the evaluation. Not surprisingly, many consultants simply accept the contract and agree to measure impacts, even knowing that this will not be possible.

Ideally, all of the issues affecting the ability of the evaluation to address the questions of concern to clients, and to achieve a satisfactory level of methodological rigor, should be discussed with clients before the evaluation contract is finalized. This is particularly important when working with clients who are not familiar with evaluation methodology and with the need to have a clearly defined design and timeline. Clients who have previously worked with individual consultants whose studies were mainly based on key informant interviews may assume that evaluations will have the same degree of flexibility where questions can be added as the consultancy progresses.

There are several points that are particularly important to clarify before the evaluation contract is finalized. First is the concept of precision and validity of the findings. It is often assumed that an easy way to reduce cost is to reduce the sample size, and it is necessary to explain to clients how smaller sample sizes will affect the validity of the findings, or the types of information that can be collected and the level of disaggregation of the analysis that will be possible. Second, it is often difficult to explain the importance of a control group (which greatly increases the cost of data collection). Many clients assume that if the conditions of the project population have improved, this proves that the project was successful. Third, a certain amount of time is required before it will be possible to assess whether different kinds of outcomes or impacts have been achieved. If the timeline of the evaluation is reduced for political or other reasons, it may be too early to say whether the project has been successful. Finally, most evaluations follow a number of precisely defined steps for planning, data collection, and analysis, and if the evaluator is asked at a late stage to advance the report submission, this may seriously affect the coverage or validity of the findings.

So, it is important to try to have the conversation with clients on these issues before the evaluation contract is finalized. However, there are many real-world situations where these issues my not arise until the evaluation is already underway.

Negotiating with Clients under These Different Scenarios

This section illustrates three questions that often have to be negotiated with clients under the scenarios discussed above.

- *The client wishes to evaluate questions that are not technically possible within the evaluation timeframe.* Many clients are not familiar with the logic of assessing outcomes and impacts and often have not thought through at what point it will be possible—for example, to measure the impact of road construction on farmers' income. A theory of change or other program theory can provide a helpful framework for this discussion. The theory of change presents graphically *program inputs* (money, equipment, staff, etc.), the *activities* (construction, community meetings, processing credits for farmers, etc.) through which these are transformed into *outputs* (road construction, provision of public transport), and how these are expected to produce *outcomes* (more goods sold in the market) and *impacts* (increased farmer production and income). An important element of the framework is that it also includes a timeline estimating when the different stages are expected to be achieved. This provides an easily understood way to show how many years must pass before different impacts can be achieved.

The theory of change framework can also identify intermediary mileposts that can be monitored to check that the program is on track to achieve its impacts. For example, as soon as the road is completed (or even partially completed) it will be possible to monitor whether farmers are able to transport more goods to market, and whether more customers can also travel to the market—both necessary steps for farmers to increase their income.

There is another political argument that will resonate with program management if the results of the evaluation have to be presented to parliament or the ministry of finance. It will be much better for the agency to show proactively why impacts cannot be measured at this early point in the project cycle, while proposing milestones that can be measured, than to claim that it will be possible to measure impacts in Year X, and then have to explain why the evaluation was not able to actually measure these impacts or that the impacts did not materialize because it was too soon.

- *The client expects an evaluation that is more methodologically rigorous than is possible within the available budget and time constraints.* Clients will often require that an evaluation should be "methodologically rigorous" or that it should ensure "high professional standards" even though, in the opinion of the evaluator, it will not be possible to achieve this with the available time and resources. It is important to clarify what the client means by "high professional standards." While the evaluator may assume the client is thinking of methodologies such as RCTs, the client may simply mean an evaluation that will be considered as acceptable to parliament or other interest holders. Often interest holders may have lower expectations. For example, they might consider that contracting a university professor to conduct the evaluation would be sufficient. So this should be clarified before starting to plan a relatively complex design.

One of the challenges when negotiating with an agency with limited experience in evaluation concerns the need for a counterfactual. Many clients assume that impact can be assessed by measuring changes before and after an intervention in the project population (Are more girls attending secondary school or more youth finding jobs? Have malnutrition rates declined?), and it is difficult to explain why a comparison group is needed to determine whether similar changes have occurred in other communities not affected by the project.

In practical terms it will often be necessary to explore with clients a range of alternative design options that can be used to assess outcomes and impacts when experimental designs are not possible or are not considered appropriate. These were discussed in "Option 1: Simplifying the Evaluation Design." For agencies that have been told by funding agencies or evaluation consultants that RCTs are the only accepted way to assess impacts, it may be a challenge to gain acceptance for alternative evaluation designs.

A first point is to explain that it is now becoming accepted that there is no single "best" evaluation design that should be used in all evaluations. There are many different kinds of evaluation questions and different questions require different designs (see "Option 1: Simplifying the Evaluation Design"). So the first step is to clarify what are the evaluation questions to be addressed. In cases where assessing attribution (To what extent has the program intervention contributed to the observed changes in outcomes for the project group?) is a key purpose of the evaluation, it will be necessary to discuss possible alternatives to the RCT (see Box 24.4). If budget or other considerations rule out the use of an RCT, the first step is to convince the client that the evaluation profession recognizes that there are alternative approaches. These should be presented, and their advantages and limitations (including costs and timing) discussed.

- *The client wishes to be able to generalize evaluation findings to a wider population than is possible within the budget and time constraints.* Assuming the evaluation shows that the program has been relatively successful in achieving at least some of its intended outcomes and impacts, one of the reasons for conducting most evaluations is to provide guidance on the conditions under which the project would be likely to be successful in other localities and working with populations with different socioeconomic characteristics. It is often difficult to explain to clients that the fact that a program works in one context does not mean that it will necessarily work elsewhere and with different groups. Pilot projects are usually implemented in places where they are most likely to be successful and they are often provided with kinds of financial, technical, and often political support that may not be available elsewhere. Also, the projects being evaluated were usually launched 3 or more years ago so that the conditions supporting their success may have changed. However, as there are often political pressures (including from funding agencies) to replicate the program on a larger scale, clients are often not receptive to advice that the positive project evaluation is not an automatic endorsement that it will work elsewhere.

It is also important to explain that many widely used evaluation designs do not provide guidance on the potential replicability of a program. For example, the logic of the RCT design means that it does not provide any guidance on the potential of the project to be successful if replicated in other contexts.

Once the client understands this limitation, it is possible to discuss other designs that can provide guidance on replicability. These include a number of mixed methods designs that, in addition to assessing attribution (perhaps combining qualitative methods or case studies with an RCT or quasi-experimental design), can also assess the factors that will help judge replicability. In most cases the methods for assessing replicability will include an element of professional judgment and it is usually not possible to provide the same level of statistical precision that can be used to assess the impact of the original project. Most of the available methods combine various quantitative and qualitative methods to identify factors that contributed to or limited the success of the project, such as the economic and educational characteristics of participants and their communities, ethnicity, geographical location, economic and other characteristics of the surrounding areas, and the local political environment. Replicability will then be assessed by combining available data on the distribution of these features in other regions with the professional judgment of interest holders and experts on potential replicability in other areas and in the current economic and political environment.

CONCLUSION AND SUMMARY

- Six strategies can be considered for reducing the costs of evaluation planning, data collection, and analysis. (It should be noted that each of these may reduce the validity of results obtained.)

- The first is to simplify the evaluation design, usually by eliminating the collection of data on the project or comparison group before the project begins (pretest) or on the comparison group after the project is implemented (posttest). In the simplest design, when data are collected on only the posttest project group, the data collection budget can be reduced by as much as 80%. However, as discussed earlier, it is often difficult to explain to clients not familiar with evaluation methodology, why reducing the budget can seriously limit the kinds of questions that can be asked, or the level of disaggregation of the findings that is possible. For example, reducing the sample size may mean that it is only possible to estimate the average impact for the total project population but not to include the previously planned comparisons between, for example, impact levels in each department or state.

- The second is to agree with clients on the elimination of nonessential information from the data collection instruments.

- The third is to maximize the use of existing documentation (secondary data). See Gates and Schwandt (Chapter 5, this volume) for more details.

- The fourth is to reduce the sample size. Although this can produce significant savings, if the sample becomes too small, there is the danger of failing to detect statistically significant project effects even when they do exist.

- The fifth is to reduce the costs of data collection through methods such as the use of self-administered questionnaires; direct observation (instead of surveys); automatic counters; inputting data through handheld devices; reducing the number of periods of observation; prioritizing informants; and hiring and training students, nurses, and other more economical data collectors. It should be noted, however, that although these methods may reduce the cost of data collection, they will not necessarily reduce or may even increase the costs of data analysis. The message is that creativity is required in finding affordable ways to collect the required information. It may not be necessary to fly a consultant from Europe to explain to the ministry of housing how to collect information on the quality of house construction; or to explain to the ministry of health how to collect information on child malnutrition. Creativity is also required when the original method of data collection is no longer possible.

- The final strategy involves the use of new information technologies (big data and information and communication technologies, such as mobile phones, tablets, and wearable electronic devices). These greatly expand the range of data collection and analysis tools available to evaluators while offering significant reductions in the costs and time required for data collection and analysis.

Most of the above strategies for reducing costs involve trade-offs because they pose threats to the validity of the evaluation findings and recommendations.

REFERENCES

Bamberger, M. (2017). *Integrating big data into the monitoring and evaluation of development programs.* UN Global Pulse and Rockefeller Foundation. Available at www.unglobalpulse.org/big-data-monitoring-and-evaluation-report

Bamberger, M., & Mabry, L. (2019). *RealWorld evaluation: Dealing with budget, time, data, and political constraints* (3rd ed.). SAGE.

Belli, R., Stafford, F., & Alwin, D. (2009). *Calendar and time diary methods in life course research.* SAGE.

Bourgois, P. (2002). Respect at work: Going legit. In S. Taylor (Ed.), *Ethnographic research: A reader* (pp. 15–35). SAGE.

Chelimsky, E. (1997). The political environment of evaluation and what it means for the development field. In E. Chelimsky & W. Shadish (Eds.), *Evaluation for the 21st century: A handbook.* Sage.

Clemmer, G. (2010). *The GIS: 20 essential skills.* ESRI Press

Dane, F. (2011). *Evaluating research: Methodology for people who need to read research.* SAGE.

Heath, C. (2004). Analyzing face-to-face interaction: Video and the visual and material. In D. Silverman (Ed.), *Qualitative research: Theory, method and practice* (pp. 283–304). SAGE.

Henry, G. (1990). *Practical sampling.* SAGE.

Kumar, K. (Ed.). (1993). *Rapid appraisal methods: Regional and sectoral studies.* World Bank.

Kumar, S. (2002). *Methods for community participation: A complete guide for practitioners.* ITDG.

Lincoln, Y. S. & Guba, E. G. (1985). *Naturalistic enquiry.* SAGE.

Patton, M. Q. (2002). *Qualitative research and evaluation methods.* SAGE.

Schwandt, T. (2005). Politics of evaluation. In S. Mathison (Ed.), *Encyclopedia of evaluation* (pp. 319–322). SAGE.

Shaddish, W. R., Cook, T. D., & Campbell, D. (2002). *Experimental and quasi-experimental designs for generalized causal influence.* Houghton-Mifflin.

Stern, E., Stame, N., Mayne, J., Davies, R., & Befani, B. (2012). *Broadening the range of designs and methods for impact evaluation* (Working paper No. 38). Department of International Development.

Teddlie, C., & Tashakkori, A. (2009). *Foundations of mixed-methods research: Integrating quantitative and qualitative approaches in the social and behavioral sciences.* SAGE.

Theis, J., & Grady, H. (1991). *Participatory rapid appraisal for community development: A training manual based on experiences in the Middle East and North Africa Region.* Save the Children/International Institute for Environment and Development.

Vaessen, J., Raimondo, E., & Bamberger, M. (2016). Impact evaluation approaches and complexity. In M. Bamberger, J. Vaessesn, & E. Raimondo (Eds.), *Dealing with complexity in development evaluation: A practical approach* (pp. 62–87). SAGE.

Wholey, J. (2010). Use of evaluation in government: The politics of evaluation. In J. S. Wholey, H. P. Hatry, & K. E. Newcomer (Eds.), *Handbook of practical program evaluation* (3rd ed.). Jossey-Bass.

Part V

CROSSCUTTING ISSUES

Chapter 25

Communicating with Interest Holders

Glenn O'Neil

CHAPTER OVERVIEW

The importance of communications for evaluation has long been recognized. Most discussion and research to date has focused on the role of communications in promoting evaluation findings. However, communications has an important role throughout the whole evaluation process: before, during, and after an evaluation. For communications to be an asset for evaluation it should be strategic and systematic; tailored toward the different needs and interests of interest holders and audiences. Early in the process, an evaluation should determine what will be communicated, when, how, and for what purpose. Communicating before an evaluation is an effective way of involving project/program staff and can include receiving and inputting into evaluation design, signaling the evaluation approach, creating awareness, developing ownership, building relationships, and managing expectations. Communicating during an evaluation, both formally and informally, is a key way to maintain relationship, communication progress, gather feedback, and facilitate a dialogue on preliminary findings. After an evaluation, communication efforts are oriented to disseminating the evaluation findings, having a dialogue about them, and encouraging their use. Different formats to communicate findings are possible through **text-based**, **interpersonal**, and **audio-visual** channels. Finally, while recognizing the potential supportive role of communications for evaluation, its potential is tempered by the nature of the evaluation, the organizational setting, and the context.

Communications is an important feature of life and society. As individuals, we are communicating constantly, either knowingly or not. It has been said that without communications, organizations would cease to exist (Mumby, 2012). The importance of communications for evaluation has been recognized by leading evaluation scholars (Bamberger et al., 2011; Patton, 2010; Weiss, 1998).

It has been said that "evaluation without communications would not be possible" (Alkin et al., 2006, p. 384). This statement holds true: The persons wanting the evaluation must communicate the need; those carrying out the evaluation must communicate its purpose and must communicate in order to have access to information and people; and finally, the evaluation findings must be communicated to their intended audiences. On this last point, it has been claimed that for an evaluation *to be* an evaluation, its findings must be communicated, heard, and generate learning and eventual change (Alkin et al., 2006; Torres et al., 2005).

It is a reasonable assumption that those involved in evaluation are already communicating. However, many communications challenges can arise in an evaluation, including misunderstandings, miscommunications, messages not received or understood, a lack of dialogue—and communication overload, as Cronbach and colleagues (1980) wrote over four decades ago in their 95 theses on evaluation reform, reform number 49: "Communication overload is a common fault; many an evaluation is reported with self-defeating thoroughness" (p. 29).

A review of the literature on communications and evaluation indicates that most discussion has focused on the role of communications in promoting evaluation findings (Alkin et al., 2006; Fox et al., 2016; Torres et al., 2005). Communications should support this aspect but it also has an important role to play throughout the whole evaluation process. To understand the possible multiple roles of communications, it is useful to think about the evaluation process in three simplified phases: before, during, and after an evaluation.

This chapter provides an overview of a systematic and strategic approach to communications for evaluation. An explanation of the evolution of communications theory and practices is provided and followed by key points to ensure that communications is an asset for evaluation. The potential roles of communications before, during, and after an evaluation are discussed in addition to the preparatory steps needed.

UNDERSTANDING COMMUNICATIONS

Throughout this chapter, communications and evaluation are considered from the viewpoint of actually carrying out an individual evaluation at the project/program level, although equally applicable for evaluation at the activity, strategy, policy, theme, organizational, or sector level. There is no focus on other aspects of communications and evaluation, such as how to communicate on evaluation itself as a concept or sector, or how evaluation units within institutions use communications to promote their services or activities (although communication activities described in this chapter can be used for these purposes).

A broad definition of **communications** is used in this chapter: "the process through which people share thoughts, ideas and feelings with each other in commonly understood ways" (Hamilton, 2013, p. 4). This definition places emphasis on the elements of sharing and common understanding, a recognition that communications today has moved on from the notion that it is only a persuasive action from a "sender" to a "receiver" (Berger, 1995). At first, communications were thought to work in this simplistic manner: an organization or individual prepares and sends their message to a public; they understand and are persuaded to do as they are told—the so-called magic-bullet theory (Bowman, 2019). However, over time the all-powerful influence of communications was reassessed and challenged by the "minimal effects" theory that focused on the variables influencing the public and thus reducing the effects of communications (Perse & Lambe, 2016). These variables included who is at the origin of the communications, what are the key **messages**, how it is presented and how often, through which **channel** is it sent, how is it understood by the given public and their motivation to pay attention, what noise interferes with the communications, and who else is also communicating at the same time (Berger, 1995; DeFleur & DeFleur, 2016).

In recent years, a focus has been on understanding how these variables can be minimized to be able to communicate effectively. One major finding has been that communications is more effective when carried out as a two-way process of dialogue, focused on achieving a mutual understanding between the involved actors (see Figure 25.1; Dozier et al., 1995; Macnamara, 2016).

Communications can be a powerful tool and there is ample evidence that if well thought out, it can be a real asset for evaluation (Alkin et al., 2006; Morris et al., 1987; Torres et al., 2005).

COMMUNICATIONS AS AN ASSET FOR EVALUATION

Drawing from the communications and evaluation literature (Alkin et al., 2006; Berger, 1995; Rossi et al., 2003; Torres et al., 2005; Windahl

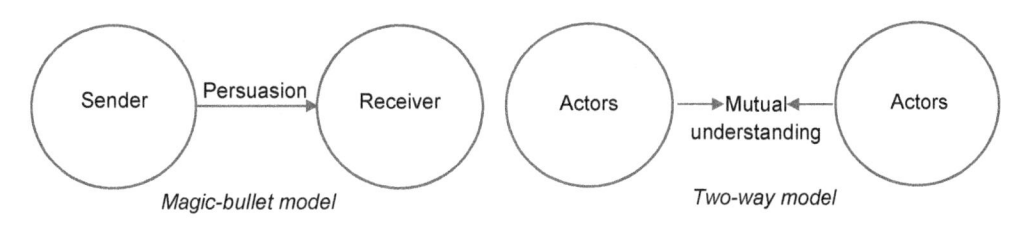

FIGURE 25.1. Evolution from magic bullet to two-way model.

et al., 2008), the key points recommended to ensure that communications is an asset for evaluation are summarized as follows:

- *Planning of communications should occur early in the evaluation process.* In the early stages of the evaluation, the desired communications should be determined. At a minimum it should be decided as to who are the **interest holders** and audiences, what are their communication needs, when should the communications occur, by whom, how, and at what cost (Alkin et al., 2006; Torres et al., 2005).

- *Ongoing collaborative communications is successful.* As emphasized in this chapter, communications is an ongoing process that continues throughout the evaluation. This type of collaborative communications has proved to be successful in facilitating learning and that evaluation findings are actually used (Rossi et al., 2003; Torres et al., 2005). Throughout the evaluation, an evaluator needs to maintain contact with the evaluation commissioner, project/program staff, and interest holders, either formally (e.g., presentations and written updates) and/or informally (e.g., discussions and oral updates).

- *Communications as a dialogue is successful.* Studies show consistently that communications can trigger change where there is a dialogue between the actors, more so than simple one-way communications (Dozier et al., 1995; Sanders & Gutiérrez-García, 2020). For example, regular and even informal communications between an evaluator and interest holders during an evaluation process is preferable to simply delivering an evaluation report at the end of the evaluation (Rossi et al., 2003; Torres et al., 2005). This is important to build into the evaluation process, such as moments where there will be a dialogue with key interest holders on the evaluation approach, process, and/or findings. The first brief case study at the end of this chapter illustrates well this point; the second brief case study illustrates the consequences of limited dialogue.

- *A combination of communications formats is required.* For any communications effort, a combination of formats is typically required to reach interest holders and audiences (Alkin et al., 2006; Rossi et al., 2003; Morris et al., 1987; Torres et al., 2005). This means for an evaluation that there needs to be additional formats than the standard written report, such as **presentations, workshops, informal discussions, multimedia reports,** and use of **data visualization,** as discussed below.

- *Communications needs to be tailored to interest holders and audiences.* Modern communications is based on the notion that different groups have different needs and as a consequence, the messages and formats need to be designed accordingly (Dozier et al., 1995; Windahl et al., 2008). For example, a detailed written report may be appropriate for policymakers, whereas it would not necessarily be the most appropriate format for conveying evaluation findings to a community group.

- *"Who" communicates is important.* The source or messenger for the communications plays an important role in how it is received by interest holders and audiences (Berger, 1995; DeFleur & DeFleur, 2016). For example, when communicating with young people, it could be more effective to work with their peers/leaders in having them lead discussions on evaluation findings, rather than by the evaluator, staff, or commissioner.

- *Interest holders and audiences will understand communications differently.* Interest holders and audiences will selectively recall and digest the evaluation messages and information that was intended for them. For example, in a case study I found that half of the instances where an evaluation triggered use by project/program staff were unexpected and not explicitly stated as recommendations in the evaluation reports (O'Neil & Bauer, 2018). In this regard, the evaluation has to consider the perspective of those for whom the communications is intended for and anticipate that reception will be selective and possibly unexpected (Alkin & King, 2017; Cousins et al., 2014; Cronbach et al., 1980; Kirkhart, 2000).

- *Audiences' interests will differ widely.* Audiences and interest holders will be more involved and seek more information and engagement on an evaluation where they feel directly concerned (Alkin et al., 2006; Morris et al., 1987; Torres et al., 2005). In this regard, an evaluation has to consider what audiences want and need rather than what an evaluation selects to communicate, while still communicating the key messages of the evaluation (see further below).

- *Communications cannot overcome all obstacles for evaluation.* There is sometimes a misunderstanding that communications will be able to overcome all obstacles for evaluation (Cronbach et al., 1980; Torres et al., 2005). For example, an evaluation may increase the quality and quantity of information on an evaluation process with the aim of overcoming staff resistance. However, it may not be access to information that is the issue but other issues such as staff disagreeing with what is being evaluated and/or the way it is being done. Communicating more would not necessarily be the solution; the evaluation's purpose and process would need to be revisited. The second brief case study at the end of this chapter also touches on this point.

COMMUNICATIONS THROUGHOUT THE EVALUATION

Communications can take various roles throughout an evaluation, as seen in the examples provided in Table 25.1 that set out some possible roles.

As an evaluator or someone involved in evaluation, you may review the above table and declare, "I am already doing all of this!" In the evaluation process, the evaluator, interest hold-

TABLE 25.1. Examples of Roles of Communications: Before, During, and After the Evaluation

Before	During	After
• Input into evaluation design • Signal evaluation approach • Create awareness • Develop ownership • Build relationships • Manage expectations	• Communicate progress • Maintain relationships • Present initial findings • Test findings • Gather feedback from interest holders	• Present findings • Dialogue on findings • Promote uptake of findings

ers, and commissioners, are constantly communicating to ensure that the evaluation progresses. This would be considered as standard project management (Fox et al., 2016). Communication activities are different in that they are planned and implemented systematically with the aim of supporting the communication needs identified (Alkin et al., 2006; Torres et al., 2005).

A question often raised when considering a more systematic and strategic approach to communications for evaluation is who will be responsible? This is often a mixture and depends upon the phase of the evaluation. When an evaluation is in its "before phase," with the **terms of reference** (TOR) or **request for proposal** (RFP) being put together, the commissioner of the evaluation normally takes the lead on communications. Once engaged, an evaluator often contributes ideas concerning aspects of communications and sets out planned communication activities in their inception report or evaluation work plan, a document prepared by the evaluator that details the methodology, schedule, and deliverables (Bamberger et al., 2011; Stockmann, 2010). During the evaluation, the evaluator is often in the forefront, communicating to facilitate access to interest holders and to provide updates, while the commissioner and the project/program staff provide support. Once the evaluation report has been published, the commissioner normally takes the lead in disseminating evaluation findings, with the support of the evaluator and project/program staff. After this promotional phase, the communications role winds down as the organization focuses on the implementation of the findings and recommendations and broader learning implications for future projects and programs (Alkin et al., 2006; Rossi et al., 2003).

The ability to use communications to support an evaluation depends largely upon the nature of the evaluation, the organizational setting, and the context in which the evaluation is taking place (Alkin et al., 2006; Torres et al., 2005). For example, an evaluation carried out in a participatory manner will be able to use communications extensively given that this type of evaluation is based on strong interaction with interest holders throughout the evaluation process and prioritizes their information needs. In the same way, a management-orientated evaluation prioritizes the information needs of decision makers so the possibility to use communications to promote findings would be more limited (Alkin et al., 2006). Nevertheless, for all types of evaluation some communications is required and the guidance provided in this chapter would still be pertinent.

Some organizations may have policies and practices that actively encourage communications to support evaluation. For example, the International Labour Organization (ILO) provides guidance on interacting and communicating with interest holders during the evaluation process and has a policy to share publicly all key evaluation reports. The ILO produces **knowledge products** from evaluations, such as meta-studies, synthesis reviews, meta-analyses, and think pieces to encourage learning. Larger evaluations may have a dissemination strategy to target a specific range of interest holders and audiences (ILO, 2014, 2017).

PREPARING TO COMMUNICATE

In the preparatory stage of an evaluation, it is useful to pose some questions on the context and organizational setting that will guide the possible role(s) for communications throughout the evaluation:

- What is the motivation for the evaluation?
- Is this a midterm, final, or other type of evaluation?
- Are staff at different levels in the organization familiar with evaluation?
- What aspects of the organizational culture could potentially impact an evaluation?
- What aspects of the external environment could potentially impact an evaluation?
- What is the anticipated involvement of internal and external interest holders?
- What evaluation policies and practices of the organization exist to support communications?
- What is the level of willingness to discuss and share results?

Reflecting on the above questions will help determine to what extent communication will be able to support the evaluation so that the planned communications can be designed. Some scholars advocate documenting the planned communications in a plan or strategy (Bamberger et al., 2011; Torres et al., 2005; Rossi et al., 2003), whereas others do not think that such formality is always needed (Alkin et al., 2006). However, all agree that some structure is needed for communications. A **communications plan of action** (see suggested template below) would normally set out the following:

- **Situation analysis**
- **Communications objectives**
- **Interest holders/audiences**
- **Communications activities**

The situation analysis is a summary of the responses to the questions posed above—notably, what are the key points to be aware of from the context and organizational setting for the communications? The communication objectives set out what are the desired achievements through communications, which would vary depending upon the situation analysis and the communication needs identified (Alkin et al., 2006; Hutchinson, 2017; Torres et al., 2005). Following are example communication objectives:

- Develop ownership for the evaluation with project/program staff and a broad range of interest holders.
- Ensure buy-in for initial findings of the evaluation among the management.
- Contribute to the integration of evaluation recommendations within a future project strategy.

The next step in planning would be to analyze the interest holders and audiences of the evaluation (Hutchinson, 2017; Morris et al., 1987). A distinction is made between these two groups. Interest holders are individuals and groups who may be affected by the evaluation or have an impact on it. Audiences are those who could benefit from information about an evaluation—for example, people working on a similar program or project. Alkin et al. (2006) distinguish between "primary" and "secondary" communications needs of interest holders and audiences. Building on this, it is helpful to think of audiences and interest holders in terms of primary and secondary (interest holders) and even tertiary (audiences):

Interest holders (primary) would normally include those who have requested the evaluation (sponsors, donors, funders, commissioners), those managing the evaluation, and staff/management of the program/project being evaluated. Persons or groups who are beneficiaries/clients of the program/project would also be considered a priority.

Interest holders (secondary) are those involved in the project/program in some way and have an interest in the evaluation results. These could include related programs, partners, or entities whose work could be affected by decisions based on the evaluation findings.

Audiences (tertiary) are those less central to the evaluation but still may want to be informed about the evaluation, its progress, and results. These could include people working in like-minded programs or bodies, potential partners or funders, and those from the broader community of interest related to the program/project—but not potentially impacted directly by the evaluation as per secondary interest holders. For example, if the evaluation is in the education field, it may be of interest to academics, industry/employee associations, and people working in education. If the evaluation is only intended for internal use, tertiary audiences would not be relevant.

Once interest holders and audiences are identified, it is helpful to establish what their main communications needs are and when they should be met (Hutchinson, 2017; Morris et al., 1987). This can be summarized in the communications plan of action. Even if it is assessed that above segmentation of interest holders and audiences is not needed, at a minimum, it is still important to determine the purpose of communications and who it is intended for (Alkin et al., 2006).

To reach the interest holders and audiences, the next step would be to plan the appropriate communications activities (also called "actions," "tools," or "tactics"). The choice of activities depends on a number of factors, notably, suitability for audiences, the level of interactivity desired, the "depth" of the information being communicated, willingness to engage publicly, and the budget available. As stated above, evaluations often need a combination of communications activities to match the different needs of the interest holders and audiences (Morris et al., 1987; Torres et al., 2005).

Planning communications activities could give the impression that the evaluation will be communicating publicly. But this doesn't have to be the case. Many communications activities are carried out internally or with a limited number of partners, depending upon the nature of the evaluation and the sensitivity of its findings (Alkin et al., 2006; Morris et al., 1987; see Love, Chapter 22, this volume, for further discussion on the role of the internal evaluator).

Many activities can be carried out at low cost—or at the cost necessary for the staff or evaluator to prepare and carry them out. These can include, for example, presentations, workshops, or posting on **social media**. However, at this stage of the planning, the commissioning organization needs to determine the budget and staff time, especially if it foresees more ambitious communications activities (Hutchinson, 2017; Morris et al., 1987). It is also important to determine who will be carrying out the activities, drafting the materials, organizing the events, and so on. Often it will be a combination of the commissioner and the evaluator with the support of project/program staff and communications staff, if available. Most evaluators and commissioners are not specialists in communications and therefore may need the support of communication specialists to implement a broader range of communications activities if required (Alkin et al., 2006; Cartland et al., 2008).

Within the communications plan of action, the main activities should be listed indicating the interest holders or audience for whom the communication is intended, which objective it is supporting, who is responsible for it, and when it should be deployed.

The template in Table 25.2 illustrates the possibility to structure and summarize the key elements of the communication plan of action. Often the plan of action would be included in the inception report or evaluation work plan. With a communication plan of action established, it is then clear to whom the evaluation will be communicating, when, how, and for what purpose.

COMMUNICATING BEFORE AN EVALUATION

The previous section described the recommended preparatory steps needed for communications in an evaluation. With these steps carried out, communications can now start before the evaluation. Communicating well in the evaluation design and planning stage has been found to be an effective way of involving project/program staff in an evaluation (Cartland et al., 2008; Stufflebeam & Coryn, 2014). There are a number of potential roles for communications before an evaluation, as listed in Table 25.1, and now described further.

Inputting into Evaluation Design

An evaluation carried out in a participatory manner can often involve interest holders in the selection of the evaluation design, scope, questions, and methods (Cousins & Chouinard, 2012; Greene, 1987; Torres et al., 2005). This can often be through an interactive exchange with interest holders. For example, the ILO (2014) encourages that interest holders are consulted when drafting the evaluation TOR on key technical issues, methodology, and timing.

Signaling the Evaluation Approach

The TOR or RFP, often released publicly, are important documents as they signal the proposed evaluation approach to interest holders and audiences. Therefore, it is an opportunity to communicate on the level of participation desired, how interest holders will be consulted, what methods will be used, and how the findings will be used (Stern, 2006).

Creating awareness about the evaluation can start early in the evaluation process—for example, through a webinar, presentation, or workshop to explain the purpose of the evaluation to interest holders. Studies have shown that if interest holders are aware of an evaluation, they are more likely to facilitate the process and eventually use its findings (Cartland et al., 2008; Stockmann, 2010).

Developing Ownership and Building Relationships

Developing ownership and building relationships can also be supported through communications, such as through workshops with interest holders as part of inputting into the evaluation design (Torres et al., 2005). Proactive communications at an earlier stage of the evaluation has been found to increase interest holder collaboration in the evaluation design process and buy-in to the evaluation in general (Cartland et al., 2008).

Managing Expectations

It is advised to communicate early to ensure that key interest holders have the same expectations of the evaluation in terms of its scope, purpose, and intended use (Cartland et al., 2008). The inception report can support shaping expectations among key interest holders. For example, the World Health Organization (2013) views the inception report as an opportunity to ensure that the evaluation is taking place on the basis of a common understanding among the evaluator, interest holders, and the evaluation commissioners.

COMMUNICATING DURING AN EVALUATION

When an evaluation is underway (i.e., data and information are being collected, analysis and report writing is carried out), communications will be going on by default as described above. There are a number of potential roles for more strategic and systematic communications during an evaluation, as listed in Table 25.1, and are now described further. Communications during an evaluation can be both structured and non-structured, formal or informal, and very dependent upon the nature of the evaluation (Rossi et al., 2003).

TABLE 25.2. Communications Plan of Action for Evaluation (with Fictional Example)

Situation analysis (summary points)

The evaluation has a broad range of interest holders and audiences that could potentially both facilitate the evaluation process and learn from the findings. Challenges are foreseen in securing the support of all interest holders, such as those based at the country level. The evaluation findings will provide an opportunity to communicate key results widely while at the same time consider messaging carefully on potentially sensitive findings. The organization's evaluation policy states that all evaluation reports are to be released publicly.

Objectives (examples)

1. Create awareness of the evaluation among primary interest holders prior to the evaluation.
2. Build relations with primary interest holders prior to and during the evaluation.
3. Facilitate the evaluation process during the evaluation with primary and secondary interest holders
4. Communicate evaluation findings widely among all interest holders to encourage use and learning.

Interest holders/audiences

Interest holders (primary)	Main communications needs	Before	During	After
Headquarters (HQ)	Be informed, see evaluation value, and use findings	X	X	X
Board	Be informed, see evaluation value, and use findings	X	X	X
Industry partners	Be informed, supportive to evaluation (process and findings)	X	X	X
Government agencies/ministries	Be informed, see evaluation value	X		X
Beneficiaries	Need for feedback on evaluation (process findings) and any follow-up		X	X

Interest holders/audiences

Interest holders (secondary)	Main communication needs	Before	During	After
Steering committees	Be informed, understand implications of evaluation (process and findings)		X	X
Field staff	Be informed, see evaluation value	X	X	X
National boards	Be informed, see evaluation value		X	X
Trade unions	See evaluation value		X	X

Audiences (tertiary)	Main communication needs	Before	During	After
Media—United States/Europe	Interesting and engaging story			X
Other primary sectors	Learn from similar sector			X
United Nations technical agencies	Learn for consideration to other industries			X
Evaluation community	Be informed of evaluation methods/challenges			X
University research departments	Implications for broader research		X	X
Consumers	Be informed of organization and evaluation findings			X

Communication activities

Activity/tool	Audience(s)	When	Which objective	By whom?
Briefing meetings and input into evaluation design	All primary interest holders	Before	1	Evaluation team
Webinar: briefing on evaluation design	All primary and secondary interest holders	Before	1	Evaluation team and commissioner
Website page—briefing on evaluation purpose and design	All audiences	Before	1	Commissioner

(continued)

TABLE 25.2. (continued)

Communication activities (continued)

Activity/tool	Audience(s)	When	Which objective	By whom?
Blog posts—updates on evaluation progress	Primary and secondary interest holders	During	1, 2, 3	Evaluation team
Feedback workshops—during field visits	Primary and secondary interest holders—field visits	During	2, 3	Evaluation team
Video report	Secondary interest holders and tertiary audiences	After	4	Evaluation team and commissioner
Press release	Tertiary audiences	After	4	Commissioner
1- to 2-page snapshot	All audiences	After	4	Commissioner
Workshops on findings	Select primary interest holders (board and HQ)	After	4	Commissioner (support of evaluation team)

Communicating Progress

Communicating progress of the evaluation to interest holders is an important aspect during the evaluation and is normally carried out by the evaluator. In a 2019 survey of American Evaluation Association members, 87% identified "Communicating findings to interest holders as the evaluation progresses" as "influential" or "very influential" in influencing evaluation use (Fleischer & Christie, 2009). In some cases, this can be informal based on ongoing discussions among an evaluator, the commissioner, and relevant project/program staff (Alkin et al., 2006). In other cases, this may be more formal with milestones established where an update is shared with interest holders, verbally or in a written form. For example, this could be the case where a working/advisory group has been established to support the evaluation and for which regular updates are scheduled (Stufflebeam & Coryn, 2014). Again it depends upon the nature of an evaluation: A management-oriented evaluation may require more formal and documented communications; a participatory-oriented evaluation may encourage more informal and undocumented communications (Alkin et al., 2006; Stufflebeam & Coryn, 2014). Both types of communications have their advantages and disadvantages. Informal communications, such as discussions with interest holders, can be more spontaneous, provide useful information as it comes available, and build relations between the evaluator and interest holders, but has a disadvantage that it is not documented and therefore cannot be reproduced and reused. Formal communications, such as written updates, can reach a broader range of interest holders but has the disadvantage that a two-way exchange to facilitate understanding would be limited (Hutchinson, 2017; Stufflebeam & Coryn, 2014; Torres et al., 2005). Written updates can also be misunderstood as finalized findings (see further below).

Maintaining Relationships

Maintaining relationships is an ongoing role in all evaluations and is usually led by the evaluator with the support of the commissioner and relevant project/program staff. This type of action could also be considered as part of the project management aspects of the evaluation (Fox et al., 2016). Communications is more so a support to this aspect—for example, by ensuring that all interest holders have access to updated information on the evaluation as a basis for a constructive relationship. There is general agreement that an evaluator needs to work actively in maintaining relationships with interest holders and this need is often underestimated, given its importance to facilitating access for the evaluator, the need to balance potentially competing interests of interest holders, and its role in contributing to a positive reception for evaluation findings (Bamberger et al., 2011; Cartland et al., 2008; Stufflebeam & Coryn, 2014; Weiss, 1998).

Presenting Initial (or Interim) Findings

Presenting initial (or interim) findings can be a key moment in this phase, depending upon the planned intention to do so. Some have found that interim reports are as influential, if not more influential, than the final report, as it can support immediate program development and improvement (Stufflebeam & Coryn, 2014). Initial findings can range from reporting on the implementation of the evaluation process to results from the early stages of data collection to high-level findings (Fox et al., 2016). It is recommended to present initial findings when an evaluation is longer term (e.g., a year or more) and/or it is playing a formative role for program development (Fox et al., 2016; Stufflebeam & Coryn, 2014). At the same time, as Alkin et al. (2006) point out, an evaluator during data collection and analysis will share their impressions and initial findings in informal discussions with project/program staff (and possibly commissioners), either intentionally or not. They advise that an evaluator needs to be aware of this and take care in what they share as even informally it still signals key messages from the evaluation. Presenting initial findings more formally (i.e., through a workshop, **webinar,** or presentation) can also be an excellent opportunity for a dialogue with interest holders, based on the notion that dialogue is an efficient way to bring about change through communications as discussed above. However, there is a risk that initial findings are understood by interest holders as final and they do not take into account that they may evolve further before they are finalized. Therefore, their interim nature has to be stated clearly (Fox et al., 2016; Torres et al., 2005). At this point, an evaluator can also start to signal any potential negative findings that have emerged, as their treatment needs early and careful attention to ensure that the findings in general are received positively (Bamberger et al., 2011; see Box 25.1). In presenting initial findings, either formally or informally, evaluators start to form the key messages they wish to communicate on their findings, as discussed below.

Testing Findings and Gathering Feedback

Testing findings and gathering feedback with interest holders signals the positive intention of the evaluator to listen and take into account their points of view (Stufflebeam & Coryn, 2014). Some argue that discussing findings as they emerge will make the user more receptive, particularly to findings that may not support their preconceptions (Morris et al., 1987). A communications activity used in this respect would be a "validation workshop" held with relevant project/program staff to discuss the findings, conclusions, and recommendations (Torres et al., 2005; Weiss, 1998). Where an evaluation is carried out over multiple locations, this can also be part of the data collection phase. Caution is needed in testing and gathering feedback on evaluation findings; the evaluator has to demonstrate that they value feedback from interest holders but can refute inputs that lack logic or merit, or compromises their independence (Stufflebeam & Coryn, 2014).

During the evaluation, an evaluator is building the key messages emerging from their evaluation findings, often doing this unconsciously. Normally in communication planning, a **messaging strategy** would be considered in the initial plan of action (Hamilton, 2013). However, when communicating evaluation results, the forming of messages can only occur when initial findings start emerging. The reason is that key messages in this phase are normally on the findings rather than on the evaluation itself. Until this point, any messages would have focused mainly on the evaluation approach and process. As the results are being formulated, this is the moment to consider what key messages to communicate from the evaluation. The challenge of communicating evaluation results is to determine what are the key messages to be conveyed from the (often) significant body of findings, conclusions, and recommendations (Hutchinson, 2017). Often it helps to do this in a systematic way through a messaging strategy:

- What is the most significant message coming out of the evaluation findings?
- What are the secondary messages (maximum of four) coming out of the evaluation findings?
- What is the supporting information for these messages?

> **BOX 25.1. Communicating Negative Findings**
>
> In the data collection and analysis phase of the evaluation, it may emerge that some results are not positive; the evaluation finds it necessary to recommend minor modifications, substantial changes, or even discontinuation of the project/program being evaluated. There is an ease in communicating "good" news and a challenge to communicating "bad" news. But evaluation has to communicate the "full picture" and there is no easy solution. Many evaluation scholars and practitioners have proposed a range of coping strategies to communicate negative findings, based on their own research and experiences (Alkin et al., 2006; Bamberger et al., 2011; Fox et al., 2016; Morris et al., 1987; Sinclair Taylor, 2013; Stufflebeam & Coryn, 2014; Torres et al., 2005). The main points of this research and experiences are summarized as follows:
>
> - *Involving interest holders and staff throughout the evaluation.* By involving the people concerned before and during the evaluation, a relationship is built with them and the progress of the evaluation is discussed constantly. In this way, a more constructive relationship will hopefully prepare for any difficult discussions and findings.
> - *Keeping interest holders' perspectives in mind.* When putting together critical findings, it is helpful for the evaluator to consider the perspective of the interest holders—notably the staff managing the project/program under evaluation. It is difficult for people to accept criticism even if it is logically set out. There is a need to find a balance between a critical tone and respect for all involved.
> - *Communicating early with staff on negative findings.* Presuming there is ongoing dialogue with the commissioner and the project/program staff, it is wise to discuss early in the evaluation as negative findings emerge or those that question preconceptions. This allows staff to digest these findings and provide extra information if needed. Early engagement and communication has been seen to reduce tensions between the evaluator and project/program staff.
> - *Presenting positive findings first.* When presenting negative findings, it is important to first mention the positive aspects of the project/program, making reference to where it is doing well. This can help ease acceptance of an evaluation's findings.
> - *Using the voice of the beneficiaries.* Often negative findings can be interpreted as the views of the evaluator that are not founded on any evidence base. The strongest voice to support findings is often the voice of beneficiaries—quoting or referring to their feedback strengthens the evaluation's credibility.
> - *Placing the emphasis on the future.* Most evaluations have a summative role, such as looking at the changes brought about by the project/program. But, in addition, virtually all have a forward-looking view in that they recommend how the project/program could be improved for the future. Ideally, negative findings should be coupled with suggested solutions for improvements.
> - *Being careful in the use of negative language.* In writing up evaluation findings, it is important to guard against the overuse of negative language. In English, phrases such as "objectives still in progress," "needs improvement," "critical feedback," or "partially achieved" are more acceptable in evaluation writing than direct negative descriptions.
> - *The poor reception of findings can be an indication of broader issues at play.* An evaluator can be surprised that when presenting findings that they view as not negative, they can receive a poor reception from interest holders and possibly be contested. It has been found that broader issues and conflicts between interest holders can be played out in an evaluation and are then reflected in how they consider evaluation findings. This can be challenging for an evaluator to mitigate and they need to be aware of context and political issues that could impact the evaluation in this respect.

Table 25.3 presents an example of a messaging strategy from an evaluation I carried out by for the international nongovernmental organization Oxfam (O'Neil & Goldschmid, 2013).

Messaging strategies are all about making choices and determining the most important points to communicate to interest holders and audiences (Hutchinson, 2017). Evaluation, like reporting from many other technical fields, is rich in details but needs to be condensed for broader consumption. It is also useful in some evaluations to determine messages for each specific audience—for example, senior management, politicians, funders, project managers, and staff. Messages provide guidance to structuring the information to communicate for all communication activities.

TABLE 25.3. Messaging Strategy for an Evaluation (Oxfam's Global Food Justice Campaign, GROW, 2013)

Key message

The most significant achievement of Oxfam's GROW campaign was persuading governments and corporations to revise food and land policies.

Secondary message 1:	Secondary message 2:	Secondary message 3:
The campaign was able to influence global land policy by lobbying the World Bank and, to a lesser extent, governments.	The biggest challenge of the campaign has been to engage with 50 million people, with only 10% of this target reached.	The campaign needs to consider where it has successfully built support and coalitions and merge these into a global movement on food.
Supportive information:	**Supportive information:**	**Supportive information:**
Public commitment secured from the World Bank; policy changes seen in 20 countries.	Five million people were reached mainly through social media actions on specific issues.	Findings show that the campaign has yet to harness and coordinate the support built through different initiatives.

COMMUNICATING AFTER AN EVALUATION

Before and during the evaluation, communications can play a key role in supporting the evaluation process as described above. With the finalization of the evaluation report, communication efforts are usually reoriented to focus on the evaluation findings: disseminating them, having a dialogue on them, and encouraging their use (Morris et al., 1987; Torres et al., 2005).

At this point, with the findings in hand, it is necessary to review the planned communications for this phase and pose the following questions:

- How widely are the evaluation findings to be disseminated?
- What level of dialogue on the results is desired?
- What communication activities have been foreseen?

It could be that during the evaluation process, the desire to communicate the evaluation findings may have increased or decreased depending upon the nature of the evaluation findings, so the planned communications would need adjusting. Stufflebeam and Coryn (2014) caution that it is not legitimate for an organization to agree to make the evaluation findings public and then once they have seen the findings, decide to release none or only part of the findings.

In this respect, organizations that frequently carry out evaluations often have a policy on making public evaluation findings. The United Nations (UN) Evaluation Group's Norms and Standards for Evaluation (2016) that guides all UN bodies in evaluation, proposes that organizations should have an explicit disclosure policy that all key evaluation products (including annual reports, evaluation plans, TOR, evaluation reports and management responses) should be publicly accessible (Standard 1.5, p. 17). At the same time, they indicate that there may be reasons for not releasing publicly findings or only partially, such as to respect the privacy of interest holders. A case study on evaluation in India found that the findings of evaluation reports for Indian government agencies are often not released publicly for these reasons (Agrawal & Rao, 2011).

Presenting Findings

As described above, different formats to communicate evaluation findings are needed for the various interest holders and audiences. Further, they will require different amounts and levels of information (Alkin et al., 2006; Stufflebeam & Coryn, 2014). Hutchinson (2017) called this "layering" (p. 26) of content with the key messages found in all formats and then the level of detail ranging from the shallow (e.g., an infographic) to medium (e.g., a presentation) to detailed (e.g., the evaluation report and appendices).

New formats for communications tools and activities suitable for presenting evaluation findings are emerging constantly. In many cases, these tools and activities can also be used before and during an evaluation (depending upon the communication needs identified). Table 25.4 lists the main communication activities and tools for communicating evaluation findings, categorized by the type of communications channel.

TABLE 25.4. Communications Activities/Tools by Channel

Text based	Interpersonal	Audiovisual
• Reports • Summaries/ snapshots • Infographics • Articles • Press releases • Social media • Interactive websites	• Presentations • Workshops • Discussions • Webinars	• Multimedia reports • Video testimonies • Podcasts • Photographs

Text-Based Tools

Text-based tools, such as interim and final evaluation reports, are often the main medium to communicate evaluation findings for many evaluations. While recognizing that different formats aside from text based are recommended to be used, care must also be taken with text-based tools to ensure that they are well written, structured, and designed to facilitate learning (Morris et al., 1987; Torres et al., 2005). The evaluation report can be complemented by other text-based tools as described below that break up the evaluation findings into more easily digestible forms of content, designed for specific audiences and/or for broader consumption (Hutchinson, 2017; Morris et al., 1987; Torres et al., 2005).

THE EVALUATION REPORT

A lot has been written about best practices for the evaluation report (Alkin et al., 2006; Evergreen, 2017; Hutchinson, 2017; Torres et al., 2005), with key points summarized as follows:

- *Brevity and clarity.* A commonly heard criticism is the density of evaluation reports as Cronbach et al. (1980) lamented of their "self-defeating thoroughness" (p. 29). Writing should be clear and concise, free of jargon and abbreviations as far as possible.
- *Applying design principles.* Elements of layout and graphic design can enhance readability and make the report more appealing to readers by using design principles such as **contrast, repetition, proximity,** and **alignment**. Elements such as **highlighted boxes, quotes, bullet-point lists, headings,** and **subheadings** can be used to break up the text and facilitate readability. For example, the Asian Development Bank (ADB) applies these design principles to its evaluation reports (*www.adb.org/site/evaluation/resources*).
- *Using data visualization.* Tables, charts, and illustrations can be useful to facilitate understanding of an evaluation report. Tables are appropriate for summarizing and comparing; illustrations, such as flowcharts, are useful for explaining a process; charts illustrate quantitative data, such as survey results.

SUMMARIES/SNAPSHOTS

Summaries/snapshots illustrate findings in several pages, often using images and graphics. This is useful in communicating the main messages (see Table 25.4) and reaching those who need only a quick overview of findings. A summary/snapshot would be different from an executive summary report in that it would aim to be even more concise and use visual elements. The ADB also produces two-page summaries of its larger evaluations (e.g., *www.adb.org/sites/default/files/evaluation-document/487496/files/eib-transport.pdf*)

INFOGRAPHICS

Infographics graphically illustrate key findings in one image, which can be a combination of charts and text. Infographics are particularly useful for disseminating findings online, notably through social media, although challenges can be seen in summarizing findings into such a format, notably that they favor quantitative data and only high-level findings can be shown. For example, the UN Development Programme regularly produces infographics to highlight evaluation findings, processes, and global achievements (*http://web.undp.org/evaluation/media-centre/infographics.shtml*).

ARTICLES

Articles in the style of newspaper articles can be written to convey the main findings or certain aspects, such as a human interest story. Articles may not always appeal to mainstream newspapers but could be used for internal or "owned" media, such as newsletters, e-newsletters, blogs, websites, and intranets.

PRESS RELEASES

Press releases announce a newsworthy item to media outlets with the anticipation that they will then publish or cover the given item. For some evaluations, an organization could decide to issue a press release announcing the publication of the evaluation findings. However, there would have to be an assessment by a communications professional of the potential newsworthiness of the evaluation to attract the interest of media outlets. Care must also be taken with the media as they are selective as to what they report on and typically focus on the negative or failures that an evaluation report could highlight (particularly for government agencies or other publicly funded bodies; Torres et al., 2005).

SOCIAL MEDIA

Social media are not only one tool but a variety of networks and platforms (e.g., Facebook, LinkedIn, YouTube, Twitter [now X]) that are useful as a means to distribute evaluation findings to broader audiences in appropriate formats, such as infographics, summaries/snapshots, videos, and photographs. Social media can also be a platform for dialogue on evaluation findings, as they facilitate direct exchanges with audiences. For example, a **blog** can be set up for the duration of the evaluation to communicate progress and findings. The Independent Evaluation Group of the World Bank regularly blog on evaluation findings, methodologies, and processes (*http://ieg.worldbank.org/blogs*). Social media evolves quickly so its effective use requires a good understanding of the latest developments and audience usage (Fox et al., 2016).

INTERACTIVE WEBPAGES

Interactive web pages display evaluation results and can be used to view findings from different perspectives and formats—for example, to display findings overlaid on a map comparing results from different locations. This crosscutting needs assessment in Iraq from 2023 displays results in an interactive website: *https://dashboards.impact-initiatives.org/irq/cross_cutting_needs_assessment*.

Interpersonal Activities and Tools

These activities and tools can be particularly effective in communicating evaluation findings as they allow a dialogue between evaluators, commissioners, and interest holders, complementing what has been understood from the text-based tools. As mentioned above, dialogue is important before and during the evaluation; after an evaluation it facilitates understanding of the findings and promotes an uptake of evaluation findings. "Who" is leading the dialogue is also important as described above. This could be the evaluator, commissioner, project/program staff, or interest holders themselves depending upon who is being reached.

PRESENTATIONS

Typically the evaluator, commissioner, or interest holder presents the evaluation findings to interest holders and the audience. Following an evaluation, multiple presentations may be required for different interest holders and audiences and adapted accordingly, depending upon the identified communication needs.

WORKSHOPS

Workshops involve a more extended interaction with interest holders, possibly for half a day or a full day. A workshop allows more time to discuss findings and can be useful for the evaluator to work with staff in determining the implications of the findings for the project/program. Workshops are also a useful format before an evaluation (e.g., for discussing the scope, purpose, and intended use of an evaluation) and during an evaluation (e.g., to discuss preliminary findings or for validation) as discussed above.

DISCUSSIONS

Discussions are a more informal activity to explain the evaluation findings and exchange views with interest holders. As for presentations, several discussions may be required with different groups. Discussions also play an important role in sharing initial impressions and findings as described above.

WEBINARS

Webinars allow for a presentation over the internet to a larger audience, potentially to several hundred people. An advantage of webinars is their ability to reach larger numbers of people in diverse locations.

Audiovisual Tools

These tools place an emphasis on the audio and visual aspects in communicating evaluation findings. These tools can be particularly effective to complement text-based and interpersonal channels, given that it has been established that audiences tend to retain more from audio and visual communications (Hamilton, 2013).

MULTIMEDIA REPORTS

Multimedia reports explain the main findings using a combination of animations, interviews, and texts. Available in either video or web format, multimedia reports are useful in engaging broader audiences and can be used in combination with other formats, such as presentations and workshops. This multimedia video report presents the findings of a 2012 evaluation of the African Climate Change Resilience Alliance: *https://youtu.be/WJteTOYB2eI*

VIDEO TESTIMONIES

Video testimonies involve filming beneficiaries, interest holders, or staff speaking about an aspect of the evaluation. They can be effective in putting forward the direct voice of people involved in or benefiting from a project/program and can be combined with other tools, such as shown during presentations or posted on websites.

PODCASTS

Podcasts are audio recordings that are presented in the form of a radio show that can be subscribed and listened to. Podcasts can be useful for profiling more in-depth discussions and aspects of the evaluation findings, such as interviews with the evaluators, brief case studies, or profiles of beneficiaries. For example, the Independent Evaluation Unit of the Green Climate Fund regularly produces a podcast on evaluation and related issues (*https://ieu.greenclimate.fund/new-from-ieu/podcasts*).

PHOTOGRAPHS

Photographs can be useful to communicate context of an evaluation setting and provide further explanation to texts. They can be both standalone (e.g., for exhibitions, launches) or incorporated in other evaluation tools (e.g., evaluation report, summaries/snapshots, social media).

More creative activities and tools are also possible to communicate evaluation findings, such as drama, poetry, dance, music, photo stories, and cartoons (Hutchinson, 2017; Torres et al., 2005).

Promoting an Uptake of Evaluation Findings

An important aspect of the after phase of evaluation is the follow-up of the evaluation's conclusions and recommendations—to what extent they will be implemented, how, and by whom. Organizations have in place various mechanisms to monitor and encourage the follow-up of recommendations. Additionally, many organizations have a focus on learning and actively encourage staff and management to consider the implications of the broader findings of evaluation for their current and future programs/projects (Bamberger et al., 2015). Communications can support this focus, by reinforcing learning for those directly involved with the evaluation and reaching those not involved but potentially interested. For example, some organizations collate **lessons learned** from evaluation and make them available to all, such as the UN Democracy Fund (*www.undeflessonslearned.org*) and the ADB (*https://lessons.adb.org*). The commissioner normally takes the lead in this aspect with the support of the evaluator as needed.

In a meta-review of evaluation use studies from 1986 to 2005, the authors concluded that "engagement, interaction, and communication between evaluation clients and evaluators is key to maximizing the use of the evaluation in the long run" (Johnson et al., 2009, p. 377), supporting the approach proposed in this chapter to communicate actively before and during an evaluation. However, it should be recognized that other factors have been identified as being influential on evaluation use, such as *context*, *organizational setting*, *decision-making characteristics*, the *policy environment*, and the *quality* of the evaluation (Contandriopoulos & Brousselle, 2012; Cousins & Leithwood, 1986; Højlund, 2014). Communicating throughout the evaluation process also facilitates learning and direct use (called "process use"; Patton, 2010). Fostering evaluation use is discussed further by Alkin and Vo (see Chapter 8, this volume).

CONCLUSION

As expanded upon in this chapter, if approached in a systematic and strategic manner, communications can be a real asset for evaluation—before, during, and after an evaluation. Those involved with evaluation should be aware of the support that communications can bring to an evaluation, while being conscious that the nature of the evaluation, the organizational setting, and the context also influence its potential role, as exemplified by the two cases (Boxes 25.2 and 25.3) that conclude this chapter.

BOX 25.2. Example of Communications Supporting an Evaluation

Shifting the Power (STP) was a 3-year project (2015–2017) funded by the United Kingdom's Department for International Development through the Start Network. STP aimed to shift power toward locally owned-and-led humanitarian response. STP was implemented by six international nongovernmental organizations (INGOs) that worked with 55 local and national NGOs in Bangladesh, the Democratic Republic of the Congo, Ethiopia, Kenya, and Pakistan. In late 2017, a five-person team was engaged to carry out a final evaluation of STP (I was the team leader; Austin et al., 2018). A participatory approach was adopted with initial briefings (in person and remotely) conducted for headquarters and country teams. A steering group was established from across the project that discussed with the team their proposed methods and approach. Planned communication activities were discussed and agreed upon with the steering group. For example, at the conclusion of each country visit, a validation workshop was held to discuss initial findings with key interest holders. Regular contact was maintained between the evaluation team leader and the STP project manager. After completion of the country visits, a presentation of global initial findings was made to the steering group with discussions and inputs provided. The findings were not without challenges; a sensitive finding was the role of the INGOs as project implementers and the perceived reluctance of some to "shift the power" to local NGOs. This was discussed with the STP project manager and the steering group to determine how best to communicate this finding.

Before completion of the evaluation, the evaluation findings were presented to over 50 project interest holders at a "Good Practices and Learnings" workshop in March, 2018, where they developed action points drawn from the evaluation. Video testimonies of STP partners taken during the country visits were used to highlight the evaluation findings at the workshop. Following the publication of the evaluation report (Austin et al., 2018), it was shared on social media and several communities of practice, including the Global Network of Civil Society Organisations for Disaster Reduction. Lessons learned from this evaluation on communications were:

- The multicultural team (members from Asia, Africa, and Europe) facilitated both a varied and appropriate style of communications.
- The participatory approach for the evaluation supported the use of communications successfully.
- The opportunities to discuss and exchange on the emerging evaluation findings strengthened the final findings.
- The use of varied communication activities and tools at different moments of the evaluation increased the opportunities for learning and use of the evaluation findings.

BOX 25.3. Example of Communications Unable to Support an Evaluation

The evaluation was commissioned by an evaluation unit of an institution on one of their crosscutting services. This service had direct implications for most programs of the institution. The evaluation aimed to evaluate the relevance, efficiency, and effectiveness of this service. A two-person evaluation team was engaged to carry out the evaluation (I was the team leader). The evaluation unit had commissioned the evaluation given the implication of this crosscutting service for most programs and that it had never been evaluated previously (the service itself had not asked for the evaluation).

The evaluation team produced an inception report that went through a formal process of approval with the crosscutting service and programs inputting into it. During the data collection, regular contact was maintained with the evaluation service but not with a broader range of interest holders. The main contact with the director of the crosscutting service was an interview as part of data collection. Staff of the crosscutting service were also interviewed as were program staff. Feedback from beneficiaries was collected through an online survey.

Once finalized, the evaluation findings were validated by the evaluation unit and distributed for comments from the crosscutting service and programs. The results were presented to the program staff who were very favorable to the findings given that it recognized their need for further coordination and support from the crosscutting service, which was backed up by the survey results from beneficiaries. Also presented with the findings, the staff of the crosscutting service, however, were surprised and not favorable given the dissatisfaction highlighted of their service by program staff and beneficiaries. When presented to the institution's executive team, the director of the crosscutting service criticized strongly the findings and rejected the follow-up plan of action formulated by the evaluation unit.

A year after the evaluation, the director of the crosscutting service was obliged to follow up on the plan of action by the institution's oversight committee. Lessons learned from this evaluation on communications were:

- The formal evaluation process of the institution was not conducive to regular and informal contact with the staff and director of the crosscutting service.
- There was no opportunity to discuss initial findings with the staff and director of the crosscutting service so they could be aware in advance of the dissatisfaction found; a more participatory approach could have partly mitigated this situation.
- There were a number of obstacles that could not be solved by communications; the crosscutting service had not commissioned the evaluation and were not favorable to it from the start; the program staff were very favorable to the evaluation's findings but could not implement its recommendations without the collaboration of the crosscutting service.

REFERENCES

Agrawal, R., & Rao, B. V. (2011). Capacity building: The Indian experience. In R. C. Rist, M.-H. Boily, & F. Martin (Eds.), *Influencing change: Building evaluation capacity to strengthen governance* (pp. 123–139). World Bank.

Alkin, M. C., Christie, C. A., & Rose, M. (2006). Communicating evaluation. In I. Shaw, J. C. Greene, & M. M. Mark (Eds.), *Handbook of evaluation: Policies, programs and practices* (pp. 384–403). SAGE.

Alkin, M. C., & King, J. A. (2017). Definitions of evaluation use and misuse, evaluation influence, and factors affecting use. *American Journal of Evaluation, 38*(3), 434–450.

Austin, L., Dizon, A. M., Ekesa, O., O'Neil, G., & Shahzad, N. (2018, April). *End of project evaluation—shifting the power*. Retrieved March 22, 2020, from www.owlre.com/wp-content/uploads/2018/08/stp_eval_report_FINAL.pdf

Bamberger, M., Rugh, J., & Mabry, L. (2011). *Realworld evaluation: Working under budget, time, data, and political constraints*. SAGE.

Bamberger, M., Vaessen, J., & Raimondo, E. (Eds.). (2015). *Dealing with complexity in development evaluation: A practical approach*. SAGE.

Berger, A. A. (1995). *Essentials of mass communication theory*. SAGE.

Bowman, N. D. (2019). Media effects: A functional perspective. In D. W. Stacks, M. B. Salwen, & K. C. Eichhorn (Eds.), *An integrated approach to communication theory and research* (pp. 223–234). Routledge.

Cartland, J., Ruch-Ross, H. S., Mason, M., & Donohue, W. (2008). Role sharing between evaluators and stakeholders in practice. *American Journal of Evaluation, 29*(4), 460–477.

Contandriopoulos, D., & Brousselle, A. (2012). Evaluation models and evaluation use. *Evaluation, 18*(1), 61–77.

Cousins, J. B., & Chouinard, J. A. (2012). *Participatory evaluation up close: An integration of research-based knowledge*. Information Age.

Cousins, J. B., Goh, S. C., Elliott, C. J., & Bourgeois, I. (2014). Framing the capacity to do and use evaluation. *New Directions for Evaluation, 141.*

Cousins, J. B., & Leithwood, K. A. (1986). Current empirical research in evaluation utilization. *Review of Educational Research, 536,* 331–364.

Cronbach, L. J., Ambron, S. R., Dornbusch, S. M., Hess, R. D., Hornik, R. C., Phillips, D. C., . . . Weiner, S. S. (1980). *Toward reform of program evaluation.* Jossey-Bass.

DeFleur, M. L., & DeFleur, M. H. (2016). *Mass communication theories: Explaining origins, processes, and effects.* Routledge.

Dozier, D. M., Grunig, L. A., & Grunig, J. E. (1995). *Manager's guide to excellence in public relations and communication management.* Routledge.

Evergreen, S. D. (2017). *Presenting data effectively: Communicating your findings for maximum impact.* Sage.

Fleischer, D. N., & Christie, C. A. (2009). Evaluation use: Results from a survey of US American Evaluation Association members. *American Journal of Evaluation, 30*(2), 158–175.

Fox, C., Grimm, R., & Caldeira, R. (2016). *An introduction to evaluation.* SAGE.

Greene, J. C. (1987). Stakeholder participation in evaluation design: Is it worth the effort? *Evaluation and Program Planning, 10*(4), 379–394.

Hamilton, C. (2013). *Communicating for results: A guide for business and the professions.* Cengage Learning.

Højlund, S. (2014). Evaluation use in evaluation systems—the case of the European Commission. *Evaluation, 20*(4), 428–446.

Hutchinson, K. (2017). *A short primer on innovative evaluation reporting.* Community Solutions Planning and Evaluation.

International Labour Organization. (2014). *Guidance note 7: Stakeholder participation.* Retrieved March 2, 2020, from ilo.org/publications/guidance-note-7-stakeholder-participation

International Labour Organization. (2017). *ILO evaluation policy.* GB.331/PFA/8. Retrieved March 2, 2020, from www.ilo.ch/wcmsp5/groups/public/---ed_mas/---eval/documents/policy/wcms_603265.pdf

Johnson, K., Greenseid, L. O., Toal, S. A., King, J. A., Lawrenz, F., & Volkov, B. (2009). Research on evaluation use: A review of the empirical literature from 1986 to 2005. *American Journal of Evaluation, 30*(3), 377–410.

Kirkhart, K. (2000). Reconceptualizing evaluation use: An integrated theory of influence. *New Directions for Evaluation, 2000,* 5–23.

Macnamara, J. (2016). *Organizational listening. The missing essential in public communication.* Peter Lang Verlag.

Morris, L. L., Fitz-Gibbon, C. T., & Freeman, M. E. (1987). *How to communicate evaluation findings.* SAGE.

Mumby, D. K. (2012). *Organizational communication: A critical approach.* SAGE.

O'Neil, G., & Bauer, M. W. (2018). Pathways to use of communication campaigns' evaluation findings within international organizations. *Evaluation and Program Planning, 69,* 82–91.

O'Neil, G., & Goldschmid, P. (2013). Oxfam's GROW campaign, mid-point external evaluation, final report. Retrieved March 22, 2020, from www.owlre.com/wp-content/uploads/2018/07/oxfam-grow-midterm-report-oct2013.pdf

Patton, M. Q. (2010). *Developmental evaluation: Applying complexity concepts to enhance innovation and use.* Guilford Press.

Perse, E. M., & Lambe, J. (2016). *Media effects and society.* Routledge.

Rossi, P. H., Lipsey, M. W., & Freeman, H. E. (2003). *Evaluation: A systematic approach.* SAGE.

Sanders, K. B., & Gutiérrez-García, E. (2020). Understanding the role of dialogue in public sector communication. In V. Luoma-aho & M. J. Canel (Eds.), *The handbook of public sector communication* (pp. 289–302). Wiley Blackwell.

Sinclair Taylor, J. (2013). *Tips for delivering negative results* [Blog post]. Retrieved March 22, 2020, from http://betterevaluation.org/blog/delivering-bad-news

Stern, E. (2006). Contextual challenges for evaluation practice. In J. Shaw, J. C. Greene, & M. M. Mark (Eds.), *Handbook of evaluation: Policies, programs and practices* (pp. 292–314). SAGE.

Stockmann, R. (Ed.). (2010). *A practitioner handbook on evaluation.* Elgar.

Stufflebeam, D. L., & Coryn, C. L. (2014). *Evaluation theory, models, and applications* (2nd ed.). Wiley Blackwell.

Torres, R. T., Preskill, H. S., & Piontek, M. E. (2005). *Evaluation strategies for communicating and reporting: Enhancing learning in organizations.* SAGE.

United Nations Evaluation Group. (2016). *Norms and standards for evaluation.* Author. Retrieved March 2, 2020, from www.unevaluation.org/document/detail/1914

Weiss, C. H. (1998). *Evaluation: Methods for studying programs and policies* (2nd ed.). SAGE.

Windahl, S., Signitzer, B., & Olson, J. T. (2008). *Using communication theory: An introduction to planned communication.* SAGE.

World Health Organization. (2013). *Evaluation practice handbook.* Retrieved March 2, 2020, from https://apps.who.int/iris/bitstream/handle/10665/96311/9789241548687_eng.pdf

Chapter 26

Information Visualization and Evaluation

Tarek Azzam
Sarah Douville
Ciara Knight
Piper Grandjean Targos
Natalie D. Jones

CHAPTER OVERVIEW

Data visualization can powerfully communicate evaluation findings. This chapter presents foundational data visualization principles to help create **effective data visualizations** with the goal of improving evaluation communication. The chapter outlines a process for creating evaluation data visualizations, which includes determining the purpose and audience for the visual (including context, specific experience, culture, accessibility, and visualcy or visual literacy); using gestalt principles of human perception; and then creating and refining the data visual (including selecting the appropriate visual, creating it, and improving the visual). Multiple examples of this process are provided throughout this chapter. Special topics in data visualization are also discussed including qualitative data visualization, interactive displays, performance monitoring and dashboard displays, and logic models.

COMMON DATA VISUALIZATION PRINCIPLES FOR EFFECTIVE COMMUNICATION

Evaluators are frequently asked to communicate complex data and findings to various interest holders. Frequently, our goal is to help interest holders understand how a program was implemented or the impacts it had. The challenge often centers on how to present information in ways that facilitate understanding for a variety of audiences. This challenge is compounded by the growing popularity of new data display formats, rapid proliferation of data visualization software options, and increased use of interactive data displays. These innovative developments can be helpful if used in the right situations. However, if used without knowledge of good data visualization principles, these displays may detract or even distort the critical messages emerging from the evaluation and its findings.

When done well, data visualization can efficiently and powerfully communicate evaluation findings, and when done poorly, they can confuse or mislead. The 2018 American Evaluation Association Evaluator Competencies emphasize the importance of using communication to "enhance the effectiveness of the evaluation" (AEA, 2018; King & Stevahn, 2020, p. 54), suggesting that effective communication is an important part of good evaluation. The purpose of this chapter is to introduce foundational data visualization principles to help create effective data visualizations to improve communication. These principles can be applied to a range of communication tools, from static graphs to interactive designs. This chapter also offers helpful guidance on how to approach the information visualization process and avoid some of its common pitfalls. Note that this chapter does *not* include a detailed explanation of the human visual system nor cover the fundamentals of data visualization. For more information on *why* the approaches outlined here are effective, we recommend *Show Me the Numbers* by Stephen Few (2012) or *Information Visualization: Perception for Design* by Colin Ware (2021).

DEFINING EFFECTIVE DATA VISUALIZATION

While many definitions of data visualization exist, this chapter defines *effective* data visualization in evaluation as the *accurate and efficient visual representation of data to facilitate understanding* (adapted from Zhu, 2007; Kirk, 2016). In this definition, *accurate* conveys that the visual should truthfully represent the underlying data; *efficient* implies that the visualized representation improves understanding without unnecessary cognitive effort; and *to facilitate understanding* includes increasing engagement, making the information memorable, and hopefully encouraging use. This definition implies that effective data visualization must successfully *communicate* the intended message accurately to be considered effective but does not necessarily mean that the visualization must "stand on its own." Context, which is often provided through descriptive narrative or facilitated by a guide (i.e., the evaluator), is also frequently needed for effective data visualization.

A critical aspect for creating an effective visualization is the context in which it will be used. Context, broadly speaking, can be operationalized in terms of purpose and audience. The *purpose* of a visual is connected to your evaluation question: What are you trying to convey to your audience? Decisions on how to hone and enhance your visual should ultimately serve this guiding question. The *audience* is also an important consideration. You should try to answer questions about who will be seeing the visual and consider how the audience might interpret the visual. Also consider how the personal experience and biases, goals, interests, values, language literacy, data and graphic literacy, accessibility, and cultural differences can affect how the information you are presenting will be received. Making your data visualization effective means crafting your message with thoughtful consideration of purpose and audience. To help support this effort, a process is needed to systematically consider and select the optimal visualization for your evaluation. Our suggested process is presented in Figure 26.1, and the next part of this chapter takes you through it step-by-step.

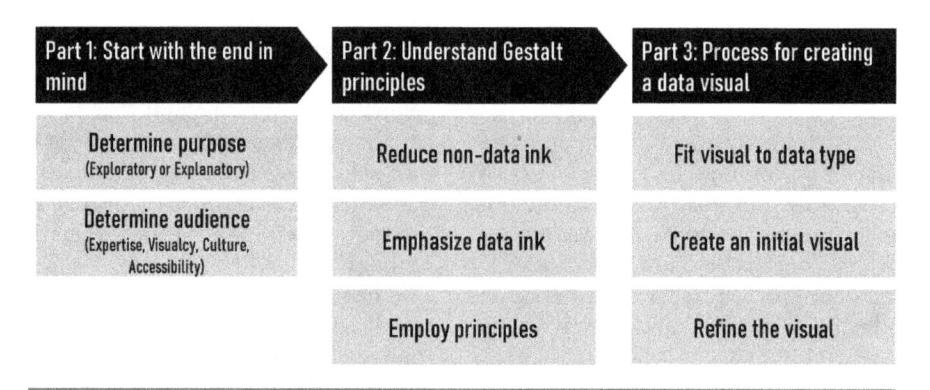

FIGURE 26.1. A process for creating a data visualization.

START WITH THE END IN MIND: DETERMINE PURPOSE AND AUDIENCE

Throughout the process of data visualization design you should consistently keep the final goal in mind: Consider the story you want to communicate and the audience you are targeting. What question(s) are you answering? What is the primary message you want your audience to understand? The highly interrelated considerations of purpose and audience have a strong impact on the data visualization you design and display medium you choose.

Purpose of the Data Visualization

Why is visualization required? In broad terms, data visualization can be used to *explore* and/or *explain* data. For example, data visualization can be used for identifying patterns in the data, simplifying complex datasets, supporting a report narrative, adding aesthetic appeal, making data relatable, or drawing and keeping the viewer's interest.

As an evaluator, you may use data visualization during the analysis stage to explore the data by inspecting scatter plots to detect outliers or trends in the data, or by using conditional formatting to color code null data fields in a spreadsheet to look for patterns of missing data and areas with high or low response averages. While some interest holders might use data visualization to explore data, especially when large amounts of data are updated frequently, you will most likely be creating data visualization to explain the data and facilitate understanding of the analysis you have already done. Explaining the data with a visual can be expanded beyond telling a story to persuading an audience or inspiring action.

To determine the primary objective of the visualization, it may be helpful to ask yourself, Will the final visual tell the entire story? If the answer is "yes," then the visual is most likely being used to explain the data. If the answer is "almost," then the visual is still likely explanatory but you may need to carefully consider adding additional cues or information in the accompanying text to help the viewer understand the message. For example, a scatter plot showing the relationship between wages and rates of homelessness might be effective for most viewers but additional information about a particular community may be needed to guide viewers toward an enhanced understanding of this relationship and its potential implications for their community.

If the final visual will *not* tell the entire story, then consider animation or interactivity to allow users to explore the data. Animation or multiple visuals that build a story can be an excellent choice when the presentation medium allows it. You may also consider interactive data visualizations, where the audience can interact with the data to conduct their own analysis or generate new questions (Azzam et al., 2013; Isenberg et al., 2013; Smith, 2013). For example, an interactive report that allows viewers to drill down into specific areas of interest or discover underlying patterns within subgroups can be very powerful. However, interactivity invites a host of special considerations that are discussed later in this chapter.

It is also important to identify who will see the visual and how their experience may influence how they interpret it. The purpose for any single visual may not perfectly reflect the purpose of the evaluation as a whole. Although often associated with evaluation reporting, data visuals may be employed for a variety of reasons throughout the evaluation process. For instance, program administrators may work together to design a logic model of the program, funders may review a detailed analysis of populations served, and community members may be provided a flier of outcomes specific to their community. Just as is the case for commissioning an evaluation, interest holders will have various reasons for expecting a data visualization, and these may not always be immediately obvious.

Audience for the Data Visualization

Who will view this data visualization? The audience may be a scientific group expecting a detailed breakdown, or a program manager expecting to post the visual on a billboard to market the program, or a host of other interested interest holders with their own unique skills and knowledge base. Is the visual effective for the target audience's culture in content, color, form, and message? Have issues related to accessibility been considered? Is the vocabulary appropriate and free of confusing technical terms or jargon? Utilizing suggestions from this chapter and pilot testing visuals prior to finalization can help address concerns such as these.

A data visualization must be developed with both the data and the audience in mind. Avoid all *unnecessary* complexity in your data visualization. When in doubt, choose the simplest chart for the data. Simple text displays or bar charts are often appropriate. Keep in mind that the *eventual* audience may not be your direct interest holder, and you should attempt to understand your audience's content expertise, visual literacy, and culture. The following highlights techniques that may be used to focus the data visualization.

Specific Expertise

In some ways, communicating effectively with data visualization is like communicating any other information; you must understand what your audience already knows about the topic so you know how much background information to include. This is more noticeable in data visualization because the emphasis on simplicity can result in fewer supporting details and the fact that visuals may be viewed separately from the text, even when text is intended to support them. Knowing this, you must carefully consider the baseline knowledge needed to interpret your visual considering the audience you expect to view it. For instance, a group of medical professionals will require less information on the causes and effects of diabetes than another viewer due to their previous training and knowledge but may need more information on the costs associated with transporting and storing fresh vegetables than the program administrator of the food bank involved in the same evaluation.

Visualcy

Visualcy—also referred to as data visualization literacy, graphical literacy, or visualization readership skill—is concerned with the interest holder's ability to interpret and make meaning from visual representations of data (Börner et al., 2019) and is a skill that must be learned (Zhu, 2007). Just as you would consider the text literacy and numeracy (mathematical literacy) of your audience as you prepare a presentation, you should consider visualcy when preparing a data visualization.

You should ask, How familiar is your audience with data and statistics? How familiar are they with these specific data? Do they know how to read and interpret different visualizations? For instance, some individuals will be very comfortable with a visualization of a network analysis, while others will not have encountered that visual before. It may be necessary to use a visual they are more familiar with or teach them how to interpret a less familiar visual. Importantly, there is no strict hierarchy of complexity in visualizations, and your specific audience may be comfortable with some visuals and need guidance with others. Just as you should not assume that an audience's strong literacy or numeracy automatically translates to strong visualcy, you should not assume that a group of statisticians familiar with scatter plots will intuitively grasp a tree map.

Culture

The culture of the audience should also be considered as part of the visualization process. *Culture* can be defined broadly as "the shared experiences of people, including their languages, values, customs, beliefs, and mores" (American Evaluation Association, 2011). Culture is critical to effective communication as it reflects worldviews in how one thinks, interprets, and communicates because it can impact one's attitudes, behaviors, decision making, and cognition. Understanding cultural context is integral to understanding your audience. Questions you might ask yourself include What are the cultural factors of the audience? What particular beliefs does the audience hold? Is there a language barrier? Are they able to understand some of the words or phrases that accompany visualizations? Are there certain visualizations (or colors, images, etc.) that may convey a negative or different connotation than what I intend? Examples include assumptions about the direction from which the audience will start reading the graph (right to left or left to right); the gender associations of pink and blue in some Western cultures; or the audience's associations with an image, such as a rainbow, which could refer to luck, ethnic diversity, or diversity of sexual identities.

Accessibility

Like culture, accessibility is related to understanding the audience of the data visualization. Making something *accessible* typically refers to ensuring that the same information is available to all people, regardless of their range of abilities. As data visualization relies heavily on visual ability, visual impairment among interest holders is an accessibility challenge that evaluators must thoughtfully navigate. Ensuring accessibility of visualizations is ethically important, but also legally important. For instance, evaluators must adhere to Section 508 compliance (*www.ada.gov/cguide.htm*) when working on government contracts.

Designing for accessibility will likely entail trade-offs in design decisions. For instance, humans recognize color exceptionally well but approximately 8.0% of men and 0.05% of women have some form of color vision deficiency (CVD; also called color blindness) and will be confused or misled by certain color combinations (Few, 2012; Ware, 2021; Wexler et al., 2017). A simple recommendation is to never rely solely on color (e.g., use data labels in addition to color).

Overall, you must consider both *who* will use the data visualization and the *intended* medium for the visual. Different elements will be more or less effective depending on how the visual will be viewed. For example, design choices should differ between a black and white printed report being mailed to funders, an animated PowerPoint presentation for community leaders, and an **interactive website** designed for the public. Importantly, you should consider how interest holders might use the visual. Will someone try to print the website in black and white to mail to funders? Will a community leader take cell phone photos of the animated visualization during the presentation? If these scenarios are likely, you may have to balance design choices, or create multiple visuals for different audiences and uses.

Remember that the data visualization is ultimately about effective communication. Intentionally considering the purpose and audience of the data visualization throughout the process can help you choose and design the most appropriate data visualization.

Basic suggestions when designing for interest holders who may have minor to moderate visual impairment are:

- Font, background colors, or visualizations should be clearly visible when printed in gray scale, so those with CVD can interpret them.
- Use large fonts and visualizations that are easily readable from the distance that the viewer will likely be viewing them.
- Use nondecorated fonts (e.g., Times New Roman, Calibri) and simple visualizations.
- Apply colors that allow sufficient contrast between fonts and backgrounds, and are viewable for those with CVD. A number of free web apps are available to help you better understand the implications of color choices and assist you in testing your designs for color-blind audiences.

Additionally, interest holders with severe visual impairments (i.e., blindness) often rely on screen-reading software to describe any visually based materials. Evaluators should design visuals, including photos, images, and logic models, to be compatible with screen readers by utilizing "alt text" functions, captioning, or by providing brief written descriptions to accompany visual depictions. While blindness or color blindness (CVD) are the concerns that typically come to mind when considering accessibility in data

---

BOX 26.1. Section 508 Compliance

Meeting Section 508 compliance can be a significant undertaking and should be considered early in the project. Rather than taking the approach of "checking the box" on compliance, we recommend familiarizing yourself with these principles as they will make your visuals more accessible overall, not just within a particular evaluation as mandated. A web search will return a number of free resources to check common accessibility concerns but these sources change frequently. The U.S. General Services Administration maintains a comprehensive website (*www.section508.gov*) and we also recommend the U.S. Department of Health and Human Services website (*www.hhs.gov/web/section-508/accessibility-checklists/index.html*) as an excellent starting point. Resources are updated frequently on this site.

visualization, keep in mind that the materials supporting the visual should also be accessible, such as providing captions in the video accompanying the visual to increase accessibility for the hearing impaired.

Creating an Optimal Visual

Once you have determined the purpose and audience of the visualization, you should consider which visualization will best communicate the evaluation findings. We suggest being question driven in the design process, which involves the careful consideration of how a visual aligns with an evaluation question. Figure 26.2 illustrates the potential alignments between different commonly asked evaluation questions and the visualizations that may optimally help communicate their answers.[1] For example, if you have data on levels of implementation from different sites (i.e., categorical data), then you would want to avoid using a line graph when visualizing this information (because line graphs are often used to illustrate change over time or a continuous variable) and use bar charts instead. The ability to match the evaluation question to the type of data available and then to the appropriate visualization is critical, since each visualization can highlight or unintentionally obscure the information you wish to display.

Additional Resources

Choosing the optimal visualization can be a daunting endeavor as different visualizations highlight different data relationships. In addition to numerous books on the selection of visualizations, countless online resources exist to help you identify, select, and then create the most appropriate chart for your data. While there is no universally agreed-upon typology of data visualizations (Börner et al., 2019), you may find the resources below helpful in selecting a visualization for your purpose and audience:

- In addition to his award-winning book *Data Visualisation: A Handbook for Data Driven Design*, Andy Kirk (2016) offers the *Chartmaker Directory* as a free resource to assist you in selecting the appropriate chart type for your data *and* software for the chart type (*http://chartmaker.visualisingdata.com*).
- Stephanie Evergreen's (2019) *Effective Data Visualization: The Right Chart for the Right Data, Second Edition*, has a chart chooser for both quantitative and qualitative data. There are also a lot of great tips in her online blog (*https://stephanieevergreen.com*).
- The Interactive Chart Chooser at Depict Data Studio by Ann Emery (n.d.) offers guidance for selecting the most appropriate chart for the data with a wealth of evaluation-specific suggestions (*https://depictdatastudio.com*).
- The Data Visualisation Catalogue developed by Severino Ribecca is an interactive library of information visualization types (*https://datavizcatalogue.com*).
- The Data Viz Project by Danish infographics company, Ferdio, organizes a comprehensive archive of data visualizations (*www.datavizproject.com*).

UNDERSTAND VISUALIZATION PRINCIPLES TO AVOID COMMON MISTAKES

The core premise in cognitive psychology is that our mind takes in stimuli, then employs filtering methods to help us interpret the world around us. These filtering methods aim to reduce our cognitive load and enhance our ability to quickly navigate our surroundings. This has implications beyond choosing the type of chart or graph to use. The driving principle in this process is to increase the use of data ink and reduce the presence of nondata ink (Tufte, 1990), thereby highlighting the intended message.

Data ink refers to any visual element—such as lines, color, or shapes—that convey data. For example, the bars in a bar graph are a form of data ink. **Nondata ink** is anything that does not contain data or information—for example, using thick lines around a figure, or having multiple black lines in a grid in a graph, or even using multiple colors in a bar graph (that do not represent additional information) are all non-

---

[1] Data visualization, like evaluation, should be guided by questions, so we have arranged a sample of data visualization types around potential evaluation questions evaluators commonly answer. This is far from a comprehensive list, and you are encouraged to visit the resources listed throughout this chapter to explore more chart types.

Evaluation Question	Visualization	Description of Visualization
How do these groups compare?		Bar charts compare the amount of something between two or more groups. A wide variety of bar charts exist, including simple, clustered, diverging, floating, and stacked (shown here).
		Pie charts indicate the proportion allocated to each group within a whole. These are best used with a few groups; consider using a bar chart or tree map to compare many groups.
		Tree maps use nested areas to show the relative proportion of subgroups and their hierarchical structure for a visual comparison of how each group compares to other parts of the whole.
		Heat maps show the relative intensity of a phenomenon between groups by varying the depth of color for each group. When groups are arranged around another variable (e.g., location or time), differences across that variable can be seen.
		Bubble charts, like bar charts, use shapes or icons to display the relative amount of something between groups. If displayed as a graph with an x–y axis, these charts can also display how they compare along other variables.
What was the change over time?		Line graphs are a simple way to demonstrate change over time, where the x-axis represents points in time, and the y-axis contains the variable of interest. Shading can be added to create area as shown here.
		Dumbbell plots show change over time for several groups, such as improvements in pretest and posttest scores by group. Another option is to place these on an x–y axis for a slope graph.
		Gantt charts show several events over time, as well as their level of completion. Timelines or marks on a calendar are simple visuals to show events over time. More information on timelines will be presented in qualitative examples.
		Histograms group data to display frequency along a given dimension or variable. For instance, binning participation by week demonstrates participation rates and changes over time. Histograms can display cycles in the data, such as an increase in enrollment at the start of each quarter.
How large was the effect?		Single numbers are sometimes the most effective way to display data. The single number can be enlarged, displayed with color, or paired with an icon to draw more attention to it.
		Pictograms are images that represent a concept. A waffle chart (shown here) is a simple type of pictogram using colored squares to show the amount of something. Other pictographs can use circles or even icons that represent a concept.
		Overlapping bar charts display the current dataset on top of a comparison group, baseline data, or other standard. Target lines (also shown here) show how the displayed data differed from a minimum standard or benchmark.

(continued)

FIGURE 26.2. Sample data visuals for common evaluation questions.

Evaluation Question	Visualization	Description of Visualization
How are things related?		Scatter plots graph data along the x–y axis, showing the relationship between two variables. Including a line of best fit or a Pearson's correlation number will show strength of this relationship.
		Parallel sets demonstrate the relative frequencies across categories, represented along vertical axes. Use more than two axes to compare multiple categories. These look similar to Sankey charts, which also show a hierarchical flow in the data.
		Concept maps use shapes, lines, and colors to display connections between topics.

FIGURE 26.2. *(continued)*

data ink visual elements (Tufte, 1990). Good data visualization emphasizes data ink, and de-emphasizes and regularizes nondata ink (Few, 2012). Data ink elements should be made visually salient (e.g., exciting, interesting) by reducing any feature of the visualization that is not data ink. Nondata ink elements should be removed when possible, as they detract from the data ink visual elements, which can confuse, mislead, and obscure the main message of the visualization. Figure 26.3 shows data from a hypothetical multisite math program to demonstrate the importance of appropriately using data ink in a graphic and choosing the appropriate chart type for the data. The visual presented in Figure 26.3a is the wrong type of chart for the data and has too much nondata ink, including thick marker lines and background shading on the legend and axis markers as two quick examples. The visual in Figure 26.3b highlights the data more effectively using data visualization principles covered in this chapter. We revisit this example later in the chapter.

The process of reducing nondata ink elements is supported by background knowledge of cognitive psychology and more specifically gestalt theory. Gestalt theory offers a representation of how cognitive filtering methods manifest in a visual domain and how they can be used to enhance data ink elements in a visualization while reducing or underemphasizing nondata ink elements. We can apply these principles to creating more effective data visualizations: helping the audience identify the important elements of a data visualization, ignore the unimportant, and easily and correctly identify the purpose of the visual (Few, 2012).

Gestalt Theory

Gestalt theory was formed in the early 20th century as a response to structuralism, association-

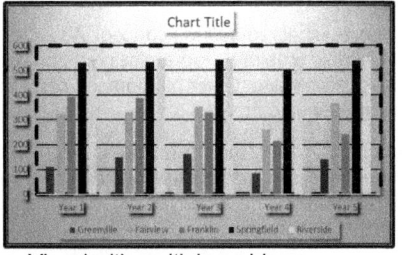

a. Visual with multiple problems

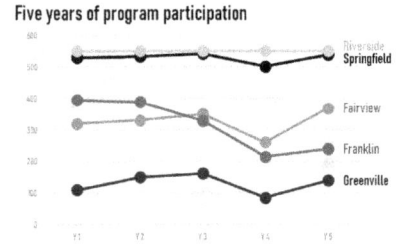

b. Better visual ready to be refined

FIGURE 26.3. Refining a visual by selecting the appropriate chart type and removing nondata ink.

ism, and empiricism (Wagemans et al., 2012). *Gestalt*—translated from German as *shape* or *pattern*—was an attempt to explain our understanding of the world through our perceptions of phenomena as parts of a larger whole. Rather than our understanding being based on the summation of individual sensations, gestalt theory suggests we tend to perceive our surroundings holistically. From this concept, a set of principles were derived to explain how we tend to see patterns. Through these principles, we can come closer to understanding our audience and how they may interpret a data visualization. This section does not cover all **gestalt principles** but highlights the most commonly used ones for creating effective visualizations (see Figure 26.4). Examples of applying the gestalt principles and improving a graph are included in the section "Process for Creating a Data Visualization."

Core Gstalt Principles Important to Data Visualizations

- *Continuity*. Objects appear as part of a group if they align with one another. That is, items found on a line or curve are perceived as more related to one another than to items not on the same line or curve. This principle is commonly observed in line charts, data tables (where cells along a column or row are linearly connected), and in bar charts (where all the bars on a single axis are considered related on some dimension).

- *Connection*. Objects that are connected by a line are perceived as part of a group. This is a common principle used in line charts. Often, a line connecting the objects is needed to draw the viewer's attention to the group, even if they are the same color or shape—in those cases, the principle of *connection* is potentially more salient to the viewer than the principle of *similarity*.

- *Similarity*. Objects with similar elements are perceived as related or part of a group. For example, in a basket of green apples and yellow onions, the apples are seen as part of the group because of their similarity of color, but also type. This is similar to a line chart, where green dots are perceived as part of the same line, distinct from yellow squares.

- *Closure*. Objects that appear to form a closed or complete figure will be perceived as part of a group, rather than as individual items. This can be used in data visualization to imply

Continuity: The black circles appear as part of a group because they fall in a linear pattern.

Connection: The circles connected by a line are seen as related to each other.

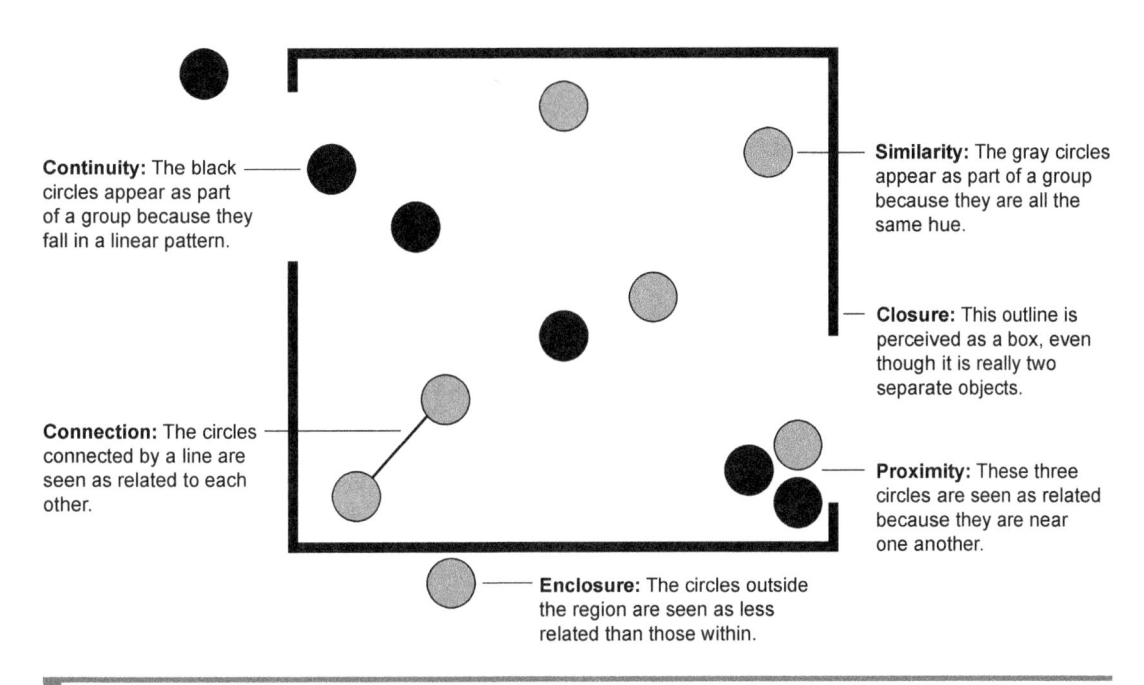

Similarity: The gray circles appear as part of a group because they are all the same hue.

Closure: This outline is perceived as a box, even though it is really two separate objects.

Proximity: These three circles are seen as related because they are near one another.

Enclosure: The circles outside the region are seen as less related than those within.

FIGURE 26.4. Common gestalt principles used in data visualizations.

the axes on a line chart (Few, 2012), and reduce nondata ink by implying a complete figure in the background without having to show it fully.

- *Proximity.* Objects near one another—and at a relative distance from other objects—are considered part of a group. This is common in data tables, as we perceive cells within a column as being related to one another, because each column is separated in space from other columns (Few, 2012).

- *Enclosure.* Objects held within a common region are perceived as grouped together. Data visualists can use this principle to draw attention to relevant groups in the data using borders and backdrop fill (Few, 2012). This principle is used in shaded sidebars for text, and to draw attention to a particular graph or region within a graph.

Employing these principles will help you reduce nondata ink in your visuals. Reducing the nondata ink emphasizes the most important elements for the viewer, making your visual more effective at clearly communicating the point. Once you have honed the purpose of the visual and identified the audience, consider these principles when creating the visual.

PROCESS FOR CREATING A DATA VISUALIZATION

Once you have a sense of your purpose and audience and know what needs to be communicated, the next step is to develop an effective data visualization. This is generally an iterative process that combines the design principles noted previously to select and then refine the visualization(s). To illustrate this process, this section follows a hypothetical dataset for a program to help guide you through the development of a data visualization, and the design choices you need to consider.

Step 1: Examine the Type of Data and Identify the Best Visualization Type

Once you know the purpose and audience for the visual, you can identify what data should be used to answer the questions. Ask yourself, What is the *most* important piece of information that needs to be communicated as clearly as possible (in other words, What is your priority?). Then, What is the second, third, and so on, most important thing to communicate? We recommend that the evaluation questions should guide the prioritization process. The most critical evaluation question(s)—possibly those answers that will lead to instrumental use of findings—may be the appropriate focus of the visualization.

Let's revisit the simple example from earlier in this chapter (see Figure 26.3) of a multisite program to improve the math performance of students. This imaginary evaluation collected data about (1) participant gender, (2) pretest math scores, (3) posttest math scores, (4) number of sessions attended by students, and (5) site attended. Consider these possible evaluation questions along with visual(s) that could be used to answer the questions.

Figure 26.5 uses the same dataset to answer each question. This demonstrates that the dataset does not determine the visual to use—the question and audience should determine the visual. Visuals should be selected carefully to make sure they are question and priority focused to effectively help answer the evaluation questions.

Step 2: Create an Initial Draft Chart

Sometimes it is useful to take the time to explore the data using visualizations. Simple sorting and filtering of a dataset; conditional formatting; or basic bar, line, or scatter charts can reveal interesting patterns or limitations (such as outliers and missing observations) that might need to be addressed, or even offer initial insights about visuals that may best fit the data.

Many visualization experts recommend hand sketching a visual for initial idea generation (Douville et al., 2021). Once you have an idea for which visualization would optimally answer the evaluation question, then visualizations are typically created using software, such as Microsoft Office (Excel, PowerPoint, Word, etc.), Adobe Creative Suite (Photoshop, Illustrator, Indesign, etc.), and Google Workspace (Sheets, Slides, Docs); through a rapidly expanding selection of data visualization software, such as Tableau and Microsoft PowerBI; or through custom code, such as Python or R. Software typically helps facilitate the visualization process but we

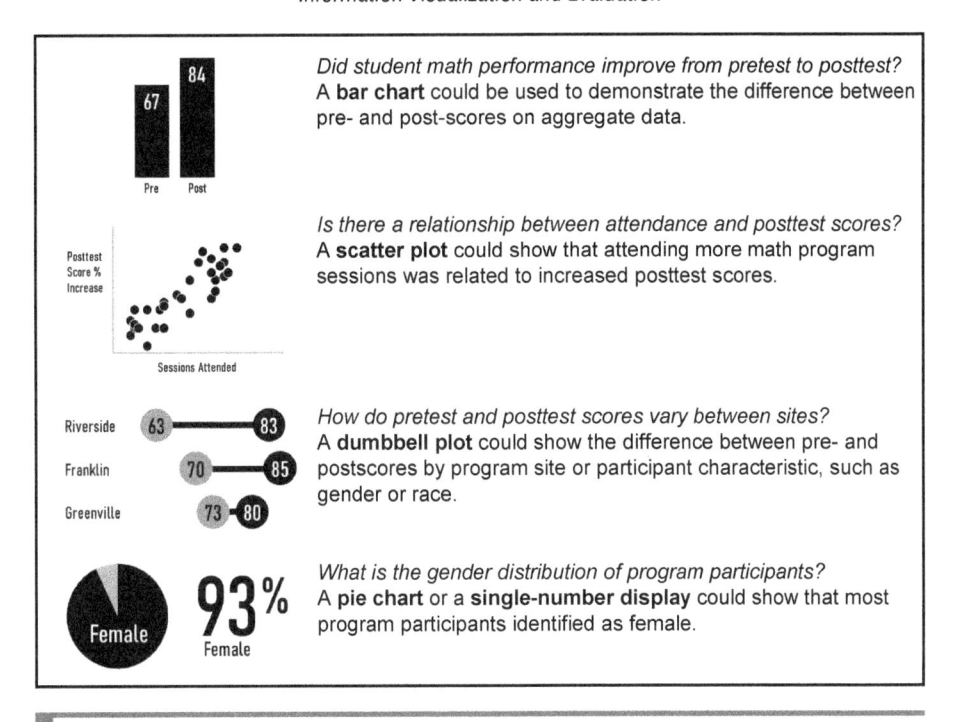

FIGURE 26.5. Different visuals display very different information to address different questions.

do not focus on software in this chapter because it frequently changes and evolves (to the point that whatever is said now will be obsolete in a few months).

As long as the visualization is appropriate for the purpose, audience, and data, then the specific software used is irrelevant for this step. That is not to imply that software decisions are not important. You need to balance your own visualization designs with client expectations, software proficiency, and budgetary needs when making software decisions. You may need to ask questions such as "Will the client need to update the visuals with new data later? Will the visuals produced by the software open on the client's computers?"

Regardless of which software(s) you select, expect that you will need to review the default settings and refine the visual to conform to best data visualization principles.

Step 3: Refine the Visual

Continuing with the example of the hypothetical multisite math program discussed above, we visualize participation by site. For this example, we refine an Excel default "clustered column" chart to show differences between categories. This chart was the default "recommended chart" in Excel (Version 2016) when we highlighted our data and selected "insert" (see Stage 0 in Figure 26.6).

Review the Visualization with the Goal of Reducing Complexity and Nondata Ink

Stage 1 of refining the visual should consider the gestalt principles. Examine the graph that is produced and work to reduce anything that is confusing, misleading, or unnecessary nondata

---

BOX 26.2. Visualization Process Varies by Software

All adjustments for this example are done in Microsoft Excel but this visual refinement process would be similar regardless of the software used. Quotation marks are used to identify the Excel terminology but these terms vary by software. Also note that the order of the adjustments vary by software and by individual designer preference.

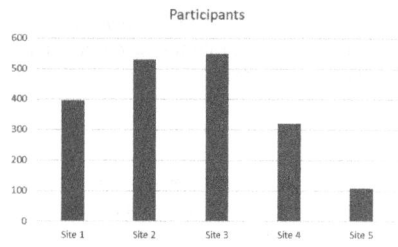

[Stage 0: Default graphic before reducing nondata ink]

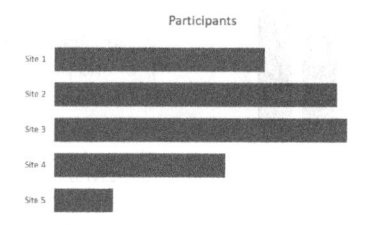

[Stage 1: Graphic after reducing nondata ink]

FIGURE 26.6. Stages 0 and 1 of refining the visual.

ink. Possible initial improvements of this image could be:

- Change the graph type to a "clustered" bar chart.
- Remove (or reduce) the grid lines.
- Remove the axis line and the "major type tick marks" between the site designation and the data bar.
- Remove the border.

Additional potential considerations:

- This default "recommended chart" started significantly cleaner in appearance than commercial software suggestions of just a few years ago but if your software defaults to effects such as shadow, mirror, or 3D, remove them unless they are absolutely necessary to communicate effectively.
- Ensure that each axis represents the appropriate range; for a numeric graph, this typically means starting a y-axis with zero. Often, the default setting does not fit with the data context and misrepresents the degree of difference between categories.
- Ensure that color use is consistent and appropriate. Different colors may denote additional information for the viewer.
- Reduce the gap width between bars to remove excess white space. This allows the viewer to visually group the bars on the principle of proximity, while leaving enough to distinguish individual bars.

Use Data Ink to Encode Relevant Information

Stage 2 focuses on ensuring that the most important information is conveyed by highlighting the data ink elements in the graphic (see Figure 26.7). Adjustments could include:

- Check that axis titles are present and clear. This includes eliminating jargon and clarifying details to make engagement easier; consider what kinds of information your audience needs to help interpret the visual. In the case of this example, it might make more sense to

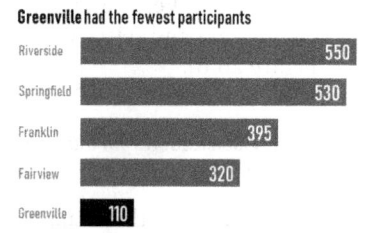

[Stage 2: Figure after encoding information — Greenville had the fewest participants: Riverside 550, Springfield 530, Franklin 395, Fairview 320, Greenville 110]

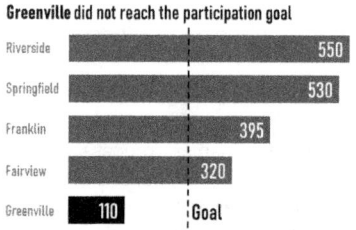

[Stage 3: Figure after adding data ink — Greenville did not reach the participation goal: Riverside 550, Springfield 530, Franklin 395, Fairview 320, Greenville 110, Goal]

FIGURE 26.7. Stages 2 and 3 of refining the visual.

replace a site designation with the actual name of the site, as anonymity was not required.
- Add data labels (if needed) to help the viewer understand the details now that the grid lines are gone. In this case, the participant numbers are now noted directly within each bar rather than by referencing the grid lines.
- Ensure that the title of the chart helps viewers grasp the intended point. In this case, the word *participants* should be replaced by the main takeaway for the viewer.
- Organize the categorical data in an appropriate manner, such as highest to lowest participation, or alphabetical by site. This improvement could be considered within the first stage as a gestalt principle but it is made here to highlight the idea that even gestalt principles should not be applied without intentionality; if interest holders are used to seeing data presented in a specific order, then maintain the order that requires the least cognitive effort for the viewer to interpret.
- Use colors to highlight significant features, such as a particular bar of interest. You can adjust color or font style in the title or data labels to indicate associated data, or possibly include a legend if required. In this case, the Greenville bar was darkened and the title adjusted to link the bar to the site.

After you have stripped out unnecessary ink and adjusted the remaining ink appropriately, you may find that *adding* ink back into the visual benefits comprehension (see Stage 3 under Figure 26.7). If practical, you should add visual details to help guide the viewer but if this addition makes the data visualization overly complicated, then ensure that the necessary context is included in accompanying text or another presentation medium. An example of adding data ink could be adding a line to indicate the goal or planned outcome level. This type of fine-tuning is often done in design or presentation software. For instance, we imported this visual from Excel into PowerPoint to add the goal line.

A simple test of your refined visual is to ask, "How would someone describe the story presented in the figure?" The likely response to the Stage 0 visual is "I need more information." However, if asked to describe the story presented in the Stage 3 visual, the response would likely be "All sites, except Greenville, met the participation goal, with Riverside having the highest participation."

While the initial visual recommended by the software was relatively clean in the example above, this is not always the case. The visualization in Figure 26.3a earlier in this chapter is this same hypothetical math program after 5 years of implementation. Although we added nondata ink to illustrate the data ink principles, poorly designed charts such as this are still common.

The line chart in Figure 26.3b is an improvement: We took the Excel recommendation of a clustered bar chart and converted it to a line graph, changed the legend to labels, and reduced the nondata ink while emphasizing the data ink. This image is now ready for final editing during which an explanatory title is added, colors are adjusted to highlight appropriate data, and explanatory text might be added to address the evaluation questions. For instance, maybe an explanation of the Year 4 dip for all sites except Riverside is needed (see Figure 26.8a), or an explanation of Fairview's performance following a natural disaster is appropriate (see Figure 26.8b), or any of the other data stories that are not clear without added context.

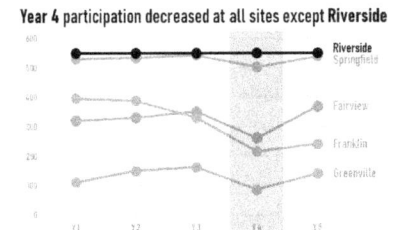

8a. Highlighting Year 4 participation drop

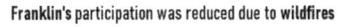

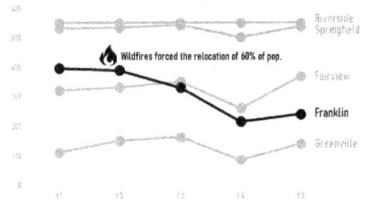

8b. Adding historical context to visual

FIGURE 26.8. Refining a visual by adding explanatory data ink.

SPECIAL TOPICS IN DATA VISUALIZATION

This part is focused on providing an overview of emerging topics in data visualization and evaluation. We provide a brief introduction to each topic along with examples and recommendations for how to potentially use visualizations within each topic area.

Qualitative Data

Visualizing qualitative data has historically received much less attention than visualizing quantitative data but there is a growing interest in identifying more techniques for visualizing qualitative data (Verdinelli & Scagnoli, 2013). As with quantitative data, qualitative visualizations should consider the audience and purpose for the visualization but must also consider the theoretical and analytical approaches inherent in qualitative data (see Rallis & Usinger, Chapter 15, this volume) to ensure that the visualization aligns appropriately with the qualitative approach.

The majority of qualitative data displays are based on quantitizing the data first and then using quantitative data visualization practices discussed in this chapter. **Quantitizing** is the "process of assigning numerical (nominal or ordinal) values to data conceived as not numerical" (Sandelowski et al., 2009, p. 2). In qualitative research, this is frequently performed by counting the frequency of certain words, themes, or specific behaviors in a qualitative data source (e.g., interview transcripts, video recording). This is often done to facilitate analysis and pattern recognition. Two common approaches to quantitizing and displaying qualitative data are **word clouds** in which keywords are displayed by size according to frequency, and **word trees** in which a hierarchical relationship is displayed of keywords followed by "branches" of associated terms and their prominence (see Figure 26.9).

While these techniques are often employed by researchers to *explore* qualitative data during the analysis process, it's important to note that the richness of qualitative data are frequently lost in these simple quantitized visuals and may not be appropriate—on their own—to help *explain* and communicate qualitative findings.

It may be more appropriate to visualize the relationships in qualitative data without quantitizing the information. For example, a type of nonquantitized data display can be created by highlighting a direct quotation through callout boxes, font color, bolding, and so on. A review conducted by Verdinelli and Scagnoli (2013) analyzed the type and frequency of use of qualitative displays in three major qualitative research journals and found that matrix, network, flowchart, boxed display, and modified Venn diagram were the most common display types. Those display types along with others common in evaluation are presented in Figure 26.10.

Other qualitative visualizations to consider include diagrams (e.g., floor plans, instructions), embedded audio or videos (e.g., websites, interactive visual reports), taxonomies, and theoretical frameworks. An example of nonquantitized data visualization, the logic model, is used extensively in the evaluation field. With its prominence and frequency of use, we have provided a section specifically devoted to this topic.

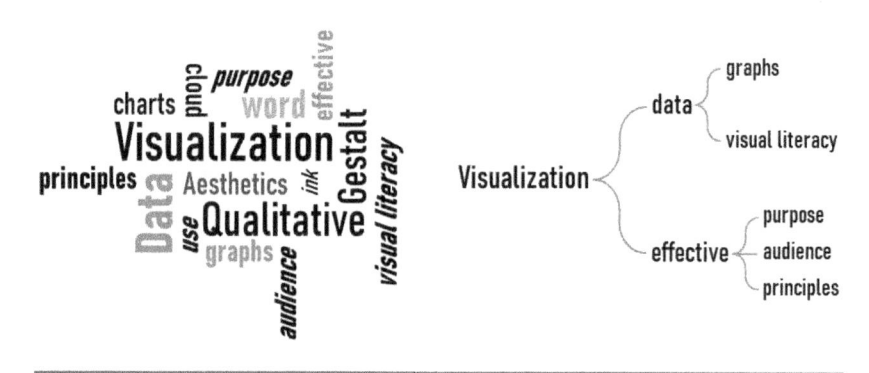

FIGURE 26.9. Example word cloud and word tree.

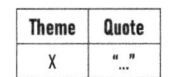

Matrix
Crossing two or more dimensions, variables, or concepts of relevance to the topic of interest.

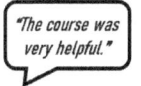

Callout Box
To highlight a specific narrative considered important and frame it.

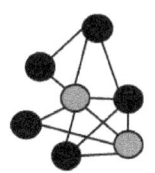

Network
Depicts relationships between themes and subthemes or categories and subcategories.

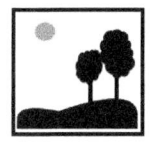

Photographs
Provide photo visuals of people, places, or objects (e.g., landscape over time, connected to a quotation).

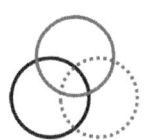

Modified Venn Diagram
Indicates shared or overlapping aspects of a concept, a category, or a process.

Icons
To succinctly represent a theme, concept, category, or variable.

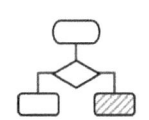

Flowchart
Illustrates directional flow and shows pathways of different groups. Related displays: logic models.

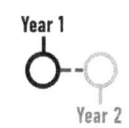

Timeline
Presents time-related information, usually in chronological order. Related displays: journey maps, Gantt charts.

FIGURE 26.10. Common qualitative data visualizations.

As the field of data visualization progresses, we hope to see a greater emphasis placed on how to effectively visualize qualitative data for its specific context and maintain its richness and detail as its being communicated to interest holders.

Beyond the Static Page: Interactive Displays and Their Considerations

Interactive data displays offer an opportunity to take advantage of available technology and move beyond a single static visual. However, developing *effective* interactive displays presents additional challenges. To help with this process, you can consider the choices you have along a continuum that ranges from using interactive displays to *explain* data to viewers to allowing them space to *explore* the data (see Figure 26.11). This continuum also roughly presents a continuum from the *least* to *most* cognitively complex visualization and a continuum from *least* to *most* engaging visualization.

This is not a strictly linear relationship and there are examples that violate this framework. For instance, a static table may be sufficient to explore a dataset. However, adding the ability to *sort* the data in that table may allow faster or deeper data exploration. This invites an additional question: "Where is *sort* on this continuum? Is it before or after *drill down*?" Again, there is no single agreed-upon typology and currently no definitive answers to this question (Börner et al., 2019; Cavaller, 2021). This model is not meant to be comprehensive and you need to carefully consider your purpose and audience when adding interactive features to a data visualization.

In general, a static image is quite versatile and has many strengths. It can be disseminated via

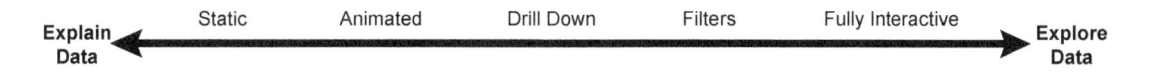

Explain Data ← Static — Animated — Drill Down — Filters — Fully Interactive → Explore Data

FIGURE 26.11. Continuum of interactivity considerations.

print but is also appropriate for web displays; the designer has great control over the viewer experience; and it is often "easier" to produce as it can be created with a wide variety of tools, including simple pen and paper. However, static images are limited in how much information can be shared without overwhelming the viewer.

As you consider which interactive features would be helpful, here are some questions that can help guide you:

- *Will the interest holder benefit from having someone "walk" them through the data and findings?* If yes, then animation might be useful in supplying the context and details of the visual in a specific order. Animation can be used to highlight important features of the data, draw attention to relationships in a specific order (e.g., showing each step in a process in a specific order), and add layers of information that build context for the viewer without overwhelming the user with one static image.

- *Will the interest holder need access to case data or direct quotes?* If yes, then allowing the viewer to drill down from aggregate data to case data is useful. This is a common way to link direct quotations to a theme when displaying qualitative data. This is also a useful way to design interactive logic models in which the user can click on, for instance, the word sites, and see a list of all program sites. Further details on interactivity specific to logic models is offered later.

- *Will interest holders need to investigate the data by group?* If yes, then allowing the user to apply filters to the data might be appropriate. For instance, a checkbox per site allows the user to see how many math sessions were held at only Site A, only Site C, or Sites A and C combined.

- *Will the interest holder have questions about the data that you have not considered?* If yes, then consider richer interactive visuals that allow them to investigate the data on their own. At this point, you may want to think of the user as an analyst. They are using the visualizations to find new insights in the data. Guidance on designing data visuals for analysis is outside the scope of this chapter but caution is advised. While the gestalt principles still apply, you have far less control over the user experience as you will not be able to add clarifying labels, add context, or guide the user (Lysy, 2013).

If you are creating an interactive data visualization that will require data updating and maintenance, you must consider whether you will be maintaining this visual or if you will train your interest holder or client to do so. As you make that decision, you must consider issues around data visualization capacity building and software choices to support the client's ability. For instance, if a small nonprofit can only afford free software licenses, you are immediately limited in your software choices. Interactive visuals are often employed when data are frequently updated. If you will be frequently updating the data, the cleaning and transformation process will likely need to be automated. This chapter does not discuss the many implications surrounding acquiring, cleaning, and properly transforming data for visualization, but you should not skip over this challenge when planning your own visualizations, even the noninteractive variety.

Consistent with the principle of choosing simplicity in data visualization, as you consider your choices along the continuum of interactivity features presented here, it is wise to stay to the left of the continuum unless the purpose and audience warrant adding interactivity. Just as not everything needs to be visualized, not everything needs to be interactive. The best rule is to choose the fewest moving parts.

Performance Monitoring, Data Dashboards, and Dashboard Reports

One common reason for requiring frequently updated data is to support **performance monitoring** within the broader umbrella of monitoring and evaluation. With an end goal of being able to manage (and improve) performance, performance monitoring is concerned with providing decision makers frequent access to key metrics that measure the program or organization's activities, outputs, or outcomes (Poister et al., 2015). Data visualizations that summarize key metrics quickly and with an emphasis on directionality or comparison to a standard (to answer questions such as "Is the process improving?") are useful in performance monitoring.

The often continuous nature of performance monitoring can lend itself to the creation of **data dashboards**, which provide a single page view of the most important data required for decision making that can be interpreted at a glance (Few, 2013). Dashboards are not simply a display of multiple data visuals on one page, nor are they a *report* or a *portal* displaying all possible data. A dashboard should display the specific data needed to act. Simplicity and the gestalt principles are key to good dashboard design. Note that interactivity is not a requirement of a data dashboard—many printed and static reports include dashboards.

Dashboard reports is a more appropriate term to use when visuals are spread across multiple pages (Smith, 2013) or when significant interaction is available within the visuals (such as drill downs and filtering). While tremendous overlap and interest holder confusion will exist, performance monitoring, data dashboards, and dashboard reports are not synonymous and care should be taken in the design decisions of each. The questions at the beginning of this chapter concerning the audience and purpose of the data visualization should be carefully considered. Even though dashboards and dashboard reports are concerned with the visual display of data, consider that flashy data visualization may not be required at all. If a simple display of numbers with context indicators will support decision making, then choose that—often, these simple displays are best at highlighting the most important and actionable information (Few, 2013).

Two newer, compact types of data visualization are well suited to dashboards (see Figure 26.12). As they continue to grow in popularity and interest holders request them, your ability to frame *what* should be measured to answer *which* questions is of utmost importance. If your work involves creating data dashboards, we highly recommend you read Stephen Few's (2013) *Information Dashboard Design*, *The Big Book of Dashboards* by Wexler et al. (2017), and Veronica Smith's (2013) chapter on the process of dashboard creation in *New Directions for Evaluation*.

Logic Model Design

Little is understood about the application of design principles to logic models to accurately represent a program's theory. Program information is organized into logic models to convey a message about the interconnections between the key components of a program theory, which includes inputs, activities, outputs, outcomes, impact, and a variety of contextual factors. Details regarding generating content and organizing it within logic models are available in Joy Frechtling's chapter (Chapter 20, this volume) on logic models.

Many logic model guidebooks tend to be limited in the range of options for visually designing logic models. Rather, they generally focus on generating content, distinguishing between logic model components, and visualizing them using a combination of lines, arrows, or boxes. Data visualization guidebooks used by evaluators do not address the application of design principles to logic models. This creates a missed opportunity for evaluators to ensure each logic model they design accurately represents and communicates the program theory. Figure 26.13 illustrates a commonly used design based on the worksheets used in the *W.K. Kellogg Foundation Logic Model Development Guide* (W.K.

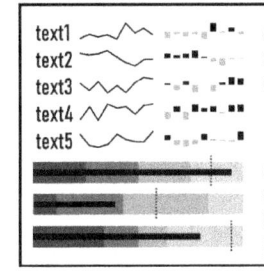

Sparklines are "data-intense, design-simple, word-size graphics" (Tufte, 2006, p. 47) that provide visual comparisons of time-series data in a condensed format (Few, 2013).

Bullet graphs are specialized bar graphs with "a single bar, an additional mark for a quantitative comparison, and shades of color in the background" to signify contextually relevant ranges such as performance goals or forecasts (Few, 2013).

FIGURE 26.12. Example visuals for a dashboard.

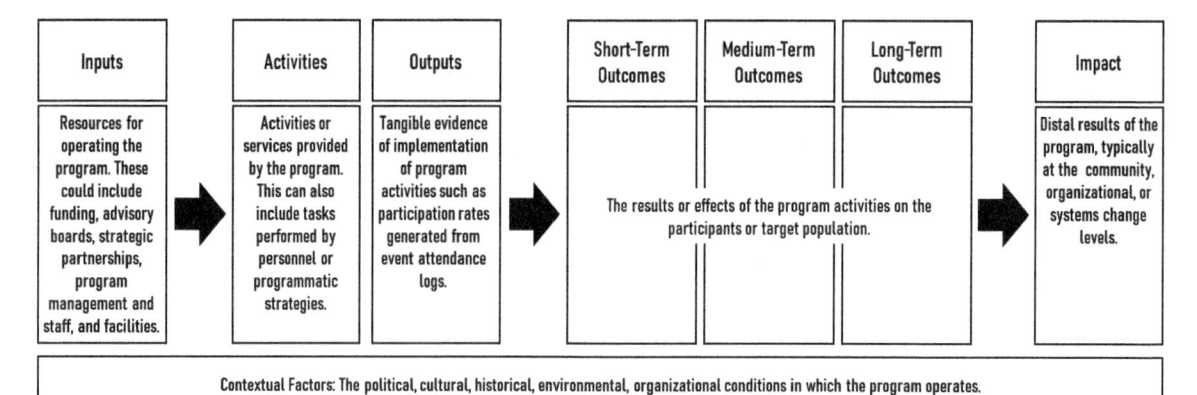

Inputs	Activities	Outputs	Short-Term Outcomes	Medium-Term Outcomes	Long-Term Outcomes	Impact
Resources for operating the program. These could include funding, advisory boards, strategic partnerships, program management and staff, and facilities.	Activities or services provided by the program. This can also include tasks performed by personnel or programmatic strategies.	Tangible evidence of implementation of program activities such as participation rates generated from event attendance logs.	The results or effects of the program activities on the participants or target population.			Distal results of the program, typically at the community, organizational, or systems change levels.

Contextual Factors: The political, cultural, historical, environmental, organizational conditions in which the program operates.

FIGURE 26.13. Common logic model design utilizing arrows and columns.

Kellogg Foundation, 2004) and defines each component.

This section covers several key considerations evaluators should address to facilitate effective communication between interest holders and evaluators. These considerations include design principles, culture, accessibility, complexity, and interactivity. They are related to logic model design as opposed to the process of creating content and drawing connections among content. Yet, they are important as they draw upon insights from audience-specific and data visualization literature.

Design Principles

Findings from Jones and colleagues (2020) highlight the importance of visual design principles to ensure logic models are developed to provide effective communication. The authors modified a common logic model design using many of the design principles in this chapter, such as using color and proximity appropriately, and reducing nondata ink. When tested, they found that a logic model presented to individuals that follows the design principles took less time to understand, increased response accuracy, and reduced the viewer's mental effort (Jones et al., 2020). This not only supports the use of design principles to guide a logic model design but it added empirical support for the use of logic models as an effective communication tool for understanding a program and its components (i.e., program theory). Figures 26.14 and 26.15 provide examples of how the gestalt principles can be used to improve the design of two different logic model frameworks.

Interactivity

Evaluators may find it appropriate to add interactive features to a logic model. This capability is supported by the broad availability of technological tools (i.e., PowerPoint, Google slides), functions within word processing programs (i.e., hyperlinks, animation, etc.), and software or applications specifically developed for creating logic models (i.e., Snow & Snow, 2017). Interactivity within logic models centers on layering information. In its simplest form, designing interactive logic models can entail adding hyperlinks to additional information about specific content areas. For instance, if an interest holder wants to see information about a specific program outcome, that outcome could be hyperlinked to additional information accessed via another page, file, or website detailing how this outcome is measured; any data collected on the outcome; or updates on its current status or progress. A more involved example combines the features of a logic model with data dashboards where the program theory is layered over real-time program performance and monitoring data relevant to the specific outcomes within the logic model. For instance, interest holders can select a specific output and see the data related to it. If an output was participation rates, then interest holders would be able to see the current

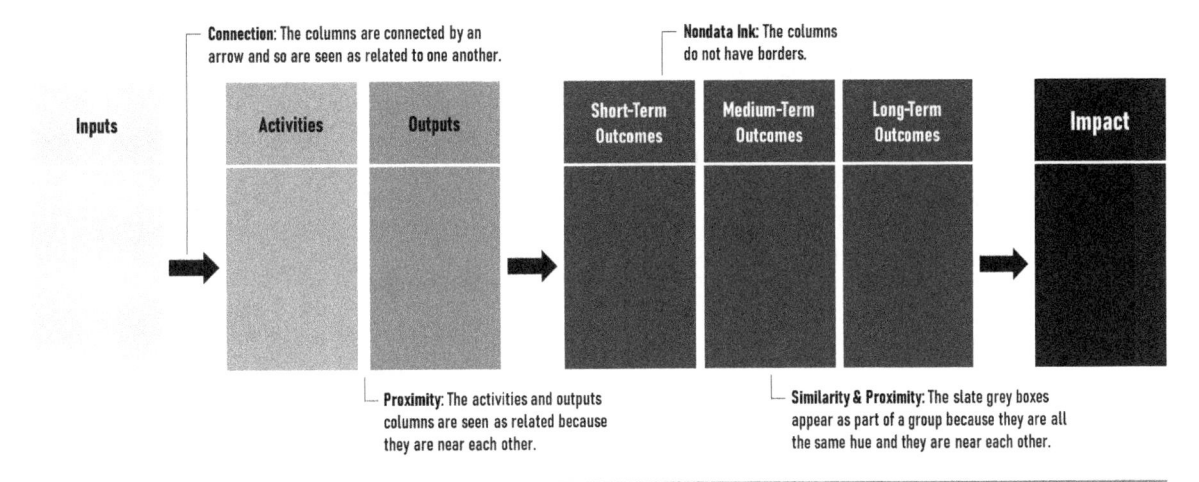

FIGURE 26.14. Design principles applied to a common logic model design with columns.

participation data from the program. A variation of this would be utilization of software that permits the user to hover over specific content of the logic model to view detailed information. Both options rely on the *drill down* interactivity technique discussed previously.

The interactive features of a logic model can be tailored to the audience. If language is a challenge, then interactivity can add translations. If literacy or visual impairment is a challenge, interactive logic models can be designed with linked audio recordings of the written information.

Interactive logic model designs may require more development time, more resources, such as software or custom software development, and greater communication with interest holders than a static logic model design, all of which

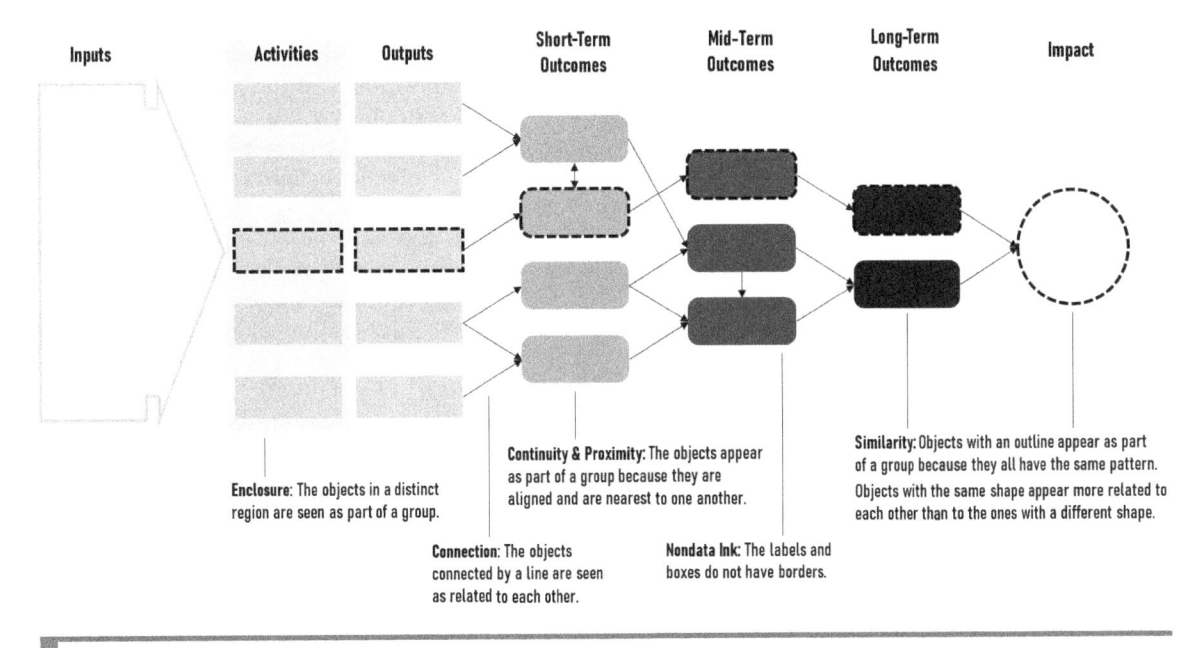

FIGURE 26.15. Design principles applied to a common logic model design with arrows and boxes.

can drastically increase an evaluation budget. Given this, evaluators should plan accordingly, and consider whether this added level of interactivity is worth the investment of time and effort.

Complexity and Culture

Programs and the people they serve are complex, so evaluators should consider how to design logic models to reflect this complexity. In addition to using design principles to guide logic model designs, the role of culture should not be overlooked as it is related to understanding the audience. Culture is represented in words, phrases, and nontextual visualizations used in logic models. Evaluators should carefully select these features to represent the culture of program staff and the community they serve. For instance, the use of inputs, outputs, outcomes, and impact as labels for logic model components are not used in the program impact model designed for the La Plazita Institute (2021; *https://laplazitainstitute.org*), which serves indigenous and Mexican communities. Instead, their logic model component labels are culturally tailored to reflect the values of their community: what it takes (i.e., inputs), what we know, what we do (i.e., activities), and what we build (i.e., outcomes and impact), which is reflective of the cultural values of the community the program serves.

Visualizations selected for logic models should not only be culturally representative but they should resonate with the staff and community that the program serves. For instance, the African American Culturally Responsive Evaluation System for Academic Settings (ACESAS) designed an Afrocentric logic model in the shape of a *Sankofa* (see Figure 26.16) as this is a well-known symbol across the African diaspora that refers to how history should guide the direction of one's future (Frazier-Anderson et al., 2012). Similarly, the La Plazita Institute impact model uses visualizations that resonate with the community (e.g., a cluster of adobe and teepee icons to represent indigenous and Mexican communities).

The ACESAS and La Plazita models do not fully align with the design principles outlined in this chapter. This is important to note because the design principles covered in this chapter are also culturally influenced as they were developed predominantly by White men for a White, Western audience. Since culture shapes how we communicate and interpret information, we suggest thoughtfully "violating" these design principles when facing conflicts between stated design principles and cultural norms.

FUTURE DIRECTIONS

There Will Be More Tools and More Types of Data Visualization

The tools and available technology for ever more complex data visualization will continue to proliferate, likely even accelerate, as the cost to collect, store, connect, and transform the data for visualization continues to decrease. With the increasing presence of data visualization, expect to have more interest holders requesting data visuals for an ever-broadening range of reasons. Some will request visuals because they are truly necessary to aid in analysis and understanding, while others will find visuals valuable in marketing the program, attracting funding, and recruiting participants. A potential downside of this rapid expansion of data visualization ability and awareness is that you may receive more requests for dashboards, automation, and "big data" analysis projects, even when such displays would be inappropriate for the questions being answered.

Data visualization is at the nexus of innovation across multiple fields; building upon overlapping knowledge from psychology, biology, journalism, technology, business, and so on. The exciting upside of this rapid expansion is that new visuals will be created that help us make sense of data in new ways. There will be a burden, however, for evaluators to keep abreast of advances in this rapidly changing field, to sort through conflicting research (and opinions!), and to be aware of pitfalls and unintended consequences. For instance, some data visualization sources state the limitations of the pie chart and strongly recommend against using them (Few, 2012; Wexler et al., 2017) but some studies *have* shown that the "pie chart is a useful tool for the display of proportions, especially when the observer is required to make comparisons involving combinations of components" (Spence & Lewandowsky, 1991, p. 75) and there are cases when they can be used effectively. Meanwhile,

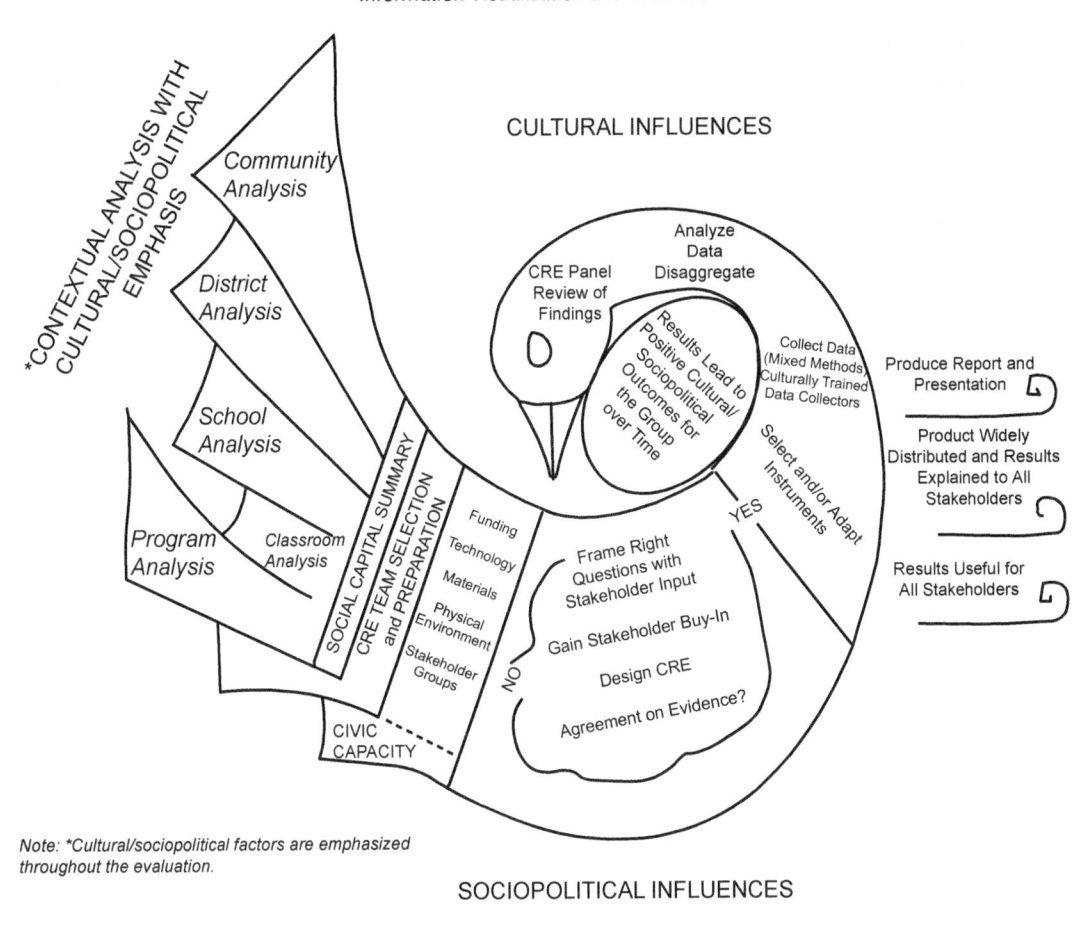

FIGURE 26.16. Sankofa-based logic model used by ACESAS. From Frazier-Anderson, Hood, and Hopson (2012). Reprinted with permission from John Wiley and Sons.

recent research by Holder and Xiong (2022) suggests that displaying data as bar charts (the format typically recommended to avoid the perils of the pie chart) may actually reinforce bias and encourage stereotyping by hiding the variability present within the data.

Evaluators Will Be Better Equipped to Design Visualizations for Multiple Audiences

Ethical guidelines for evaluation practice include ensuring transparency in our communication. Yet visualization literature and sources that evaluators may use often do not address expertise, visualcy, culture, and accessibility—all of which are critical for effective communication. Moreover, neglecting these audience-specific characteristics can have serious ethical and legal ramifications. With this, evaluators should ensure they are equipped with training and tools to design visualizations accordingly.

There Will Be More Interest in Visualizing Qualitative and Mixed Methods Data

With the growing emphasis on the many ways of knowing, particularly within cultural contexts, and a realization that an overreliance on quantitative data limits evaluation potential, expect more emphasis on collecting and analyzing qualitative and mixed methods data. With this increased interest and the computing power to process qualitative data, expect more interest in techniques to visualize qualitative data and to blend mixed method findings into visual displays.

Evaluators Will Be Better Able to Harness Data Visualization for Our Own Analysis, Not Just Communication

Currently, data visualization is most often presented in the final stages of communication, in telling the story, but as technology and data visualization tools continue to expand in ways that support analysis and not just communication, we should expect to see a shift toward using data visualization to assist sense making within data exploration (Batch & Elmqvist, 2018). This trend can help evaluators understand data faster and better, not just help us share that understanding with others.

CONCLUSION AND FINAL THOUGHTS

As an evaluator, you can use your knowledge of data and design principles to help interest holders make sense of the data, support meaningful decision making, and increase the potential for utilization. However, we want to reinforce that data visualization in evaluation is still fundamentally about effectively communicating the often complex answers to evaluation questions. This chapter offers suggestions for how to potentially improve visualizations to help engage and inform interest holders but the hard work of identifying the relevant evaluation questions, collecting and analyzing the data, and understanding your audience is still necessary before creating your visualization. We hope that when you reach the visualization stage that the product produced reflects the quality of the evaluation itself.

REFERENCES

American Evaluation Association. (2011). *Statement on cultural competence in evaluation.* Retrieved August 25, 2021, from *www.eval.org/ccstatement*

American Evaluation Association. (2018). *The 2018 AEA evaluator competencies.* Retrieved August 8, 2021, from *www.eval.org/About/Competencies-Standards/AEA-Evaluator-Competencies*

Azzam, T., Evergreen, S., Germuth, A. A., & Kistler, S. J. (2013). Data visualization and evaluation. *New Directions for Evaluation, 2013*(139), 7–32.

Batch, A., & Elmqvist, N. (2018). The interactive visualization gap in initial exploratory data analysis. *IEEE Transactions on Visualization and Computer Graphics, 24*(1), 278–287.

Börner, K., Bueckle, A., & Ginda, M. (2019). Data visualization literacy: Definitions, conceptual frameworks, exercises, and assessments. *Proceedings of the National Academy of Sciences of the United States, 116*(6), 1857–1864.

Cavaller, V. (2021). Dimensional taxonomy of data visualization: A proposal from communication sciences tackling complexity. *Frontiers in Research Metrics and Analytics, 6,* 1–22.

Douville, S., Grandjean Targos, P. T., Jones, N., Knight, C., & Azzam, T. (2021). Data visualization process and challenges: Key thoughts from data *visualization experts* [Conference session]. American Evaluation Association Annual Conference, Virtual.

Emery, A. (n. d.). *Interactive chart chooser.* Depict Data Studio. Available at *https://depictdatastudio.com/charts*

Evergreen, S. D. (2019). *Effective data visualization: The right chart for the right data* (2nd ed.). SAGE.

Few, S. (2012). *Show me the numbers* (2nd ed.). Analytics Press.

Few, S. (2013). *Information dashboard design: Displaying data for at-a-glance monitoring* (2nd ed.). Analytics Press.

Frazier-Anderson, P., Hood, S., & Hopson, R. K. (2012). Preliminary consideration of an African American culturally responsive evaluation system. In S. Lapan, M. Quartaroli, & F. Riemer (Eds.), *Qualitative research: An introduction to methods and designs* (pp. 347–372). Jossey-Bass.

Holder, E., & Xiong, C. (2022). Dispersion vs disparity: Hiding variability can encourage stereotyping when visualizing social outcomes. *IEEE Transactions on Visualization and Computer Graphics, 29*(1).

Isenberg, T., Isenberg, P., Chen, J., Sedlmair, M., & Möller, T. (2013). A systematic review on the practice of evaluating cisualization. *IEEE Transactions on Visualization and Computer Graphics, 19*(12), 2818–2827.

Jones, N. D., Azzam, T., Wanzer, D. L., Skousen, D., Knight, C., & Sabarre, N. (2020). Enhancing the effectiveness of logic models. *American Journal of Evaluation, 41*(3), 452–470.

King. J., & Stevahn, L. (2020). Presenting the 2018 AEA evaluator competencies. *New Directions for Evaluation, 2020*(168), 49–61.

Kirk, A. (2016). *Data visualisation: A handbook for data driven design.* SAGE.

La Plazita Institute. (2021, July 31). About us. Retrieved August 8, 2021, from *https://laplazitainstitute.org*

Lysy, C. (2013). Developments in quantitative data display and their implications for evaluation. *New Directions for Evaluation, 139,* 33–51.

Poister, T. H., Hall, J. L., & Aristigueta, M. P. (2015). *Managing and measuring performance in public and nonprofit organizations: An integrated approach* (2nd ed.). Jossey-Bass.

Sandelowski, M., Voils, C. I., & Knafl, G. (2009). On quantitizing. *Journal of Mixed Methods Research, 3*(3), 1–13.

Smith, V. S. (2013). Data dashboard as evaluation and research communication tool. *New Directions for Evaluation, 140,* 21–45.

Snow, M. E., & Snow, N. (2017). Interactive logic models: Using design and technology to explore the effects of dynamic situations on program logic. *Evaluation Journal of Australasia, 17*(2), 20–28.

Spence, I., & Lewandowsky, S. (1991). Displaying proportions and percentages. *Applied Cognitive Psychology, 5*(1), 61–77.

Tufte, E. (1990). *Envisioning information.* Graphics Press.

Tufte, E. R. (2006). *Beautiful evidence.* Graphics Press.

Verdinelli, S., & Scagnoli, N. I. (2013). Data display in qualitative research. *International Journal of Qualitative Methods, 12,* 359–381.

Wagemans, J., Elder, J. H., Kubovy, M., Palmer, S. E., Peterson, M. A., Singh, M., & von der Heydt, R. (2012). A century of gestalt psychology in visual perception: I. Perceptual grouping and figure–ground organization. *Psychological Bulletin, 138*(6), 1172–1217.

W.K. Kellogg Foundation. (2004). *W.K. Kellogg Foundation's LM development guide.* W.K. Kellogg Foundation. Available at *www.wkkf.org/resource-directory/resources/2004/01/logic-model-development-guide*

Ware, C. (2021). *Information visualization: Perception for design* (4th ed.). Elsevier.

Wexler, S., Shaffer, J., & Cotgreave, A. (2017). *The big book of dashboards: Visualizing your data using real-world business scenarios.* Wiley.

Zhu, Y. (2007). Measuring effective data visualization. In G. Bebis, R. Boyle, B. Parvin, D. Koracin, N. Paragios, S. M. Tanveer, . . . T. Malzbender (Eds.), *Advances in visual computing: ISVC 2007 lecture notes in computer science* (Vol. 4842, pp. 652–661). Springer-Verlag.

Chapter 27

Exemplary Evaluations in a Multicultural World

Stewart I. Donaldson

> We need to discover the root causes of success, rather than the root causes of failure.
> —David Cooperrider

CHAPTER OVERVIEW

Systematically studying success and the strengths of evaluations and evaluands, while sometimes difficult, unnatural, and nontraditional, can provide important insights about the opportunities and challenges of evaluation practice in these rapidly changing post-COVID pandemic times. The focus of this chapter is to understand what diverse evaluators consider exemplary evaluation in a multicultural world at this point in our history across various regions of the global evaluation landscape. I discuss how exemplary evaluation is defined and explore exemplary professional evaluation practice, exemplary evaluation theory, and exemplary research on evaluation (ROE). It is my hope that as our world and evaluation practice continues to evolve rapidly in the years ahead, professional evaluators will continue to redefine and update definitions and criteria for exemplary evaluations, and use these as an aspiration to strive for, and when occasionally obtained, learn from and celebrate as a global evaluation community.

The year 2015 was declared the International Year of Evaluation in São Paulo, Brazil (Donaldson & Donaldson, 2016). A global movement to strengthen evaluation capacity throughout the world was underway. More than 80 evaluation conferences were planned throughout the world in 2015 to take stock of the global evaluation community and to develop an agenda focused on using evaluation to develop more effective and equitable societies across the globe (Donaldson, 2022a; Donaldson & Picciotto, 2016).

An evaluation torch was passed from event to event to signify that all of the events were connected and that cumulative knowledge would be developed, synthesized, and discussed at a culminating event. The EvalPartners Second Global Forum (the 80th event) was held in the Parliament of Nepal in Kathmandu to reflect on what had been learned across the 80 events during the International Year of Evaluation and to launch a 2016–2020 Global Evaluation Agenda.

The 73rd event was the American Evaluation Association's (AEA) Annual Conference in Chicago, Illinois. In an effort to make a unique contribution to the yearlong discussion a decision was made to create a space in Chicago and online (for the first time at the AEA conference) to learn about the root causes of evaluation success. The assumption was there was much to learn from all regions of the world from examples of high-quality, ethically defensible, culturally responsive evaluation practices that have clearly contributed to decision-making processes, program improvement, policy formulation, effective and humane organizations, and to the enhancement of the public good. Evaluation professionals, sponsors, and users were inspired and energized to spotlight and focus in depth on what has gone well in evaluation from their diverse perspectives. The event turned out to be the largest gathering to date for AEA (and possibly the largest evaluation conference of the year and maybe ever) with more than 5,000 registrants (more than 3,500 in Chicago and 1,500 online) focused on the theme of "Exemplary Evaluations in a Multicultural World: Learning from Evaluation Successes Across the Globe (see Donaldson, 2022a; Donaldson et al., 2022).

Unfortunately, describing the many examples of evaluation success in countries at all points along the development continuum and the potential root causes of each is beyond the scope of this chapter. But there were some key themes that emerged from this extensive discussion that have continued to gain attention during the years since and seem worth highlighting in this chapter with an eye toward improving evaluation practice in the years ahead in post-COVID pandemic times. Those themes include the processes used by the participants to define exemplary evaluation, efforts to make evaluation practice more exemplary, and calls for more exemplary evidence-based evaluation theories. Each of these themes is explored in some depth throughout the remainder of the chapter.

DEFINING EXEMPLARY EVALUATIONS

Let me begin this section by briefly describing an experience I suspect many professors of evaluation can relate to. One of the most reoccurring and common experiences I've had teaching evaluation over the past 25 years has been students asking for examples or exemplars to emulate. No matter how well I describe evaluation concepts, principles, approaches, theories, or methods, many of my evaluation graduate students strongly desire to learn from an example of a "successful" evaluation. This immediately challenges me to select evaluations I can defend as "successful" or exemplary. I know whatever I select will strongly influence the content of their term papers, projects, and exams for the course. I would much rather teach them how to do an evaluation and see what creatively emerges. Replicating what I select as exemplary has the risk of restricting their creativity and leading to less thoughtful, innovative, and deep work. Nevertheless, "professor, please show me an exemplary evaluation to emulate."

So, I decided to ask my evaluation colleagues from around the world for help in 2015 by asking them to showcase exemplars from their evaluation practice. I encouraged them to share with their peers evaluations that they had done or knew about that they would rate as exemplary. In many instances I could see them struggling with the same issues I have faced while performing this evaluative exercise. Many asked me what do you mean by exemplary. My typical response was please share an example of an evaluation that *you* would give a 7 on a 7-point scale. Not a 6, 5, or above-average rating. Not a 4 or average rating. And especially not a below-average evaluation that you would rate as a 3, 2, or 1. It seemed to be as difficult for them as it has been for me all these years.

The challenge I observed was to feel comfortable giving a rating of 7, which requires that all of the values you hold about what is exemplary in evaluation practice must be fully met to the highest degree, and the arguments you need to defend these value judgments must be bulletproof. How often have you felt that strongly about any evaluation? Most of us believe all evaluation work, including our own, has both strengths and weaknesses. However, the exercise inspired my colleagues to discuss how often they naturally focus on the problems in evaluation practice or the deficits of an evaluation (especially in the context of meta-evaluation; Scriven, 1991), how our evaluation methods largely focus on the average (mean, median, or mode), and how difficult it is to systematically evaluate success or defend exemplars. It also was clear that it quickly became an exercise in expressing our values, and how values often differ in various regions of the world and across cultures. For example, U.S. evaluators seemed to put much less value on monitoring than evaluators working in developing countries who seem to highly value both monitoring and evaluation activities. Evaluators working in Europe seem to appreciate and account for national culture more than evaluators primarily focused on practicing in a large country like the United States, Canada, or Australia. Finally, many evaluators working in developing countries seem to value having indigenous evaluators working in collaboration with evaluators from outside their region (see Ofir & Kumar, 2013).

So what were some of the values that participants seemed to focus on when they were arguing that their work, or at least aspects of their work, was exemplary evaluation? Not surprisingly the program evaluation standards of use (see Alkin & Vo, Chapter 8, this volume), accuracy (see Peck & Snyder, Chapter 13, this volume), and how we value immediately rose to the surface (Gates & Schwandt, Chapter 5, this volume)—that is, it was clear that many participants decided to frame their exemplary work using the values put forward in the third edition of the *Program Evaluation Standards* (Yarbrough et al., 2011). In addition to the standards, excelling on the AEA Guiding Principles (2018b) was a related framework that people used to measure their work against and make the case that aspects of their work were exemplary in light of these values and principles:

1. *Systematic inquiry.* Evaluators conduct data-based inquiries that are thorough, methodical, and contextually relevant.
2. *Competence.* Evaluators provide skilled professional services to interest holders.
3. *Integrity.* Evaluators behave with honesty and transparency in order to ensure the integrity of the evaluation (e.g., see Morris, Chapter 7, this volume).
4. *Respect for people.* Evaluators honor the dignity, well-being, and self-worth of individuals and acknowledge the influence of culture within and across groups (e.g., see Atkinson, Chapter 6, this volume).
5. *Common good and equity:* Evaluators strive to contribute to the common good and advancement of an equitable and just society (e.g., see Donaldson, 2022b; Julnes & Rog, 2015).

Many of the participants seemed interested in the multicultural nature of the conference, conference theme, and the multicultural nature of the international year of evaluation. This discussion seemed to emphasize that values to determine what is exemplary are often shaped by the evaluation context (Rog, 2012), including culture and one's cultural background. These values were acknowledged to often diverge across national cultures, and other times be diverse within a national culture, such as the United States. They have continued to be addressed at evaluation conferences around the world. For example, in 2022, the theme of the African Evaluation Association Conference was "Evaluation That Leaves No-One Behind: Empowering Progress towards the Africa We Want Amidst the COVID-19 Pandemic and other Crises and Opportunities Facing Us." The European Evaluation Society Conference focused on "Evaluation at a Watershed: Actions and Shifting Paradigms for Challenging Times." The Australasian Evaluation Society Conference theme was "Weaving Evaluation into the Whole," whereas the Canadian Evaluation Society theme was "Diversity, Our Interwoven Experiences." In the same year, the AEA theme was "Reshaping Evaluation Together." Within each of these conference themes and subthemes, as well as themes at the many other voluntary organizations for professional evaluation (VOPEs) conferences, specific values and criteria for what makes an evaluation exemplary at a particular point in time in a geographic region are often clearly expressed.

One of the valuable resources that is referenced often as a guide for measuring exemplary multicultural or culturally responsive evaluation is the AEA Statement on Cultural Competence (AEA, 2011). This statement is discussed as an exemplary guide for ensuring that evaluators strive for exemplary culturally responsive evaluation practice. It is based on the notion that:

> Cultural competence is a stance taken toward culture, not a discrete status or simple mastery of particular knowledge and skills. A culturally

competent evaluator is prepared to engage with diverse segments of communities to include cultural and contextual dimensions important to the evaluation. Culturally competent evaluators respect the cultures represented in the evaluation throughout the process. (p. 1)

Figure 27.1 provides a summary of the other values and principles expressed in the statement. While its original focus was on diverse cultures within the United States, one of the great opportunities often discussed is how to better use and adapt the statement when working with diverse cultures in other regions of the world (see Atkinson, Chapter 6, this volume).

There are a wide range of emerging issues and themes discussed in reference to how to define exemplary evaluations in 2015 and beyond or what aspects of evaluation practice are most important to address for evaluation work to be exemplary. For example, some of the common

---

AMERICAN EVALUATION ASSOCIATION

The American Evaluation Association (AEA) Public Statement on Cultural Competence in Evaluation

Summary
The complete Statement can be found at http://www.eval.org/ccstatement

The AEA Public Statement on Cultural Competence in Evaluation (a) affirms the significance of cultural competence in evaluation and (b) informs the public of AEA's expectations concerning cultural competence in the conduct of evaluation. The concepts in this statement apply to all evaluations. However, because this statement was written for a U.S. audience, care should be used in employing these guidelines outside the U.S.

What is culture? Culture is the shared experiences of people, including their languages, values, customs, beliefs, and mores. It also includes worldviews, ways of knowing, and ways of communicating. *Culturally significant factors encompass, but are not limited to, race/ethnicity, religion, spirituality, social class, caste, language, lineage, disability, sexual orientation, age, gender, geographic region, and socioeconomic circumstances.* It is important to note that while these factors include culture they are not fixed and can change over time.

Evaluations reflect culture. Culture shapes all evaluation regardless of type (process, outcome, impact, etc.), setting (government, academia, business, etc.), or evaluand (policy, practice, teaching, etc.). Culture impacts all phases of evaluation—including staffing, development, and implementation of evaluation efforts as well as communicating and using evaluation results. Culture shapes the ways in which evaluation questions are conceptualized, which in turn influences what data are collected, how the data will be collected and analyzed, and how data are interpreted. Those who engage in evaluation do so from perspectives that reflect their values, their ways of viewing the world, and their culture. Evaluations cannot be culture free.

What is cultural competence? Cultural competence is a stance taken toward culture, not a discrete status or simple mastery of particular knowledge and skills. Cultural competence is a "process" or a sensibility cultivated throughout a lifetime. It requires awareness of self, reflection on one's own cultural position, awareness of others' positions, and the ability to interact genuinely and respectfully with others.

Why is cultural competence in evaluation important? Cultural competence in evaluation is important for three main reasons. First, the evaluation team is ethically responsible to be culturally competent in order to produce work that is honest, accurate, respectful of stakeholders, and considerate of the general public welfare. Second, cultural competence supports validity by insuring that diverse voices and perspectives are honestly and fairly represented, which in turn, helps to make valid inferences and interpretations. Third, evaluation is steeped in theories that are, themselves shaped by cultural values and perspectives; therefore, it is important to scrutinize theories in order to understand how they describe societal issues, and how to address them.

Essential Practices for Cultural Competence.

- *Acknowledge the complexity of cultural identity.* Culturally competent evaluators recognize, respond to, and work to reconcile differences between and within cultures and subcultures.
- *Recognize the dynamics of power.* Culturally competent evaluators work to avoid reinforcing cultural stereotypes and prejudice in their work.
- *Recognize and eliminate bias in social relations.* Culturally competent evaluators are thoughtful and deliberate in their use of language and other social relations in order to reduce bias when conducting evaluations.
- *Employ culturally congruent epistemologies, theories, and methods.* Culturally competent evaluators seek to understand how the constructs are defined by cultures and are aware of the many ways epistemologies and theories can be utilized, how data can be collected, analyzed and interpreted, and the diversity of contexts in which findings can be disseminated.
- *Continue self-assessments.* Regularly monitor the extent to which you can serve as an open, responsive instrument given relevant attributes of an evaluation context.

FIGURE 27.1. AEA public statement on cultural competence in evaluation. Reprinted with permission from the AEA.

themes aimed at making evaluation practice more exemplary discussed at evaluation gatherings throughout the world have been:

1. How do we bridge the gap between the supply side of evaluation (the evaluation community) and the demand side (the need of policy and decision makers)?
2. What should be the priorities for a global evaluation agenda in post-COVID times?
3. How do we best make evaluation more gender responsive?
4. How do we best design equity-focused evaluations to help develop more equitable societies?
5. What are the best practices for using big data, data visualization, and new technologies in evaluation practice?
6. In what ways can we best advance values of environmental sustainability, diversity–equity–inclusion, social justice, and social betterment in contemporary evaluation practice?

Discussion of how to use evaluations to develop more equitable societies has led to even deeper discussions of exemplary ethics in evaluation and how to avoid conflicts of interest, and exemplary approaches for dealing with the undue influence of power, privilege, and funding sources in evaluation practice (Donaldson & Picciotto, 2016). For example, Greene (2016) argues to think evaluatively (see Archibald et al., Chapter 3, this volume) and is perhaps foremost to ask how well a program's resources are reaching those least well served, and to ask whether a program is affording equity in access, experience, and accomplishments to all. Kirkhart (2016) argues that all evaluation is implicitly involved with equity and privilege because these concepts are linked to determinations of validity, and validity concerns are central to the integrity of evaluation. Schwandt and Gates (2016) suggested we need to push exemplary evaluation into the domain of normative undertaking that tackles the questions "Are we doing the right thing?" and "What makes this the right thing to do?" as opposed to being content with current practice concerned with the question of "Are we doing things right?"

The discussion of how to measure and use our collective values to define exemplary evaluation in a multicultural world is alive and well as evaluation practice has been transformed by the global pandemic and more recently the poly crisis (e.g., Lawrence et al., 2022). A very tangible result of this discussion is that many of the VOPEs from around the world have developed a systematic evaluation process based on the collective values of their membership to identify and celebrate exemplary evaluations and evaluators, often on an annual basis. This collective process of determining exemplary evaluation is commonly known as VOPE awards, usually given at an annual awards ceremony or luncheon. Renger and Donaldson (2024) also found that in addition to many VOPEs, funders of evaluation (e.g., National Science Foundation) and other public evaluation organizations (e.g., United Nations Development Programme Independent Evaluation Office; U.S. Office of Management and Budget) celebrate exemplar evaluation with regular awards.

The AEA has a long history of giving awards for exemplary evaluation. For a few years the awards program was paused to give the AEA Board time to rethink the criteria and process for determining exemplary evaluations and evaluators. The program resumed guided by these new criteria and using a detailed and systematic peer review evaluation process to select the exemplary evaluations and evaluators of the year in the categories of exemplary contributions to evaluation theory, practice, service, advocacy and use, enhancing the public good, ROE, and outstanding new evaluator, as well as the most exemplary evaluation of the year. The criteria that have been used to date for the most exemplary evaluation include:

- An award is given for the successful completion of a single evaluation project that can essentially stand alone as an example of high-quality evaluation.
- The quality judgment will reflect both the methodology of the project and the usefulness of the findings.
- Taken as a whole, the evaluation should be considered exemplary of its kind and a potential model for other evaluators doing similar kinds of work.

- Example standards: Joint Committee's Program Evaluation Standards, Personnel Evaluation Standards, Student Evaluation Standards, or other relevant standards.
- An award is open to an evaluation study in any area of evaluation (e.g., environmental, the arts, foundations).

Some prominent examples of AEA's most exemplary evaluations include the 2000 Fort Bragg Evaluation (Bickman, 1996; Bickman et al., 2000), the 2002 Colorado Healthy Communities Initiative Evaluation (Conner et al., 1999), and the 2012 Paris Declaration Evaluation (Patton, 2018). The complete list of exemplary evaluations honored by AEA can be viewed on the AEA website (*www.eval.org/About/Awards/Past-Award-Winners*). One way of understanding what evaluation communities collectively value in their region of the world and consider exemplary evaluation is to carefully study the nomination letters, letters of support, and the nature of the evaluation or evaluation activity that has earned the exemplary evaluator or evaluation of honor.

Exemplary Professional Evaluation Practice

The globalization of evaluation marked by the rapid expansion of the number of VOPEs and attempts to improve evaluation practice all around the world illustrate the importance and emphasis that is currently being placed on professionalizing evaluation practice. It was discovered during the International Year of Evaluation in 2015 that an estimated 227 VOPEs represented 141 countries and more than 52,000 members (Donaldson & Donaldson, 2016). But, it was also noted often that the demand for evaluation services seems to far exceed the supply of professional evaluators who are highly trained, specifically in evaluation, and hold membership and regularly attend regional or national VOPE annual meetings or conferences like the annual AEA conference. This is believed to be creating a situation nationally as well as in most other parts of the world where many, if not most, people conducting evaluations are not trained in evaluation and have little or no access to the cumulative knowledge base that ideally should inform evaluation practice. This state of affairs seems to be motivating a strong push for more professionalization and evaluator preparation education and training worldwide—that is, one key to more exemplary evaluation practice in the future is expanding what works to best prepare evaluators to perform well in practice.

It was reported that in many parts of the world VOPEs were leading efforts to develop and approve a clearly defined set of evaluator competencies. It is believed these competencies are needed to create an awareness of what is required to provide exemplary evaluation services in their region. Once practitioners are made aware of what competencies they should be striving to develop, tailored professional development opportunities in the region are often provided by VOPEs and/or universities. Some of the exemplary VOPE evaluator competency frameworks that have been approved and showcased (see Galport, 2022) were provided by:

- International Board of Training, Performance, and Instruction (2006)
- United Nations Evaluation Group (2008)
- Visitors Studies Association (2008)
- Gesellschaft fur Evaluation (2008)
- Canadian Evaluation Society (2010)
- Aotearoa New Zealand Evaluation Association (2011)
- European Evaluation Society (2011)
- International Development Evaluation Association (2012)
- Australasian Evaluation Society Inc. (2013)
- United Kingdom Evaluation Society (2013)

Each of these frameworks attempts to guide practitioners to develop the required knowledge and skills needed to perform exemplary evaluations in their region with all of its important multicultural dimensions considered. It should be noted that most of these frameworks seem to be based on criteria focusing on what is adequate competency rather than exemplary, although the intention seems to be to develop more evaluators with the capabilities needed to provide exemplary evaluation services. Furthermore, many contemporary evaluations are carried out by evaluation teams, not individual evaluators, which the competency frameworks focus on. Future efforts to understand how to develop exemplary evaluation teams and the team competencies critical for producing exemplary evaluations might be a promising new direction for the field.

One glaring gap in the global evaluation practice landscape in 2015 was that one of the first and largest VOPEs with more than 7,500 members, the AEA, had not developed and approved an evaluator competency framework. While there had been years of discussion and debate about professionalizing evaluation in the United States (see Altschuld & Engle, 2015; Bickman, 1999; Donaldson, 2018), no real progress toward professionalization had been achieved despite the success and the many exemplars noted above by many of the newer and smaller VOPEs.

This inspired 2015 AEA president Stewart Donaldson to facilitate discussions and ask the question, "Is it time to revisit possible paths that AEA could take to enable more exemplary evaluation practice?" These discussions resulted in the AEA Board being willing to support the formation of a task force to determine whether the association was ready to invest time and energy in developing and approving an evaluator competency framework, perhaps the first significant step toward professionalizing evaluation in the United States. The 2015 AEA Evaluator Competency Task Force, chaired by Jean King, was formed and spent 3 years engaging evaluators in the United States and across the globe to determine the appropriate domains and subdomains critical for training aspiring evaluators to be prepared to provide exemplary evaluation services (see King, Chapter 2, this volume).

After three decades of vigorous discussions about professionalizing evaluation in the United States (see Altschuld & Engle, 2015; Bickman, 1999), the board of the AEA voted for the first time to approve a set of general evaluator competencies in 2018 (see King, Chapter 2, this volume):

1.0 *Professional domain.* Focuses on what makes evaluators distinct as a profession.
2.0 *Methodology domain.* Focuses on technical aspects of evidence-based, systematic inquiry for valued purposes.
3.0 *Context domain.* Focuses on understanding the unique circumstances, multiple perspectives, and changing settings of evaluations and their users/interest holders.
4.0 *Management domain.* Focuses on determining and monitoring work plans, timelines, resources, and other components needed to complete and deliver an evaluation study.
5.0 *Interpersonal domain.* Focuses on human relations and social interactions that ground evaluator effectiveness for professional practice throughout evaluation.

A more detailed graphic of the new AEA Evaluator Competencies (2018a) and a summary of the process that was used to develop and build support for their approval is provided in Figure 27.2. In many respects this process and ultimate product might be considered exemplary and has provided a set of competencies that evaluation training programs of all types (e.g., degree, certificate, and professional development) can use to educate, train, and develop the next generation of evaluator practitioners (also see Cho et al., 2022).

While AEA and the other VOPEs listed above can now celebrate their progress toward professionalizing evaluation in their region of the world, the Canadian Evaluation Society (CES) has moved well beyond just having an evaluator competency framework, and their progress toward professionalizing evaluation in Canada is often viewed as an exemplar.

After decades of debate about professionalization within the Canadian evaluation community, the CES officially launched a credentialed evaluator (CE) professional designation in June 2009 with the goal of promoting ethical, high-quality, and competent evaluation in Canada. Through the CES Professional Designation Program (PDP), which was founded on the three pillars of standards, competencies, and a code of ethics, CES contributed to the professionalization of evaluation, while also enhancing the reputation of the field among CES members and prospective clients (Fierro et al., 2016; Love, 2015). The CES PDP aspires to increase the identification of practitioners as professional evaluators and the recognition of evaluation as a distinct profession; enhance the evaluation knowledge, skills, and professional development of applicants as well as the alignment between the CES competencies for Canadian Evaluation Practice and educational curricula; and increase the value of and demand for the CE designation.

The 2018 AEA
Evaluator Competencies

Our two-part charge from the AEA Board:

1 Frame an initial draft set of competencies that builds on foundational documents and is the next step in professionalizing.

2 Engage AEA members in conversation about what makes evaluators distinct as practicing professionals, arriving at a set of competencies that: serves as a roadmap for guiding evaluator education & training • encourages members to engage in critical self-reflection about strengths & limitations & find appropriate ways to expand & improve their practice • reflects the kinds of services evaluators are called upon to perform in multiple contexts • recognizes the interdependence & overlap of the domains • illustrates—as much as evaluation theory—who we are!

NOTE: We're discussing program evaluation only—not policy, product, or personnel.

Four ideas summarizing our intent

Pragmatic
Our intent was to do something useful—to move forward!

We worked to frame the competencies within the context of AEA's core values—including social justice & the public good.

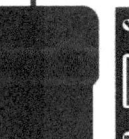

These competencies are meant to be changed, edited, adapted.

Inclusive
We spent three years on this process—receiving a great deal of feedback & working hard to respond.

This is not a series of revisions by a small group of insiders, but rather the result of a long & thoughtful process that reached out in many ways.

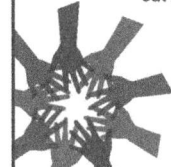

A proposed *NDE* volume will provide grounding & grist for next steps.

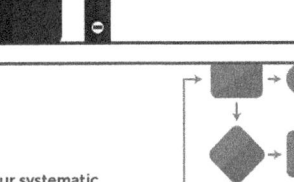

Intentional
Our systematic, design-driven process—like a modified Delphi—engaged members in a holistic effort with multiple perspectives & multiple forms of feedback.

The survey was the final step in an iterative process, a tool to gather member input & feedback.

Dynamic
There's motion here! The AEA Competencies are unlike the Program Evaluation Standards or the AEA Guiding Principles. These competencies are a document for engaging members through multiple forms of outreach.

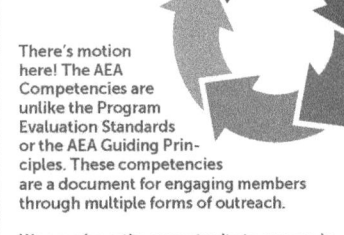

We now have the opportunity to engage in community conversations.

2015 AEA CONFERENCE (CHICAGO) World Café-style listening post (gathered feedback on general competency domains, potential uses of competencies, & members' concerns about AEA proceeding to endorse a set of foundational competencies) • Listening posts at Wednesday & Friday evening receptions

Open solicitation of feedback on the AEA website (www.eval.org) that continued through 2018

Membership engagement sponsored by the Competencies Task Force (2015-2018)

FIGURE 27.2. AEA Evaluator Competencies. Reprinted with permission from the AEA.

1.0
DOMAIN
PROFESSIONAL PRACTICE

focuses on what makes evaluators distinct as practicing professionals

Professional practice is grounded in AEA's foundational documents, including the Program Evaluation Standards, the AEA Guiding Principles, and the AEA Statement on Cultural Competence.

The competent evaluator...

1.1 Acts ethically through evaluation practice that demonstrates integrity and respects people from different cultural backgrounds and indigenous groups.
1.2 Applies the foundational documents adopted by the American Evaluation Association that ground evaluation practice.
1.3 Selects evaluation approaches and theories appropriately.
1.4 Uses systematic evidence to make evaluative judgments.
1.5 Reflects on evaluation formally or informally to improve practice.
1.6 Identifies personal areas of professional competence and needs for growth.
1.7 Pursues ongoing professional development to deepen reflective practice, stay current, and build connections.
1.8 Identifies how evaluation practice can promote social justice and the public good.
1.9 Advocates for the field of evaluation and its value.

2.0
DOMAIN
METHODOLOGY

focuses on technical aspects of evidence-based, systematic inquiry for valued purposes

Methodology includes quantitative, qualitative, and mixed designs for learning, understanding, decision making, and judging.

The competent evaluator...

2.1 Identifies evaluation purposes and needs.
2.2 Determines evaluation questions.
2.3 Designs credible and feasible evaluations that address identified purposes and questions.
2.4 Determines and justifies appropriate methods to answer evaluation questions, e.g., quantitative, qualitative, and mixed methods.
2.5 Identifies assumptions that underlie methodologies and program logic.
2.6 Conducts reviews of the literature when appropriate.
2.7 Identifies relevant sources of evidence and sampling procedures.
2.8 Involves stakeholders in designing, implementing, interpreting, and reporting evaluations as appropriate.
2.9 Uses program logic and program theory as appropriate.
2.10 Collects data using credible, feasible, and culturally appropriate procedures.
2.11 Analyzes data using credible, feasible, and culturally appropriate procedures.
2.12 Identifies strengths and limitations of the evaluation design and methods.
2.13 Interprets findings/results in context.
2.14 Uses evidence and interpretations to draw conclusions, making judgments and recommendations when appropriate.

AEA Evaluator Competencies

SPRING-SUMMER 2016 A series of virtual and in-person focus group discussions using a structured guide with leadership & members of TIGs & affiliates • Targeted efforts to engage international members, who make up 20% of AEA's membership (reviewed proposed domains, specific items for each domain, & discussed pros & cons of defining evaluator competencies) • A guide for AEA Affiliate leaders to use at their annual meetings to solicit member feedback

2016 AEA SUMMER INSTITUTE (ATLANTA) Follow-up listening post

2016 AEA CONFERENCE (ATLANTA) Second series of listening posts

DECEMBER 2016 an aea365 week on the draft competencies in highlighting the dedicated feedback link on the AEA website

2016

FIGURE 27.2. *(continued)*

3.0
DOMAIN
CONTEXT

focuses on understanding the unique circumstances, multiple perspectives, and changing settings of evaluations and their users/stakeholders

Context involves site/location/environment, participants/stakeholders, organization/structure, culture/diversity, history/traditions, values/beliefs, politics/economics, power/privilege, and other characteristics.

The competent evaluator...
- 3.1 Responds respectfully to the uniqueness of the evaluation context.
- 3.2 Engages a diverse range of users/stakeholders throughout the evaluation process.
- 3.3 Describes the program, including its basic purpose, components, and its functioning in broader contexts.
- 3.4 Attends to systems issues within the context.
- 3.5 Communicates evaluation processes and results in timely, appropriate, and effective ways.
- 3.6 Facilitates shared understanding of the program and its evaluation with stakeholders.
- 3.7 Clarifies diverse perspectives, stakeholder interests, and cultural assumptions.
- 3.8 Promotes evaluation use and influence in context.

4.0
DOMAIN
PLANNING & MANAGEMENT

focuses on determining and monitoring work plans, timelines, resources, and other components needed to complete and deliver an evaluation study

Planning and management include networking, developing proposals, contracting, determining work assignments, monitoring progress, and fostering use.

The competent evaluator...
- 4.1 Negotiates and manages a feasible evaluation plan, budget, resources, and timeline.
- 4.2 Addresses aspects of culture in planning and managing evaluations.
- 4.3 Manages and safeguards evaluation data.
- 4.4 Plans for evaluation use and influence.
- 4.5 Coordinates and supervises evaluation processes and products.
- 4.6 Documents evaluation processes and products.
- 4.7 Teams with others when appropriate.
- 4.8 Monitors evaluation progress and quality and makes adjustments when appropriate.
- 4.9 Works with stakeholders to build evaluation capacity when appropriate.
- 4.10 Uses technology appropriately to support and manage the evaluation.

5.0
DOMAIN
INTERPERSONAL

focuses on human relations and social interactions that ground evaluator effectiveness for professional practice throughout the evaluation

Interpersonal skills include cultural competence, communication, facilitation, and conflict resolution.

The competent evaluator...
- 5.1 Fosters positive relationships for professional practice and evaluation use.
- 5.2 Listens to understand and engage different perspectives.
- 5.3 Facilitates shared decision making for evaluation.
- 5.4 Builds trust throughout the evaluation.
- 5.5 Attends to the ways power and privilege affect evaluation practice.
- 5.6 Communicates in meaningful ways that enhance the effectiveness of the evaluation.
- 5.7 Facilitates constructive and culturally responsive interaction throughout the evaluation.
- 5.8 Manages conflicts constructively.

SEPTEMBER 2017 Member survey on the content of the latest draft (roughly 1200 responses/16% response rate, including nearly 1100 separate comments)

2017 AEA CONFERENCE (WASHINGTON, DC) Two sessions to gather additional feedback from members

2017

FIGURE 27.2. *(continued)*

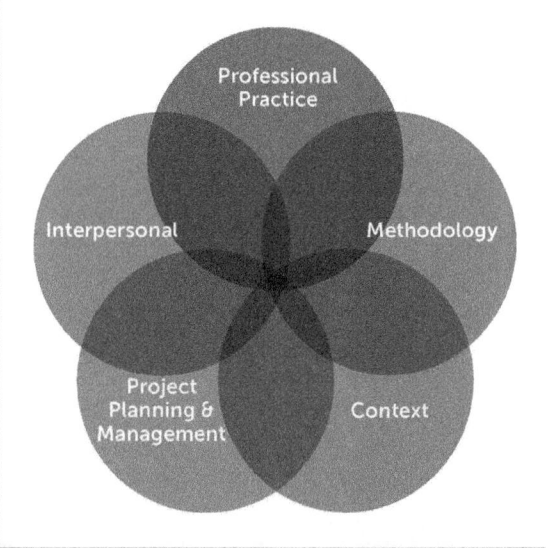

The AEA Evaluator Competencies

AMERICAN EVALUATION ASSOCIATION

What they are:

A common language & set of criteria to clarify what it means to be included in the definition of evaluator.

A way to make clear to everyone the important characteristics of professional evaluation practice & to challenge us to create pathways for engaging all types of people in becoming evaluators.

An inclusive approach that helps provide multiple clear pathways for entry into the practice.

The second of three steps in approaching the professionalization of the field:

1. Review foundational documents & reach out globally to learn from others.
2. Use the knowledge from Step 1 to develop & validate a set of AEA competencies grounded in member engagement (THIS IS WHERE WE ARE).
3. Begin to define how to recognize evaluator competencies.

A *guidemap* for the future.

Competency domains: Professional Practice, Interpersonal, Methodology, Project Planning & Management, Context

What they are not:

These are not perfect & never will be.

They're not a way of excluding qualified people from the field.

They're not a way of addressing systematic challenges in the professionalization of the field.

They're not a credentialing or assessment system—those are separate issues, for future consideration.

MAY 2018 Submission to the AEA Board for approval along with a proposed process for the competencies' routine revision/updating

JUNE 2018 A proposal for a *New Directions* volume to present the competencies, much as AEA's Guiding Principles were originally presented

ONWARD!

2018

FIGURE 27.2. *(continued)*

To partly model exemplary evaluation practice, the CES commissioned a formative evaluation of the PDP by an evaluation center outside of Canada, in the hopes of obtaining an objective and systematic evaluation of their progress to date and recommendations for improvement. It was found that there were more than 350 CES CEs. Based on online surveys with 1,070 participants (706 CES members, 336 former CES members, and 28 nonmembers) and interviews with CES board members, credentialing board members, commissioners of evaluations, employers of evaluators, potential partners for CES, and vocal critics of the PDP, an interesting set of program strengths, weaknesses, opportunities, and potential threats to the program emerged. Several of the key findings included:

- One hundred percent of university respondents were using evaluation competencies in their curriculum.
- Ninety percent of the evaluators were aware of the PDP.
- Seventy-four percent of the CEs reported that the maintenance requirement improved their skills as evaluators.
- Sixty percent of the CEs said the credential improved their exposure as an evaluator.
- An action plan was developed based on the findings and recommendations of the formative evaluation, and serious improvements were made to the program demonstrating an exemplary level of evaluation use.

A more detailed summary of the key findings of the formative evaluation of the CES PDP are presented in the infographic in Figure 27.3.

The development and improvement of the CES PDP program illustrates the momentum the global evaluation community has toward professionalizing evaluation in a way that enables more exemplary evaluation practice. Another related development that occurred during some of the International Year of Evaluation Convenings in 2015 was that the European Evaluation Society announced it was going to follow the lead of CES and begin piloting a new Voluntary Peer Review Evaluator Credentialing System (Picciotto, 2015). This system is now the second major effort by a VOPE to professionalize evaluation through credentialing. LaVelle and Donaldson (2021) describe how these credentialing efforts by VOPEs in combination with the growth of evaluation professional development, certificate, and degree programs being offered by universities represent a substantial effort to address the current state of affairs in evaluation practice preparation, and to develop the capacity for more exemplary evaluation practice in the future.

EXEMPLARY EVIDENCE-BASED EVALUATION THEORY

The AEA evaluator professional practice competency domain focuses on what makes evaluators distinct as practicing professionals. One important subdomain encourages evaluators to select and use evaluation theories appropriately to guide their evaluation practice.

Alkin (2012) explained how evaluation theories offer evaluators a set of rules, prescriptions, prohibitions, and guiding frameworks that specify what a good or proper evaluation is and how evaluation should be done (see also Mark, Chapter 4, this volume; Alkin & Christie, 2022).

Evaluation theory is often pointed out to be an important dimension of evaluation that separates evaluation from research. Shadish (1998) focused his AEA Presidential Year and Conference on the importance of evaluation theory for guiding exemplary evaluation practice. Shadish strongly argued that:

- All evaluators should know evaluation theory because it is central to our professional identity.
- It is what we talk about more than anything else.
- It gives rise to our most trenchant debates.
- It gives us the language we use for talking to ourselves and others.
- It encompasses what evaluators care about most.
- Perhaps most important, it is what makes us different from other professions.
- It is important to make evaluation theory the very heart of our identity.
- Every profession needs a unique knowledge base. For evaluation, evaluation theory is that knowledge base.

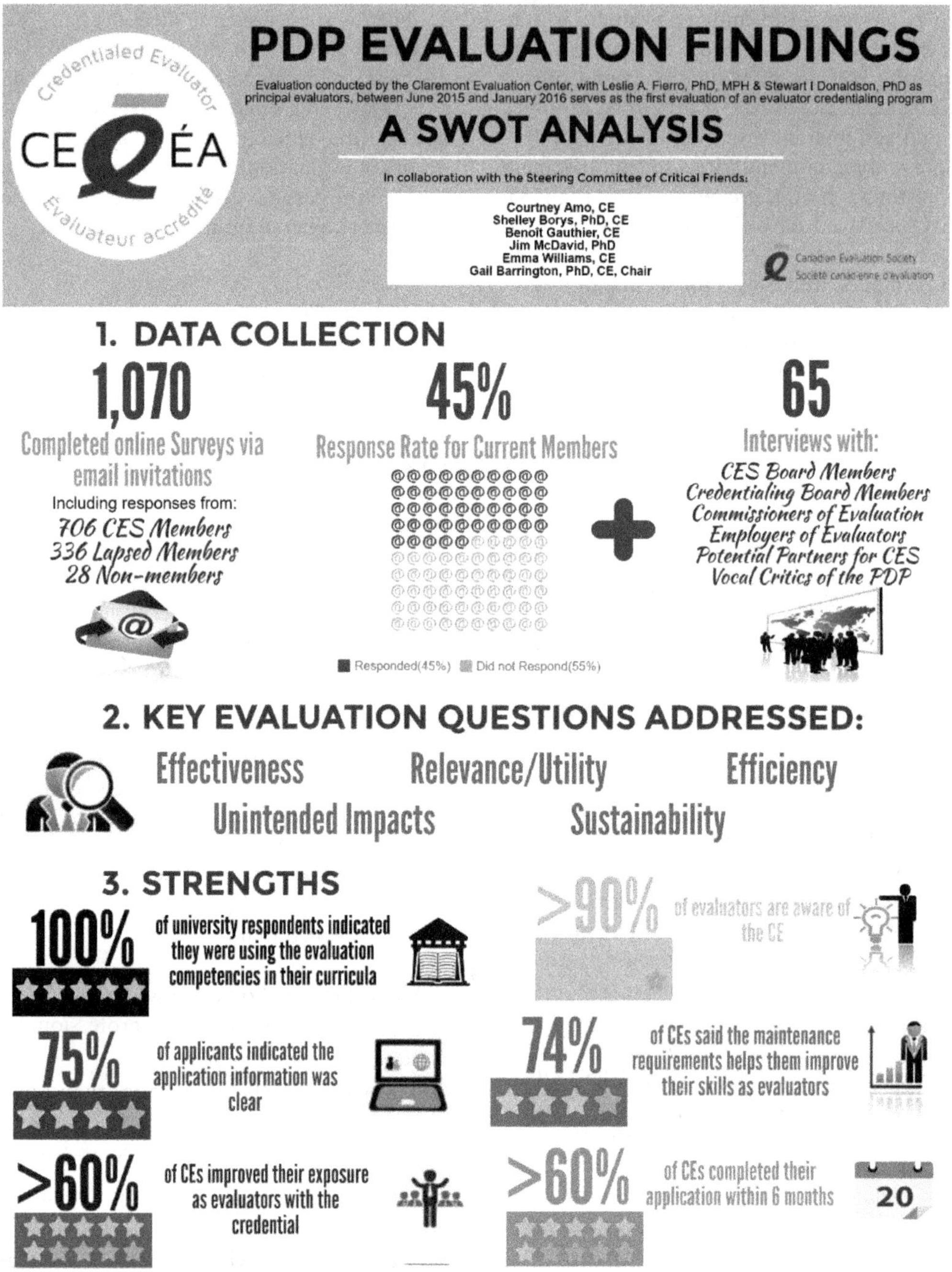

FIGURE 27.3. Canadian Evaluation Society PDP evaluation findings. Reprinted with permission from the Canadian Evaluation Society.

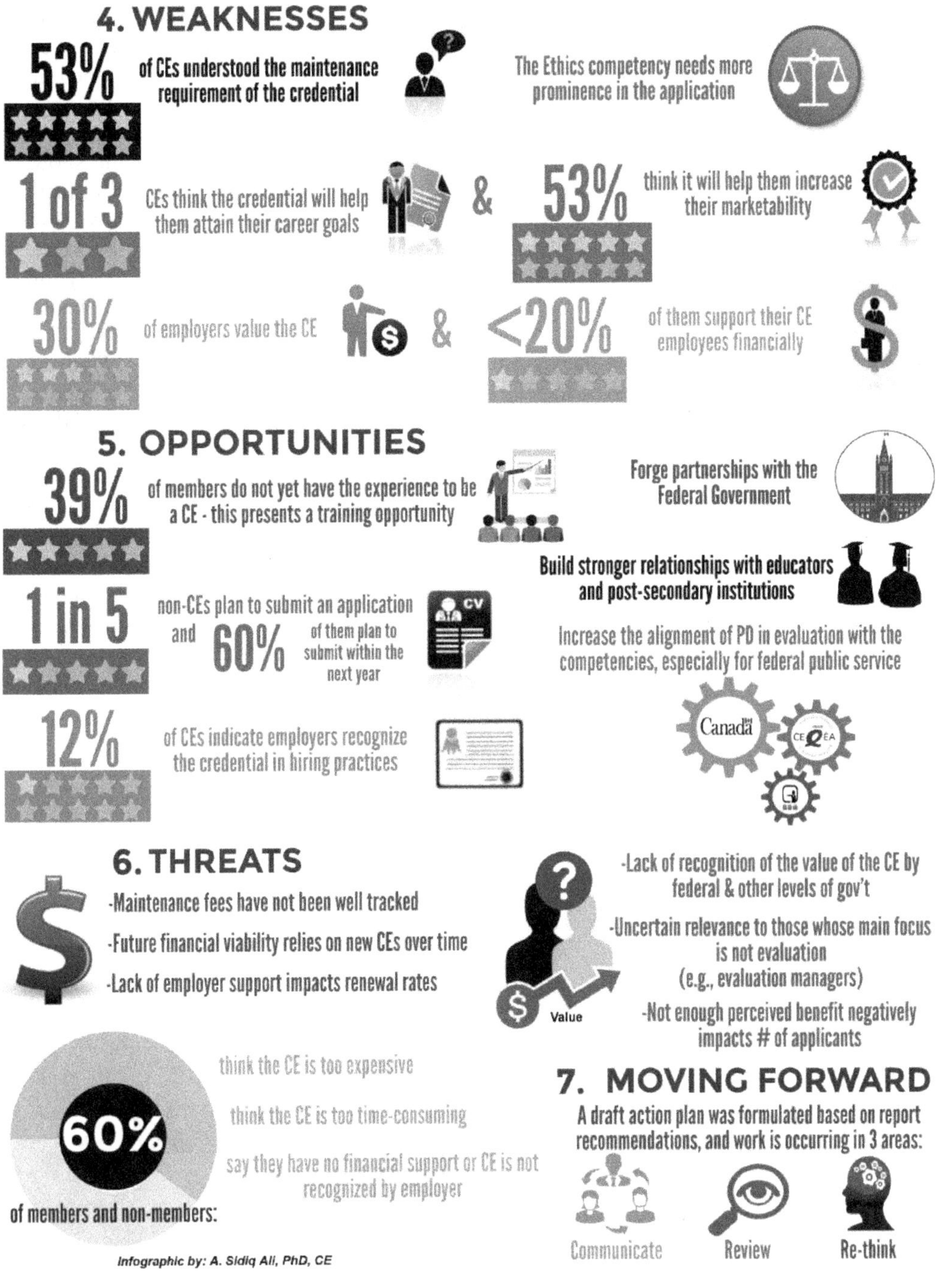

4. WEAKNESSES

53% of CEs understood the maintenance requirement of the credential

The Ethics competency needs more prominence in the application

1 of 3 CEs think the credential will help them attain their career goals

53% think it will help them increase their marketability

30% of employers value the CE

<20% of them support their CE employees financially

5. OPPORTUNITIES

39% of members do not yet have the experience to be a CE - this presents a training opportunity

Forge partnerships with the Federal Government

1 in 5 non-CEs plan to submit an application and **60%** of them plan to submit within the next year

Build stronger relationships with educators and post-secondary institutions

Increase the alignment of PD in evaluation with the competencies, especially for federal public service

12% of CEs indicate employers recognize the credential in hiring practices

6. THREATS

- Maintenance fees have not been well tracked
- Future financial viability relies on new CEs over time
- Lack of employer support impacts renewal rates

- Lack of recognition of the value of the CE by federal & other levels of gov't
- Uncertain relevance to those whose main focus is not evaluation (e.g., evaluation managers)
- Not enough perceived benefit negatively impacts # of applicants

60% of members and non-members:
- think the CE is too expensive
- think the CE is too time-consuming
- say they have no financial support or CE is not recognized by employer

7. MOVING FORWARD

A draft action plan was formulated based on report recommendations, and work is occurring in 3 areas:

Communicate   Review   Re-think

Infographic by: A. Sidiq Ali, PhD, CE

FIGURE 27.3. *(continued)*

The proliferation of evaluation theories over the past two decades has made it difficult for evaluators to understand and master the wide range of options. This has led to a series of frameworks or organizing schemes to help practicing evaluators understand the central issues related to each evaluation theory, and to help evaluators compare and contrast evaluation theories to determine which one(s) are likely to be most effective and useful for guiding their evaluation practice.

One of the earliest evaluation theory frameworks focused on how evaluation theory had evolved over time, passing through stages of a focus on seeking truth in social problem solving, to pursuing useful and pragmatic approaches, to integrative theories that try to cumulate knowledge about evaluation practice by building on the lessons learned from previous applications of evaluation theory (Shadish et al., 1991). Donaldson and Scriven (2003) updated this framework by asking some of the theorists featured in the prior framework and a diverse group of new evaluation theorists to provide their visions for how to best achieve exemplary evaluation practice in the new millennium. Several years later Alkin and Christie (2012) developed an evaluation theory tree with three main branches of use-oriented theories, method-oriented theories, and valuing-oriented theories and showed how the theorists on each branch had influenced one another's ideas. This comparative evaluation theory tree was later criticized by Mertens and Wilson (2018) for leaving out a very important group of evaluation theories and theorists that focused their work on social justice. The revised evaluation theory tree shown in Figure 27.4 has a fourth branch to represent the importance of theories and efforts to promote social justice in evaluation practice.

Many of the discussions about the evaluation theory tree in recent years have focused on the social justice branch, and whether social justice should remain on Alkin and Christie's (2012) valuing branch or be represented on its own branch elevating it to the same level as use, methods, and valuing. This new spotlight on social justice theories has encouraged evaluators

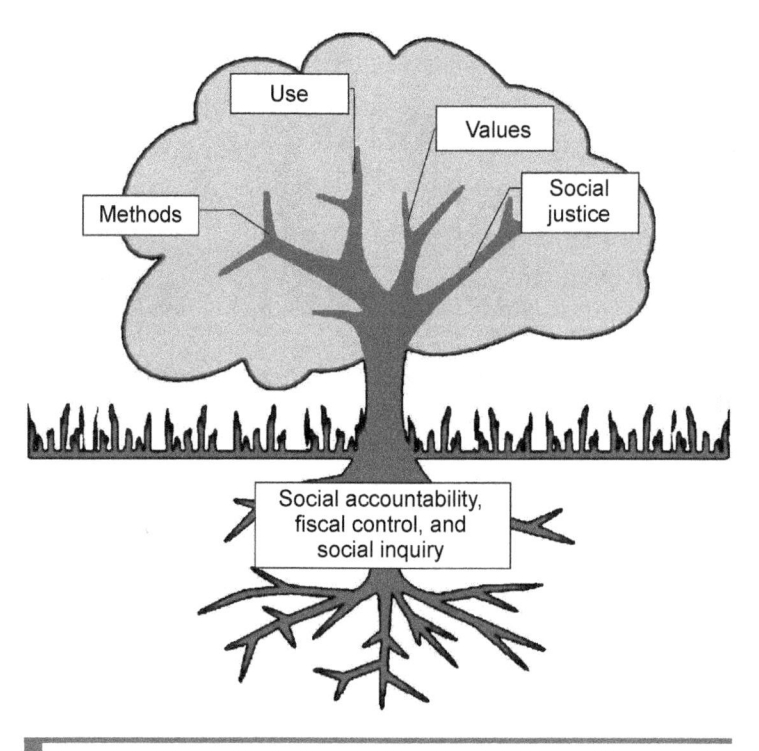

FIGURE 27.4. Four-branch evaluation theory tree. From Mertens and Wilson (2018). Copyright © 2018 The Guilford Press. Reprinted by permission.

to think more deeply about how they might improve their evaluation practice and make their work more socially just. For example, in an article in the *American Journal of Evaluation*, Caldwell and Bledsoe (2019) ask the question, Can social justice live within the structural racism present in the field of evaluation? They highlighted evaluation theories and literature that intellectually protests and positions paradigm shifts for more equity in the evaluation profession, provides a new framework for professional behavior modification as a strategy for the extinction of structural racism in evaluation, and asserts that social justice can only be realized when structural racism is eradicated. Lively discussions of how to improve evaluation theory, practice, and the profession are one critical avenue for advancing our field.

While comparing and contrasting evaluation theories in a way that leads to the best guidance possible in evaluation practice has long been advocated as a path to exemplary evaluation, one clear limitation of most of the evaluation theories we have to date are that they are based on practitioner prescriptions rather than research and evidence-based practice. This state of affairs has led to calls for more ROE in the last decade in an effort to develop more evidence-based theories to guide evaluation practice (Alkin & Christie, 2022; Julnes & Rog, 2007; Mark, 2008; Mark et al., 2011).

Many examples of exemplary ROE studies were discussed at the AEA conference in 2015 and at evaluation conferences around the world since. The AEA Awards Program has honored a number of prolific researchers who have made significant contributions to advancing exemplary ROE, including to William R. Shadish (1998), Marvin Alkin (2012), Michael Quinn Patton (2018), and J. Bradley Cousins (2018). In 2019, a new volume was published to illustrate exemplary contributions to growing our knowledge base through ROE, with a specific focus on honoring the research contributions of J. Bradley Cousins (Chouinard & Amo, 2019). Recent empirical research exemplars on topics such as organizational learning, participatory evaluation, and evaluation capacity building are presented and discussed in detail. Furthermore, it is important to point out that some of the most widely cited articles in evaluation have been ROE studies that have examined the evidence base supporting widely used evaluation theories, such as empowerment (Miller & Campbell, 2006) and theory-driven evaluation (Coryn et al., 2011). In summary, one promising path for enhancing exemplary evaluation practice in the future is the development of more evidence-based evaluation theories to effectively guide evaluator decisions in complex practice situations (see Mark, Chapter 4, this volume).

CONCLUSION

Systematically studying evaluation success and the strengths of evaluations and evaluands, while sometimes difficult and unnatural, can provide insights that complement our more traditional knowledge and focus on the average evaluation or effect size of an evaluand, evaluation problems and deficits, and the challenges of global evaluation practice. The focus on exemplary evaluation in a multicultural world during the International Year of Evaluation in 2015, and during the years that have followed, has taught us about the common and diverse values evaluators use to determine what is considered exemplary evaluation in their region of the world. It is my hope that in the future, evaluators will think of exemplary evaluation as an aspiration to strive for, realizing its attainment might be rare but certainly worth learning from and celebrating as a developing global evaluation community.

REFERENCES

Alkin, M. (2012). *Evaluation roots: A wider perspective of theorists' views and influences*. SAGE.

Alkin, M., & Christie, C. A. (2012). An evaluation theory tree re-examined. In M. Alkin (Ed.), *Evaluation roots: A wider perspective of theorists' views and influences* (pp. 11–58). SAGE.

Alkin, M., & Christie, C. A. (2022). *Evaluation roots: Theory influencing practice* (3rd ed.). Guilford Press.

Altschuld, J. W., & Engle, M. (2015). Accreditation, certification, and credentialing: Relevant concerns for US evaluators. *New Directions for Evaluation, 145*.

American Evaluation Association. (2011). *Cultural competence statement*. Available at http://eval.org/Community/Volunteer/Statement-on-Cultural-Competence-in-Evaluation

American Evaluation Association. (2018a). *Evaluator competences*. Available at http://eval.org/Portals/0/Docs/AEA%20Evaluator%20Competencies.pdf

American Evaluation Association. (2018b). *Guiding principles for evaluators*. Available at http://eval.org/Portals/0/AEA_289398-18_GuidingPrinciples_Brochure_2.pdf

Bickman, L. (1996). A continuum of care: More is not always better. *American Psychologist, 51*(7), 689–701.

Bickman, L. (1999). AEA, bold or timid? *American Journal of Evaluation, 20*(3), 519–520.

Bickman, L., Lambert, E. W., & Andrade, A. R. (2000). The Fort Bragg continuum of care for children and adolescents: Mental health outcomes over 5 years. *Journal of Consulting and Clinical Psychology, 68*(4), 710–716.

Caldwell, L. D., & Bledsoe, K. (2019). Can social justice live in a house of structural racism? A question for the field of evaluation. *American Journal of Evaluation, 40*(1), 6–18.

Cho, M., Castleman, A. M., Umans, H., & Mwirigi, M. O. (2022). Measuring evaluator competencies: Developing and evaluating the evaluator competencies assessment tool. *American Journal of Evaluation, 44*(3), 474–494.

Chouinard, J. A., & Amo, C. (2019). *Growing the knowledge base in evaluation: The contributions of J. Bradley Cousins*. Information Age.

Connor, R. F., Tanjasiri, S. P., & Easterling, D. (1999). *Communities tracking their quality of life: An overview of community indicators project of the Colorado Healthy Communities Initiative*. The Colorado Trust.

Coryn, C. L. S., Noakes, L. A., Westine, K., & Schroter, D. C. (2011). A systematic review of theory-driven evaluation practice from 1990 to 2009. *American Journal of Evaluation, 32*(2), 199–226.

Cousins, J. B. (2018). Evaluation of Gamgard: A tool to identify gaming risks to vulnerable players under "normal" playing conditions. University of Ottawa. Available from: https://crecs.uottawa.ca/sites/crecs.uottawa.ca/files/gamgard_evaluation_report.pdf

Donaldson, S. I. (2018). Where do we stand? Recent AEA member views on professionalization. *Evaluation and Program Planning, 72*, 152–161.

Donaldson, S. I. (2022a). *Introduction to theory-driven program evaluation: Culturally responsive and strengths-focused applications*. Routledge.

Donaldson, S. I. (2022b). Riding shotgun down evaluations' highways: A tribute to the legacy of George Julnes. *American Journal of Evaluation, 43*(2), 298–300.

Donaldson, S. I., & Donaldson, S. I. (2016). Visions for using evaluation to develop more equitable societies. In S. I. Donaldson & R. Picciotti (Eds.), *Evaluation for an equitable society*. Information Age.

Donaldson, S. I., Donaldson, S. I., & Renger, J. A. (2022). Evaluation in the United States of America. In R. Stockmann, W. Mayer, & L. Szentmarjay (Eds.), *The Institutionalization of Evaluation in the Americas* (pp. 355–377). Palgrave Macmillan.

Donaldson, S. I., & Picciotto, R. (2016). *Evaluation for an equitable society*. Information Age.

Donaldson, S. I., & Scriven, M. (Eds.). (2003). *Evaluating social programs and problems: Visions for the new millennium*. Erlbaum.

Fierro, L. A., Galport, N., Hunt, A., Codd, H., & Donaldson, S. I. (2016). *Evaluation of the Canadian Evaluation Society Credentialed Evaluator Designation Program*. Claremont Evaluation Center Evaluation Report.

Galport, N. (2022). *Professionalizing evaluation: Exploring competencies and professional development*. Evaluation Report, Claremont Evaluation Center, Claremont Graduate University.

Greene, J. C. (2016). Advancing equity: Cultivating an evaluation habit. In S. I. Donaldson & R. Picciotto (Eds.), *Evaluation for an equitable society* (pp. 49–66). Information Age.

Julnes, G., & Rog, D. J. (Eds.). (2007). Informing federal policies on evaluation methodology: Building the evidence base for method choice in government sponsored evaluation. *New Directions for Evaluation, 113*.

Julnes, G., & Rog, D. J. (2015). Actionable evidence in context: Contextual influences on adequacy and appropriateness of method choice in evaluation. In S. I. Donaldson, C. A. Christie, & M. M. Mark (Eds.), *Credible and actionable evidence: The foundation of rigorous and influential evaluations* (2nd ed., pp. 221–258). SAGE.

Kirkhart, J. C. (2016). Equity, privilege, and validity: Traveling companions or strange bedfellows? In S. I. Donaldson & R. Picciotto (Eds.), *Evaluation for an equitable society* (pp. 109–132). Information Age.

LaVelle, J., & Donaldson, S. I. (2021). Opportunities and challenges ahead for university-based evaluation education programs, faculty, and students. *American Journal of Evaluation, 42*(3), 428–438.

Lawrence, M., Janzwood, S., & Homer-Dixon, T. (2022). *What is a global polycrisis?* Version 2.0. Discussion Paper 2022-4. Cascade Institute. Available at https://cascadeinstitute.org/technical-paper/what-is-a-globalpolycrisis

Love, A. (2015). Building the foundation for the CES professional designation program. *Canadian Journal of Program Evaluation, 29*(3), 1–20.

Mark, M. M. (2008). Building a better evidence base for evaluation theory. In N. Smith & P. L. Brandon (Eds.), *Fundamental Issues in Evaluation* (pp. 111–134). Sage.

Mark, M. M., Donaldson, S. I., & Campbell, R. (2011). *Social psychology and evaluation*. Guilford Press.

Mertens, D. M., & Wilson, A. T. (2018). *Program evaluation theory and practice: A comprehensive guide*. Guilford Press.

Miller, R. L., & Campbell, R. (2006). Taking stock of empowerment evaluation: An empirical review. *American Journal of Evaluation, 27*(3), 296–319.

Ofir, Z., & Shiva Kumar, A. K. (2013). Evaluation in developing countries: What make it different? In S. I. Donaldson, T. Azzam, & Connor, R. (Eds.), *Emerging practices in international development evaluation* (pp. 11–23). Information Age.

Patton, M. Q. (2018). Metaevaluation: Evaluating the evaluation of the Paris Declaration. *Canadian Journal of Program Evaluation, 27*(2), 147–171.

Picciotto, R. (2015). *The Voluntary Evaluator Peer Review (VEPR) initiative*. European Evaluation Society.

Renger, J., & Donaldson, S. I. (2024). *Reimagining meta-evaluation: A participatory approach to increase use*. Manuscript submitted for publication.

Rog, D. J. (2012). When background becomes foreground: Toward context-sensitive evaluation practice. *New Directions for Evaluation, 135,* 25–40.

Schwandt, T. A., & Gates, E. F. (2016). What can evaluation do? An agenda for evaluation in service of an equitable society. In S. I. Donaldson, & R. Picciotto (Eds.), *Evaluation for an equitable society* (pp. 67–82). Information Age.

Scriven, M. (1991). *Evaluation thesaurus* (4th ed.). SAGE.

Shadish, W. R. (1998). Evaluation theory is who we are. *American Journal of Evaluation, 19*(1), 1–19.

Shadish, W. R., Jr., Cook, T. D., & Leviton, L. C. (1991). *Foundations of program evaluation: Theories of practice*. SAGE.

Yarbrough, D. B., Shulha, L. M., Hopson, R. K., & Caruthers, F. A. (2011). *The program evaluation standards: A guide for evaluators and evaluation users* (3rd ed.). SAGE.

Glossary

Acceptability: the extent to which a given program is agreeable, palatable, or satisfactory to interest holders.

Accountability: outcomes and accountability; producing results within the context of existing policies, standards, and measures of accountability; did the program or initiative accomplish its objectives?

Action research: Kurt Lewin's conceptualization of research as a series of steps that involve data collection, planning, action, and changes in behavior. In turn, changes in behavior are evaluated and the results used as inputs for the next cycle of planning, action, change, and evaluation.

Activities: the components that describe what the treatments or services a program is providing. They are the actions taken to move toward the program's goals and outcomes.

Adaptation: a form of modification characterized by thoughtful and deliberate alteration to the design or delivery of a program to improve its fit or effectiveness in a given context.

Adoption: the intention, initial decision, or action to try or employ an innovation or evidence-based practice.

American Evaluation Association (AEA) Guiding Principles for Evaluators: the core values of the AEA, intended as a guide to the professional ethical conduct of evaluators. The five Guiding Principles address systematic inquiry, competence, integrity, respect for people, and common good and equity.

Annualized/annualization: the process by which the value of a long-term durable asset can be divided over its useful life, taking into account depreciation and the opportunity cost of investing capital in the asset instead of alternative investments.

Anonymous datasets: all personally identifiable data are either removed or encrypted in these datasets.

Appropriateness: The perceived fit, relevance, or compatibility of the program for a given problem, practice setting, provider, or consumer.

Artificial intelligence (AI): the intelligence of machines (computers) in contrast to humans.

Assignment variable/forcing variable: in regression discontinuity designs, the assignment variable is a quantitative variable that is used to assign individuals to treatment or comparison conditions. Usually, individuals on one side of a prespecified cut point are assigned to treatment while individuals on the other side are not.

Audiences: those individuals or groups that could benefit from information about the progress and results of an evaluation.

Average cost per participant: the total cost of an intervention divided by the number of participants.

Axiological assumptions: paradigmatic assumptions that deal with the nature of ethics.

Balance tests: statistical tests for whether baseline characteristics between program participants and members of the comparison group are similar (i.e., not statistically significantly different) before the program began.

Baselines: the number or frequency before the intervention.

Behavioral function of internal evaluation: the influence that participation in evaluation exerts on the behavior of those involved in the evaluation process. The individuals delivering a program as well as those receiving a program are affected by the recognition that they are involved in an evaluation.

Benefit–cost analysis: an analysis of the costs of an intervention relative to the economic estimate of the social value of the intervention in monetary terms, or the benefits of the outcomes of the intervention.

Best-case and worst-case scenario testing: a type of sensitivity analysis applying extreme values of assumptions to determine best-case and worst-case scenarios to determine if such scenarios are acceptable.

Big data: Large and usually complex data that can include structured data that usually grows over time.

Bivariate analysis: an umbrella term for the analysis of two variables at once for the purpose of determining the relationship between the two variables.

Blog: a regularly updated website or web page, typically by an individual or small group, that is written in an informal or conversational style.

Bootstrapping: a method of estimating a sampling distribution for statistical testing using random resampling within the observed sample.

Break-even analysis: a type of sensitivity analysis to determine the levels of assumptions required to change the result of an analysis. For example, to determine at what point would a cost-effectiveness ranking change, or at what point would the benefits of an intervention exactly equal its costs to determine if such values are plausible.

Business lens: the perspective or viewpoint through which business decisions and strategies are analyzed and made. It involves considering various factors such as market trends, financial performance, competitive landscape, customer needs, and organizational goals.

Calendar time: time taken to complete a task counted in calendar days, weeks, or months.

Campbell, Donald: an evaluation theorist, perhaps best known for his advocacy of experimental and quasi-experimental methods to assess the outcomes of a program, and for the concepts of *internal* and *external validity* (see entries).

Capacity building: enhancing interest holders' skills and ability to conduct evaluation and improve program planning and implementation.

Categorical variable: a variable that can only take on a set number of discrete values. Values often, but not always, represent nonnumeric, mutually exclusive categories, such as race, gender, college major, and so on.

Causal analysis: a category of analytic methods that seek to establish how a change in one variable (often participation in a program) causes another variable (usually the outcome of interest) to change.

Certificate of Confidentiality: a certificate issued by the National Institutes of Health or by other U.S. Department of Health and Human Services agencies. Its purpose is to ensure that identifiable research information is protected from forced or compelled disclosure in civil, criminal, administrative, legislative, or other proceedings, whether federal, state, or local. Such a certificate helps to minimize risks to subjects by adding an additional level of protection for maintaining confidentiality of private information.

Channel: the medium selected to carry a communications message.

Channel, audiovisual: all actions, tactics, or tools that are mainly made up of sound and images.

Channel, interpersonal: all actions, tactics, or tools that involve face-to-face communications (in person or virtually).

Channel, text based: all actions, tactics, or tools that are mainly made up of written communications.

Clock time: time taken to complete a task that is usually counted in hours independent of the calendar.

Closely bound internal evaluator: an internal evaluator who works under contract and reports to the management of the organization. Although the evaluator is not an employee of the organization in the usual sense, the reporting relationships and contractual arrangements do not give the evaluator independence from the organization.

Cluster analysis: a data-driven, algorithmic approach to identifying groups that are not otherwise readily identifiable and that minimize within-group heterogeneity and maximize between-group heterogeneity.

Coarsened exact matching (CEM): an algorithmic approach to constructing a comparison group that uses multiple characteristics and where the treatment–comparison imbalance of one characteristic has no effect on the imbalance of another; a type of *multidimensional matching*.

Coding: the process of assigning descriptive labels to data to organize and discover relationships and patterns. The labels or codes may be chosen inductively or deductively.

Cohort design: a type of interrupted time series model where cohorts of individuals who participate in the program of interest are compared with different cohorts that did not participate in the program.

Collaboration members: specific individuals (possessing unique characteristics) who work jointly with the evaluator(s) to help with particular tasks in order to achieve the evaluation vision.

Collaborative evaluation: an approach where evaluators work with interest holders to design and conduct evaluations, ensuring the process is inclusive and the findings are relevant.

Collaborative evaluators: individuals who are in charge of the evaluation but create an ongoing engagement between evaluators and interest holders, contributing to stronger evaluation designs, enhanced data collection and analysis, and results that interest holders understand and use.

Communications: the process through which people share thoughts, ideas, and feelings with one another in commonly understood ways.

Communications activities: actions, tactics, or tools to carry the messages to interest holders and audiences.

Communications objectives: statements of what is desired to be achieved through the communications.

Communications plan of action: a plan that sets out what will be communicated, when, how, and for what purpose.

Community-based participatory research (CBPR): a collaborative approach to research that equitably involves all partners in the research process and recognizes the unique strengths that each brings.

Community knowledge: community members' collective knowledge about their own community capacity, needs, aspirations, respect, and values.

Community ownership: ownership that values and facilitates community control, use, and sustainability.

Comparative effectiveness research (CER): research that seeks to assist consumers, clinicians, purchasers, and policymakers to make informed decisions to improve health care at both the individual and population levels.

Comparative interrupted time-series design (CITS): a comparison-group evaluation design that uses the projection of a preprogram trend to estimate a counterfactual.

Comparison group evaluation design: a quasi-experimental evaluation design that involves using a comparison group's outcomes to estimate a counterfactual; types include posttest-only comparison group design, pretest–posttest comparison group design, comparative interrupted time-series design, and regression discontinuity design.

Competencies: in evaluation, they are the skills, knowledge, and abilities required to perform a quality evaluation study.

Complexity and systems evaluation: approaches that consider the complex and interconnected nature of programs and their contexts.

Conflict of interest: a conflict between the private interests and official responsibilities of a person in a position of trust.

Confounder: a factor that influences both selection into the program and the relevant outcome. Failure to account for a confounder will likely lead to biased estimates of program effects.

Constructivist: a worldview associated with qualitative approaches; the stance that there are multiple meanings or realities and that there should be purposeful attempts to represent these multiple realities through the qualitative analysis and a descriptive process.

Context: the combination of factors accompanying the implementation and evaluation of a project that might influence its results, including culture, geographical location, timing, political and social climate, and economic conditions.

Contextual factors are factors that are out of control of the program but may help or hinder achievement of the outcomes. Context can include both current context and historical context, as previous experiences may color how participants perceive a current experience.

Contingency model: a Contingency Model, in the context of evaluation, specifies how different approaches to evaluation should be undertaken depending on particular situational attributes, such as stage or intended use.

Convergent/parallel design: one of the core mixed methods designs, also referred to as a simultaneous or parallel design, where qualitative and quantitative data sources are collected separately and concurrently and through an integration process (e.g., joint display) examines an issue or answer a question using qualitative and quantitative perspectives.

Correlational analysis: an analysis that establishes a relationship between two variables; however, the existence of this relationship is insufficient to claim causation.

Cost-effectiveness analysis: an analysis of the effects of its intervention relative to its costs. A cost-effectiveness analysis is comparative in nature, and can compare interventions on their costs relative to their effects on the same, single outcome.

Cost-effectiveness ratio: the ratio of the average cost per participant to the average effectiveness per participant, or cost per unit of outcome.

Cost–feasibility analysis: an analysis of the costs of an intervention compared to a budget constraint. This analysis can be performed in conjunction with other types of feasibility, such as political feasibility, or the feasibility of successful implementation.

Cost–utility analysis: an extension of cost-effectiveness analysis to incorporate multiple outcomes, comparing interventions based on their costs relative to the overall well-being that is generated from multiple outcomes.

Counterfactual: the scenario that would have occurred in the absence of the intervention, used as a comparison to determine the intervention's impact.

Covariate: a variable that can influence the relationship between the primary independent variable of interest and the dependent variable. However, covariates are usually not the primary independent variable of interest.

Covariate balance: whether program participants and comparison group individuals exhibit similar characteristics prior to exposure to the program or intervention.

Criteria: dimensions of value or performance that provide a basis for evaluative judgments.

Critical friends: evaluators view *program staff members, program as in control* of the evaluation; empowerment evaluators serve as critical friends or coaches to help keep the process on track, rigorous, responsive, and relevant.

Critical realism: a school of philosophy that, as espoused by *Donald Campbell* (see entry), posits that there is an external world independent of our construction of it, but that our perceptions of it are fallible and mediated by perceptual, cognitive, and social processes.

Cross-sectional data: data collected at a single point in time or over a short period from multiple subjects, such as individuals, groups, or organizations. This type of data provides a snapshot of a particular phenomenon or population at a specific moment.

Culturally responsive evaluation (CRE): an evaluation theory that emphasizes the importance of cultural context, power dynamics, program history, and interest holders views and values, including the lived experience of intended beneficiaries.

Cut-point design: (*see* Regression discontinuity)

Dashboard reports: a method of presenting data in which visuals are spread across multiple pages or when significant interaction is available within the visuals (such as drill-downs and filtering).

Data: the basic units or building blocks of information. Data can be found in many forms: images, sounds, written words, spoken words, documents, numbers, smells, and actions. Grouped into patterns (analyzed and synthesized), data become information to be interpreted. Note that the word *data* is plural; a single unit is *datum*.

Data dashboards: a method of displaying the most important data needed for decision making in a single page view.

Data ink: ink in a graphic that contains nonredundant data or information.

Data source, primary: data that evaluators collect themselves for the purposes of a specific evaluation. May include data sources such as surveys, interviews, and document reviews.

Data source, secondary: data that evaluators acquire from another source that was originally collected for purposes other than the present evaluation. Popular secondary data sources include administrative data from state departments of education, U.S. Census data, and large datasets collected by governments or agencies.

Data structure: a dataset with a separate row for each unit of observation and time period. The number of observations in long data for a program evaluation with multiple time points will be equal to the number of program participants multiplied by the number of time points for which data were collected.

Data structure, wide a dataset with a single row for each unit of observation. The number of observations in wide data for a program evaluation with multiple time points will be equal to the number of program participants. Multiple time points are represented as separate variables within a single observation.

Data visualization: the accurate and efficient visual representation of data to facilitate understanding.

Dataset: a collection of variables for a given set of observations, organized in a tabular format.

Dataset, longitudinal: data that follow participants over multiple time periods. In program evaluation, longitudinal data usually includes a time point prior to the start of the intervention and at the end of the intervention but can include multiple time points between or even further beyond the end of the intervention.

Decision-making characteristics: the elements that are considered when making decisions.

Deductive and inductive thinking: reasoning processes involved in reaching a conclusion. With inductive reasoning you begin with details or particular experiences and move to more general statements leading toward theory. Deductive reasoning begins with theory and uses specifics to support or test its applicability. In short, inductive reasoning is a bottom-up approach, while deductive reasoning is top-down.

De-identified dataset: often used interchangeably with *anonymization*. De-identified health data can be shared making it HIPPA compliant.

Democratic participation: participation open to the community and open and fair decision making.

Descriptive analysis: a category of data analysis used to investigate characteristics of programs, participants, and other relevant program features.

Design, alignment: placing text or other design elements on a page so they line up (e.g., use of bullet points with the same distance from the page margin).

Design, bullet-point list: a list of items with a bullet point (large dot) in front of each work/phrase.

Design, contrast: distinguishing elements in a document by different colors and fonts.

Design, heading: a title at the start of a chapter or section.

Design, highlighted box: a text box to highlight specific content of a report.

Design, proximity: putting related design elements close to each other (e.g., a table close to the text that describes it).

Design, quotes: a sentence or phrase from a text, speech, or interview transcript quoting an individual.

Design, randomized: in the context of experiments, refers to a method where subjects or experimental units are randomly assigned to different treatment groups. This approach helps ensure that the groups are comparable and that the results are not biased by confounding variables.

Design, repetition: reusing the same or similar elements in a document (e.g., same style of graphs, the font, headings, or tables).

Design, subheading: a title at the start of a subchapter or subsection.

Design-based tradition: composed of randomized controlled trials and regression discontinuity designs, the design-based tradition uses manipulation of access to the program in order to produce equivalent treatment and comparison groups.

Design feasibility: assessing whether a proposed design or solution is practical, achievable, and cost-effective. It involves evaluating technical, economic, and operational aspects to determine whether the design can be successfully implemented.

Development: training (such as workshops or seminars) or any other mechanism (e.g., mentoring) to enhance educational learning and self-improvement.

Developmental evaluation: an approach that engages with social innovators to support adaptation of interventions in complex dynamic systems.

Dialogue: discussion about the "taking stock" ratings; one of the most important parts of the empowerment evaluation approach used to clarify issues; evidence used to support viewpoints; "sacred cows" are surfaced and examined; process of specifying the reason or evidence for a rating provides the group with a more efficient and focused manner of identifying what needs to be done next, during the planning for the future steps of the process.

Difference-in-differences (DID): a model that compares pre–post differences in outcomes for program participants minus the same pre–post difference for comparison group individuals.

Differential attrition: a threat to internal validity; different rates of follow-up data collection for treatment and control groups, resulting in nonequivalent groups; also referred to as experimental mortality.

Direct (or instrumental) use: when the findings of an evaluation are employed in decisions or actions, such as a decision to fund a program expansion or actions that modify an ongoing program.

Discounting: the process of adjusting costs and benefits that occur at different points in time to present value in a single time period to account for the time value of money by applying a discount rate.

Ecological momentary assessments (EMA): a research methodology that involves repeatedly sampling a person's current behaviors and experiences in their natural environment.

Economic evaluation: an umbrella term that refers to methods for systematically analyzing both inputs and outcomes in an evaluation framework, comprising cost analysis, cost–feasibility analysis, cost-effectiveness analysis, cost–utility analysis, and cost–benefit analysis.

Effect size: a statistical calculation that measures the strength of the relationship between two variables.

Effective data visualization: a method of communicating the intended message accurately.

Empathy: display of sensitivity, understanding, and a thoughtful response toward the feelings or emotions of others.

Empowerment: development of a sense of self-efficacy; removing obstacles limiting the attainment of established goals.

Empowerment evaluation: an approach that aims to increase the capacity of program interest holders to plan, implement, and evaluate their own programs.

Empowerment evaluator: someone who follows the precepts of empowerment evaluation, developed by David Fetterman and colleagues. This approach to evaluation sets out as a key goal for evaluation the empowerment of the interest holders who participate in the conduct of an evaluation.

Enhanced Evaluability Assessment (EEA): a modification of the Systematic Screening and Assessment (SSA) method, implemented by the Centers for Disease Control and Prevention, for identifying innovative programs for evaluation. The process aims to reduce the time typically needed for the SSA and the subsequent evaluation by having much of the process conducted by staff, using abbreviated approaches to conducting the evaluations, and selecting sites for evaluation that have existing data.

Epistemological assumptions: paradigmatic assumptions that deal with the nature of knowledge.

Equality: according to *Merriam-Webster*, the quality or state of being equal.

Equity: according to *Merriam-Webster*, justice according to natural law or right; specifically, freedom from bias or favoritism.

Ethical practices: standards of professional conduct that guide behavior in evaluation, ensuring actions are fair, transparent, and respectful and align evaluation ethical standards.

Ethics: dealing with what is good and bad and with moral duty and obligation.

Ethnographic methods: research methods that involve observing and interviewing people in their natural environments to understand their cultures and behaviors.

Evaluability assessment: a process to determine whether a program is ready for evaluation and if an evaluation will be useful and feasible.

Evaluands: the specific objects or entities, usually a program or system, being evaluated. In the context of program evaluation, evaluands can include interventions, policies, projects, or specific components of a program.

Evaluation capacity building (ECB): an intentional process to increase individual motivation, knowledge, and skills, and to enhance a group or organization's ability to conduct or use evaluation.

Evaluation dashboard: use of baselines, milestones, goals, and actual performance data to determine the degree of progress or program improvement.

Evaluation equity framework: a framework based on an equity perspective that is used to develop an evaluation.

Evaluation failure: when there are null effects of a program but a valid test of the program did not occur because the data collected and/or the data analysis are not well aligned with the targets for measurement suggested by the program theory.

Evaluation report: a document that reports the findings, conclusions, and recommendations of an evaluation.

Evaluation science: the systematic study of how well efforts to change the world work in practice.

Evaluation synthesis: drawing an overall judgment of performance based on criteria and evidence.

Evaluation theory: a kind of *theory* (*see* entry) that specifies why and how evaluation is to be done, and how the activities an evaluation engages in should lead to the intended goals of the evaluation. An evaluation theory may also specify how evaluation goals, activities, and process should vary across contexts.

Evaluation theory tree: a graphical representation of relationships among evaluation theories/theorists, with *three branches* (*see* entry) representing the predominant focus of a given theory; a creation of Alkin and Christie.

Evaluation use: helping people use evaluation to inform decision making, program planning and implementation, and strategic planning.

Evaluative judgment: a claim about the value of something based on evidence and values.

Evaluative reasoning: cognitive and social processes used to determine and justify claims about the value of something.

Evaluative thinking: a cognitive and relational process, motivated by an attitude of inquisitiveness and a belief in the value of evidence, that involves identifying assumptions, posing thoughtful questions, marshaling evidence to make judgments, pursuing deeper understanding, and making logically aligned, contextualized decisions in preparation for action.

The Evidence Act: The Foundations for Evidence-Based Policymaking Act of 2018, which requires federal agencies to develop evidence to support policymaking.

Evidence-based intervention: program, practice, process, policy, and guidelines that have proven efficacy or effectiveness in a population and setting.

Evidence-based strategies: the knowledge base of researchers and scholars (used in conjunction with community knowledge).

Exact matching: a model in which program participants are matched with comparison individuals who share the same characteristics but did not participate in the program.

Exhaustive: possible values of a variable comprise all possible values of that variable in the sample.

Explanatory sequential design: as a core mixed methods design, this design has an overarching aim of explaining the quantitative findings through subsequentially collected qualitative data (see Chapter 18, Figure 18.2).

Exploratory analysis: an approach to analyzing data sets to find patterns or relationships without having a specific hypothesis in mind.

Exploratory sequential design: a mixed-methods design that helps the evaluator "explore" relevant program processes or outcomes through the use of qualitative methods. Quantitative methods (e.g., surveys) are then used to determine whether the qualitative findings are more broadly present in a larger sample/population.

External validity or generalizability: the extent to which an evaluation's findings (based on a subset of study participants) can be applied to other persons, settings, or times.

Fidelity: the degree to which an intervention was implemented as it was prescribed in the original protocol or as it was intended by the program developers.

Fishing: looking for patterns in measures without guidance from a theory, a logic model, or a hypothesis.

508 compliance: with reference to Section 508 of the Rehabilitation Act (29 U.S.C. §798, Electronic and Information Technology), it focuses on federal agencies in the developing, procuring, maintaining, or using electronic and information technology. Agencies are required to give access to employees and members of the public with disabilities similar to that provided to individuals without disabilities.

Five components of evaluation theory: social programming, knowledge construction, valuing, use, and practice, according to Shadish, Cook, and Leviton.

Fixed cost: a cost that is the same regardless of the number of participants in an intervention.

Fixed-effect model: a model that allows evaluators to compare observations within a unit (e.g., school, state, year) only with each other and controls for any observed or unobserved characteristics that affect all observations within the same unit.

Flexibility: the ability to pivot or shift gears concerning an evaluation approach or specific applications based on resources, needs, and skills of participants.

Focus on action planning: identifying points of action to improve program implementation.

Foreshadowing: a narrative device that hints at what is to come as the story unfolds. As an evaluator, you lay the groundwork in the design and throughout in your thick descriptions.

Formative evaluation: a term introduced by Edward Suchman to refer to an evaluation of a program during its developmental or formative phases. These phases usually include establishing the need for the program, initial design and operational plan of the program, pilot testing and monitoring program implementation, and assessing the immediate and shorter-term results of the program.

Frequency distribution: the range and frequency of values that a variable takes.

Fundamental problem of causal inference: individuals cannot be observed as having participated in a program (or receiving a treatment) and also having not participated in the program at the same time.

Gantt charts: a horizontal bar chart that shows a project's planned schedule and its tasks or events over time. Named after the developer Henry Gantt, it is a graphical representation of activity against time that helps project professionals monitor progress.

Generalizability: extent to which a finding from a sample holds is true for the population of interest.

Gestalt principles: a set of principles to explain our understanding of the world through our perceptions of phenomena as parts of a larger whole.

Getting-to-outcomes: a 10-step approach to empowerment evaluation (complements the three-step approach).

Government Performance and Results Act: the Government Performance and Results Act of 1993, which requires U.S. federal agencies to engage in performance management activities such as setting goals, measuring results, and reporting progress.

Health equity: the state in which everyone has a fair and just opportunity to attain their highest level of health.

High-risk evaluations: evaluations that focus on highly sensitive topics or circumstances, such as issues of finance, malfeasance, continued relevance or mandate, and the effectiveness and/or cost–benefit of a program. It is important that high-risk evaluations be objective, both in fact and in perception, and conducted with the highest ethical standards and technical expertise. External evaluators usually conduct high-risk evaluations to avoid any question of bias.

History: a threat to internal validity; historical events, trends, or forces that influence outcomes of interest.

Hybrid effectiveness–implementation designs: research designs that combine elements of both effectiveness and implementation studies in order to shorten the length of time between studies that establish that a program works in real-world settings and studies that focus on establishing effective strategies for implementing, sustaining, and scaling those interventions.

Ignorability assumption: the assumption that missingness in data can be treated as random.

Impact: the change in an outcome that is attributable to the program.

Impact evaluation: an assessment of the changes that can be attributed to a particular intervention, such as a project, program, or policy.

Implementation cost: the additional costs associated with implementing a program, including costs associated with the particular program, the implementation strategy used, and the location of service delivery.

Implementation failure: when there are null effects of a program but a valid test of the program did not occur because the program was not implemented as intended.

Implementation outcomes: the effects of deliberate and purposive actions to implement new treatments, practices, and services, which serve as indicators of implementation success, indicators of implementation processes, and key intermediate outcomes in relation to service system or clinical outcomes in treatment effectiveness or quality of care.

Implementation strategies: the methods or techniques used to improve adoption, implementation, sustainment, and scale-up of programs.

Improvement: better program performance; build on successes and reevaluate areas meriting attention.

Inception report: a report required by many evaluation contracts after the initial phase of the evaluation to present the methodology and to identify any factors that may limit the consultant's ability to fully comply with the terms of reference.

Inclusion: involvement and participation from diverse members of the community; contributions come from all levels and walks of life.

Independent consultant: an external expert hired to provide objective evaluation services.

Independent evaluation: an evaluation in which the evaluator has no role in developing or operating the program being evaluated.

Infographics: a visual representation of information or data.

Informal discussion: a conversation to share and exchange information with no formal agenda.

Informational function of internal evaluation: the information that internal evaluation provides as a result of its evaluations. It includes data gathering, analysis, synthesis, reporting and communicating findings, and knowledge management and mobilization.

Ingredients method: a method for estimating the costs of an intervention by documenting the actual ingredients or resources used to achieve a particular effect, regardless of who pays for or provides each resource.

Inputs: resources brought to a program, typically funding sources or the experiences and knowledge of the individuals and institutions involved.

Institutional review board (IRB): a committee that reviews the methods proposed for research to ensure that they are ethical.

Instrumental use: using evaluation findings to inform decision making, improve program effectiveness, or guide policy changes. It emphasizes practical application rather than just producing reports.

Instrumentation bias: a threat to internal validity caused by systematic errors in measurement tools; the influence of changing measures or data collection procedures on outcomes.

Integrated data platforms: software programs bringing together many different sources of information from administrative records, secondary data, phone records, and audio and visual data into a common format so that new and existing data sources can be compared in ways that were previously not possible. Many applications use artificial intelligence to identify new patterns and associations in the data.

Integration: the mixing of qualitative and quantitative data strands. This can take place during multiple stages of the study (e.g., the design, collection, analysis, and/or interpretation of findings).

Intended use by intended users: a phrase that captures the goal of Michael Patton's utilization-focused evaluation. That approach is open to most any evaluation theory or method, as long as its application in the particular situation is ethical, consistent with professional standards, and leads to intended use by users.

Interactive data displays: a visual representation of data that allows users to actively manipulate and explore the information through interactive elements such as filtering, zooming, or selecting specific data points.

Interactive website: a website that allows users to interact and select content in different ways.

Interest holder: a person with an interest or a stake in the program, process, or product being evaluated. The primary interest holder is typically the person or group that commissioned the evaluation.

Interest holder approaches to evaluation: methods that involve interest holders in the evaluation process to ensure their perspectives and needs are considered.

Interest holder involvement/engagement: an evaluation team's inclusion of interest holders, particularly those with lived experiences of the conditions being served by the program being evaluated or of the program itself.

Internal audit: serves the function of reducing risk and improving the efficiency of an organization by providing assurances about the effectiveness of risk management, internal fiscal controls, reliability of reporting, and governance processes. Internal auditors are employees of the organization that they are auditing.

Internal evaluation: an evaluation conducted by individuals within the organization running the program.

Internal evaluation function: the generic term to describe the internal evaluation capability of an organization, irrespective of the model being used. In other words, a small organization with a few part-time evaluators and a large internal evaluation unit in a government agency are both examples of organizations that have internal evaluation functions, albeit different types.

Internal validity: according to the American Psychological Association, "the degree to which a study or experiment is free from flaws in its internal structure and its results can therefore be taken to represent the true nature of the phenomenon."

Internet of things (IOT): a network of devices that can connect and exchange data with one another and the cloud. IOT devices can include mechanical and digital machines, consumer objects, and smart home devices.

Interrupted time-series (ITS) design: a quasi-experimental design in which a potential outcome is measured repeatedly over time, with observations both before and after the introduction of a treatment (such as a new program). Analyses can assess whether and how much the outcome variable changed after introduction of the treatment.

Involvement: participation in the process; level of involvement varies among everyone who collaborates in an effort.

Joint display: a figure or table in which the researcher arrays both qualitative and quantitative data so that the two sources of data can be directly compared.

Knowledge products (evaluation): outputs (meta-studies, synthesis reviews, meta-analyses, and think pieces) that are designed to share knowledge and encourage learning.

Latent class analysis: a data-driven, algorithmic approach to identifying groups that are defined by categorical data and not otherwise readily identifiable.

Learning: determining what is working about a program and what is not to determine what actions are needed to improve program outcomes.

Lesson learned: An experience distilled from a project that should be actively taken into account in future projects.

Level 1 questionnaire: a questionnaire that asks for participants' immediate reactions to the event. Donald Kirkpatrick's four-level model offers a sequential framework to evaluate training. The model can be applied to evaluate various aspects of programs.

Limited datasets: a type of protected health information that does not contain direct identifiers about individuals. There are very specific federal rules of what can be included in this dataset.

Lived expertise: the knowledge and insights gained from personal experience, often used in participatory and empowerment evaluations.

Logic models: visual representations that show the relationships between a program's resources, activities, outputs, and outcomes.

Logic of evaluation: determining value-based criteria and standards, generating evidence, and reporting or synthesizing evaluative judgments; also called *valuing logic*.

Longitudinal data: data collected from the same subjects repeatedly over a period of time.

Machine learning: a type of artificial intelligence that allows computers to learn from data and improve their performance over time.

Marginal cost: the cost of one additional participant in an intervention.

Market price: a valuation of an input/resource/ingredient or an outcome determined by the equilibrium set by a market comprising many buyers and sellers.

Matching: the set of matching models allows the evaluator to select comparison individuals who share similar (or exactly the same) characteristics as individuals who participate in the program.

Matrix sampling: a sampling technique where a large set of questions or test items is divided into smaller subsets, and different subsets are administered to different groups of participants, allowing for comprehensive data collection while minimizing the testing burden on individuals by not requiring them to answer all questions.

Maturation: a threat to internal validity (see entry) whereby one's conclusions about the effect of a program on an outcome may be inaccurate because of naturally occurring changes among program participants, such as improvements that may occur as the participants age.

Mean reversion: the tendency for individuals who experience a period of abnormally high or low values of the outcome to revert back nearer to their long-term average in the following time periods.

Measure: a value representing a program outcome, implementation, or other characteristic of participants.

Measure, interval: a continuous measure in which the distance between two equally spaced values has the same meaning regardless of where those values are located on the variable scale. There is not necessarily a meaningful zero value for the measure.

Measure, nominal: a measure representing a particular characteristic with no numeric meaning or meaningful order.

Measure, ordinal: a measure that contains categories that can be assigned a rank order. The distance between two equally spaced values does not need to have the same meaning across the range of possible values. For example, the distance between strongly agree and agree on a 4-point Likert scale does not necessarily reflect the same difference in agreement as the difference between agree and disagree.

Measure, outcome: measure that the program is intended to influence.

Measure, process or implementation: measure that describes program implementation, such as the extent to which a program was implemented as intended, dosage, or program quality.

Measure, ratio: a continuous measure in which the distance between two equally spaced values has the same meaning regardless of where those values are located on the variable scale. There must be a meaningful zero value for the measure.

Mediational analyses: analyses, often multivariate statistical in nature, that assess whether a variable is serving as a *mediator* (*see* entry) in the relationship between program and outcome.

Mediators: in a program evaluation context, short- or intermediate-term outcomes that change because of the program and that in turn bring about change in longer-term outcomes.

Member checking: a process for checking on the trustworthiness of qualitative data. It involves asking interviewees to review and approve the transcript of the interview and, in some cases, the analysis of the set of interviews.

Message: key information to be communicated.

Messaging strategy: the selection and prioritization of key information to be communicated.

Meta-evaluation: the evaluation of an evaluation (or set of evaluations). The evaluation theorist *Michael Scriven* (*see* entry) is among the advocates of meta-evaluation, in his case as one factor to counter potential bias that can affect an evaluation.

Meta-model: a kind of theory of evaluation theories, such as Shadish, Cook, and Leviton's *five-components of evaluation theory* (see entry) model and Alkin and Christie's *evaluation theory tree* (see entry).

Milestones: important points or events in the project, such as the final report. Milestones typically require no time, even though time is spent preparing for them.

Missing at random (MAR): data that are missing in a pattern that can be explained by observed values of other variables, but conditional on observed variables, cannot depend on unobserved variables.

Missing completely at random (MCAR): data that are missing in a pattern that is completely independent of other variables. Patterns of missingness cannot be explained by either observed or unobserved variables.

Missing not at random (MNAR): data that are missing in a pattern that is not measured by the researcher. In other words, the reason for the data missing is directly related to the unobserved data.

Missing observations: observations that are expected to be in a dataset but are not included. In the case of missing observations, the entire row is missing. This is distinct from missing values where the row is included but the value of a particular variable or variables is blank.

Missing values: cells that are empty for a given observation in a dataset—that is, values of a variable that are unknown.

Mission: the group's consensus concerning their mission, purpose, or values.

Mixed methods research: research in which the investigator collects and analyzes data, integrates the findings, and draws inferences using both qualitative and quantitative approaches or methods in a single study or a program of inquiry.

Model for collaborative evaluations (MCE): a comprehensive framework for guiding collaborative evaluations in a precise, realistic, and useful manner; the model has a systematic structure and revolves around a set of six interactive components specific to conducting collaborative evaluations, providing a basis for decision making.

Moderators: in the context of program evaluation, elements that change the relationship between the program and an outcome (e.g., age would be a moderator if a program is helpful for younger participants but not for older participants).

Modification: changes to the content or method of a program that are not specified in the protocol.

Monte Carlo analysis: a simulation method used to predict variability in possible outcomes taking into account random variation in aspects of the model—in this case, a cost–benefit estimate.

Moral courage: the willingness to take action for principled reasons despite the risk of adverse consequences.

Multidimensional matching: a comparison group matching strategy that involves matching on multiple characteristics; an example is *coarsened exact matching* (see entry).

Multimedia report: a presentation that integrates different formats, such as video, images, and graphics.

Multiphase/complex design: a type of mixed methods design that can combine multiple core designs to create a more complex or multifaceted design. Examples of a complex design include multilevel, fully integrated, and experimental designs.

Multivariate regression: a set of statistical techniques that allow researchers to control for observable characteristics that are likely to bias estimated program effects.

Mutually exclusive: possible values of a measure do not overlap.

Natural language model: a statistical model that analyzes human language patterns to predict the likelihood of a sequence of words in a sentence. Language models are a core component of natural language processing (NLP), which is a branch of artificial intelligence (AI) that gives machines the ability to understand human language.

Natural language processing: a field of artificial intelligence that focuses on the interaction between computers and human language.

Needs assessment: an exploratory analysis that assesses the nature, magnitude, and distribution of a social problem to determine whether an intervention is needed as well as what type of intervention may best fit the actual problem. The needs assessment systemically studies and assesses the discrepancy between current conditions and desired conditions, keeping in mind that desired conditions need to be carefully discussed and understood by all relevant interest holders.

Negotiation and balance of power: negotiating the balance of power among team members and the evaluator to determine each step of the evaluation process.

Nested design: a type of experimental design that considers two or more factors, with one factor found within another. In a nested design, each level of the nested factor occurs only within one level of the other factor, and not across all levels.

Noncompliance: occurs when individuals are assigned to the treatment condition (or comparison condition) but then are not placed into their assigned condition.

Nondata ink: ink in a graphic that contains redundant information or does not contain data or information.

Nondisclosure agreement (NDA): a legal contract between parties that restricts the sharing of confidential information. They are commonly used to protect sensitive data during evaluations or collaborations.

Nonprobability sampling: the process of selecting a sample from a population in which each member of that population does not have a known, nonzero chance of being selected for the sample. Participants are not sampled at random and the resulting sample is not representative of the target population.

Nonresponse bias: This concept refers to a situation in which the nonrespondents differ from those who respond or that the nonrespondents would respond in a different way from those who do respond.

Nonspecialist evaluators: may include senior managers, team leaders, and professionals from other fields who are systematically educated to acquire evaluative thinking and evaluation skills, and then to apply evaluation to enhance their own work. Nonspecialists initiate and support internal evaluation and its use, while retaining their principal roles and continuing their respective professional work.

Null hypothesis: the hypothesis that there is no statistical difference between two groups on a given outcome measure. In the case of program evaluation with an outcomes analysis, a null hypothesis is likely to be that there is no difference between the treatment and comparison groups on the outcome the intervention is intended to influence.

Observation: a row in a dataset representing a unit of observation (e.g., an individual program participant or even an individual program participant at a given time period). In a quantitative dataset, observations are represented as rows.

One-group pretest–posttest design: a reflexive evaluation design where one group's pre- and postprogram outcomes are compared to estimate impacts.

Ontological assumptions: paradigmatic assumptions that deal with the nature of reality.

Open-ended questions: questions without predetermined answers; they allow participants to choose their own words in their responses in the form of sentences or short paragraphs.

Opportunity cost: the economic value of a resource based on what is given up by using the resource for a particular purpose, or the value of its next best alternative use.

Organizational interventions: interventions that affect individuals, groups, or the entire organization by promoting positive outcomes and preventing or reducing problems. Organizational interventions typically affect more than one level at once (e.g., individuals, teams, departments) and affect the way work is designed, structured, and managed. Feedback from internal evaluation is an integral part of the design and implementation of organizational interventions. Paradoxically, the fact that an organization has an internal evaluation function and uses evaluation feedback on itself is an organizational intervention.

Organizational learning: using data to inform decision making, and implement program practices; using information/data to help organizations learn from their experience (building on successes, learning from mistakes, and making midcourse corrections).

Organizational setting: the factors within an organization that could influence its results, including structure, hierarchy, culture, policies, and practices.

Outcome: the set of social conditions that a program is expected to change.

Outcome evaluation: an evaluation that focuses on assessing the results or outcomes of a program. It examines whether the intended outcomes were achieved and often involves measuring changes in specific indicators.

Outcome measure: a quantitative measure of a social condition that the program is expected to change. A program may have multiple relevant outcome measures. These measures are used in outcome evaluations.

Outcome monitoring: periodic measurement and reporting of indicators of the status of the outcomes for program participants that the program is accountable for improving.

Out-of-range values: values of a variable that are either impossible or highly unlikely.

Output: the direct product of a program.

Overlap: in matching models, refers to whether program participants and individuals in the comparison group overlap in their estimated probability of participating in the program.

Parallel trends: a validity check that shows that average outcomes for the treatment and comparison groups mirror each other in periods prior to program exposure.

Parsimony: in measurement, having the best possible measure that requires the least amount of measuring.

Participant focus and ownership: honor the perspectives, voices, and knowledge of those most impacted, including program participants or recipients, who are often voiceless in the evaluation process; facilitate ownership among key interest holders.

Participatory evaluation: an approach that involves interest holders in the evaluation process, from design to data collection and analysis.

Participatory evaluators: evaluators and program staff members who *jointly share* control of the evaluation.

Patterns: sets of characteristics, traits, or activities that are arranged or organized according to some rule that identifies them as related. Patterns are observed: as you see them in the data, you interpret and begin to construct themes.

Peer review: a method to help ensure the trustworthiness of the analysis of qualitative data. It involves a reanalysis of the data by a colleague or peer and then an identification and potential resolution of discrepancies.

Penetration: the integration of a practice within a service setting and its subsystems.

Perfect collinearity: a condition in which the value of one variable can be explained with 100% certainty using another variable or combination of other variables in a regression model.

Performance measurement: the process of collecting, analyzing, and reporting data on the performance of a program or organization.

Performance measurement systems: measurement systems that track aspects of a program over time. These usually include program activities, program products ("outputs"), and outcomes (as far down the chain of outcomes as is possible). In *Joseph Wholey's* (*see* entry) evaluation theory, performance measurement systems are designed to enable program managers to manage better, presumably leading to better programs and outcomes over time.

Performance monitoring: the process of collecting, tracking, and analyzing data—compared to indicators—to evaluate a program, system, or process over time.

Persons with lived experiences: persons who have experienced the phenomenon in question; they have either faced the challenges in question in real life beyond educational awareness or they have behaved in a similar manner to participants.

Perspective taking: for a qualitative evaluator, recognizing the point of view you hold and that you can look beyond to perceive or understand the alternative viewpoints others in your study may hold.

PERT chart: a PERT chart, which stands for Program Evaluation and Review Technique chart, is a visual project management tool that maps out a project's tasks and dependencies, allowing users to estimate the overall project timeline by identifying critical paths and visualizing how different tasks relate to each other.

Pipeline design: when a project is implemented in phases (e.g., the installation of a water and sanitation system in an impoverished area with 100,000 inhabitants, which may be implemented over several years), it may be possible to use individuals, families, or communities where the system will be installed in Year 2 as the comparison group for families that receive the services in Phase 1. This will work well only if subjects in Phase 2 have similar characteristics as those in Phase 1, and if it is not possible for Phase 2 families to access benefits during the implementation of Phase 1.

Planning for the future: generating goals, strategies, and credible evidence to determine whether the strategies are being implemented and whether they are effective; goals are directly related to the activities selected in the taking stock step.

Plausibility: the logical or reasonable connection between an intervention and its expected outcomes. It assesses whether the proposed cause-and-effect relationship makes sense.

Podcast: an episodic series of spoken word digital audio files that a user can download to a personal device for easy listening.

Policy-analytic contingency theories of evaluation: advocate for the thoughtful consideration of the decision and action space that is likely to exist after the evaluation, and for selecting evaluation methods most likely to provide useful information for that context.

Policy environment: the interests, priorities, groups, organizations, and existing policies external to the organization that can influence a project, program, strategy, or evaluation.

Postpositivist: a worldview associated with quantitative approaches. The stance that researchers have the ability to be objective and that the truth underlying experiences can be measured with a certain degree of accuracy, since there is a single and shared reality.

Posttest-only comparison group design: a comparison group evaluation design whose postprogram mean outcome is compared to the treatment group's postprogram mean outcome.

Potential outcomes framework for causal inference: an effect expressed as the difference between the potential outcome that would appear with exposure to the program and the potential outcome that would appear without exposure to the program.

Power analysis: a statistical method to calculate necessary sample size for an evaluation using significance criterion, estimated effect size, and desired power level. Alternatively, a method to calculate the minimum detectable effect size using sample size, significance criterion, and desired power level.

PRA: originally referring to *participatory rural appraisal*, now used as a generic term referring to wide range of participatory research techniques used in urban as well as rural areas. All approaches are based on empowering the community to conduct its own analysis of its needs, rather than having an outside expert conduct the needs assessment. There are a wide range of methods, all of which work through community groups that use techniques such as social maps, timelines, causal analysis, and power analysis. A number of techniques can be used to help reconstruct baseline data but most are qualitative and cannot be used to provide precise numerical estimates of, for example, changes in income or access to services.

Practical empowerment evaluation: evaluation designed to enhance program performance and productivity; controlled by program staff, participants, and community members; focus is on practical problem solving, as well as programmatic improvements and outcomes (similar to *formative evaluation*; *see* entry).

Practical participatory evaluation: focused on use, not empowerment, and specifically on producing evaluation findings that can be used for immediate program improvement; rooted in organization learning theory and designed to support program or organizational decision making and problem solving.

Practical wisdom: doing the right thing, at the right time, for the right reason; or doing the right thing in the special circumstances of performing the job.

Pragmatic: a worldview associated with mixed methods approaches. This stance has an orientation toward problem solving, with an emphasis on identifying practical solutions and methods that can provide the best answer to a research or evaluation question.

Pragmatic measures: measures that possess desirable properties that makes them more likely to be widely used, such as usefulness (e.g., informs clinical or organizational decision making), compatibility (e.g., fits organizational activities), acceptability (e.g., low cost), and ease of use (e.g., uses accessible language, brief).

Praxeological assumptions: paradigmatic assumptions that deal with the nature of human action.

Presentation: a speech or talk to present a topic to a group of people.

Press release: a document of newsworthy content intended for the media for the purpose of providing information, an official statement, or an announcement.

Pretest–posttest comparison group design: a comparison group evaluation design that uses a pretest and posttest comparison group difference to estimate a counterfactual.

Primary data: firsthand information or data collected by researchers for a specific purpose; also known as *raw data* or *firsthand information*.

Priority: level of importance placed on each data source or type of data.

Probability sampling: the process of selecting a sample from a population in which each member of that population does not have a known, nonzero chance of being selected for the sample. The resulting sample is intended to be representative of the target population.

Probity: honesty, wholeness, integrity, and grounded in strong moral principles.

Process evaluation: examination of what a program is, the activities undertaken, who receives services or other benefits, the consistency with which the program is implemented in terms of its design and across sites, and other such aspects of the nature and operation.

Process use: assumes the more that people are engaged in conducting their own evaluations, the more likely they are to believe in them because the evaluation findings are theirs; makes them more likely to make decisions and take actions based on their evaluation data; represents much of the rationale or logic underlying empowerment evaluation in practice; it cultivates ownership by placing the approach in community and staff members' hands.

Program Assessment Rating Tool: the Program Assessment Rating Tool, used by the U.S. Office of Management and Budget to assess the performance of federal programs.

Program effect/program impact: the portion of the change in outcomes among program participants that can be uniquely attributed to the program.

Program equity framework: this framework is based on an equity perspective during program development and implementation.

Program evaluability: assesses whether a program is ready for evaluation. It considers factors such as program clarity, available data, and interest holder support.

Program evaluation review technique (PERT) chart: a flowchart or network diagram used by project managers to create schedules. Developed by the Navy in 1958, it is a visual representation of a project's timeline that helps break down tasks, estimate duration, and identify dependencies. It is a more modern version of the Gantt chart.

Program Evaluation Standards: guidelines developed by the American Evaluation Association that ensure evaluations are useful, feasible, ethical, and accurate.

Program failure: when the underlying program theory is wrong and the evaluation correctly shows that the program did not have the intended effect.

Program feasibility: the extent to which a program can be successfully used or carried out within a particular setting or population.

Program implementation: the process of putting a planned program into action.

Program logic model: a visual representation of how a program is expected to work. It outlines inputs, activities, outputs, outcomes, and impacts in a logical sequence.

Program stage: view of a program as passing through various stages of maturity, metaphorically, akin to *in utero*, baby, toddler, adolescent, and adult. An evaluation theory that attends to program stage offers different evaluation goals and methods as a function of program stage.

Program theory: some form of model, often presented as a diagram, that describes the anticipated or actual operations of a program, typically including at least the component or key activities of a program, the program's desired long-term outcomes, and steps in between.

Propensity score: An individual's propensity score is the estimated probability that the individual participates in the program given their observable characteristics.

Propensity score matching: a comparison group matching strategy that uses multidimensional matching to a greater extent and uses regression analysis where many characteristics are used to predict treatment group membership.

Psychological contract: an unwritten agreement concerning the nature of the relationship between two parties and the steps that will be taken to ensure that mutual expectations are met.

Purposive sampling: a qualitative research technique that involves selecting a specific group of people or units for analysis. Also known as judgmental sampling, selective sampling, or subjective sampling.

Qualification: background qualifications; level of knowledge and skills needed to achieve a task, project, and/or initiative.

Qualitative comparative analysis: the unit of analysis is the case, rather than an individual subject. Cases may be individuals, households, organizations, or even countries.

Qualitative data: descriptive information that captures qualities or characteristics that cannot be measured numerically.

Qualitize: the process of transforming qualitative data into quantitative data. One example of this is factor analysis.

Quantitative data: information that can be expressed numerically, meaning it can be counted, measured, and given a numerical value.

Quantitize: the process of transforming quantitative (nominal or ordinal) data into qualitative data. This is often done to represent the frequency of themes or ideas that emerge from qualitative data.

Quasi-experimental design: an analytical method that forms treatment and control groups through a process other than random assignment. The design approximates a counterfactual; types include reflexive and comparison group designs.

Random assignment/randomization: refers to the process of placing individuals into either intervention or comparison conditions based on a random chance process, such as a coin flip.

Randomized controlled trials (RCTs): the assignment of participants (or aggregate units, such as schools) to conditions at random. The groups are compared on outcome measures to estimate the effect of the experimental contrast, which might involve a treatment versus a control group, or Treatment A versus Treatment B, or many other variations.

Randomized design: a design in which participants are randomly assigned to certain conditions (e.g., treated and non-treated conditions).

Ranking variable: (*see* **Running variable**)

Rapid cycle evaluation: a method that involves quick, iterative assessments to test and refine program components.

Reactivity: (*see* **Testing bias**)

Real time evaluation: an approach that provides immediate feedback during program implementation to allow for timely adjustments.

Real world evaluation: an approach, as developed by Michael Bamberger and Linda Mabry, that adapts evaluation methods to the budget, time, data, and political constraints and complexities of real-world settings.

Realist evaluator: as commonly used, someone following the evaluation approach developed by Pawson and Tilley, which attempts to identify the mechanisms triggered by a program and the contexts in which the mechanism(s) lead(s) to particular outcomes.

Reflective practice: deliberate thinking about action with a view to its improvement. It involves reflection in action and on action in order to understand the situation, engage relationally with others, pivot when necessary, and take intentional action through praxis.

Reflexive design: a quasi-experimental evaluation design that involves using the same group for treated and counterfactual outcomes; types include a one-group pretest–posttest and interrupted time-series design.

Regression: a statistical measure of the relationship between two or more variables.

Regression artifact: also known as *regression to the mean*; a threat to internal validity; program targets are chosen for being exceptional in some way, either at the top or the bottom of a distribution, and are therefore likely to "regress" to the mean.

Regression discontinuity (RD): an evaluation design that places individuals into either the participant or nonparticipant group based on whether the individual's value of a quantitative assignment variable is above or below a specific cut point.

Regression to the mean: (*see* **Regression artifact**)

Reliability: the extent to which a measure produces the same result for the same construct regardless of who is administering the measure and on whom or what it is being administered.

Reporting guidelines: guidelines that describe important elements of an evaluation or study that should be reported to improve transparency and promote others' ability to replicate or improve upon studies, programs, or implementation strategies.

Representative sampling: A representative sample is a subset of a larger group that accurately reflects the characteristics of the larger group. It is a type of statistical sampling that allows researchers to use data from a sample to make conclusions about the population from which the sample is taken.

Request for proposal (RFP): a formal request for evaluators to prepare a response to a planned evaluation and can be combined with elements of *terms of reference* (*see* entry).

Reshape: reorganize data from wide to long or from long to wide while maintaining unique identifiers from the original format.

Rigor: when the evaluator strictly follows closely established standards for the evaluation research in which they are engaged.

Rubric: a tool or set of guidelines used to promote the consistent measure of the attainment of expectations against a consistent set of criteria.

Running variable: the variable used in a regression discontinuity design where a cutoff point determines assignment into a treatment or comparison group; also referred to as ranking variable.

Sample: a subset of a target population selected to be part of an evaluation.

Sample, nonprobability: a sample from a population in which each member of that population does not have a known, nonzero chance of being selected for the sample. Participants are not sampled at random and the resulting sample is not representative of the target population.

Sample, probability: a sample from a population in which each member of that population has a known, nonzero chance of being selected for the sample. Participants are sampled at random and the resulting sample is representative of the target population. With appropriate research design, estimates from a probability sample can be generalized to the target population.

Scriven, Michael: an influential evaluation theorist known for explicating the underlying steps in making an evaluative conclusion and for his advocacy of goal-free evaluation, attention to the real needs of intended beneficiaries (through a form of *needs assessment*; *see* entry), and *meta-evaluation* (*see* entry).

Secondary data: data that have already been collected and made available for researchers to use in their own research; they have been collected by someone other than the primary user.

Selection bias: a threat to internal validity; people who choose to participate in a program differ from those who do not in ways that influence their outcomes.

Sensitivity analysis: an analysis of the robustness of results to changes in assumptions.

Shadow pricing: a series of methods for estimating social value of resources or outcomes not traded on a market based on revealed or stated preferences.

Simple interrupted time-series design: a reflexive evaluation design where one group's preprogram outcome trend is projected and compared to postprogram outcomes to estimate impacts.

Single-dimensional matching: a comparison group matching strategy that involves using a single trait on which to match treatment and comparison groups.

Situation analysis: analysis of internal and external factors that could impact on the communications and the evaluation. (*see* **Communications plan of action**)

Social justice: addressing social inequities in society; aimed at making a fair and just society.

Social media: websites, platforms, and applications that enable users to create and share content or to participate in social networking.

Social support: developing productive networks in order to find solutions in a collaborative manner; management of relationships with others in order to establish a safety net; sense of belonging and a holistic view of social-related issues.

Stakes: role-specific concerns and interests.

Standards: levels of value or performance.

Statistical power: the likelihood that a study will detect an effect when there is one; also known as sensitivity. A power analysis can be used to estimate the minimum sample size required for an experiment.

Statistical precision: how close repeated measures of an estimator are to each other. It also refers to the accuracy with which an estimator estimates the true value of what is being estimated.

Storytelling in evaluation: using qualitative methods in evaluation to tell the story from various angles: developmentally, formatively, or summative.

Stratification: in propensity score matching models, the process that separates individuals into groups based on their propensity scores (e.g., deciles) and comparing differences between individuals within each group.

Summaries/snapshots: a summary of evaluation findings, conclusions, and recommendations in several pages, often using images and graphics.

Summative evaluation: an evaluation conducted after a program has been implemented to assess its overall effectiveness.

Survey fatigue: a phenomenon that results in (1) item nonresponse when a survey is too long and those taking it do not complete it, or (2) unit nonresponse when respondents are overwhelmed more broadly by requests to take surveys and do not respond at all.

Sustainability: the extent to which a program is maintained or institutionalized within a setting.

SWOTS: strengths, weaknesses, opportunities, and threats.

Systematic screening and assessment method (SSA): a strategy for identifying innovations or interventions that warrant further evaluation. It involves systematically screening potential intervention candidates and assessing their promise for effectiveness before conducting full evaluations.

Taking stock: group prioritizes activities and rates how well they are doing; group engages in a dialogue about their self-assessment, which informs the next step in the process, planning for the future.

Target population: the population to which evaluation findings are intended to generalize.

Technical rationality: a positivist epistemology of professional knowledge and practice; the dominant epistemology of practice, in which professional activity consists of instrumental problem solving made rigorous by the application of scientific theory and technique.

Terms of reference (evaluation): a document that defines the purpose, objectives, and the scope of the evaluation and outlines the responsibilities of those involved.

Testing bias: a threat to internal validity; the influence of being tested on outcomes; also referred to as *reactivity*.

Theme: conveys what an evaluator has learned from their analyses. The word or statement organizes the categories and conveys the messages observed across categories. A declarative statement that captures an aspect of the story the data are telling.

Theory: according to Shadish, Cook, and Leviton, a body of knowledge that organizes, categorizes, describes, predicts, explains, and otherwise aids in understanding and controlling a topic.

Theory of action: the espoused operating theory about how a program or organization works.

Theory of change: a guiding description or illustration of how and why a particular change is desired and includes a clear description of the mechanism through which the change is expected to occur within a specific context.

Theory of use: the actual program reality; the observable behavior of interest holders.

Thick description: a foundational concept originally coined by Clifford Geertz, meaning that the evaluator has provided sufficient details of the setting (physical surroundings, nature of actions or events taking place, time, effects of actions, people present and involved, words spoken, and interactions) so that the reader can see what the evaluator sees and understand how the evaluation reached their interpretation (the reader may not agree with the evaluator's interpretation, but they can see where it came from!).

Threats to internal validity: factors that can lead to incorrect conclusions about the causal relationship between an intervention and its outcomes.

Three branches: use, methods, and valuing, from Alkin and Christie's *evaluation theory tree* (*see* entry).

Time trends: a form of bias that occurs when natural changes over time occur in ways that could potentially be misattributed to participation in the program of interest.

Timing: when the qualitative and quantitative data are collected in a mixed-methods evaluation; this may occur concurrently or sequentially.

Total cost: the sum of the value of all resources used in an intervention (price multiplied by quantity), above and beyond business as usual and regardless of who pays for or provides those resources.

Transdiscipline: a discipline (like statistics or logic) that, according to Michael Scriven, has standalone status as a discipline *and* is also used as a methodological or analytical tool in several other disciplines.

Transformative empowerment evaluation: focus on liberation from predetermined conventional roles and organizational structures or "ways of doing things"; empowerment is a more explicit and apparent goal; highlights the psychological, social, and political power of liberation; people learn how to take greater control of their own lives and the resources around them.

Transformative participatory evaluation: draws on principles of emancipation and social justice.

Transformative worldview: an approach to mixed methods that explicitly acknowledges a cultural or social position that aims to identify power dynamics that privilege or oppress different groups and work toward social justice through collaborative and participatory practices.

Transparency: the full and open documentation and display of all decisions and actions taken during a study so that others can see and understand what the evaluator did to collect, analyze, interpret, and report their findings. Transparency begins with the design, which details what the evaluator is doing, why, and with whom. Put simply, being transparent means that you are not hiding your research design and processes.

Triangulation: using multiple data sources to verify or to determine the accuracy of some findings.

Trimming: part of the propensity matching process in which once propensity scores are predicted for all study participants, the evaluator would typically compare the distribution of propensity scores for both the program participant group and the comparison sample in order to remove individuals from either group with propensity scores that are either too high or too low to be matched to the other group.

Trust: confidence in or reliance on the sincerity, credibility, and reliability of people involved in the collaboration; a high level of trust is required for a successful collaboration; trust takes time to build and is easily eliminated.

Unit of analysis: the level at which an intervention is implemented.

Unit of observation: the level at which data are collected.

Univariate analysis: an umbrella term for a one-way analysis of a single variable.

Unobserved treatments: a form of bias referring to external forces that affect outcomes for program participants at the same time as, but independent from, the program.

Utilization-focused evaluation: an approach to evaluation that focuses on intended use by intended users from the beginning and throughout an evaluation, including follow-up to enhance use.

Validity: the extent to which a measure actually reflects or represents the underlying construct that it purports to measure.

Value neutrality: standpoint that an evaluator's social, moral, or political values should not influence the process or results of an evaluation.

Values: deeply held convictions about what matters to individuals and groups.

Valuing: process of reaching warranted claims about the value of something.

Variable: an attribute of an observation, such as a quantity or category. In a quantitative dataset, variables are represented as columns.

Variable cost: a cost that varies with the number of participants in an intervention.

Video testimonies: individuals or groups video recorded speaking on a particular theme or topic.

Virtual data collection: gathering data through online tools and platforms, rather than in-person methods.

Visualcy: a learned data visualization literacy, graphical literacy, or visualization readership skill concerned with the viewer's ability to interpret and make meaning from visual representations of data.

Voluntary Organizations for Professional Evaluation (VOPES): groups that promote the practice and use of evaluation to improve policies and programs.

Webinar: a seminar or presentation conducted over the internet.

Weighting: in propensity score matching models, the procedure where outcomes of comparison individuals with a higher probability of being a program participant are given more weight.

Wholey, Joseph: an evaluation theorist, perhaps best known for his advocacy of *performance measurement systems* (*see* entry) for results-oriented management and for his work on *evaluability assessment* (*see* entry).

Word clouds: a visual display of qualitative data in which keywords are displayed by size according to frequency, with more frequent words displayed larger than less frequent words.

Word trees: a visual display of qualitative data using a branching structure to show how key words are connected to other words.

Work breakdown structure: as defined by the Project Management Institute, a decomposition of the total scope of work to be carried out by the project team to accomplish the project objectives and create the required deliverables.

Workshop: a meeting at which a group of people engage in discussions and activities on a particular subject.

Worldview: what researchers or evaluators consider to be the sources of knowledge and the validity or truthfulness of that knowledge. Some worldviews are positivism, postpositivism, interpretivism, critical theory, and pragmatism.

Yield: the ratio of the average effectiveness per participant to the average cost per participant, or the effects per dollar.

Youth participatory action research (YPAR): research conducted to ensure that the ideas and perspectives of youth are included in the evaluation design discussions.

Author Index

Aarons, G. A., 236, 239, 240
Abadie, A., 338, 339
Abadie, R., 404
Abma, T. A., 296
Abouelmehdi, K., 316
Adams, J., 91
Agrawal, R., 502
Ahmed, S., 407
Akiba, C. F., 233
Albrecht, L., 245
Ali, A. S., 545
Alkin, M. C., 8, 57, 59, 60, 61, 62, 63, 69, 73, 74, 75, 76, 80, 94, 95, 134, 142, 143, 144, 145, 146, 148, 152, 153, 157, 164, 197, 303, 354, 437, 491, 492, 493, 494, 495, 496, 499, 500, 501, 502, 503, 506, 534, 543, 546, 547, 558, 563, 572
Allan, S., 90
Allen, J. D., 233, 234, 235
Allison, G. S., 276
Allport, G., 59
Altschuld, J. W., 22, 88, 538
American Association for the Advancement of Science, 170
American Evaluation Association, 18, 19, 24, 26, 27, 28, 29, 82, 95, 105, 116, 130, 131, 132, 133, 139, 149, 162, 370, 395, 426, 430, 447, 509, 510, 512, 534, 538
American Evaluation Association Evaluation Policy Task Force, 3–4, 268
American Heart Association, 461

Amo, C., 544, 547
Anderson, A. A., 385
Anderson, M. B., 46
Andrews, S., 48
Annie E. Casey Foundation, 102
Archibald, T., 7, 18, 36, 38, 40, 41, 42, 43, 50, 59, 142, 181, 198, 383, 536
Argyris, C., 168, 192, 198
Armstrong, K., 102
Arnold, M. E., 184
Arrowsmith, M. E., 243
Asch, S., 59
Athey, S., 340
Atkinson, D. D., 8, 13, 534, 535
Atukpawu-Tipton, G., 15
Austin, L., 506
Austin, P. C., 338
Ayoo, S., 20
Azzam, T., 10, 13, 88, 90, 96, 119, 127, 239, 309, 344, 368, 416, 472, 511

Babbie, E. R., 313, 319, 325
Báez, J. C., 366
Baizerman, M., 441
Baker, A., 37
Baker, D. J., 318, 319
Baldridge, E., 49
Ballard, A., 68
Bamberger, M., 11, 12, 268, 347, 365, 377, 379, 399, 405, 411, 421, 422, 466, 470, 471, 475, 477, 478, 483, 491, 494, 495, 500, 501, 505, 569

Bandura, A., 48
Barnett, M., 238
Barnett, W. S., 273
Baron, J., 40
Barretto-Cortez, E., 190
Barrington, G. V., 12, 420, 421, 445, 446, 447, 448, 449, 451, 452, 454, 455, 456, 457, 458, 459, 463, 544
Barroga, E., 120
Baskerville, N. B., 241
Batch, A., 530
Bauer, M. S., 244
Bauer, M. W., 370, 494
Baumann, A. A., 236
Baur, V. E., 296
Becker-Haimes, E. M., 235
Bédécarrats, F., 40
Beidas, R. S., 235, 239, 240, 244
Belfield, C. R., 274, 283, 284, 285
Bell, S. H., 263, 273, 400
Belli, R., 481
Bennett, G., 37
Berger, A. A., 492, 493
Bertanha, M., 337
Bertino, E., 316
Berwick, D. M., 243, 244
Bhaskar, R. A., 63
Bhattacharyya, O., 241, 242, 243
Bickman, L., 9, 11, 14, 15, 22, 40, 47, 59, 61, 67, 230, 231, 233, 234, 235, 293, 347, 365, 372, 377, 379, 383, 384, 395, 400, 406, 408, 411, 466, 537, 538
Biesta, G., 41

Author Index

Bingham, R. D., 263
Black, P., 368
Bledsoe, K. L., 184, 547
Block, P., 136
Bloom, H. S., 273, 341
Boardman, A. E., 272, 282
Boateng, D., 401
Bogin, V., 405
Boisvert, Y., 20
Bond, C., 414
Bond, G. R., 235
Börner, K., 512, 514, 523
Boruch, R., 40, 142
Borys, S., 544
Boss, R. W., 136
Bosserman, C., 182
Bourdeau, B., 89
Bourgois, P., 476
Bowden, A. B., 9, 274, 284, 285
Bower, P., 407
Bowman, C., 197
Bowman, N. D., 492
Boyce, A., 83, 90
Boyd, M. R., 241
Boyle, S., 142
Bradford, A., 165
Bragge, P., 245
Brock, T. C., 304
Bromley, E., 134
Brookfield, S. D., 38, 40, 41, 42, 46, 47, 48
Brothers, K. B., 291
Brown, C. H., 242, 243
Brown, J., 48
Brown, R. D., 137
Bruner, B., 37
Bruns, E. J., 233
Bryman, A., 345, 368
Bryson, J. M., 43
Buchanan, H., 149
Buchanan-Smith, M., 14
Buckley, J., 7, 38, 41, 44, 47, 49, 51
Buddin, R., 335
Buffenstein, I., 404, 406
Bunce, A. E., 239
Bunger, A. C., 241, 245
Burke, J. G., 239
Burns, J., 311
Bussières, A. E., 239

Cabassa, L. J., 236
Caldwell, L. D., 547
Caliendo, M., 339
Cameron, J., 459, 461
Campbell, D. T., 15, 59, 61, 62, 63, 64, 65, 67, 68, 69, 71, 72, 73, 74, 80, 104, 552, 555
Campbell, R., 75, 142, 197, 547
Campbell-Patton, C. E., 165, 171, 172

Canadian Association of Management Consultants, 448
Canadian Evaluation Society, 23
Canadian International Development Agency, 193, 195
Cane, J., 239
Card, D., 340
Carden, F., 37
Carr, W., 371
Carter, S., 274
Cartland, J., 496, 497, 500
Cartwright, N., 40, 67
Caruthers, F. A., 25
Cascini, F., 408
Casey, M. A., 378
Cavaller, V., 523
Cave, G., 273
Center for Evaluation Innovation, 4, 71
Centers for Disease Control and Prevention, 384
Centers for Medicare and Medicaid Services, 109
Chambers, D. A., 236, 238
Chambers, R., 40, 46, 190, 195
Chamorro-Premuzic, T., 112, 118
Chavis, D., 168
Chelimsky, E., 82, 96, 97, 171, 172, 467
Chen, H. T., 30, 61, 64, 74, 142, 257, 383, 384
Chinman, M., 200
Cho, M., 538
Chouinard, J. A., 75, 191, 192, 497, 506, 547
Christensen, J., 289
Christie, 558, 563, 572
Christie, C. A., 59, 61, 62, 73, 76, 80, 142, 143, 164, 168, 499, 543, 546, 547
Cioffi, C. C., 14
Clandinin, D. J., 289
Clark, B., 126, 128, 130
Clark, H., 385
Clark, V. L. P., 368
Clark, W. C., 168
Clarke, M., 407
Clemmer, G., 481
Coffey, T., 407
Cohen, B. H., 320
Cohen, J., 313
Cohn, R., 126, 128
Coldwell, M., 383
Colquhoun, H., 245
Connell, J. P., 261
Connolly, F. M., 289
Connor, R. F., 537
Cook, J. M., 239
Cook, T. D., 61, 62, 104, 559, 563, 571

Cooksy, L. J., 132
Cooper, C. L., 405
Cornwall, A., 190
Coryn, C. L. S., 64, 75, 83, 97, 164, 497, 499, 500, 501, 502, 547
Couch, K. A., 273
Cousins, J. B., 75, 142, 145, 182, 184, 185, 190, 191, 192, 193, 197, 494, 497, 506, 547
Covert, R. W., 22
Cowan, J., 368
Craig, P., 241
Cram, F., 71
Creswell, J. D., 366, 371
Creswell, J. W., 119, 345, 347, 349, 358, 359, 366, 368, 371
Cronbach, L. J., 59, 61, 74, 161, 170, 492, 494, 503
Cronin, G., 48
Crowe, T., 234
Curran, G. M., 241, 244, 245

Dahler-Larsen, P., 38
Daigneault, P., 190
Damschroder, L. J., 239
Dane, A. V., 235
Dane, F., 475
Daries, J. P., 316
Dart, J., 91
Datta, L., 82, 95, 197
Davidoff, F., 242, 243
Davidson, E. J., 38, 42, 69, 81, 82, 86, 91, 92, 96, 97
Davidson, J., 15, 91
Davies, R., 68, 88, 91
De Bono, E., 43, 49
de Laat, B., 438
De Lancer Julnes, P., 68
Dean-Coffey, J., 106
Dearing, J. W., 233
Deaton, A., 40, 67
DeFleur, M. H., 492, 493
DeFleur, M. L., 492, 493
Degtiar, I., 400
Delaney, L., 197
Dennis, M. L., 404
Deutsch, M., 59
DeVellis, R. F., 256
Di Stefano, G., 46
Diamond, P. A., 282
Dickinson, P., 91
Dickinson, W. B., 358
Dillman, D. A., 378
Dionisio, C. S., 372
Doherty, L., 407
Donaldson, S., 4, 5, 197
Donaldson, S. I., (1), 6, 13, 40, 61, 64, 131, 134, 151, 167, 372, 532, 533, 534, 536, 537, 538, 543, 544, 546

Donaldson, S. I. (2), 532, 533, 537
Dong, N., 314
Doorenspleet, R., 358
Dopp, A. R., 238
Douglas, H., 95
Douville, S., 518
Dozier, D. M., 492, 493
Dragoset, L., 313
Drake, R. E., 235
Dreber, A., 404
Duffin, J., 169
Dunbar, J., 240
DuPre, E. P., 235
Durlak, J. A., 235
Dyson, L., 90, 91

Earl, L., 142, 190, 192, 193
Earl, S., 37
Easterling, D., 231, 233
Eccles, M. P., 168, 241, 242, 243, 244
Edmondson, A. C., 49
Eisman, A. B., 238
Elfeky, A., 407
Elmqvist, N., 530
Emerson, R. W., 183
Emery, A. K., 48, 514
Engle, M., 538
Epple, D., 335
Epstein, D., 4, 261
Epstein, R. M., 24
Erickson, F., 302, 303
Escoffery, C., 236
European Evaluation Society, 24
Evergreen, S. D., 503, 514

Feagin, J. R., 291
Felbinger, C. L., 263
Feldon, D. F., 349
Feng, A., 104
Fetterman, D. M., 9. 36, 75, 134, 182, 183, 184, 190, 192, 196, 197, 198, 199, 200, 202, 203, 557
Fetters, M. D., 349
Few, S., 510, 513, 516, 518, 525, 528
Feynman, R. P., 170
Fielding, N. G., 346
Fields, J., 169
Fierro, L. A., 538, 544
Findley, M. G., 400
Finley, E. P., 236
Fitzpatrick, J. L., 19, 430
Fleischer, D. N., 499
Flottorp, S. A., 239
Forsner, T., 239
Foster-Fishman, P., 14
Fournier, D. M., 39, 81, 82, 86
Fox, C., 492, 494, 499, 500, 501, 504

Fraser, M. W., 267
Frazier-Anderson, P., 528, 529
Frechtling, J. A., 11, 14, 42, 61, 68, 89, 209, 215, 232, 233, 256, 257, 258, 268, 289, 383, 384, 385, 395, 525
Frey, B. S., 228
Frierson, H. T., 66, 70, 104, 105, 113
Funnell, S. C., 384
Furlong, P., 358

Gajda, R., 184
Galiani, S., 400
Gallagher, H. A., 315
Galport, N., 21, 537
Gantt, H., 559
Gargani, J., 90
Gaskell, G., 370
Gates, E. F., 7, 36, 59, 64, 82, 83, 84, 86, 90, 91, 92, 96, 134, 141, 285, 486, 534, 536
Gaunt, D. M., 407
Gauthier, B., 544
Gaventa, J., 43, 190, 192, 193, 195
Gawande, A., 45, 462
Geertz, C., 299, 301, 571
Gennetian, L. A., 400
George, J., 368
Gertner, A. K., 236, 239
Gibson, J. L., 187
Gillespie, D. F., 239
Gillies K., 407
Glasgow, R. E., 240
Glisson, C., 242, 244
Gloudemans, J., 184
Goffman, E., 401
Goldschmid, P., 501
Gollwitzer, P. M., 45
Goodman, S. N., 102, 263
Goodman-Bacon, A., 340
Gopalan, M., 64
Gosfield, J., 173
Government Accountability Office, 89
Grady, H., 481
Graham, J. A., 184
Grathwohl, C., 165
Gravel, K., 239
Green, A. E., 239
Green, B. L., 184, 410
Green, M. C., 304
Greene, J. C.,40, 61, 82, 83, 89, 90, 142, 497, 536
Greiner, L. E., 446
Grimshaw, J. M., 240, 241, 242, 244
Griñó, L., 38
Grob, G. F., 81, 97
Groves, R. M., 410

Gruijters, S. L. K., 414
Guba, E. G., 69, 358, 482
Guerere, C., 184
Gueron, J. M., 273
Guest, G., 347
Guetterman, T. C., 345, 349
Guijt, I., 182, 190, 192, 193, 194, 195
Gullickson, A. M., 36
Guo, S., 267
Gutiérrez-García, E., 493
Guttentag, M., 164

Hadorn, S., 136
Hahn, S., 44, 45, 47
Haley, A. D., 241
Hall, J. N., 86
Hall, M., 447
Hallberg, K., 341
Hamilton, C., 492, 500, 505
Hamilton, G., 273
Hamm, R. F., 237
Handley, M. A., 242, 243
Harbatkin, E., 10, 121, 223, 256, 315, 326, 331, 344, 371, 401, 405
Harman, E., 88, 90, 96
Hart, N., 3
Hartshorn, A., 408
Hassall, K., 84
Hausman, J. A., 282
Hausmann-Stabile, C., 239
Health Insurance Portability and Accountability Act (HIPAA), 154
Heath, C., 477
Hedberg, B., 192
Heflinger, C. A., 230, 231, 233, 235
Heider, C., 87
Hemmings, A., 291, 306
Hendra, R., 371
Henry, G., 474
Henry, G. T., 10, 86, 315, 331
Hepi, M., 82
Hern, R., 126
Hicks, T., 184
Hill, A., 371
Hilliard, A. G. III, 70
Hitchcock, J. H., 368
Hoagwood, K. E., 9, 240
Hobson, K. A., 5
Hoffman, T. C., 231, 232, 245
Hogan, R. L., 272
Højlund, S., 506
Holder, E., 529
Holland, P. W., 334
Hollands, F. M., 274, 276, 278, 280, 281
Holzer, M., 68
Hood, S., 70, 104, 113, 529
Hooley, C., 245
Hoomans, T., 238

Hoover, A., 371
Hopson, R. K., 25, 70, 168, 529
House, E. R., 35, 36, 39, 43, 69, 73, 85, 134, 142, 162, 288, 291
Housing First, 83
Hovmand, P. S., 239
Howe, K. R., 73, 85, 134, 142, 162
Huberman, M., 192
Hughes, E. F., 145
Huijg, J. M., 239
Hundert, E. M., 24
Hurteau, M., 43, 84
Hutchinson, K., 495, 496, 499, 500, 501, 502, 503, 505
Hwalek, M. A., 446, 449, 458
Hwang, S., 242

Iacus, S. M., 267
Imbens, G. W., 337, 338, 339, 340
Independent Consulting Topical Interest Group Committee, 446
Ingle, M. D., 22
Inouye, T. E., 106
Institute of Development Studies, 193
Institute of Management Consultants, 448
International Labour Organization, 495, 497
International Organization for Cooperation in Evaluation, 24
INTRAC, 15
Ioannidis, J. P. A., 238
Isaacs, D., 48
Isenberg, T., 511
Isett, K. R., 244
Ison, R., 96
Ivankova, N. V., 350

Jackson, E. T., 190
Jackson, R. E., 70
Jacob, R., 279, 280
Jacob, S., 20, 190
Jacobs, J. A., 239
Jacobs, L., 127
James, A., 40, 41
James, C., 383
Jensen, H. J., 168
Jessani, N., 37
Johannesson, M., 404
Johnson, K., 15, 145, 505
Joint Committee on Standards for Educational Evaluation, 183
Jones, N. D., 10, 119, 309, 368, 416, 472, 526
Jordan, G. B., 215, 232, 383, 384, 395
Jorgensen, D. L., 401
Julnes, G., 86, 94, 97, 534, 547
Jupp, D., 190

Kafai, Y. B., 349
Kaftarian, S., 182, 184, 198
Kahneman, D., 35, 46, 170
Kamstra, P., 361
Kane, M., 239
Kassam, Y., 190
Katz, S., 48
Kavalci, E., 408
Kay, P., 209
Kazdin, A., 223
Kee, K. F., 233
Kellaghan, T., 164
Kelley, H. H., 129
Kelling, G. L., 260
Kelsey, M. D., 406
Kemmis, S., 371
Kendall, P. C., 237
Kern, F. G., 346
Khadjesari, Z., 232
Kidder, R. M., 138
Kilicel, D., 408
King, G., 267
King, J., 90, 91, 92, 144, 510
King, J. A., 5, 6, 7, 13, 19, 20, 21, 22, 23, 24, 25, 29, 36, 50, 142, 159, 162, 173, 395, 441, 494, 538
Kirk, A., 510, 514
Kirk, M. A., 232, 233
Kirkhart, J. C., 536
Kirkhart, K., 494
Kirkpatrick, D. L., 298, 562
Klasnja, P., 240
Klauss, R., 22
Klein, G., 170
Klerman, J. A., 261
Knowlton, L. W., 215, 384
Lincoln, Y. S., 69, 358, 482
Lipmanowicz, H., 47
Lipsey, M. W., 404
Liscow, Z., 274
Little, R. J. A., 321
Liu, Y., 402
Lobb, R., 239
Logan, T., 410
Long, M., 4
Losby, J. L., 213
Loud, M. L., 438
Love, A. J., 12, 37, 149, 187, 426, 427, 428, 431, 432, 435, 440, 496, 538
Luellen, J. K., 62, 105
Luke, D. A., 239, 242
Luluquisen, M., 182, 190, 192, 195
Lyon, A. R., 233
Lysy, C., 524

Mabry, L., 137, 466, 470, 471, 475, 477, 478, 483, 569
Maclean, J. C., 235

Macnamara, J., 492
Madaus, G. F., 57, 164
Majone, G., 85
Malone, S., 238
Management and Service Science, 168
Mancha, A., 457
Mandell, D. S., 239
Manswell-Butty, J. A. L., 66
Manzi, J., 261, 263
Marett, G., 161
Mark, M. M., 7, 11, 15, 74, 75, 76, 80, 88, 96, 142, 384, 543, 547
Marquart, J. M., 128
Marsh, D., 358
Martens, K. S. R., 91
Martz, W., 89, 184
Mason, J., 292
Mason, S., 14
Mastenbroek, E., 358
Masters, G., 103
Matanguihan, G. J., 120
Mathisen, W., 192
Mathison, S., 91, 92, 164, 426, 432, 439, 441
Matlen, B. J., 406
Matthias, C., 21
Maxwell, B., 383
Maxwell, J. A., 345, 359
Maynard, R. A., 273, 314
Mayne, J., 438
Mazzucca, S., 241, 242
McCandless, K., 47
McCrary, J., 337
McDavid, J., 544
McDonald, D., 449
McEwan, P. J., 271
McKegg, K., 82
McLagan, P. A., 24
McLaughlin, J. A., 215, 232, 383, 384, 395
McMillen, J. C., 239
McNall, M., 14
Merriam-Webster, 102, 125
Mertens, D. M., 22, 41, 62, 63, 71, 73, 142, 546
The Methodology Committee of the Patient-Centered Outcomes Research Institute (PCORI), 245
Mettert, K., 232
Metz, A., 231, 233
Metzger, R. O., 446
Meyer, W., 162
Michie, S., 231, 239, 240, 245
Michielutte, R., 65
Miciak, M., 461
Milgram, S., 59
Miller, C. J., 241
Miller, J., 112, 118
Miller, R., 197

Miller, R. L., 75, 141, 142, 143, 144, 147, 157, 547
Mills, E. J., 352
Miner, M., 170
Mittapalli, K., 359
Mittman, B. S., 168
Monette, D. R., 370
Montrose-Moorhead, B., 14
Moore, M. A., 278
Morabito, S. M., 184, 185
Morell, J., 47, 169, 170
Morgan, D. L., 358
Morgan, S. L., 335
Morin, K. H., 414
Morris, L. L., 492, 493, 494, 496, 500, 501, 502, 503
Morris, M., 8, 126, 127, 128, 130, 133, 162, 370, 447, 534
Morrison-Métois, S., 14
Morrow, N., 41
Moskos, P., 134
Mosteller, F., 40
Moyer, K., 121
Muessig, K., 233
Mulgan, G., 87
Mulkern, V., 210
Mumby, D. K., 491
Munger, K. M., 71
Murnane, R. J., 271
Murray, D., 452, 454
Myller, R., 262

Nadeem, E., 245
National Cancer Institute, 236, 239
National Commission for the Protection of Human Subjects of Biomedical and Behavioral Research, 291
National Equity Project, 102
National Research Council, 371
Nay, J., 209
Nelson, C. A., 168
Neta, G., 245
Neuman, W. L., 371
Newcomer, K. E., 3, 164
Newman, D. L., 137
Nguyen, M. X. B., 233, 244
Niewolny, K. L., 48
Nkwake, A. M., 41
Nunns, H., 39

Oakden, J., 91, 92
Office for Human Research Protection, 370
Office of Management and Budget, 111, 370
Ofir, Z., 87, 534
Ogden, T., 104
Olsen, R. B., 400
Olsson, T. M., 400, 406

O'Neil, G., 12, 13, 121, 377, 416, 494, 501
O'Neil, P., 126
Online Public Health, 102
Onwuegbuzie, A. J., 358, 368
Oral History Project Team, 75
Oregon State University, 132
Organisation for Economic Co-operation and Development, 87
Orr, L. L., 273, 400
Osborne, J. W., 320
O'Sullivan, R. G., 182, 184, 185, 188
Overbeck, G., 239
Oxford Policy Management, 90

Palinkas, L. A., 237, 239, 244
Pankaj, V., 48
Pardridge, W. M., 168
Parsons, B. A., 72
Partelow, S., 111
Patient Centered Outcomes Research Institute, 245
Patrizi, P., 171
Patton, M. Q., 7, 8, 18, 19, 20, 22, 30, 36, 37, 59, 74, 75, 94, 121, 134, 142, 143, 163, 165, 170, 171, 172, 173, 174, 197, 198, 303, 366, 384, 477, 491, 506, 537, 547, 561
Paul, R., 39
Pauly, E., 273
Pawson, R., 167
Payne, L., 68
Peck, L. R., 9, 261, 263, 264, 267, 289, 309, 332, 371, 395, 400, 534
Peersman, G., 83, 89
Pence, B. W., 233
Perrin, B., 130, 136
Perry, C. K., 241
Perse, E. M., 492
Peters, G. J. Y., 414
Pham, L. D., 10, 63, 256, 310, 311, 314, 323, 371, 405
Phillips, C. C., 215, 384
Phillips, J., 273
Phillips, K. W., 112
Picciotto, R., 20, 134, 162, 532, 536, 543
Pinnock, H., 245
Pinzon-Salcedo, L. A., 96
Plano Clark, V. L., 119, 345, 347, 349, 358, 359
Pleger, L. E., 128, 136
Podems, D., 25
Poes, M., 15
Pohlmann, T., 42
Poister, T. H., 524
Porter, T. M., 273
Portney, S. E., 379

Poth, C. N., 371
Powell, B. J., 9, 221, 233, 238, 239, 240, 241, 260, 331, 332, 368, 378, 422
Power, T. J., 235
Prasad, V., 238
Preskill, H., 37, 47, 48, 142, 366, 367, 377
Pritchard, I. A., 291
Proctor, E. K., 232, 233, 235, 237, 238, 239, 240, 242, 245
Project Management Institute, 366
Proshansky, H., 59
Pyburn, R., 48

Quade, E. S., 273
Quadrant Conseil, 36
Quistorff, B., 400

Rallis, S. F., 10, 292, 299, 300, 301, 302, 303, 309, 344, 345, 522
Ramalingam, B., 47
Ramirez, G. G., 14
Rao, B. V., 502
Rassel, S. M., 22, 25
Ravitz, J., 196
Rawls, J., 73
Rawson, H., 170
Reeves, P., 238
Reich, S. M., 40, 67
Reichardt, C. S., 65, 345
Reid, A. M., 83
Renger, J., 6, 536
Renger, R., 89
Reynolds, A. J., 285
Reynolds, M., 83, 91, 96
Rice, M., 422
Riley, W. T., 240
Rincones-Gómez, R., 184, 185, 186, 188, 189, 190
Robert Wood Johnson Foundation, 102, 103, 104
Roberts, S. L. E., 238
Rodríguez-Campos, L., 9, 182, 184, 185, 186, 188, 189, 190, 191
Rog, D. J., 9, 14, 68, 72, 172, 210, 226, 231, 232, 261, 384, 400, 534, 547
Rogal, S. S., 241, 244
Rogers, A., 441
Rogers, P., 383, 384
Rogers, P. J., 384
Rolston, H., 273
Rose, S., 400
Rosenbaum, P. R., 338, 339
Ross, L. F., 126, 127
Rossi, P. H., 59, 61, 104, 160, 272, 309, 311, 312, 326, 331, 334, 337, 339, 368, 492, 493, 495, 497

Rossman, G. B., 292, 299, 300, 301, 302, 303
Rubin, D. B., 334, 338, 339
Rudiger, A., 104
Rugh, J., 4
Russ-Eft, D. F., 11, 12, 69, 312, 365, 366, 367, 370, 371, 372, 375, 377, 379, 399
Russell, R. S., 272
Russon, C., 187
Rutman, L., 209
Ryan, K., 184

Sabo Flores, S., 190, 194, 202
Sager, F., 136
Saldaña, J., 299, 300
Saldana, L., 238
Sandelowski, M., 358, 522
Sanders, J., 22, 188
Sanders, K. B., 493
Sawhill, J. C., 66
Saxe, G. N., 15, 407
Scagnoli, N. I., 522
Scheirer, M. A., 74
Schmidt, R., 209
Schneider, B. H., 235
Schoeffel, G. J., 410
Schoenwald, S. K., 235
Schön, D. A., 43, 171, 192, 198, 384
Schroeter, D., 42
Schwabish, J., 104
Schwandt, T. A., 7, 24, 36, 41, 43, 50, 59, 64, 82, 83, 84, 85, 86, 87, 92, 95, 96, 133, 134, 141, 173, 285, 467, 486, 534, 536
Schwindt, O., 256
Scriven, M., 22, 35, 36, 38, 39, 40, 47, 59, 61, 63, 68, 72, 73, 74, 80, 81, 82, 83, 85, 86, 88, 89, 92, 93, 95, 101, 141, 164, 165, 167, 168, 169, 184, 197, 368, 432, 533, 546, 563, 570, 572
Sechrest, L., 14
Seiber, J. E., 291
Sette, C., 192
Severens, J. L., 238
Shadish, W. R., 56, 58, 59, 61, 62, 80, 105, 160, 161, 163, 167, 174, 262, 263, 482, 543, 547, 559, 563, 571
Shadish, W. R., Jr., 56, 58, 59, 60, 62, 63, 69, 70, 71, 75, 77, 546
Shand, R., 9, 238, 277, 279, 284
Shanker, S., 21
Sharrock, G. O., 7, 41, 44, 45, 47, 49, 50
Shaw, I. F., 164
Sheldon, T., 169
Shelton, R. C., 238
Shinkfield, A. J., 184
Shipman, S., 89, 92
Shiva Kumar, A. K., 534
Shonhe, L., 104
Shotland, R. L., 96
Shulha, L. M., 25, 75, 145, 182, 190, 193
Sielbeck-Bowen, K. A., 71
Sigel, I. E., 95
Sinclair Taylor, J., 501
Singer, E., 371
Skelton-Wilson, S., 14
Skinner, K., 68, 210, 211
Sleezer, C. M., 69, 377
Smith, J. D., 241
Smith, K. V., 417
Smith, M. F., 210
Smith, N. L., 57
Smith, V. S., 511, 525
Snell-Johns, J., 197
Snow, M. E., 526
Snow, N., 526
Snowden, D., 44
Snyder, R. B., 9, 289, 309, 332, 371, 395, 534
Somers, M. A., 341
Soneson, E., 410
Sox, H. C., 102, 263
Spangenberg, J. H., 168
Spear, P., 132
Spector, J. M., 168
Speiglman, R., 132
Spence, I., 528
Stacy, R., 44
Stake, R. E., 59, 69, 70, 86, 92, 170, 244, 366, 432
Standish, T., 371
Stanick, C. F., 240
StataCorp, 327, 328, 329
Stein, J., 166
Stern, A., 107
Stern, E., 91, 469, 497
Stetler, C. B., 241
Stevahn, L., 5, 6, 19, 20, 21, 23, 29, 510
Stewart, R. E., 239, 240
Stick, S. L., 350
Stockdill, S. H., 36
Stockmann, R., 162, 494, 497
Stone, D., 462
Straub, V. L., 446, 449, 458
Struening, E., 164
Stuart, E. A., 339, 400
Stufflebeam, D. L., 57, 88, 164, 184, 497, 499, 500, 501, 502
Suchman, E. A., 383, 431
Suppes, P., 161
Sweeney, C., 173
Sweetman, D., 359
Symonette, H., 21, 27

Takeuchi, L., 88
Tashakkori, A., 344, 345, 358, 482
Taut, S., 153
Taylor, B. W., III, 272
Taylor, M. J., 232
Teasdale, R. M., 83, 87, 88
Tebes, J. K., 291
Teddlie, C., 344, 358, 482
Teixeira, S., 118
Teresi, J. A., 414
Teslia, I., 422
Thabane, L., 414
Theis, J., 481
Thew, G. R., 417
Thomas, D. S., 166
Thomas, N. M., 42
Thomas, V. G., 72
Thomas, W. I., 166
Thomke, S., 263
Tipton, E., 406
Torres, R. T., 377, 492, 493, 494, 495, 496, 497, 499, 500, 501, 502, 503, 504, 505
Torres-Cuello, M. A., 96
Tovey, T. L., 42
Townsend, A., 168
Trevisan, M. S., 68, 210, 211
Treweek, S., 407
Trochim, W. M. K., 38, 47, 239
Tsaltskan, V., 408
Tucker, S. A., 5, 19, 25
Tufte, E. R., 104, 514, 516, 525
Turner, K., 241
Turner, S. F., 346
Tuxworth, E., 19
Tversky, A., 170

Ulrich, W., 91, 96
Umbach, P. D., 371
UNICEF, 195
United Nations Evaluation Group, 82, 502
United Way of America, 384
University of Southern California, 132
University of Washington, 132
Upshur, C. C., 190
Urban, J. B., 42
Urdang, L., 166
U.S. Bureau of Labor Statistics, 445
U.S. Census Bureau, 445
U.S. Centers for Disease Control and Prevention, 104, 106
U.S. Department of Education, 271
U.S. Department of Health and Human Services, 132
Usinger, J., 10, 309, 344, 522

Vaca, S., 22
Vaessen, J., 226, 470

Vale, L., 238
Van der Weile, T., 192
van't Hof, S., 91
VanderWeele, T. J., 334
Vaughn, A., 244
Veale, J., 184
Verdinelli, S., 522
Viano, S., 318, 319
Vo, T. V., 437
Volkov, B. B., 37, 38, 142, 426, 427, 430, 435, 439, 441
Vonnegut, K., Jr., 134

W. K. Kellogg Foundation, 106, 118, 215, 232, 384, 385, 387, 525–526
Wagamese, R., 461
Wagemans, J., 517
Walker, R., 127
Wallerstein, N., 118, 366
Walser, T. M., 68, 210, 211
Walsh-Bailey, C., 241
Waltz, T. J., 240
Wandersman, A., 182, 184, 197, 198
Ware, C., 510, 513
Webster's New World Dictionary, 165
Wehipeihana, N., 82
Weiner, B. J., 237, 238
Weiss, C. H., 36, 61, 75, 141, 143, 149, 289, 291, 383, 491, 500
Welsh, J., 184
Wensing, M., 241, 242, 244
Wexler, S., 513, 525, 528
What Works Clearinghouse, 337
Wheatley, M. J., 49
White House, 102, 104
Whitmore, E., 142, 190, 193
Wholey, J. S., 59, 63, 66, 67, 68, 71, 72, 73, 74, 209, 210, 214, 384, 393, 467, 566, 573
Wieber, F., 45
Wilcox, Y., 24
Wildavsky, A., 427, 428, 433
Wilder Research, 384
Willett, J. B., 271
William, D., 368
Williams, B., 91
Williams, J., 544
Williams, N. J., 240
Williamson, D., 66
Willoughby, L., 401
Wilson, A. L., 48
Wilson, A. T., 41, 62, 63, 71, 73, 546
Wilson-Grau, R., 91
Wiltsey Stirman, S., 236, 241
Wind, T., 37
Windahl, S., 492, 493
Wingate, L., 42
Winship, C., 335
Wittink, M. N., 346
Wolfenden, L., 242
Wood, D., 45
Woodward, R. B., 256
Workgroup for Intervention Development and Evaluation Research, 245
World Bank, 273
World Health Organization, 497
Worthen, B. R., 19, 20, 22

Xiong, C., 529

Yamey, G., 239
Yarbrough, D. B., 19, 25, 82, 129, 130, 134, 135, 149, 370, 447, 534
Yeh, S. S., 184
Yin, R. K., 244, 371
York, P., 411

Zatzick, D., 239
Zhu, Y., 510, 512
Ziegler, J., 50
Zimmer, R., 335
Zimmerman, B., 44
Zimmerman, L., 239, 240
Zukoski, A., 9, 182, 190, 192, 195
Zwarenstein, M., 241, 242, 243

Subject Index

Note. *f*, *t*, or *n* in a page number indicates a figure, a table, or a note.
Bold in a page number indicates a glossary term.

Acceptability, 237, 241, **551**. *See also* Implementation outcomes
Acceptability of Intervention Measure, 237
Access to data. *See also* Data; Data collection
 addressing budget constraints, 473
 addressing data constraints, 478–481
 real-world evaluation approach and, 466, 468*t*
 threats to validity and, 481–482
Accessibility, 399, 408–409, 513–514
Accountability
 community consultation and, 183
 definition of, **551**
 empowerment evaluation and, 199, 201–202
 ethics and, 134, 135
 evaluation as practice and, 171–172, 173
 independent consulting and, 447
 internal evaluation and, 428, 437–438
 overview, 4
 roles of internal evaluators and, 432–433
Accounting processes, 452, 455. *See also* Billing practices; Budget; Money management
Accuracy, 134, 135, 510
Action planning, 193, 194*f*, 195–196

Action research, 428, **551**
Activities. *See also* Tasks
 budget cuts and, 421–422
 communications and, 495, 496, 498*t*–499*t*, 502–503, 503*t*
 data visualization and, 526*f*, 527*f*
 definition of, **551**
 empowerment evaluation and, 200–201, 201*f*, 203
 evaluability assessment (EA) and, 211, 216, 217*f*, 219*t*, 221, 222*t*, 223–224
 evaluative thinking and, 38–39, 38*f*
 internal evaluation and, 438–439, 441–443, 442*t*
 logic models and, 385, 385*f*, 386*f*, 387*f*, 388*f*, 389*f*, 391, 392*f*, 394*f*
 negotiating with clients and, 484
 outcome evaluation and, 257*f*, 258*f*
 site selection and, 401–402
 storytelling in evaluation and, 290–291
Actual performance, 91, 202, **551**. *See also* Performance
Adaptation, 236, 447, **551**. *See also* Fidelity
Adherence, 235, 354. *See also* Fidelity; Implementation outcomes
Administrative data, 479–480. *See also* Records review
Adoption, 233, **551**. *See also* Implementation outcomes

Advisory groups or committees, 116, 117, 438
Advocacy, 95, 110
Agendas, 122, 220
Alignment, 39–40, 39*f*, 40*f*, 51, 503, **556**
All-things-considered approaches, 92
Alpha transdiscipline, 164. *See also* Transdiscipline
American Association for the Advancement of Science (AAAS), 170
American Evaluation Association (AEA), 161–163, 532–543, 539*f*–542*f*. *See also* American Evaluation Association (AEA) Guiding Principles for Evaluators
American Evaluation Association (AEA) competencies for program evaluators, 26–29, 27*t*, 28*t*, 29*t*, 532–543, 539*f*–542*f*
American Evaluation Association (AEA) Guiding Principles for Evaluators
 community consultation and, 183
 competencies and, 19, 25–29, 26*f*, 27*t*, 28*t*, 29*t*, 31
 definition of, **551**
 ethics and, 125, 130–134, 135, 136, 139
 evaluation as practice and, 173
 evaluation planning and, 370

581

American Evaluation Association (AEA) Guiding Principles for Evaluators *(cont.)*
  history and current status of competencies and, 22–23
  overview, 5–6, 8, 13, 19
  sociopolitical factors and, 95
Analytic strategies, 121. *See also* Data analysis
Angoff procedure, 91
Annualized/annualization, 278, 551
Anonymous datasets, 410, 551
Applied social science methods, 160–161
Appraisal of value, 85. *See also* Valuing
Appropriateness, 85, 237–238, 241, 551. *See also* Implementation outcomes
Archaeologist role of internal evaluators, 433*t*, 435. *See also* Internal evaluators
Art, 160*f*, 170, 174*t*
Articles, 503–504, 551. *See also* Communications
Artifacts, 292, 293, 295, 298. *See also* Document review
Artificial intelligence (AI), 14, 398, 408, 551
Assessment of value, 85. *See also* Valuing
Assignment variable/forcing variable, 330, 336, 551–552
Assumptions
  assumption audit, 41–42
  evaluative thinking and, 39*f*, 40*f*, 41–42, 51
  promoting a culture of evaluative thinking and, 46–48
Assumptions and belief preservation principle, 46–48, 51
Attrition, 401, 412. *See also* Participants
Audiences. *See also* Communications; Interest holders
  communications plan of action and, 495, 498*t*–499*t*
  data visualization and, 510, 511–514, 515*f*–516*f*, 529
  definition of, 552
  evaluability assessment (EA) and, 224
  overview, 496
  real-world evaluation approach and, 467
  tailoring communications to, 493–494
  valuing and, 93
Audio recordings, 235

Audiovisual channel, 553
Audiovisual tools, 505. *See also* Communications
Audit and monitoring studies, 244
Authorization, 399, 402–404
Average cost per participant, 279, 552. *See also* Cost; Participants
Awareness building, 110
Axiological assumptions, 41, 552

Backstage activities, 401–402
Balance tests, 337, 552
Balanced scorecards, 384
Bar graphs, 326, 329*f*, 330, 515*f*, 519*f*, 520, 520*f*
Baselines, 479–481, 552
Behavioral function of internal evaluation, 427–428, 552. *See also* Internal evaluation
Belief preservation, 46–48, 51
Beneficiaries, 117. *See also* Interest holders
Benefit–cost analysis. *See also* Economic evaluation
  definition of, 552
  economic evaluation and, 283
  overview, 10, 271, 272*t*, 274, 282, 285
Benefits in terms of costs, 85
Benefits of valuing, 96–97. *See also* Valuing
Best-case and worst-case scenario testing, 282–283, 552
Bias
  data visualization and, 510
  equity in evaluation and, 114
  internal evaluation and, 429, 429*t*
  meta-evaluation and, 69
  quantitative data analysis and, 338, 339–340, 341, 342
  real-world evaluation approach and, 483
  recruitment and, 404–405
  resource planning and, 399
  selection bias and, 63, 262, 335–336, 570
  site selection and, 400–401
  testing bias, 262, 571
Big data. *See also* Data
  addressing budget constraints, 470–471, 471*f*, 473, 477–478
  definition of, 552
  overview, 410–411
  resource planning and, 398
Billing practices, 447–448, 451–452, 453*t*, 454*t*, 455, 461*t*, 462. *See also* Money management
Bivariate analysis, 333*t*, 334, 552

Blog, 504, 552. *See also* Communications
Bootstrapping, 283, 552
Box-and-whisker plot, 327*f*, 334
Break-even analysis, 282–283, 450, 552
Bubble charts, 515*f*
Budget. *See also* Cost
  addressing budget constraints, 469–478, 471*f*, 474*t*–475*t*, 486–487
  budget cuts and, 421–422
  equity in evaluation and, 115–116, 119
  evaluation planning and, 377–379
  independent consulting and, 459, 461*t*
  mixed methods design and, 347
  money as a resource and, 399
  monitoring implementation expenses, 422
  negotiating with clients and, 483–486
  overview, 419–421, 420*t*
  real-world evaluation approach and, 465–466, 468*t*, 469–478, 471*f*, 474*t*–475*t*
  resource planning and, 398, 399
  storytelling in evaluation and, 302–303
  threats to validity and, 481–482
  time budgets, 412–413
Bullet graphs, 525*f*
Bullet-point list design, 503, 556
Business lens. *See also* Ethics
  definition of, 552
  independent consulting and, 447–448
  starting up as an independent consultant, 448–456, 451*t*, 452*t*, 453*t*, 454*t*, 456*t*
Business name, 449
Business plan, 449, 450, 462

Calendar time, 411, 416–417, 481, 552. *See also* Time factors
Calloutbox data visualization, 523*f*
Campbell, Donald, 63–65, 71–73, 552
Canadian Evaluation Society (CES), 20*n*, 23, 25, 538, 543, 544*f*–545*f*
Capacity building. *See also* Evaluation capacity building (ECB)
  community consultation and, 183
  definition of, 552
  empowerment evaluation and, 199
  evaluation planning and, 367

exemplary evaluations and, 547
goal of fostering evaluation use and, 142
participatory evaluation and, 192
program equity framework and, 110–111
Case studies, 244, 476
Categorical variable, 319, 552
Catholic Relief Services (CRS), 44–50
Causal analysis. *See also* Data analysis; Quantitative data analysis
 definition of, 552
 exploratory analysis and, 331
 overview, 10, 325, 384
 potential outcomes framework and, 334–341
 quantitative data collection and analysis and, 310, 323, 334
Causal explanations, 47, 384
CDC framework, 112–113
Census data, 473
Center for Culturally Responsive Evaluation and Assessment (CREA) framework, 113
Central tendency, 333t, 334
Certificate of Confidentiality, 370, 552
Change agent role of internal evaluators, 433t, 434. *See also* Internal evaluators
Change over time, 515f
Channel, 492, 553. *See also* Communications
Channel, audiovisual, 553
Channel, text-based, 553
Checklists, 45, 88–89, 93–97
Cleaning, data, 320–323
Clients, 116–118, 483–486. *See also* Interest holders
Clinical trials, 401
Clock time, 411–412, 553. *See also* Time factors
Closely bound internal evaluation contractors model of internal evaluation, 436t, 439. *See also* Internal evaluation
Closely bound internal evaluator, 439, 553
Closing procedures, 443
Closure gestalt principle, 517–518, 517f. *See also* Gestalt principles
Cluster analysis, 267, 553
CMS framework for health equity, 109, 110
Coarsened exact matching (CEM), 267, 553
Codes of conduct, 448. *See also* Ethics

Coding
 definition of, 553
 mixed methods design and, 360
 nominal variables and, 318–319
 pilot testing and, 414
 storytelling in evaluation and, 299–301
Cognitive values, 82. *See also* Values
Cohort design, 340, 553
Collaboration. *See also* Collaborative evaluation; Community consultation; Interest holders
 communications and, 493
 community-based participatory research (CBPR) approach and, 118
 equity in evaluation and, 118
 evaluation use and, 153
 independent consulting and, 458
 interest holders and, 310–311
 internal evaluation and, 439
 participatory evaluation and, 194, 194f, 195, 196
Collaboration members, 185, 187, 553
Collaborative evaluation. *See also* Collaboration
 community consultation and, 184–190, 186f, 203–204
 definition of, 185, 553
 evaluation as practice and, 172
 example of, 191
 framework of, 185–190, 186f
 group dynamics, 190
 overview, 9, 184–185, 203–204
Collaborative evaluators, 182, 185, 188, 190, 553
Collaborative inquiry, 49. *See also* Inquiry
Collaborators, 112
Commitment, 185, 186f, 187, 191
Common good and equity principle, 133–134, 139, 534
Communication plan, 312. *See also* Communications
Communications. *See also* Audiences; Data visualization; Dissemination of results; Interest holders; Reporting
 after an evaluation, 502–506, 503t
 as an asset for evaluation, 492–494
 before an evaluation, 497
 budget and, 378
 collaborative evaluation and, 185, 186f, 187, 191
 community consultation and, 184
 data visualization and, 12–13

definition of, 553
during an evaluation, 497, 499–501, 502t
equity in evaluation and, 116, 121
ethics and, 128, 129
evaluability assessment (EA) and, 225–226
evaluation planning and, 367, 377, 377t, 378
evaluation use and, 153
examples of, 506–507
interest holders and, 312
overview, 491–492, 493f, 506
participatory evaluation and, 192, 194f
preparing to communication, 495–497, 498t–499t
program equity framework and, 110, 113, 114
throughout the evaluation, 494–495, 494t
valuing and, 93–94
Communications activities, 495, 496, 503t, 553. *See also* Communications Activities; Communications
Communications objectives, 495, 553. *See also* Communications
Communications plan of action, 312, 495–496, 498t–499t, 553. *See also* Communications; Situation analysis
Community consultation. *See also* Collaboration; Consultation; Interest holders
 collaborative evaluation and, 184–190, 186f
 to control approaches to evaluation, 182–183
 empowerment evaluation and, 196–203, 200f, 201f, 202f
 Guiding Principles and, 183
 overview, 181–182, 203–204
 participatory evaluation and, 190–196, 194f
 shared methods and skills, 184
Community engagement, 9, 181–182, 186, 189, 192. *See also* Interest holders
Community knowledge, 183, 199, 553
Community leaders, 513
Community ownership, 198–199, 553. *See also* Ownership
Community-based participatory research (CBPR), 118, 553
Community-oriented evaluation, 436
Comparative effectiveness research (CER), 101–102, 553. *See also* Equity

Comparative interrupted time-series design (CITS), 263, 265t, 266f, 341, 553. *See also* Interrupted time-series (ITS) design
Comparison group evaluation design. *See also* Quasi-experimental evaluation designs
  data visualization and, 515f
  definition of, 554
  impact evaluation and, 265t, 267
  overview, 337–341
Competencies
  AEA competencies for program evaluators, 26–29, 27t, 28t, 29t, 532–543, 539f–542f
  cultural competence, 162, 534–535, 535f
  definition of, 554
  development of, 19–22, 24–26, 25t, 26f
  ethics and, 130–131, 139
  evaluation as a profession and, 161–163
  evaluation as practice and, 173
  evaluation identity kaleidoscope and, 161–163
  exemplary evaluations and, 534, 539–543, 539f–542f
  history and current status of, 22–24
  overview, 5–7, 13, 18–19, 30–31, 539f–542f
  program theory and logic models and, 395–396
  use of, 19–22, 29–30, 30t
Competencies Task Force (CTF), 5
Complexity and systems evaluation, 13, 528, 554
Concept maps, 384, 516f
Conceptual development, 413, 413t
Conclusions, 112
Conduct lens, 447, 554. *See also* Ethics
Confidentiality
  authorization and, 403
  ethics and, 127–128
  records review and, 410
  storytelling in evaluation and, 292
Confirmability, 482f
Conflicts of interest, 126, 131–132, 554. *See also* Ethics
Confounder, 337–341, 554
Connection gestalt principle, 517, 517f. *See also* Gestalt principles
Construct validity, 482f. *See also* Validity
Constructivist perspective, 358–359, 554

Consultation, 137, 445–446, 478. *See also* Community consultation; Independent consultant
Context. *See also* Contextual factors; Organizational context; Political factors; Real-world evaluation approach
  communications and, 494–495, 506
  context contingencies, 172
  contextual viability, 134
  data visualization and, 510
  definition of, 554
  evaluability assessment (EA) and, 213, 221
  evaluation as practice and, 172
  evaluation planning and, 367
  evaluation theory and, 71–72
  valuing and, 94–95
Context competency domain of the AEA Competency Task Force. *See also* American Evaluation Association (AEA) Guiding Principles for Evaluators; Competencies
  evaluation as a profession and, 162
  exemplary evaluations and, 538, 541f, 542f
  overview, 26, 26f, 28, 28t, 31
Contextual factors, 385f, 386, 386f, 387f, 388f, 389f, 394f, 554. *See also* Context
Contingency models, 73–74, 77, 172, 554
Continuity gestalt principle, 517, 517f. *See also* Gestalt principles
Contrast design, 503, 556
Contrasting groups procedure, 91
Controlled before-and-after designs, 243
Convergent/parallel design, 347, 348–350, 348f, 554. *See also* Mixed methods design
Correlational analysis. *See also* Data analysis; Quantitative data analysis
  definition of, 554
  overview, 10, 325, 341–342
  quantitative data collection and analysis and, 310, 323, 334
Cost. *See also* Cost analysis; Economic evaluation; Implementation outcomes; Summative evaluation
  budget and, 419–421, 420t, 422, 469–478, 471f, 474t–475t, 486–487
  combining costs and effects, 280–283, 281t

  equity in evaluation and, 108, 119, 122
  evaluation planning and, 377–379
  overview, 270–271, 275–280, 280t
  program implementation and, 231, 238–239
  resource planning and, 398
  storytelling in evaluation and, 293
  valuing and, 96
Cost analysis. *See also* Cost; Cost-effectiveness analysis; Economic evaluation
  overview, 271, 272t
  skills inventory and, 417f
Cost–benefit evaluation, 173
Cost-effectiveness analysis. *See also* Cost analysis; Economic evaluation
  combining costs and effects, 280–283, 281t
  definition of, 554
  overview, 10, 270–271, 272t, 274, 285, 286
Cost-effectiveness ratio, 280–282, 281t, 554
Cost–feasibility analysis, 10, 271, 272t, 554. *See also* Economic evaluation
Cost–utility analysis, 10, 271, 272t, 285, 554. *See also* Economic evaluation
Counterfactual
  definition of, 554
  impact evaluation and, 262, 263–264, 263f, 264f, 266f, 267
  overview, 9, 254–255, 334
  potential outcomes framework and, 335
  selection bias and, 335
Courage, 138, 447
Covariate balance, 339, 554
Covariates, 338, 554
COVID-19 pandemic, 21, 427, 439, 442, 536
Credentials, 149
Credibility
  evaluation use and, 149
  evaluative thinking and, 40
  program equity framework and, 112
  real-world evaluation approach and, 482f
  selecting internal or external evaluation and, 430f, 432
  storytelling in evaluation and, 306
  valuing and, 96

Criteria
  definition of, 554
  logic of evaluation and, 86
  overview, 86, 87, 97
  selecting, 86–89, 90
  valuing and, 93–94
Critical approach, 371–372
Critical friend, 199–200, 555
Critical incidents, 481
Critical race theory, 359
Critical realism, 63, 555
Critical systems heuristics technique, 91–92
Critical theory, 82
Critical thinking, 39
Criticism, 82
Cross-sectional data, 316–317, 555
Crowdsourcing, 88, 90
Cultural competence, 162, 534–535, 535f. *See also* Competencies; Cultural context
Cultural context. *See also* Multicultural context
  culturally responsive evaluation (CRE) and, 70
  data visualization and, 510, 512–513, 528, 529f
  equity in evaluation and, 105–106, 107, 109, 114–115, 121
  ethics and, 131
  evaluation as practice and, 173
  overview, 87
  sources of values used in evaluative judgments and, 89
Cultural responsiveness, 85
Culturally responsive evaluation (CRE), 66, 70–71, 72, 555
Culturally responsive professional practice, 82
Culture, organizational, 37, 44–50, 51
Curiosity, 49–50. *See also* Inquiry
Cut-point design. *See* Regression discontinuity (RD)

Dashboard reports, 525, 555. *See also* Evaluation dashboard
Data. *See also* Access to data; Big data; Data analysis; Data collection; Interpretation of data; Primary data; Qualitative data; Quantitative data; Secondary data
  addressing data constraints, 478–481
  data screening and cleaning and, 320–323
  data structure, 316–317, 317f
  definition of, 555
  dependability of, 442–443, 482f
  integrity and, 442–443
  internal evaluation and, 442–443
  management of, 292–293, 294t, 316
  overview, 292
  planning for quantitative analysis and, 316
  preparation of, 308–310
  program equity framework and, 110
  quality of, 401
  real-world evaluation approach and, 478–481
  as a resource, 399–411
  security of, 316, 323
  sources of, 398
  types of for creating a data visualization, 518
  understanding, 316
Data analysis. *See also* Data; Exploratory data analysis; Interpretation of data; Quantitative data analysis
  addressing budget constraints, 476–477, 486–487
  communications and, 500, 501
  community consultation and, 184
  economic evaluation and, 282
  empowerment evaluation and, 197
  equity in evaluation and, 121
  ethics and, 128, 370
  evaluability assessment (EA) and, 222–224, 222t
  evaluation planning and, 368, 370–372
  explanatory sequential designs and, 351f
  logitistical factors, 369
  mixed methods design and, 361
  multiphase/complex designs and, 356f, 357f
  overview, 308
  participatory evaluation and, 194f, 195, 196
  planning for innovations in, 410–411
  program equity framework and, 113
  quantitative data and, 309
  secondary data and, 409–410
  skills inventory and, 417–418, 417f
  storytelling in evaluation and, 298–302, 300f
  time as a resource, 414
Data collection. *See also* Access to data; Data; Quantitative data collection
  accessibility and, 408–409
  addressing budget constraints, 470, 476–477, 486–487
  addressing data constraints, 479
  addressing time constraints, 478
  authorization and, 402–404
  budget cuts and, 422
  communications and, 500, 501
  community consultation and, 184
  data as a resource and, 399–411
  data security, 316
  economic evaluation and, 276–277, 277t, 282
  empowerment evaluation and, 197
  equity in evaluation and, 115, 119–121
  ethics and, 127–128, 370
  evaluability assessment (EA) and, 214–215, 218, 219t, 221–222
  evaluation planning and, 368, 370–372
  financial resources and, 421
  logitistical factors, 369, 408
  methodologies of, 120–121
  mixed methods design and, 345–346
  outcome evaluation and, 258–259
  overview, 308–310, 404–408
  participatory evaluation and, 194f, 195, 196
  pilot testing and, 414
  planning for innovations in, 410–411
  primary data collection, 399–409
  program equity framework and, 113
  program implementation and, 235, 241
  quantitative data and, 308–309, 318–319, 323
  real-world evaluation approach and, 465–466, 478
  recruitment and, 404–406
  resource planning and, 398, 399
  secondary data and, 409–410
  site selection and, 400–402
  storytelling in evaluation and, 292–298, 294t, 299, 300f, 305–306
  support needed for, 409
  time as a resource, 411–417, 413t
Data dashboards, 525, 525f, 555. *See also* Evaluation dashboard
Data elicitation, 370, 371–372. *See also* Data collection
Data ink, 514, 516, 520–521, 520f, 521f, 555. *See also* Data visualization
Data screening and cleaning, 320–323
Data source, primary, 323, 555. *See also* Primary data

Data source, secondary, 323, 555. *See also* Secondary data
Data structure, 316–317, 317*f*
Data structure, long, 316, 555
Data visualization. *See also* Communications
  avoiding common mistakes and, 514, 516–518, 516*f*, 517*f*
  creating, 518–521, 519*f*, 521*f*
  definition of, 555
  emerging topics in, 522–528, 522*f*, 523*f*, 525*f*, 526*f*, 527*f*, 529*f*
  future directions in, 528–530
  logic model design and, 525–528, 526*f*, 527*f*
  overview, 12–13, 493, 509, 510, 510*f*, 530
  presenting findings and, 503
  principles of, 509–510
  purpose and audience and, 511–514, 515*f*–516*f*
Databases
  data collection and data analysis and, 409–410
  evaluability assessment (EA) and, 219*t*
  evaluation planning and, 371
  mixed methods design and, 361
Dataset, long, 317, 555
Dataset, wide, 317, 555
Datasets. *See also* De-identified dataset
  addressing budget constraints, 471
  data screening and cleaning and, 321
  data visualization and, 518
  definition of, 555
  graphical analysis and, 330
  planning for quantitative analysis and, 316
  secondary data and, 410
Deadlines, 465–466. *See also* Time factors
Decision making
  communications and, 506
  equity in evaluation and, 121
  evaluability assessment (EA) and, 222–223
  evaluation as practice and, 171
  evaluation use and, 145, 152, 154
  evaluative thinking and, 36–37, 43–44, 51
  participatory evaluation and, 194, 194*f*, 196
  resource planning and, 398–399
  selecting internal or external evaluation and, 429–432, 430*f*, 431*f*

storytelling in evaluation and, 299
values and, 82
Decision-making characteristics, 13, 506, 555. *See also* Decision making
Deductive and inductive thinking, 298–299, 305, 555
De-identified dataset, 410, 556. *See also* Datasets
Deliberative approaches, 92, 436
Democratic participation, 183, 199, 204, 436, 556
Dependability of data, 442–443, 482*f*. *See also* Data
Descriptive analysis. *See also* Data analysis; Quantitative data analysis
  definition of, 556
  exploratory analysis and, 330
  overview, 10, 75, 311, 324, 331–334, 333*t*, 341
  quantitative data collection and analysis and, 310, 323
Design, alignment, 503, 556. *See also* Alignment
Design, bullet-point list, 503, 556
Design, contrast, 503, 556
Design, evaluation. *See* Evaluation design
Design, heading, 503, 556
Design, highlight box, 503, 556
Design, program. *See* Program design
Design, proximity, 503, 556
Design, quote, 503, 556
Design, randomized, 556
Design, repetition, 503, 556
Design, subheading, 503, 556
Design characteristics, 122. *See also* Evaluation design
Design feasibility, 209, 556
Design principles, 370, 371, 503, 526. *See also* Evaluation design
Design-based tradition, 337, 556
Development, 188, 556
Developmental evaluation
  definition of, 556
  embedded internal evaluator model of internal evaluation and, 436
  evaluation as practice and, 172, 173
  overview, 13, 390
Dialogue, 201, 203, 493, 556. *See also* Communications
Difference-in-differences (DID), 311, 340–341, 556
Differential attrition, 262, 336, 556
Differentiation, program. *See* Program differentiation

Direct (or instrumental) use, 64, 556. *See also* Instrumental use
Direct costs, 420–421, 422. *See also* Cost
Direct data, 235. *See also* Data collection
Direct observation, 239. *See also* Observations
Disaggregation, 474*t*
Discipline, 160*f*, 163–165, 174*t*
Discounting, 278, 279, 556
Discussions, 504–505. *See also* Communications
Dispersion, 333*t*, 334
Dissemination of results. *See also* Communications; Findings of evaluations; Reporting
  empowerment evaluation and, 197
  equity in evaluation and, 116, 121
  ethics and, 129
  evaluability assessment (EA) and, 225–226
  interest holders and, 312
  internal evaluation and, 443
  participatory evaluation and, 194*f*, 195, 196
  presenting findings and, 502–505, 503*t*
  program equity framework and, 110, 113, 114
  program implementation and, 245
  storytelling in evaluation and, 302–305
Diversity–equity–inclusion, 536
Document review. *See also* Records review
  data collection and data analysis and, 409–410
  economic evaluation and, 276, 277*t*
  evaluability assessment (EA) and, 214–218, 217*f*, 219*t*
  evaluation planning and, 371
  literature searches, 184
  program implementation and, 239
  storytelling in evaluation and, 293, 298, 302–303
Documentation, 137, 218–221, 219*t*, 276
Dose, 235. *See also* Fidelity; Implementation outcomes
Dumbbell plots, 515*f*, 519*f*

Ecological momentary assessments (EMA), 410–411, 556
Economic costs, 273, 274. *See also* Cost

Economic equity, 21. *See also* Equity
Economic evaluation. *See also* Benefit–cost analysis; Cost; Cost analysis; Cost-effectiveness analysis; Cost-feasibility analysis; Cost–utility analysis; Summative evaluation
  combining costs and effects, 280–283, 281*t*
  definition of, 557
  enhancing evaluation with, 283–286, 284*t*, 285*t*
  history of, 272–274
  overview, 270–272, 272*t*, 275–280, 276*t*, 277*t*, 280*t*, 286
  purpose of, 274–275
Effect size, 313–314, 474*t*, 515*f*, 557
Effective data visualization, 509, 510, 557. *See also* Data visualization
Effectiveness criteria, 87. *See also* Criteria
Effectiveness outcomes, 239, 241, 309. *See also* Outcomes
Effectiveness–implementation designs, hybrid, 244–245, 559
Efficacy criteria, 87. *See also* Criteria
Efficiency criteria, 87, 474*t*, 510. *See also* Criteria
Embedded internal evaluator model of internal evaluation, 436–437, 436*t*. *See also* Internal evaluation
Empathy, 183, 188, 557
Empirical theory, 75
Empowerment, 557
Empowerment evaluation
  advantages of, 197
  collaborative evaluation and, 188
  community consultation and, 182, 196–204, 200*f*, 201*f*, 202*f*
  definition of, 197, 557
  disadvantages of, 197–198
  embedded internal evaluator model of internal evaluation and, 436
  evaluation as practice and, 172
  example of, 203
  exemplary evaluations and, 547
  features of, 198–202, 200*f*, 201*f*, 202*f*
  framework of, 198
  group dynamics, 203
  overview, 9, 77, 196–197, 203–204
Empowerment evaluator, 70, 198, 199–201, 203, 557
Empowerment evaluators or critical friends, 71, 557

Empowerment theory, 198, 557
Enclosure gestalt principle, 517*f*, 518. *See also* Gestalt principles
Engagement, 110, 310–312
Enhanced evaluability assessment (EEA), 213–214, 557
Entry/contracting stage of evaluation, 126–127, 135–136, 154–155
Environmental factors
  environmental sustainability, 15
  exemplary evaluations and, 536
  interviewing and, 293, 295
  logic models and, 391
  storytelling in evaluation and, 295–296
Epistemic values, 82. *See also* Values
Epistemological assumptions, 557
Equality, 82, 102–103, 103*f*, 557
Equitable Evaluation framework, 113
Equity
  competencies and, 21
  conducting equity-focused program evaluations, 114–118
  culturally responsive evaluation (CRE) and, 70
  definition of, 102, 102*t*, 557
  ethics and, 133–134, 139
  exemplary evaluations and, 536
  framework of in evaluation work, 106–121
  interest holders and, 14
  overview, 4, 8, 13, 87, 101–103, 102*t*, 103*f*
  planning the evaluation and, 121–123
  program equity framework and, 109–113
  reflection in evaluation and, 104–106
  values and, 82
Established requirements criteria, 87. *See also* Criteria
Ethical practices, 8, 557. *See also* Ethics
Ethics
  authorization and, 403
  competencies and, 29
  definition of, 557
  evaluation planning and, 370
  evaluative judgment and, 85
  independent consulting and, 447–448
  overview, 3, 125–126
  preventing and responding to challenges and, 135–138, 139
  professional guidance for, 130–135
  recruitment and, 405

stages in evaluation and, 126–130
  storytelling in evaluation and, 293, 301–302, 306
  values and, 83, 93
Ethnicity, 115
Ethnographic methods, 13, 239, 289, 476, 557. *See also* Storytelling in evaluation
  collecting preliminary data on the feasibility of conducting an evaluation, 221–222
  communicating the findings from, 225–226
  definition of, 557
  developing follow-up options, 224–225
  documenting the program as implemented, 218–221, 219*t*
  documenting the program design, 214–218, 217*f*
  example of, 227–228
  history and background of, 209–210
  impact evaluation and, 261
  involving interested parties and intended users, 214
  logic models and, 393, 395
  overview, 9, 67, 68, 208, 209, 226–228, 384
  program implementation and, 232
  steps in, 211–224, 217*f*, 219*t*, 222*t*
  when to conduct, 210–211
Evaluands, 171, 211, 411, 557
Evaluation accountability. *See* Accountability
Evaluation activities. *See* Activities
Evaluation capacity building (ECB). *See also* Capacity building; Evaluative thinking
  definition of, 557
  exemplary evaluations and, 547
  internal evaluation and, 441
  overview, 7, 36, 38–39, 51
  power of inquiry and, 40–42
  promoting a culture of evaluative thinking and, 44–50
Evaluation competencies. *See* Competencies
Evaluation consultant. *See* Consultation; Independent consultant
Evaluation dashboard, 202, 203, 557. *See also* Dashboard reports; Data dashboards
Evaluation design. *See also* Evaluation planning
  addressing budget constraints, 469–478, 471*f*, 474*t*–475*t*
  communications and, 497

Evaluation design *(cont.)*
  constraints affecting, 466–469, 468*t*
  data collection and data analysis and, 370–372
  data visualization and, 513
  economic evaluation and, 285–286
  equity in evaluation and, 121–123
  ethics and, 127
  evaluation as practice and, 171
  overview, 365–366, 380–381
  program equity framework and, 112, 113, 119–120
  program implementation and, 241–245
  real-world evaluation approach and, 465–469, 468*t*
  resource planning and, 398–399
  skills inventory and, 417*f*
  storytelling in evaluation and, 299, 300*f*, 301–302
Evaluation equity framework, 111, 557. *See also* Equity
Evaluation facilitator role of internal evaluators, 433*t*, 434, 443. *See also* Internal evaluators
Evaluation failure, 230, 557
Evaluation goals. *See* Goals
Evaluation identity kaleidoscope
  evaluation as a discipline and transdiscipline, 163–165
  evaluation as a profession and, 161–163
  evaluation as art and, 170
  evaluation as practice and, 170–173, 171*f*
  evaluation as science and, 165–169
  overview, 159–160, 160*f*, 173–174, 174*t*
Evaluation planning. *See also* Evaluation design
  addressing budget constraints, 486–487
  authorization and, 402–404
  budget cuts and, 421–422
  communications and, 493, 495–497, 498*t*–499*t*
  data collection and data analysis and, 308–310, 370–372, 410–411
  data screening and cleaning and, 320–323
  engaging interest holders and, 310–312
  financial resources and, 377–379, 419–421, 420*t*
  interest holders and, 310–312
  logic models and, 390

  overview, 308–310, 365–366, 380–381, 401, 422–423
  personnel as a resource and, 417–419, 418*f*, 419*f*
  planning the people, 374–377, 376*t*
  planning the work and schedule, 372–374, 373*f*, 374*t*, 375*f*, 375*t*
  quantitative analysis and, 312–316, 323–324
  recruitment and, 404–408
  resource planning and, 398–399
  risk and, 379–380, 380*t*
  scope of the evaluation effort, 366–370, 369*t*
  secondary data and, 409
  selecting internal or external evaluation and, 429–432, 430*f*, 431*f*
  site selection and, 400–402
  software and, 422
  tasks and time and, 413–417, 413*t*
  time as a resource, 411–417, 413*t*
  understanding data and, 316–320, 317*f*, 318*f*
Evaluation policy, 154. *See also* Policy
Evaluation practice. *See* Practice
Evaluation questions. *See also* Questioning
  calendar time and, 411
  communications and, 497
  data visualization and, 514*n*, 515*f*–516*f*, 518
  equity in evaluation and, 115, 120
  ethics and, 125
  overview, 8–11
  PDP evaluation findings and, 544*f*
Evaluation report, 503, 558. *See also* Communications; Reporting
Evaluation science, 160*f*, 165–169, 558
Evaluation synthesis, 13, 92–94, 558. *See also* Valuing
Evaluation theory. *See also* Evaluation theory tree; Five components of evaluation theory; Program theory; Theory
  adequacy of theories, 144
  definition of, 558
  evaluation use theory, 143–144
  exemplary evaluations and, 543, 546–547, 546*f*
  future of, 74–77, 76*f*
  goal of fostering evaluation use and, 142
  guiding evaluation practice with, 71–74

  importance of, 57–58
  meta-models and, 58–62, 60*f*
  overview, 3, 7, 11, 55–57
  preparing evaluators, 5
  quasi-experimental evaluation designs, 65, 65*f*
  review of specific evaluation theories, 62–71, 65*f*
Evaluation theory tree. *See also* Evaluation theory; Methods; Three branches; Use; Valuing
  combining theories and, 73
  current version of, 76, 76*f*
  definition of, 558
  discipline of evaluation and, 164
  exemplary evaluations and, 546–547, 546*f*
  goal of fostering evaluation use and, 142
  overview, 59–61, 60*f*, 75, 76*f*, 80, 164
  Shadish et al. model and, 80
  social justice and, 62
Evaluation training. *See* Training
Evaluation units, 437–438
Evaluation use. *See also* Use
  adequacy of theories, 144
  community consultation and, 183
  definition of, 558
  evaluation use theory, 143–144
  evaluation use theory and, 143–145
  evaluator actions and, 145–156, 146*t*
  goal of fostering, 142–143
  guidelines for, 144–147, 146*t*
  observable actions and, 147–156
  for other contexts, 156
  overview, 141–142, 145, 156–157
  research on, 145–147, 146*t*, 157
Evaluation work plan. *See* Work plan
Evaluative judgment. *See also* Valuing
  definition of, 558
  overview, 84–85, 86, 93–94
  sources of values used in, 89
  valuing and, 94–95, 97
Evaluative reasoning, 85, 558
Evaluative thinking. *See also* Evaluation capacity building (ECB)
  capacity building and, 142
  community involvement approaches and, 181–182
  definition of, 558
  as a foundational philosophical concept, 39–40
  logic models and program theory and, 383

overview, 7, 18, 35–39, 38f, 51
power of inquiry and, 40–44, 42f
promoting a culture of, 44–50
Evaluators. *See also* Competencies; Independent consultant; Internal evaluators; Roles of evaluators
analyze the data and determine evaluability, 222–224, 222t
collaborative evaluation and, 189
communications and, 494–495, 494t
conducting equity-focused program evaluations, 114–118
data visualization and, 13, 530
empowerment evaluation and, 199–200
equity in evaluation and, 107–108, 122
ethics and, 129–130, 139
evaluation as a profession and, 161–163
evaluation as practice and, 172–173
evaluation competencies, 5–7
evaluation identity kaleidoscope and, 160f
evaluation planning and, 368–369, 374–377, 376t
evaluation science and, 166
evaluation theory and, 543
evaluation use and, 145–156, 146t, 157
evaluator involvement in program development, 14
exemplary evaluations and, 537–543, 539f–542f
interviewing and, 293, 295
logic models and, 390–391, 393, 395–396
mixed methods design and, 347
observable actions and, 147–156
overview, 15–16, 18
participatory evaluation and, 193–194, 195
planning for innovations in data collection and analyses, 410–411
planning for quantitative analysis and, 323
preparing evaluators, 4–5
preventing and responding to challenges and, 135–138, 139
program implementation and, 239
program theory and, 395–396
records review and, 410
resource planning and, 399
selecting internal or external evaluation and, 430–432, 430f, 431f

skills inventory and, 417–418, 417f
storytelling in evaluation and, 291, 292, 293, 295
time estimates and, 416–417
today's context of, 3–4
valuing and, 7–8, 93–94, 97
Evidence, 89–91
Evidence, credible. *See* Credibility
The Evidence Act, 3–4, 558
Evidence sources, 86, 93–94
Evidence-based evaluation theory, 543, 546–547, 546f
Evidence-based intervention mapping, 558
Evidence-based interventions, 111, 558
Evidence-Based Policymaking Act of 2018. *See* The Evidence Act
Evidence-based strategies
community consultation and, 183
definition of, 558
empowerment evaluation and, 199
evaluative thinking and, 37, 51
values and, 82
Exact matching, 338, 558
Exemplary evaluations, 532–543, 535f, 539f–542f, 547
Exhaustive, 318, 558
Expectations
collaborative evaluation and, 185, 186f, 187, 191
communications and, 497
evaluability assessment (EA) and, 215–216, 221
evaluation planning and, 368
identifying in evaluation planning, 366–367
resource planning and, 399
Experimental designs
equity in evaluation and, 119
evaluation planning and, 371
impact evaluation and, 261–263, 263f, 265t
preparing evaluators, 5
program implementation and, 241, 242–243
Expert opinions criteria. *See* Experts
Experts
data visualization and, 512
equity in evaluation and, 107–108, 116, 117
internal evaluation and, 439
negotiating with clients and, 486
overview, 87
Explanatory sequential design, 347, 350–352, 351f, 558. *See also* Mixed methods design

Exploratory data analysis. *See also* Data analysis; Quantitative data analysis
definition of, 558
overview, 10, 324, 326–331, 327f–329f, 341–342
quantitative data collection and analysis and, 310, 323
Exploratory mixed method design, 352–353, 352f, 355f, 356f, 357f
Exploratory sequential design, 352, 354, 558
External evaluations, 12, 173, 429–432, 430f, 431f
External validity or generalizability. *See also* Validity
access to the intervention and, 338
definition of, 558
overview, 63, 400
pilot and feasibility testing and, 414
potential outcomes framework and, 335
real-world evaluation approach and, 482f, 483
site selection and, 400–401

Falsifiable logic model, 261. *See also* Logic models
Feasibility. *See also* Implementation outcomes
definition of, 558
ethics and, 134
evaluability assessment (EA) and, 221–224
evaluation design and, 241
evaluation use and, 149–150
feasibility testing, 413–414, 413t
mixed methods design and, 347
program implementation and, 238
quantitative data analysis and, 325
randomized controlled trials (RCTs) and, 336
storytelling in evaluation and, 293
Feedback, 438–439, 461–462, 500–501, 502t
Feminist theories, 82, 359
Fidelity. *See also* Implementation; Implementation outcomes
definition of, 558
descriptive analysis and, 331
example of, 234
multiphase/complex designs and, 354
program implementation and, 233–236

Fidelity *(cont.)*
    sources of values used in
        evaluative judgments and, 89
    storytelling in evaluation and,
        291
Fieldwork, 292, 402. *See also* Data
    collection
Financial resources, 419–422,
    420t, 430f. *See also* Budget;
    Resources
Financial sustainability, 448–449,
    462. *See also* Budget; Money
    management
Findings of evaluations. *See also*
        Dissemination of results;
        Evaluation use; Reporting
    communicating negative findings,
        501
    data visualization and, 509–510
    empowerment evaluation and,
        197
    equity in evaluation and, 116
    ethics and, 128
    follow-up of conclusions and
        recommendations and,
        505–506
    mixed methods design and, 344
    participatory evaluation and,
        194f, 195, 196
    presentation of, 502–505, 503t
    program equity framework and,
        112
    storytelling in evaluation and,
        301, 302–305
    testing, 500–501, 502t
Fiscal control, 546–547, 546f
Fishing, 256–257, 558
Five components of evaluation
    theory, 58–59, 80, 559. *See also*
    Evaluation theory
508 compliance, 378, 558–559
Fixed cost, 279–280, 559. *See also*
    Cost
Fixed-effect model, 341, 559
Flexibility, 193, 437, 559
Flowcharts in data visualization,
    523f
Focus, 367–369, 369t, 428
Focus groups
    evaluation planning and, 372,
        378
    incentives for, 378
    program implementation and,
        239
    storytelling in evaluation and,
        293, 296, 303
Focus on action planning, 193, 559
Follow-up of conclusions and
    recommendations, 505–506
Forcing variable, 330, 336, **551–552**
Foreshadowing, 302, 559

Formative evaluation
    definition of, **559**
    evaluation as practice and, 173
    evaluation planning and, 368
    evaluation use theory and,
        143–144
    interest holders and, 310
    internal evaluation and, 431, 432,
        436
    overview, 68, 254–255
    storytelling in evaluation and,
        290–291
Fostering evaluation use framework.
    See Evaluation use
Framework for Program Evaluation
    in Public Health, 112–113
Frequency distribution, 319–320,
    332–333, 559
Front-stage activities, 401–402
Full-time equivalent (FTE) cost,
    377. *See also* Cost
Fundamental problem of causal
    inference, 334–335, 559
Funding, 398, 399. *See also* Budget
Future planning, 219t, 501. *See also*
    Planning for the future

Gantt charts
    definition of, **559**
    evaluation planning and, 374,
        375t
    monitoring implementation
        expenses and, 422
    overview, 515f
    personnel as a resource and,
        418–419, 419f
Gap analysis, 122–123
General elimination method (GEM),
    47
Generalizability
    definition of, **559**
    equity in evaluation and, 108
    negotiating with clients and,
        485–486
    number of participants and,
        406–407
    planning for quantitative analysis
        and, 313
Geographic information system
    (GIS), 481
Gestalt principles, 516–518, 517f,
    519–520, 559
GetReal Trial Tool, 401
Getting-to-outcomes, 200, 559
Goals. *See also* Mission/mission
        statement; Outcomes; Purpose
    data visualization and, 510
    definition of, **559**
    empowerment evaluation and,
        201, 202f, 203
    equity in evaluation and, 121–122

evaluability assessment (EA) and,
    209–210, 215, 219t, 222–224,
    222t
evaluation as practice and,
    171–172
evaluation planning and,
    367–369, 369t
fostering evaluation use and,
    142–143
outcome evaluation and, 257
outcome monitoring and,
    260–261
sources of values used in
    evaluative judgments and, 89
storytelling in evaluation and,
    289–291
Government Performance and
    Results Act (GPRA), 3–4, 210,
    559
Graphical analysis, 326–331,
    327f–329f, 334, 341. *See also*
    Exploratory data analysis
Great Society programs, 18–19
Group dynamics, 190, 195–196,
    203
Group interviews, 219. *See also*
    Focus groups; Interviews
Guidelines. *See also* Reporting
        guidelines
    collaborative evaluation and, 185,
        186f, 187–188, 191
    program implementation and,
        245
    for selecting internal or external
        evaluation, 429–432, 430f,
        431f
Guiding Principles. *See* American
    Evaluation Association
    (AEA) Guiding Principles for
    Evaluators

Heading design, 503, **556**
Health equity, 109, 110, 559. *See
    also* Equity
Heterogeneous groups, 296
Highlight box design, 503, **556**
High-risk evaluations, 429–430, 559
Hiring, 376
Histograms, 326, 327f, 330, 515f
Historical factors, 262, 367, 481,
    559
Homogeneous groups, 296, 474t
Honest broker role of internal
    evaluators, 433, 433t. *See also*
    Internal evaluators
Hybrid effectiveness–
    implementation designs,
    244–245, 559
Hybrid internal evaluation model,
    436t, 438–439. *See also*
    Internal evaluation

Icons in data visualization, 523f
Identification strategy
    collaborative evaluation and, 185, 186–187, 186f, 191
    criteria and, 88
    definition of, 560
    participatory evaluation and, 192
Ignorability assumption, 321, 560
Immigration status, 109. *See also* Cultural context
Impact evaluation. *See also* Impacts; Outcome evaluation
    definition of, 560
    ethics and, 137–138
    evaluability assessment (EA) and, 210–211, 261
    overview, 9, 255, 261–269, 263f, 264f, 265t, 266f, 311
    potential outcomes framework and, 334–341
    quantitative data collection and analysis and, 309, 334–341
Impacts. *See also* Impact evaluation; Summative evaluation
    addressing data constraints, 479
    data visualization and, 526f, 527f
    definition of, 560
    economic evaluation and, 284
    internal evaluation and, 437–438
    logic models and, 385f, 386, 386f, 387f, 388f, 389f, 394f
    negotiating with clients and, 484
    outcome monitoring and, 260–261
    overview, 254–255
    quantitative data collection and analysis and, 309
    real-world evaluation approach and, 483–484
Implementation. *See also* Implementation outcomes; Program implementation
    constraints affecting, 466–469, 468t
    evaluation theory and, 67
    explanatory sequential designs and, 351
    internal evaluation and, 438–439
    outcome monitoring and, 261
    overview, 422–423
    participatory evaluation and, 193
    real-world evaluation approach and, 465–469, 468t
    selecting internal or external evaluation and, 431–432
    sources of values used in evaluative judgments and, 89
Implementation cost, 231, 238–239, 560. *See also* Cost
Implementation failure, 230, 560

Implementation measure, 314–315. *See also* Measure, process or implementation; Measures
Implementation outcomes. *See also* Acceptability; Adoption; Appropriateness; Cost; Feasibility; Fidelity; Implementation; Penetration; Program implementation; Sustainability
    definition of, 560
    effectiveness outcomes and, 239
    extent and quality of program implementation and, 232–237
    overview, 232–233
Implementation strategies, 560. *See also* Implementation; Program implementation
Improvement
    authorization and, 403
    community consultation and, 183
    definition of, 560
    empowerment evaluation and, 198
    evaluation as practice and, 171–172
    participatory evaluation and, 192, 193
    roles of internal evaluators and, 432
Incentives for participants, 378, 404–405. *See also* Participants
Inception report, 467, 560
Inclusion
    AEA competencies for program evaluators, 539f
    community consultation and, 204
    definition of, 560
    empowerment evaluation and, 199
    equity in evaluation and, 122
    evaluation use and, 150–151
    exemplary evaluations and, 536
    interest holders and, 14
Incorporation, 451t
Independent consultant. *See also* Consultation; Independent consultant
    definition of, 560
    ethics and, 447–448
    finding a market niche, 456–457
    getting work, 457–459
    overview, 12, 445–446, 462, 463
    personality traits associated with, 446–448
    starting up as, 448–456, 451t, 452t, 453t, 454t, 456t
    survival skills, 459, 461–463
Independent evaluation, 173, 311, 437–438, 560

Independent internal evaluation unit model of internal evaluation, 436t. *See also* Internal evaluation
Indirect costs, 420–421. *See also* Cost
Indirect data, 235. *See also* Data collection
Inductive thinking, 298–299, 305, 555
Inequality, 103
Inequity, 70. *See also* Equity
Infographics, 503, 560. *See also* Communications
Informal discussion, 493, 560. *See also* Communications
Informants, key. *See* Key informants
Information specialist role of internal evaluators, 433t, 434. *See also* Internal evaluators
Informational function of internal evaluation, 427–428, 560. *See also* Internal evaluation
Informed consent, 403
Informed decision making, 43–44, 51. *See also* Decision making
Ingredients method, 275–280, 277t, 280t, 560
Innovation, 150–151, 509
Inputs
    data visualization and, 526f, 527f
    definition of, 560
    evaluability assessment (EA) and, 216, 217f
    logic models and, 385, 385f, 386f, 387f, 388f, 389f, 391, 394f
    negotiating with clients and, 484
    outcome evaluation and, 257f, 258f
Inquiry. *See also* Questioning
    evaluation science and, 168–169
    evaluation theory tree and, 60f
    evaluative thinking and, 36, 40–44, 42f, 51
    promoting a culture of evaluative thinking and, 44–50
    spectrum of, 42, 42f
    values and, 82, 88
Institutional development, 417f
Institutional review board (IRB)
    authorization and, 403
    definition of, 560
    ethics and, 130, 132–133
    evaluation planning and, 365–366
    overview, 125–126
    recruitment and, 405
    resource planning and, 398
    storytelling in evaluation and, 301
    time as a resource, 412

Instrumental use, 209, 560. *See also*
  Direct (or instrumental) use
Instrumentation, 113, 417*f*
Instrumentation bias, 262, 560
Insurance, 455–456, 456*t*
Integrated data platforms, 473,
  560–561
Integration
  convergent/parallel designs and,
    348*f*
  definition of, 561
  evaluation theory and, 72–73, 77
  mixed methods design and, 346,
    361
  multiphase/complex designs and,
    357*f*
  values and, 88
Integrity
  ethics and, 131–132, 139
  evaluation use and, 150–151
  exemplary evaluations and, 534
Intended use by intended users, 74,
  214, 561
Intent, 539*f*
Interactions, 262
Interactive data displays, 523–524,
  523*f*, 526–528, 527*f*, 561. *See
  also* Data visualization
Interactive evaluation, 172
Interactive logic model designs,
  526–528, 526*f*, 527*f*. *See also*
  Logic models
Interactive websites, 504, 513, 561.
  See also Communications
Interest holder approaches to
  evaluation, 13, 561. *See also*
  Interest holders
Interest holder involvement/
  engagement. *See also* Interest
  holders
  communications and, 494
  definition of, 561
  evaluation planning and, 372
  logic models and, 391–393, 392*f*
  overview, 311
Interest holders. *See also* Audiences;
  Communications; Community
  consultation; Interest holder
  involvement/engagement
  collaborative evaluation and, 186,
    189
  communicating negative findings,
    501
  communications plan of action
    and, 495, 498*t*–499*t*
  communications throughout the
    evaluation and, 494–495
  community interest holders, 181
  data visualization and, 511,
    513–514, 524, 526

definition of, 561
descriptive analysis and, 332
engaging, 310–312, 323
equity in evaluation and, 115,
  116–118
ethics and, 125, 126–127, 128,
  129, 130–132, 136, 138, 139
evaluability assessment (EA) and,
  214, 215–216, 219*t*, 221–222,
  222*t*
evaluation planning and, 368–
  369, 369*t*, 374–377, 376*t*
evaluation use and, 141–142, 148,
  151–153, 154–155
exploratory mixed method design
  and, 352–353
goal of fostering evaluation use
  and, 142
initial or interim findings and,
  500
logic models and, 390, 391–393,
  392*f*
multiphase/complex designs and,
  356
multiple perspectives and, 43
negotiating with clients and,
  483–486
overview, 14, 496
participatory evaluation and,
  192, 193, 194, 194*f*, 195
program equity framework and,
  112, 113
program implementation and,
  231, 237–238, 240–241
quantitative data collection and
  analysis and, 309, 310–312
scope of the evaluation effort and,
  366–367
sources of values used in
  evaluative judgments and, 89
storytelling in evaluation and,
  290–291
tailoring communications to,
  493–494
valuing and, 83, 93–94, 95–96,
  97
Intermediate outcomes, 257*f*,
  258, 258*f*, 259, 260. *See also*
  Outcomes
Internal audit, 12, 427, 561
Internal departmental model/
  internal evaluation unit
  model of internal evaluation,
  437–438. *See also* Internal
  evaluation
Internal evaluation. *See also* Internal
  evaluators
  characteristics of, 428–432, 429*t*,
    430*t*, 431*f*
  definition of, 561

developing effective internal
  evaluation capability, 440–
  441, 440*t*
evaluation as practice and, 173
evaluative thinking and, 37–38
guidelines for selecting, 429–432,
  430*f*, 431*f*
models of, 435–439, 436*t*
overview, 12, 427–428, 443–444
resource management and,
  441–443, 442*t*
strengths and limitations of,
  428–429, 429*t*
Internal evaluation function,
  435–436, 561. *See also* Internal
  evaluation
Internal evaluators. *See also*
  Evaluators; Internal evaluation
  developing effective internal
    evaluation capability, 440–
    441, 440*t*
  evaluative thinking and, 37–38
  models of internal evaluation and,
    435–439, 436*t*
  overview, 426–427, 443–444
  roles of, 432–435, 433*t*
Internal validity. *See also*
  Maturation; Threats to internal
  validity; Validity
  definition of, 561
  impact evaluation and, 261–262
  overview, 63, 242
  potential outcomes framework
    and, 335, 336–337
  real-world evaluation approach
    and, 481–483, 482*f*
International Development Research
  Centre (IDRC), 37
International Labour Organization
  (ILO), 495
International Organization for
  Cooperation in Evaluation
  (IOCE), 24
Internet of things (IOT), 410–411,
  561
Interpersonal competency domain
  of the AEA Competency Task
  Force. *See also* American
  Evaluation Association
  (AEA) Guiding Principles for
  Evaluators; Competencies
  evaluation as a profession and, 162
  exemplary evaluations and, 538,
    541*f*, 542*f*
  overview, 26, 26*f*, 29, 29*t*, 31
Interpretation of data. *See also*
  Data; Data analysis
  convergent/parallel designs and,
    348*f*
  ethics and, 128

explanatory sequential designs and, 351f
mixed methods design and, 361
multiphase/complex designs and, 356f, 357f
storytelling in evaluation and, 298–302, 300f
Interpretivist perspective, 371–372
Interrupted time series (ITS), **561**
Interrupted time-series (ITS) design
 access to the intervention and, 337, 339–340
 definition of, **561**
 impact evaluation and, 265t
 overview, 65, 65f
 program implementation and, 243
Interval measures, 317–318, 318f, 319, **562**. *See also* Measures
Intervention access, 337–341
Intervention design, 213
Interviews. *See also* Data collection
 addressing budget constraints, 470
 addressing data constraints, 479
 authorization and, 402, 403
 evaluability assessment (EA) and, 218, 219–221
 evaluation planning and, 372
 explanatory sequential designs and, 351
 mixed methods design and, 344, 360
 skills inventory and, 417f
 storytelling in evaluation and, 292, 293, 295–296, 303
 time estimates and, 414
Involvement, 188, **561**

Joint displays, 349, **561**
Judgment, evaluative. *See* Evaluative judgment
Justice. *See* Social justice

Kaleidoscope. *See* Evaluation identity kaleidoscope
Kernel density plot, 327f
Key informants
 addressing budget constraints, 477
 addressing data constraints, 480
 addressing time constraints, 478
 evaluability assessment (EA) and, 220
 internal evaluation and, 430
Knowledge construction
 culturally responsive evaluation (CRE) and, 70
 discipline of evaluation and, 164

evaluation as practice and, 171–172
evaluation theory and, 58, 65
interest holders and, 310–311
knowledge-generating evaluation, 173
program implementation and, 241
Knowledge mobilization, 443
Knowledge products (evaluation), 495, **561**
Knowledge use, 164

Latent class analysis, 267, **562**
Leadership
 data visualization and, 513
 empowerment evaluation and, 197
 internal evaluation and, 440
 logic models and, 390–391
 participatory evaluation and, 192
 program implementation and, 241
 promoting a culture of evaluative thinking and, 49
 skills inventory and, 417
Learning
 definition of, **562**
 empowerment evaluation and, 199
 evaluation use and, 150–151
 overview, 4
 participatory evaluation and, 192, 193
Learning to Action Discussions (LADs) tool, 44, 45
Legal factors, 89, 430f
Lessons learned, 505–506, **562**
Letter or memo of confirmation, 441
Level 1 questionnaire, 298, **562**. *See also* Surveys
Limited datasets, 410, **562**
Limited liability company (LLC), 451t
Line graph, 329f, 334, 515f, 521
Linear-fit plot, 328f
Literature searches, 184. *See also* Document review
Lived expertise, 14, 119, 372, **562**
Locus of control, 190, 195–196, 203
Log frames, 384
Logic models. *See also* Program logic model; Program theory
 benefits and drawbacks of incorporating in an evaluation, 395
 data visualization and, 511, 522, 525–528, 526f, 527f, 529f
 definition of, **562**
 developing, 390–393, 392t

evaluability assessment (EA) and, 215, 216–218, 217f
evaluator competencies and, 395–396
outcome evaluation and, 257, 257f, 258f, 259–260, 261
overview, 11, 61, 68, 383–390, 385f, 386f, 387f, 388f, 389f, 396
program implementation and, 232
selecting internal or external evaluation and, 431–432
storytelling in evaluation and, 299, 300f
uses of, 393–395, 394f
valuing and, 86–93
Logic of evaluation, 86, **562**
Logistical factors, 368, 369, 408
Long data structure, 316, 555
Long dataset, 317, 555
Longitudinal data, 311, 337–338, **562**
Long-term outcomes, 257f, 258, 258f, 259–260, 432. *See also* Outcomes

Machine learning, 13, **562**
Magic-bullet model of communication, 492, 493f. *See also* Communications
Management, 49, 445–446
Management consultant role of internal evaluators, 433t, 434. *See also* Internal evaluators
Managers
 internal evaluation and, 440, 442–443
 roles of internal evaluators and, 432–433, 435
Marginal cost, 279–280, **562**. *See also* Cost
Market price, 275, 277–278, **562**
Matching, 339, **562**
Matrix data visualization, 523f
Matrix sampling
 definition of, **562**
 financial resources and, 421
 storytelling in evaluation and, 299, 300f
Maturation, 63, 262, 337–338, **562**. *See also* Internal validity
Mean reversion, 338, **562**
Measure, outcome, **562**. *See also* Outcome measure
Measure, process or implementation, 311, 314–315, **563**
Measurement, 88, 224, 317–319, 318f, 410. *See also* Measures

Measures. *See also* Implementation measure; Interval measures; Measurement; Nominal measures; Ordinal measures; Outcome measure; Parsimony; Process measure; Ratio measures; Reliability; Validity
  data as a resource and, 401
  definition of, 562
  descriptive analysis and, 331–332
  exploratory analysis and, 326
  levels of measurement and, 317–319, 318f
  overview, 255–257
  pilot testing and, 414
  planning for quantitative analysis and, 314–315, 316–317, 317f
  quantitative data and, 308–309
Mediational analyses, 67, 563
Mediators, 67, 563
Member checking, 372, 563
Merit, 89, 141
Messages, 492, 563. *See also* Communications
Messaging strategy, 500, 501, 502t, 563
Meta-evaluation, 40, 69, 563
Meta-models, 58–62, 60f, 80, 563
Methodological assumptions, 563
Methodology, 127. *See also* Methods
Methodology competency domain of the AEA Competency Task Force. *See also* American Evaluation Association (AEA) Guiding Principles for Evaluators; Competencies
  evaluation as a profession and, 162
  exemplary evaluations and, 538, 540f, 542f
  overview, 26, 26f, 27–28, 27t, 31
Methods. *See also* Evaluation theory tree; Practice
  addressing budget constraints, 472
  communications and, 497
  community consultation and, 184
  evaluation as practice and, 171
  evaluation identity kaleidoscope and, 160–161, 160f, 174t
  evaluation theory and, 55, 59, 60, 60f, 62, 76f
  exemplary evaluations and, 546–547
  goal of fostering evaluation use and, 142
  independent consulting and, 460t
  internal evaluation and, 442
  mixed methods design and, 361

  negotiating with clients and, 485–486
  review of specific evaluation theories, 62–71
  social science methods, 160–161
Methods lens, 447, 563. *See also* Ethics
Milestones, 369–370, 373–374, 374t, 375f, 375t, 563
Misalignment, 39–40, 39f, 40f, 51
Missing at random (MAR) data, 321, 563
Missing completely at random (MCAR) data, 321, 563
Missing data, 320–321, 334–335, 410, 563
Missing not at random (MNAR) data, 321, 563
Missing observations, 320–321, 563
Missing values, 320–321, 563
Mission/mission statement, 200, 200f, 203, 258–259, 563. *See also* Goals; Purpose
Mixed methods design
  addressing budget constraints, 470, 475
  convergent/parallel designs, 347, 348–350, 348f
  culturally responsive evaluation (CRE) and, 70
  data visualization and, 529–530
  definition of, 563
  equity in evaluation and, 119–120
  evaluation planning and, 368
  explanatory sequential designs, 347, 350–352, 351f
  exploratory mixed method design, 352–353, 352f, 355f, 356f, 357f
  future directions in, 360
  issues in the use of, 358–360
  multiphase/complex designs, 347, 353–358, 355f, 356f, 357f
  negotiating with clients and, 486
  overview, 10–11, 160–161, 344–347, 361
  program implementation and, 239
  threats to validity and, 482–483
  tools in, 360
Model for collaborative evaluations (MCE), 185–190, 186f, 563. *See also* Collaborative evaluation
Model-based tradition, 563
Modeling, 49
Moderators, 67, 564
Modification, 236, 564. *See also* Fidelity
Modified Venn diagrams in data visualization, 523f

Money management. *See also* Budget; Funding
  independent consulting and, 447–448, 462
  resource planning and, 399
  starting up as an independent consultant and, 448–449, 451–452, 453t, 454t, 455
Monitoring. *See also* Outcome monitoring
  empowerment evaluation and, 201–202, 202f
  evaluation as practice and, 173
  exemplary evaluations and, 534
  program implementation and, 231
Monte Carlo analysis, 283, 564
Moral courage, 125, 138, 564
Moral values, 82. *See also* Values
Most significant change technique, 91
Multicultural context, 532–533. *See also* Cultural context
Multidimensional matching, 267, 564
Multimedia report, 493, 505, 564. *See also* Communications
Multiphase/complex design, 347, 353–358, 355f, 356f, 357f, 564. *See also* Mixed methods design
Multiple perspectives, 43, 51. *See also* Perspective taking
Multiple-arm trials, 242
Multiple-case studies, 244
Multisite datasets, 410. *See also* Datasets
Multivariate regression, 338, 564
Mutually exclusive, 310, 318, 326, 564

Narrative analysis, 289. *See also* Qualitative data; Storytelling in evaluation
National Equity Project framework, 111
Natural language model, 410–411, 564
Natural language processing, 13, 564
Navigator role of internal evaluators, 433, 433t. *See also* Internal evaluators
Nearest neighbor matching, 338
Needs, 89, 472–473
Needs assessment, 69, 87, 88–89, 326, 564
Negative findings, 501, 507. *See also* Findings of evaluations
Negotiating with clients, 483–486
Negotiation and balance of power, 193, 564

Nested design, 401, **564**
Network data visualization, 523*f*
Networking, 458, 462–463
New information technology, 477–478, 486–487. *See also* Technology
Nominal measures, 317, 318–319, 318*f*, **562**. *See also* Measures
Noncompliance, 336, **564**
Nondata ink, 514, 516, 519–520, **564**. *See also* Data visualization
Nondisclosure agreement (NDA), 214, **564**
Nonprobability sampling, 313, **564**, **570**. *See also* Sampling
Nonprofit corporation, 451*t*
Nonresponse bias, 371, **564**
Nonspecialist evaluators, 439, **564–565**
Null hypothesis, 313–314, **565**
Number cruncher role of internal evaluators, 433*t*, 434. *See also* Internal evaluators

Objectives, 215, 217*f*, 219*t*, 222–223, 222*t*, 289–291. *See also* Goals
Objectivity, 482*f*
Observable actions, 144, 147–156, 157
Observation in a dataset, 316, 321, 326, **565**
Observations. *See also* Data collection
  addressing budget constraints, 470, 477
  definition of, **565**
  evaluability assessment (EA) and, 219*t*, 221
  program implementation and, 235, 239, 241, 243–244
  site selection and, 401
  storytelling in evaluation and, 292, 293, 296–297, 303
Office of Management and Budget (OMB), 412
Office space, 451, 452*t*
One-group pretest-posttest design, 263, **565**
Ontological assumptions, **565**
Open-ended questions, 298, **565**. *See also* Surveys
Opportunist principle, 44–45, 51
Opportunities, 379–380, 380*t*
Opportunity costs, 273, **565**. *See also* Cost
Optimal visualization, 514. *See also* Data visualization
Ordinal measures, 317–318, 318*f*, 319, **562**. *See also* Measures

Organizational context
  authorization and, 400–404
  communications and, 494–495, 506
  definition of, **565**
  developing effective internal evaluation capability, 440–441, 440*t*
  evaluability assessment (EA) and, 219*t*
  evaluation use and, 150–151, 154, 155–156
  internal evaluation and, 427–428, 429*t*, 437, 440–441, 440*t*
  real-world evaluation approach and, 466, 467, 468*t*
  roles of internal evaluators and, 432
  selecting internal or external evaluation and, 431–432
Organizational interventions, 428, **565**
Organizational learning
  community consultation and, 183
  definition of, **565**
  empowerment evaluation and, 199
  exemplary evaluations and, 547
  internal evaluation and, 443
  participatory evaluation and, 192
Organizational support, 440, 440*t*
Outcome evaluation. *See also* Impact evaluation; Outcomes
  definition of, **565**
  evaluability assessment (EA) and, 210–211
  evaluation as practice and, 173
  overview, 255, 257–261, 257*f*, 258*f*, 268–269
Outcome harvesting, 91
Outcome maps, 384
Outcome measure. *See also* Measures; Outcomes
  definition of, **565**
  descriptive analysis and, 334
  overview, 311
  planning for quantitative analysis and, 314, 315
Outcome monitoring, 260–261. *See also* Monitoring; Outcomes
  definition of, **565**
  exploratory analysis and, 330
  overview, 332
  quantitative data collection and analysis and, 309
Outcomes
  data as a resource and, 401
  data visualization and, 511, 526*f*, 527*f*
  definition of, **565**

descriptive analysis and, 332
economic evaluation and, 284–285
evaluability assessment (EA) and, 216, 217*f*, 219*t*, 221, 222*t*, 223–224
interest holders and, 311
internal evaluation and, 437–439
logic models and, 385, 385*f*, 386*f*, 387*f*, 388*f*, 389*f*, 391, 394*f*
multiphase/complex designs and, 353, 356
negotiating with clients and, 484
outcome monitoring and, 260–261
overview, 254–255
potential outcomes framework and, 334–335
quantitative data collection and analysis and, 309
selecting internal or external evaluation and, 432
Out-of-range values, 322, **565**
Outputs
  data visualization and, 526*f*, 527*f*
  definition of, **565**
  evaluability assessment (EA) and, 216, 217*f*, 221
  logic models and, 385, 385*f*, 386*f*, 387*f*, 388*f*, 389*f*, 394*f*
  negotiating with clients and, 484
  outcome evaluation and, 257*f*, 258*f*
  outcome monitoring and, 260–261
  overview, 257
Overlap, 339, **565**
Overlapping bar charts, 515*f*
Ownership
  communications and, 495, 497
  community consultation and, 181, 182–183
  empowerment evaluation and, 198–199
  ethics and, 129
  evaluation as practice and, 173
  interest holders and, 312
  participatory evaluation and, 193
Ownership structure, business, 449, 451*t*

Paperwork Reduction Act (PRA), 412
Parallel design, 347, 348–350, 348*f*, 554. *See also* Mixed methods design
Parallel sets, 516*f*
Parallel trends, 340, **565**
Parsimony, 256–257, **565**

Participant focus and ownership, 193, 565. *See also* Ownership; Participants
Participants. *See also* Participatory evaluation; Recruitment
 accessibility and, 408–409
 addressing budget constraints, 470
 attrition and, 412
 evaluability assessment (EA) and, 221–222
 evaluation planning and, 374–377, 376t, 378
 incentives for, 378
 logic models and, 392f
 multiphase/complex designs and, 354
 number of, 406–407
 recruitment and retention (R&R) and, 406–408
 resource planning and, 399
 retention and, 406
 selecting, 401, 404–405
 storytelling in evaluation and, 290, 291, 301–302, 303, 306
Participatory evaluation. *See also* Participants
 addressing data constraints, 480–481
 advantages of, 192
 community consultation and, 182, 190–196, 194f, 203–204
 definition of, 190, 565
 disadvantages of, 192
 embedded internal evaluator model of internal evaluation and, 436
 evaluation as practice and, 172, 173
 exemplary evaluations and, 547
 features of, 192–196, 194f
 logic models and, 390–391
 overview, 9, 190–191, 203–204
Participatory evaluators, 182, 192, 566. *See also* Evaluators; Participatory evaluation
Participatory rural appraisal (PRA) group interview methods, 477, 480–481, 567
Participatory system dynamics modeling, 239
Partnership, 117, 451t. *See also* Interest holders
Part-time internal evaluator model of internal evaluation, 436, 436t. *See also* Internal evaluation
Patterns, 292, 566
Patton, Michael Quinn, 74, 75
Peer review, 372, 566

Penetration, 236–237, 566. *See also* Implementation outcomes
Perfect collinearity, 320, 566
Performance, 86, 93–94, 192. *See also* Actual performance
Performance measurement, 13, 566
Performance measurement systems, 67, 566
Performance monitoring, 524–525, 566
Permissions. *See* Authorization
Personal values, 137–138, 429t. *See also* Values
Personality traits, 447–448, 462
Person-loading chart, 418, 418f, 420
Personnel. *See also* Staff
 budget and, 419–420, 420t, 422
 internal evaluation and, 428, 429, 440
 person loading and, 418, 418f
 as a resource, 399, 417–419, 417f, 418f, 419f, 420t
 resource planning and, 398
 roles of internal evaluators and, 432–433
 selecting internal or external evaluation and, 430, 430f
 skills inventory and, 417–418, 417f
Persons with lived experiences, 106–107, 566. *See also* Equity
Perspective taking
 communicating negative findings, 501
 definition of, 566
 evaluation as practice and, 173
 evaluative thinking and, 51
 multiple perspectives, 43
 storytelling in evaluation and, 290–291
PERT chart. *See* Program evaluation and review technique (PERT) chart
Photo voice. *See* Data collection
Photographs
 addressing budget constraints, 477
 data visualization and, 523f
 presenting findings and, 505
 storytelling in evaluation and, 292, 295
Pictograms, 515f
Pie charts, 515f, 519f
Pilot testing
 internal evaluation and, 438–439
 negotiating with clients and, 485
 overview, 413–414, 413t
 selecting internal or external evaluation and, 431–432
Pipeline design, 469–470, 566

Planning, program. *See* Program planning
Planning an evaluation. *See* Evaluation planning
Planning and management competency domain of the AEA Competency Task Force, 26, 26f, 28–29, 28t, 31, 538, 541f, 542f. *See also* American Evaluation Association (AEA) Guiding Principles for Evaluators; Competencies
Planning for the future, 201, 202f, 203, 566
Planning resources. *See* Resources
Plausibility, 208, 211, 212, 214, 215, 224, 225, 226–227, 566
Podcasts, 505, 566. *See also* Communications
Policy. *See also* Sociopolitical factors
 communications and, 506
 data visualization and, 513
 evaluability assessment (EA) and, 210
 evaluation planning and, 378
 evaluation use and, 154
 evaluation use theory and, 143
 program equity framework and, 110
 quantitative data collection and analysis and, 309
Policy environment, 13, 506, 566. *See also* Policy
Policy-analytic contingency theories of evaluation, 74, 566
Political factors. *See also* Sociopolitical factors
 communications and, 506
 interviewing and, 293, 295
 negotiating with clients and, 484–485
 real-world evaluation approach and, 466, 467, 468t
 values and, 82, 89, 95, 172–173
Population data, 313
Populations of interest, 115, 117–118, 215–216. *See also* Interest holders; Target population
Portfolio logic model, 393, 394f. *See also* Logic models
Positivist perspective, 371
Postpositivist perspective, 247–248, 371, 566–567
Posttest-only comparison group design, 265t, 567
Potential outcomes framework for causal inference, 334–341, 567
Power, 21, 70, 127, 184, 193. *See also* Equity
Power analysis, 313–314, 405, 567

Power Cube tool, 43
PRA (participatory rural appraisal), 477, 480–481, 567
Practical empowerment evaluation, 197, 567. *See also* Empowerment evaluation
Practical participatory evaluation, 191, 567. *See also* Participatory evaluation
Practical strategies for culturally competent evaluation, 112–113
Practical wisdom, 43, 567
Practice. *See also* Methods
  collaborative evaluation and, 185, 186f, 187, 191
  discipline of evaluation and, 164
  evaluation as, 160f, 170–173, 171f, 174t
  evaluation theory and, 59, 71–74
  exemplary evaluations and, 534, 536
  five-component model and, 80
  practicing principle, 46, 51
Pragmatic measures, 240, 567
Pragmatic worldview, 359, 371, 539f, 567
Praxeological assumptions, 567
Pre-evaluation. *See* Evaluability assessment (EA)
Prescriptive model, 74–75
Presentation. *See also* Communications
  data visualization and, 513
  definition of, 567
  of initial or interim findings, 500
  overview, 493, 502–505, 503t
  presenting findings and, 502–505, 503t
Press releases, 504, 567. *See also* Communications
Pretest–posttest comparison group design, 264f, 265t, 470, 567
Primary data. *See also* Data
  data collection, 399–409
  data screening and cleaning and, 322
  definition of, 567
  overview, 311
  planning for quantitative analysis and, 314, 323
  resource planning and, 398
  sources of, 323, 555
Priority
  definition of, 567
  empowerment evaluation and, 200–201, 201f, 203
  mixed methods design and, 345, 358
Privacy, 403. *See also* Confidentiality

Privilege, 70
Probability sampling, 313, 567, 570. *See also* Sampling
Probe–sense–act approach, 44
Probity, 291, 568
Process evaluation. *See also* Descriptive analysis
  definition of, 568
  evaluation as practice and, 173
  exploratory analysis and, 330
  overview, 331
  quantitative data collection and analysis and, 309
Process measure, 311, 314–315, 563. *See also* Measure, process or implementation; Measures
Process use, 198, 568
Professional development, 5, 462
Professional evaluators. *See also* Competencies; Evaluators
  evaluation identity kaleidoscope and, 160f, 174t
  exemplary evaluations and, 537–543, 539f–542f
  overview, 161–163
Professional practice competency domain of the AEA Competency Task Force. *See also* American Evaluation Association (AEA) Guiding Principles for Evaluators; Competencies
  evaluation as a profession and, 162
  exemplary evaluations and, 538, 540f, 542f
  overview, 26–27, 26f, 27t, 31
Professional standards and values, 82, 83, 93, 129, 130–135, 136. *See also* Ethics; Values
Professionalization and Competencies Working Group, 5
Program access, 335–337
Program Assessment Rating Tool, 3–4, 210, 568
Program components/strategies, 222t, 223. *See also* Activities
Program design, 214–218, 217f, 225, 231
Program development, 14, 108–113, 224
Program differentiation, 235. *See also* Fidelity; Implementation outcomes
Program documents. *See* Document review
Program effect/program impact, 334, 568
Program equity framework, 109–113, 114–118, 568. *See also* Equity

Program evaluability, 209, 568
Program evaluation, 4–5, 8–11, 80
Program evaluation and review technique (PERT) chart
  definition of, 566
  evaluation planning and, 374, 374t, 375f
  personnel as a resource and, 419
Program evaluation review technique (PERT), 568
Program Evaluation Standards
  competencies and, 19, 26–27
  definition of, 568
  ethics and, 134–135
  overview, 5–6, 13
Program failure, 230, 568
Program implementation. *See also* Implementation; Implementation outcomes; Implementation strategies
  barriers and facilitators to, 239–240
  costs of, 238–239
  definition of, 568
  economic evaluation and, 284
  evaluability assessment (EA) and, 218–222, 219t, 222t
  evaluation design and, 241–245
  extent and quality of, 232–237
  informing future efforts and, 245
  interest holders' perceptions and, 237–238
  multiphase/complex designs and, 353–356, 355f
  outcome monitoring and, 261
  overview, 9, 230–231, 245–246
  program being evaluated and, 231–232
  storytelling in evaluation and, 291, 302–303
  sustainability, 238
  theory of change and, 231–232
Program improvement evaluations. *See* Improvement
Program logic model. *See also* Logic models
  definition of, 568
  evaluability assessment (EA) and, 215, 216–218, 217f
  outcome evaluation and, 257, 257f, 258f, 259–260
  program implementation and, 232
  storytelling in evaluation and, 299, 300f
Program management, 225, 311, 416
Program participants. *See* Participants
Program planning, 41, 416–417. *See also* Evaluation planning

Program staff. *See* Staff
Program stage, 73–74, 210–211, 214, 568. *See also* Stage model
Program theory. *See also* Evaluation theory; Logic models
  benefits and drawbacks of incorporating in an evaluation, 395
  criteria and, 89
  definition of, 568
  evaluation science and, 167
  evaluation theory and, 64
  evaluator competencies and, 395–396
  number of participants and, 406
  outcome evaluation and, 257
  overview, 11, 61–62, 64, 383–385, 396
  program implementation and, 230, 232
  storytelling in evaluation and, 289, 305
Progress of the evaluation, 499
Project management, 134, 417–418, 422
Project planning and management competency domain of the AEA Competency Task Force, 162
Propensity score, 267, 339, 471, 568
Propensity score matching, 267, 339, 568
Proposals, 370, 459, 460t–461t, 466. *See also* Request for proposals (RFP)
Propriety, 134–135
Proximity design, 503, 556
Proximity gestalt principle, 517f, 518. *See also* Gestalt principles
Psychological contract, 136, 568
Psychological safety principle, 49–50, 51
Public roles, 95–96. *See also* Interest holders
Publicity agent role of internal evaluators, 433t, 435. *See also* Internal evaluators
Purpose. *See also* Goals; Mission/mission statement
  data visualization and, 510, 511–514, 515f–516f
  evaluability assessment (EA) and, 211–212, 213
  evaluation planning and, 367–369, 369t
  interest holders and, 310
  outcomes and, 258–259
  sample size and, 474t
  storytelling in evaluation and, 289–291
Purposive sampling, 421, 568

Qualification, 183, 188, 568
Qualitative approaches. *See also* Qualitative data; Storytelling in evaluation
  addressing budget constraints, 477
  community consultation and, 184
  data collection and, 309
  generating data, 292–298, 294t
  negotiating with clients and, 486
  overview, 289
  program implementation and, 239
  threats to validity and, 482–483
Qualitative comparative analysis, 469–470, 569
Qualitative data. *See also* Data; Mixed methods design; Qualitative approaches
  addressing budget constraints, 475–477
  constructivist and postpositivist perspectives and, 358–359
  convergent/parallel designs and, 348, 348f, 349–350
  data visualization and, 522–523, 522f, 523f
  definition of, 569
  equity in evaluation and, 119–120
  explanatory sequential designs and, 350–352, 351f
  mixed methods design and, 344–347, 352–353, 352f
  multiphase/complex designs and, 353–356, 355f, 356f, 357f
  overview, 361
  sources of, 89–91
Qualitize, 346, 358–359, 569
Quality assurance, 173, 231
Quality of delivery, 235. *See also* Fidelity; Implementation outcomes
Quantitative approaches. *See also* Quantitative data
  addressing budget constraints, 477
  community consultation and, 184
  negotiating with clients and, 486
  overview, 10, 312–316, 323–324
  preparing evaluators, 5
  program implementation and, 239
  threats to validity and, 482–483
Quantitative data. *See also* Data; Mixed methods design; Quantitative approaches; Quantitative data analysis; Quantitative data collection
  constructivist and postpositivist perspectives and, 358–359
  convergent/parallel designs and, 348, 348f, 349–350
  definition of, 569
  equity in evaluation and, 119–120
  explanatory sequential designs and, 350–352, 351f
  exploratory mixed method design and, 352–353, 352f
  mixed methods design and, 344–347
  multiphase/complex designs and, 353–356, 355f, 356f, 357f
  overview, 361
  sources of, 89–91
Quantitative data analysis. *See also* Data analysis; Quantitative data
  correlational and causal analysis, 334
  descriptive analysis, 331–334, 333t
  exploratory analysis, 326–331, 327f–329f
  impact evaluation and, 334–341
  overview, 325–326, 341–342
  potential outcomes framework and, 334–341
Quantitative data collection. *See also* Data collection; Quantitative data
  data screening and cleaning and, 320–323
  evaluation planning and, 372
  overview, 308–310, 316–320, 317f, 318f, 323–324
Quantitize, 346, 358–359, 522, 569
Quasi-experimental evaluation designs. *See also* Comparison group evaluation design
  definition of, 569
  equity in evaluation and, 119
  evaluation planning and, 371
  impact evaluation and, 263–267, 264f, 265t, 266f
  internal validity and, 262
  overview, 13–14, 65, 65f, 337–341
  preparing evaluators, 5
  program implementation and, 241, 242–243
Questioning. *See also* Evaluation questions; Inquiry; Interviews; Reflective practice
  culturally responsive evaluation (CRE) and, 70
  equity in evaluation and, 119
  evaluative thinking and, 37, 51
  program equity framework and, 113
  spectrum of inquiry and, 42, 42f
  storytelling in evaluation and, 295
  valuing and, 93–94

Quibbler role of internal evaluators, 433*t*, 435. *See also* Internal evaluators
Quote design, 503, 556

Racial equity, 21. *See also* Equity
Random assignment/randomization, 222, 261, 336, 401, **569**
Randomized controlled trials (RCTs)
  credible evidence and, 40
  definition of, **569**
  economic evaluation and, 273
  overview, 67
  program implementation and, 241, 242–243
  selection bias and, 336–337
Randomized design, 13–14, 242–243, 265*t*, 336, 556, **569**
Rank order, 319
Ranking variable, 264*f*, 266, **570**
Rapid appraisal, 14–15, 195
Rapid cycle evaluation, 14–15, **569**
Rapid feedback evaluation, 68
Rapid program information, 211–212
Ratio measures, 317–318, 318*f*, 319, 563. *See also* Measures
Reactivity. *See* Testing bias
Readiness, 384
Real time evaluation, 14–15, **569**
Real world evaluation, 12, **569**
Realist evaluator, 71, 173, **569**
Reality testing, 170
Real-world evaluation approach
  addressing budget constraints, 469–478, 471*f*, 474*t*–475*t*
  addressing data constraints, 478–481
  addressing time constraints, 478
  evaluation as practice and, 173
  negotiating with clients and, 483–486
  overview, 465–466, 486–487
  threats to validity and, 481–483, 482*f*
  types of challenges and, 466–469, 468*t*
Recommendations, 224
Records review. *See also* Document review
  addressing budget constraints, 473, 477, 486
  addressing data constraints, 479
  time estimates and, 415
Recruitment. *See also* Participants
  evaluation planning and, 376
  number of participants and, 406–407
  overview, 401
  resource planning and, 398

retention and, 406
selecting participants, 404–405
Recruitment and retention (R&R), 406–408. *See also* Participants; Recruitment
Referrals, 457–458, 462
Reflective practice
  definition of, **569**
  equity and, 104–106
  evaluation as practice and, 170–171, 172–173
  evaluative thinking and, 37, 43, 51
  independent consulting and, 459, 461
  overview, 37
Reflexive evaluation design, 263, 265*t*, **569**
Reflexivity, 172–173
Regression, 337, 339, **569**
Regression artifact, 262, **569**
Regression discontinuity (RD)
  definition of, **569**
  exploratory analysis and, 330–331
  impact evaluation and, 265*t*, 266, 266*f*
  selection bias and, 336–337
Relationship building, 149–150, 497, 499–500
Relationship-based evaluations, 172, 429
Relevance, 85, 87, 237–238, 430*f*
Reliability, 256, 371, 482*f*, **569**
Remote sensors, 481
Repetition design, 503, 556
Replicability, 322, 486
Reporting. *See also* Communications; Dissemination of results; Findings of evaluations
  descriptive analysis and, 332
  equity in evaluation and, 116, 121
  ethics and, 128, 129, 370
  evaluability assessment (EA) and, 225–226
  evaluation planning and, 368, 370
  of initial or interim findings, 500
  interest holders and, 312
  internal evaluation and, 438, 443
  overview, 493
  presenting findings and, 502–505, 503*t*
  program implementation and, 245
  storytelling in evaluation and, 302–305
  time as a resource, 415–416
Reporting guidelines, 245, **570**. *See also* Dissemination of results; Findings of evaluations; Guidelines

Representation, 117–118. *See also* Target population
Representative sampling, 421, **570**
Request for an evaluation, 441
Request for proposals (RFP)
  communications and, 494, 497
  definition of, **570**
  evaluability assessment (EA) and, 211, 215
  evaluation planning and, 370
  independent consulting and, 456, 459, 460*t*–461*t*
  scope of the evaluation effort and, 366
  writing the proposal, 370
Research design, 313
Reshape, 317, **570**
Resilience, 447
Resistance, 116–117
Resource economy, 89
Resources
  addressing budget constraints, 469–478, 471*f*, 474*t*–475*t*
  data as a resource, 399–411
  data visualization and, 514
  economic evaluation and, 275–276, 284
  equity and, 103
  ethics and, 134
  evaluability assessment (EA) and, 219*t*, 222*t*, 223
  evaluation planning and, 377–379
  financial resources, 419–422, 420*t*
  independent consulting and, 447–448
  internal evaluation and, 441–443, 442*t*
  overview, 398–399
  personnel as a resource, 399, 417–419, 417*f*, 418*f*, 419*f*, 420*t*
  program equity framework and, 110
  real-world evaluation approach and, 466, 468*t*
  time as a resource, 399, 411–417, 413*t*
Respect for people principle
  ethics and, 132–133, 139
  exemplary evaluations and, 534
  storytelling in evaluation and, 301–302
Responsive evaluation, 173
Results frameworks, 37, 82, 83, 384
Retention of participants, 406–408. *See also* Participants
Retrospective evaluations, 465–466
Retrospective surveys, 480
Rigor, 291, 481–482, 485, **570**
Risks, 96–97, 379–380, 380*t*
Robert Wood Johnson Foundation (RWJF), 104

Roles of evaluators. *See also* Evaluators
  evaluator involvement in program development, 14
  internal evaluation and, 12, 429, 429*t*, 432–435, 433*t*
  overview, 11
  preparing evaluators, 4–5
  roles of managers and, 432–433, 435
  storytelling in evaluation and, 288
Rubrics, 91, 92, 296–297, 570
Rule-governed approaches, 92
Running variable, 264*f*, 266, 570

Safe-to-fail experiments, 44
Safety monitoring, 401
Salience, 406–407
Sample. *See also* Sample size; Sampling
  definition of, 570
  descriptive analysis and, 333
  equity in evaluation and, 115
  nonprobability sampling, 313, 564, 570
  overview, 313
  probability sampling, 313, 567, 570
Sample size. *See also* Sample; Sampling
  addressing budget constraints, 470, 472, 473–476, 474*t*–475*t*, 486
  equity in evaluation and, 115, 121
  planning for quantitative analysis and, 314
  threats to validity and, 483
Sampling. *See also* Sample
  addressing budget constraints, 470, 472, 473–476, 474*t*–475*t*, 486
  convergent/parallel designs and, 350
  data as a resource and, 400
  economic evaluation and, 282
  explanatory sequential designs and, 351–352
  financial resources and, 421
  pilot and feasibility testing and, 414
  planning for quantitative analysis and, 313–314
  site selection and, 400–401
  skills inventory and, 417*f*
  time estimates and, 414, 415
Sandwich ECB model, 46
Satellite images, 481
Scaffolding principle, 45–46, 51

Scatter plots, 326, 328*f*, 330, 511, 516*f*, 519*f*
Scheduling. *See also* Time factors
  evaluability assessment (EA) and, 219–220
  evaluation planning and, 373–374, 374*t*, 375*f*, 375*t*
  independent consulting and, 460*t*, 461*t*, 462
Science, 160*f*, 165–169, 174*t*. *See also* Evaluation science
Scope of evaluations
  collaborative evaluation and, 187
  communications and, 497
  evaluability assessment (EA) and, 212–214
  planning, 366–370, 369*t*
Screening, data, 320–323
Scriven, Michael, 63, 68–69, 71–73, 570
Secondary data. *See also* Data
  addressing data constraints, 480
  data collection and data analysis and, 399, 409–410
  data screening and cleaning and, 322
  definition of, 570
  overview, 311
  planning for quantitative analysis and, 314, 323
  resource planning and, 398
  sources of, 323, 555
Section 508 compliance, 513
Selection bias, 63, 262, 335–336, 570. *See also* Bias
Self-administered instruments, 477, 486. *See also* Surveys
Self-assessment, 61
Self-awareness, 137
Self-confidence, 447
Self-reflection, 137–138, 172–173
Sensitivity analysis, 278, 282, 283, 570
Shadow pricing, 275, 277–278, 282, 570
Short-term outcomes, 257*f*, 258–259, 258*f*, 260, 432, 439. *See also* Outcomes
Similarity gestalt principle, 517, 517*f*. *See also* Gestalt principles
Simple interrupted time-series design, 263, 264*f*, 570. *See also* Interrupted time-series (ITS) design
Single-dimensional matching, 267, 570
Single-number display, 515*f*, 519*f*
Site selection, 212, 213, 399, 400–402
Site visits, 218, 219–221

Situation analysis, 172, 495, 498*t*–499*t*, 570. *See also* Communications plan of action
Skills inventory, 417–418, 417*f*, 456–457. *See also* Personnel
Social accountability, 60*f*, 546–547, 546*f*
Social constructivism, 70
Social impact, 87, 150–151. *See also* Impacts
Social inquiry, 60*f*, 546–547, 546*f*. *See also* Inquiry
Social justice
  community consultation and, 183
  competencies and, 21
  definition of, 570
  empowerment evaluation and, 197, 199
  equity in evaluation and, 122
  evaluation theory tree and, 62
  exemplary evaluations and, 536, 546–547, 546*f*
  mixed methods design and, 359
  participatory evaluation and, 191
  real-world evaluation approach and, 466
  values and, 82
Social learning principle, 48–49, 51
Social media, 298, 504, 570
Social programming, 58, 70, 80, 164
Social psychology, 59–60, 60*f*
Social science methods, 160–161
Social support, 188, 570–571
Societal factors, 105–106
Sociopolitical factors. *See also* Policy; Political factors
  data visualization and, 528, 529*f*
  equity in evaluation and, 105–106
  evaluation as practice and, 172–173
  evaluation science and, 166
  valuing and, 95
Software packages. *See also* Technology
  community consultation and, 184
  data analysis and, 222
  data screening and cleaning and, 322
  data visualization and, 518–519
  economic evaluation and, 278
  evaluation planning and, 409, 419, 422
  logic models and, 218
  mixed methods design and, 360
  scheduling and, 220
Sole proprietorship, 451*t*
Sparklines, 525*f*
Specialized knowledge, 173, 430*f*

Spy role of internal evaluators, 433t, 434. *See also* Internal evaluators
Staff. *See also* Interest holders; Personnel
  budget and, 419–420, 420t
  communications and, 494–495, 501
  competencies and, 21
  data collection and, 127
  empowerment evaluation and, 197–198
  equity in evaluation and, 106
  evaluability assessment (EA) and, 214, 219–222, 225
  evaluation planning and, 376, 377–378
  evaluation theory and, 75
  evaluative thinking and, 43, 44–50
  internal evaluation and, 429, 429t, 430, 430f, 432–433
  observations and, 297
  participatory evaluation and, 182, 195, 196
  starting up as an independent consultant and, 454, 454t
  valuing and, 93
Stage model, 74, 126–130, 154–155. *See also* Program stage
Stakeholders, 96, 374–377, 375f, 376t. *See also* Interest holders
Stakes, 83, 571. *See also* Values
Standards
  definition of, 571
  logic of evaluation and, 86
  setting, 91–92
  sources of values used in evaluative judgments and, 89
  valuing and, 93–94, 97
Stated program objectives criteria, 87. *See also* Criteria
Statistical conclusion validity, 482f. *See also* Validity
Statistical power
  attrition and, 412
  definition of, 571
  evaluability assessment (EA) and, 223
  number of participants and, 406
  overview, 401
  planning for quantitative analysis and, 313–314
  recruitment and, 404–405
  sample size and, 475t
  threats to validity and, 483
Statistical precision, 472, 474t–475t, 571
Statistical testing, 414, 417–418, 417f. *See also* Data analysis

Statistics, 5, 512. *See also* Quantitative data
Stereotypes, 114
Storytelling in evaluation. *See also* Data collection; Qualitative approaches
  analysis and interpretation and, 298–302, 300f
  definition of, 571
  framing the story, 289–292, 289f
  generating data, 292–298, 294t
  overview, 10, 288–289, 305–306
  portraying the program story, 302–305
Stratification, 339, 571
Strengths, weaknesses, opportunities, and threats (SWOTs), 187, 189–190, 544f–545f, 571
Study within a trial (SWAT), 407
Subheading design, 503, 556
Summaries/snapshot, 503, 571. *See also* Communications
Summative evaluation. *See also* Cost; Impacts; Outcomes
  definition of, 571
  evaluation as practice and, 173
  evaluation planning and, 368
  evaluation use and, 143–144, 156
  interest holders and, 310
  overview, 9, 68, 254, 255
  selecting internal or external evaluation and, 431, 432
Supervision, 235–236
Survey fatigue, 571
Surveys. *See also* Data collection
  addressing budget constraints, 470, 473, 477
  addressing data constraints, 479, 480
  budget and, 420
  convergent/parallel designs and, 348, 349
  equity in evaluation and, 120
  evaluation planning and, 371, 378
  incentives for, 378
  mixed methods design and, 360
  outcome evaluation and, 258–259
  planning for quantitative analysis and, 315
  program implementation and, 235, 241
  storytelling in evaluation and, 293, 298
  time estimates and, 414
Sustainability
  community consultation and, 183
  community involvement approaches and, 182

  definition of, 571
  economic evaluation and, 273–274
  evaluation science and, 168–169
  evaluation use and, 150–151
  exemplary evaluations and, 536
  overview, 87
  program implementation and, 231, 238
  valuing and, 85
Synthesis, 13, 92–94, 558. *See also* Valuing
Systematic inquiry. *See also* Inquiry
  ethics and, 130, 139
  evaluation as practice and, 171
  evaluation science and, 166–167
  exemplary evaluations and, 534
  values and, 82
Systematic screening and assessment method (SSA), 213–214, 571
Systems evaluation, 13, 528, 554
Systems science approaches, 239

Taking stock, 200–201, 201f, 203, 571
Target population. *See also* Interest holders; Populations of interest
  definition of, 571
  equity in evaluation and, 117–118, 120
  evaluability assessment (EA) and, 215–216, 222t, 223
  exploratory analysis and, 330
  quantitative data collection and analysis and, 309, 325
Tasks. *See also* Activities; Data analysis; Data collection; Reporting
  budget cuts and, 421–422
  independent consulting and, 460t
  person loading and, 418, 418f
  skills inventory and, 417–418, 417f
  time and, 413–417, 413t
  time estimates and, 416–417
Teams and teamwork
  evaluability assessment (EA) and, 225–226
  evaluation planning and, 374–377, 376t, 377t
  independent consulting and, 459, 460t
  internal evaluation and, 436–437
  participatory evaluation and, 192, 194, 194f, 195, 196
Technical factors, 119–120
Technical rationality, 43, 571
Technology
  addressing budget constraints, 477–478, 486–487
  data collection and, 409

Subject Index

Technology *(cont.)*
 data visualization and, 518–519, 528
 evaluation as, 160f, 169–170, 174t
 logic models and, 218
 mixed methods design and, 360
Template for Intervention Description and Replication Checklist, 232
Terminator role of internal evaluators, 433t, 435. *See also* Internal evaluators
Terms of reference (TOR)
 communications and, 497
 communications throughout the evaluation and, 494
 definition of, 571
 internal evaluation and, 441–442, 442t
 real-world evaluation approach and, 467
Testing bias, 262, 571. *See also* Bias
Testing findings, 500–501, 502t
Text-based channel, 553
Text-based tools, 503–504. *See also* Communications
Theme, 300–301, 357f, 571
Theory. *See also* Evaluation theory
 definition of, 571
 economic evaluation and, 284
 goal of fostering evaluation use and, 142
 overview, 55–56
 program implementation and, 233
Theory of action, 198, 275, 289, 571
Theory of change
 addressing budget constraints, 472–473
 definition of, 571
 descriptive analysis and, 331–332
 logic models and, 387–388, 387f, 388f, 389f, 390
 negotiating with clients and, 484
 program implementation and, 231–232
 selecting internal or external evaluation and, 431–432
 storytelling in evaluation and, 289, 289f, 299, 300f, 305
Theory of use, 198, 571
Theory tree. *See* Evaluation theory tree
Theory-driven evaluation, 383–384, 385. *See also* Logic models; Program theory
Thick description, 299, 301, 303, 571–572
Thomas theorem, 166
Threats, 379–380, 380t

Threats to internal validity, 9, 572. *See also* Internal validity
Threats to validity, 466, 481–483, 482f
Three branches, 60–61, 60f, 164, 572. *See also* Evaluation theory tree
Time factors. *See also* Scheduling
 addressing data constraints, 481
 addressing time constraints, 478
 data collection and, 411–412
 evaluation planning and, 369–370, 373–374, 374t, 375f, 375t
 evaluation question and, 411
 financial resources and, 421
 internal evaluation and, 429, 429t
 negotiating with clients and, 483–486
 real-world evaluation approach and, 465–466, 468t, 478
 resource planning and, 398, 399
 tasks and, 413–417, 413t
 time as a resource, 399, 411–417, 413t
 time budgets, 412–413, 416–417
 time estimates and, 416–417
 time trends, 337, 481, 572
Time tracking, 452
Timelines in data visualization, 523f
Timing, 345–346, 368, 572
Top-down approach, 49, 480
Total cost, 279, 572
Training
 collaborative evaluation and, 188
 competencies and, 5–6, 21, 30
 evaluation planning and, 376–377
 evaluation use and, 157
 logitistical factors, 369
 preparing evaluators, 4–5
 program implementation and, 235–236
 promoting a culture of evaluative thinking and, 44–50
Transdiscipline, 36, 160f, 163–165, 174t, 572
Transferability. *See* External validity or generalizability
Transformative empowerment evaluation, 197, 572. *See also* Empowerment evaluation
Transformative participatory evaluation, 191, 572. *See also* Participatory evaluation
Transformative worldview, 359, 572
Transparency
 community consultation and, 204
 definition of, 572
 evaluation use and, 150–151
 interest holders and, 310–311

 overview, 291
 storytelling in evaluation and, 299, 306
Travel, 378, 420, 421
Tree maps, 515f
Trend graph, 329f
Trial conduct, 401
Triangulation
 addressing budget constraints, 470
 definition of, 572
 economic evaluation and, 276
 equity in evaluation and, 119–120
 evaluation planning and, 372
 storytelling in evaluation and, 297
Trimming, 339, 572
Trust
 collaborative evaluation and, 188
 community consultation and, 182–183
 culturally responsive evaluation (CRE) and, 70
 definition of, 572
 independent consulting and, 447
 participatory evaluation and, 194
Two-arm trials, 242, 263
Two-way model of communication, 492, 493f. *See also* Communications
Type of evaluation, 143–144, 145

Unit cost, 377. *See also* Cost
Unit of analysis, 315–316, 401, 413, 572
Unit of observation, 315–316, 572
United Way framework, 110–111
Univariate analysis, 332–333, 572
Unobserved treatments, 337, 572
Use. *See also* Evaluation theory tree; Evaluation use
 culturally responsive evaluation (CRE) and, 70
 evaluability assessment (EA) and, 214, 222t
 evaluation theory and, 59, 60, 60f, 62, 76f
 evaluation use theory, 143–144
 exemplary evaluations and, 546–547
 follow-up of conclusions and recommendations and, 505–506
 mixed methods design and, 361
 overview, 141–142
 review of specific evaluation theories, 62–71
 storytelling in evaluation and, 290–291
Utility, 96, 129, 134

Utilization validity, 482f, 483. *See also* Validity
Utilization-focused evaluation
  definition of, **572**
  evaluation as practice and, 171–173, 171f
  goal of fostering evaluation use and, 142
  overview, 74, 75, 121

Validity. *See also* External validity or generalizability; Internal validity
  data as a resource and, 400
  definition of, **572**
  evaluation planning and, 371
  evaluation theory and, 63, 65
  internal evaluation and, 442–443
  overview, 255–256
  potential outcomes framework and, 335, 336–337
  program implementation and, 242
  real-world evaluation approach and, 481–483, 482f
  valuing and, 96
Value neutrality, 82, **573**
Values. *See also* Valuing
  combining theories and, 73
  data visualization and, 510
  definition of, **573**
  ethics and, 137–138
  evaluation use and, 150–151
  evaluative thinking and, 36
  exemplary evaluations and, 534–535, 536, 546–547, 546f
  overview, 81–84, 88, 97
  sources of, 89
  storytelling in evaluation and, 306
Values lens, 447, **573**. *See also* Ethics
Valuing. *See also* Evaluation theory tree; Evaluative judgment; Values
  benefits and risks of, 96–97
  considerations for, 93–97
  culturally responsive evaluation (CRE) and, 70
  definition of, **573**
  discipline of evaluation and, 164
  evaluation science and, 167, 168
  evaluation theory and, 58–59, 60, 60f, 62, 69, 76f
  evaluation use and, 141
  evaluative thinking and, 36
  identifying sources of evidence and, 89–91
  logic and related methods, 86–93
  overview, 7–8, 81–82, 84–85, 97
  selecting criteria and, 86–89
  setting standards and, 91–92
  social justice and, 62
  synthesis and, 92–93
  values assessment, 88–89
Variable, 316, 326, **573**
Variable cost, 279–280, **573**. *See also* Cost
Variable distributions, 319–320
Video recordings, 235, 477
Video testimonies, 505, **573**. *See also* Communications
Virtual data collection, 13, **573**

Visualcy, 512, **573**. *See also* Data visualization
Visualization, data. *See* Data visualization
Voluntary evaluation peer-review (VEPR) process, 24
Voluntary Organizations for Professional Evaluation (VOPEs)
  competencies and, 23–24
  definition of, **573**
  exemplary evaluations and, 534, 536, 543
  overview, 4

War on Poverty, 18–19
Webinars, 500, 505, **573**
Weight and sum, 92
Weighting, 88, 339, **573**. *See also* Values; Valuing
Wide dataset, 317, 555
Word clouds, 522, 522f, **573**
Word trees, 522, 522f, **573**
Work breakdown structure (WBS), 372–373, 372f, **573**. *See also* Evaluation planning
Work plan, 419–421, 420t, 442
Workshops, 493, 504, **573**. *See also* Communications
Worldview, 366–367, **573**
Worst-case scenario testing. *See* Best-case and worst-case scenario testing
Worth, 89, 141

Yield, 280, **573**
Youth participatory action research (YPAR), 118, **573**

About the Editors

Debra J. Rog, PhD, is a Vice President for Social Policy and Economics Research at Westat and President of its nonprofit affiliate, The Rockville Institute. Throughout her career, Dr. Rog has directed numerous evaluation studies of homeless and housing interventions and systems, mental health and substance abuse interventions, public health programs and initiatives, and criminal justice initiatives, among other areas. She is a recognized expert in evaluation practice and applied research design. Dr. Rog is Associate Director for Faculty Affairs at The Evaluators' Institute and past president of the American Evaluation Association (AEA). She has been recognized for her evaluation work by the National Institute of Mental Health, the AEA, the Eastern Evaluation Research Society, and the Knowledge Utilization Society.

Leonard Bickman, PhD, is Professor Emeritus of Psychology at Vanderbilt University, former Director of the Center for Evaluation and Program Improvement at Peabody College, and Research Professor at Florida International University. Dr. Bickman is a nationally recognized leader in program evaluation and mental health services research on children and adolescents. He is past president of the AEA and the Society for the Psychological Study of Social Issues. Dr. Bickman's contributions have been recognized with the Outstanding Evaluation Award from the AEA, the Award for Distinguished Contributions to Research in Public Policy from the American Psychological Association, and the Secretary's Award for Distinguished Service from the U.S. Department of Health and Human Services, among other honors.

Contributors

Marvin C. Alkin, PhD, School of Education and Information Studies, University of California, Los Angeles, Los Angeles, California

Thomas Archibald, PhD, Department of Agricultural, Leadership, and Community Education, Virginia Tech University, Blacksburg, Virginia

Donna Durant Atkinson, PhD, Behavioral Health and Health Policy, Westat, Rockville, Maryland

Tarek Azzam, PhD, Department of Education, University of California, Santa Barbara, Santa Barbara, California

Michael Bamberger, PhD, International Initiative for Impact Evaluation, Seattle, Washington

Gail Vallance Barrington, PhD, Writer and Evaluation Advisor, Calgary, Canada

Leonard Bickman, PhD, Department of Psychology, Florida International University, Miami, Florida

A. Brooks Bowden, PhD, Graduate School of Education, University of Pennsylvania, Philadelphia, Pennsylvania

Jane Buckley, MEd, Independent Consultant, West Henrietta, New York

Stewart I. Donaldson, PhD, Claremont Evaluation Center and The Evaluators' Institute, Claremont Graduate University, Claremont, California

Sarah Douville, MBA, Independent Consultant, Montclair, California

David M. Fetterman, PhD, Fetterman and Associates, Claremont, California

Joy Frechtling, PhD, Education Studies, Westat, Rockville, Maryland

Emily F. Gates, PhD, Department of Measurement, Evaluation, Statistics, and Assessment, Boston College, Chestnut Hill, Massachusetts

Erica Harbatkin, PhD, Department of Educational Leadership and Policy Studies, Anne Spencer Daves College of Education, Health, and Human Services, Florida State University, Tallahassee, Florida

Gary T. Henry, PhD, College of Education and Human Development, School of Education, and the Joseph R. Biden, Jr. School of Public Policy and Administration, University of Delaware, Newark, Delaware

Kimberly Eaton Hoagwood, PhD, Department of Child and Adolescent Psychiatry, New York University Langone Health, New York, New York

Natalie D. Jones, PhD, Center for Evaluation and Assessment, Gevirtz Graduate School of Education, University of California, Santa Barbara, Santa Barbara, California

Jean A. King, PhD, Department of Organizational Leadership, Policy, and Development, University of Minnesota, Minneapolis, Minnesota

Ciara Knight, PhD, Sankofa Consulting, Seattle, Washington

Henry M. Levin, PhD, Department of Economics and Education, Teachers College, Columbia University, New York, New York

Arnold Love, PhD, Arnold Love and Associates, Toronto, Canada

Melvin M. Mark, PhD, Department of Psychology, Pennsylvania State University, University Park, Pennsylvania

Michael Morris, PhD, Department of Psychology, University of New Haven, West Haven, Connecticut

Glenn O'Neil, PhD, Owl RE, Commugny, Switzerland

Michael Quinn Patton, PhD, Utilization-Focused Evaluation, Pine City, Minnesota

Laura R. Peck, PhD, Income Security and Economic Mobility Domain, MEF Associates, Alexandria, Virginia

Lam D. Pham, PhD, Department of Educational Evaluation and Policy Analysis, North Carolina State University, Raleigh, North Carolina

Byron J. Powell, PhD, Center for Dissemination and Implementation and Center for Mental Health Services Research, Brown School, Washington University in St. Louis, St. Louis, Missouri

Sharon F. Rallis, EdD, Department of Education Policy and Reform, University of Massachusetts, Amherst, Amherst, Massachusetts

Liliana Rodríguez-Campos, PhD, Department of Educational and Psychological Studies, University of South Florida, Tampa, Florida

Debra J. Rog, PhD, Social and Economic Policy Research, Westat, Rockville, Maryland

Darlene F. Russ-Eft, PhD, Department of Technology Leadership and Innovation, Purdue University, West Lafayette, Indiana

Thomas A. Schwandt, PhD, Department of Educational Psychology, University of Illinois at Urbana–Champaign, Champaign, Illinois

Robert Shand, PhD, School of Education, American University, Washington, DC

Guy O'Grady Sharrock, MSc, Catholic Relief Services, Baltimore, Maryland

R. Bradley Snyder, MPA, EdM, New Amsterdam Consulting, Inc., Scottsdale, Arizona

Piper Grandjean Targos, MA, Ascending Edge Creative Evaluation, Evergreen, Colorado

Janet Usinger, PhD, College of Education and State Extension Specialist, University of Nevada, Reno, Reno, Nevada

Anne T. Vo, PhD, Department of Health Systems Science, Kaiser Permanente Bernard J. Tyson School of Medicine, Pasadena, California

Ann P. Zukoski, DPh, Center for Health Promotion, Minnesota Department of Health, St. Paul, Minnesota